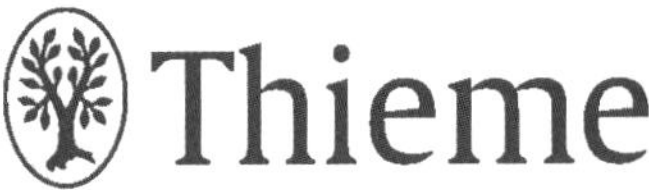
Thieme

Pediatric Cardiology

Symptoms—Diagnosis—Treatment

Nikolaus A. Haas, MD
Supervising Physician
Hospital for Congenital Heart Diseases
Heart and Diabetes Center NRW
Bad Oeynhausen, Germany

Ulrich Kleideiter, MD
Supervising Physician
Christophorus Clinics
Hospital for Pediatrics and Adolescent Medicine
Coesfeld, Germany

484 illustrations

Thieme
Stuttgart • New York • Delhi • Rio de Janeiro

Library of Congress Cataloging-in-Publication Data

Haas, Nikolaus A., author.
[Kinderkardiologie. English]
Pediatric cardiology : symptoms, diagnosis, treatment / Nikolaus A. Haas, Ulrich Kleideiter; translator, Melanie Nassar; illustrators, Rose Baumann, Heike H?bner.
p. ; cm.
Includes bibliographical references and index.
ISBN 978-3-13-174941-3 (alk. paper)
I. Kleideiter, Ulrich, author. II. Title.
[DNLM: 1. Child. 2. Heart Diseases. 3. Infant. 4. Adolescent. 5. Cardiology–methods. WS 290]
RJ421
618.92'12–dc23

2014046350

This book is an authorized translation of the German edition published and copyrighted 2011 by Georg Thieme Verlag, Stuttgart. Title of the German edition: Kinderkardiologie: Klinik und Praxis der Herzerkrankungen bei Kindern, Jugendlichen und jungen Erwachsenen.

Translator: Melanie Nassar, Bethlehem, Palestine

Illustrators: Rose Baumann, Schriesheim; Heike Hübner, Berlin

Thieme Publishers Stuttgart
Rüdigerstrasse 14, 70469 Stuttgart, Germany
+49 [0]711 8931 421, customerservice@thieme.de

Thieme Publishers New York
333 Seventh Avenue, New York, NY 10001 USA
+1 800 782 3488, customerservice@thieme.com

Thieme Publishers Delhi
A-12, Second Floor, Sector-2, Noida-201301
Uttar Pradesh, India
+91 120 45 566 00, customerservice@thieme.in

Thieme Publishers Rio, Thieme Publicações Ltda.
Edifício Rodolpho de Paoli, 25° andar
Av. Nilo Peçanha, 50 – Sala 2508,
Rio de Janeiro 20020-906 Brasil
Tel: +55 21 3172-2297 / +55 21 3172-1896

Cover design: Thieme Publishing Group
Typesetting by DiTech Process Solutions Pvt. Ltd., India
Printed in Germany by appl druck, Wemding

ISBN 9783131749413

Also available as e-book:
eISBN 9783131749512

Important note: Medicine is an ever-changing science undergoing continual development. Research and clinical experience are continually expanding our knowledge, in particular our knowledge of proper treatment and drug therapy. Insofar as this book mentions any dosage or application, readers may rest assured that the authors, editors, and publishers have made every effort to ensure that such references are in accordance with **the state of knowledge at the time of production of the book.**

Nevertheless, this does not involve, imply, or express any guarantee or responsibility on the part of the publishers in respect to any dosage instructions and forms of applications stated in the book. **Every user is requested to examine carefully** the manufacturers' leaflets accompanying each drug and to check, if necessary in consultation with a physician or specialist, whether the dosage schedules mentioned therein or the contraindications stated by the manufacturers differ from the statements made in the present book. Such examination is particularly important with drugs that are either rarely used or have been newly released on the market. Every dosage schedule or every form of application used is entirely at the user's own risk and responsibility. The authors and publishers request every user to report to the publishers any discrepancies or inaccuracies noticed. If errors in this work are found after publication, errata will be posted at www.thieme.com on the product description page.

Some of the product names, patents, and registered designs referred to in this book are in fact registered trademarks or proprietary names even though specific reference to this fact is not always made in the text. Therefore, the appearance of a name without designation as proprietary is not to be construed as a representation by the publisher that it is in the public domain.

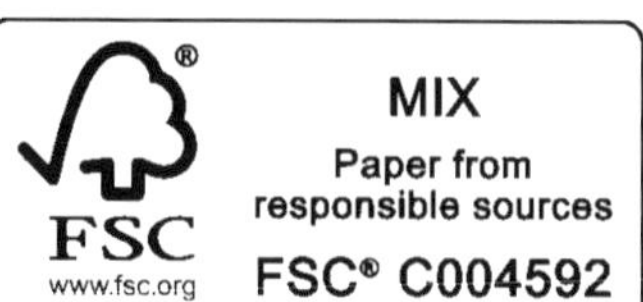

Contents

Part IV Treatment

Part V Appendix

Preface

Yet another textbook on pediatric cardiology...

Based on the positive feedback from many colleagues, students, nurses, and, above all, from the many contacts made during international meetings, we were encouraged to consider an English version of our textbook on pediatric cardiology and congenital heart defects. In this book, we present a practice-based overview of pediatric cardiology that will assist caregivers when making diagnoses and treatment decisions. Our primary aim always is to provide adequate scientific information from this exciting field combined with clear and simple practice-oriented advice on what to do and how to do it in any given circumstances. We hope that we have succeeded...

Pediatric cardiology today should involve far more than just the diagnostics and treatment of congenital and acquired heart disease in children. Pediatric cardiology has developed into a highly specialized field comprising the interdisciplinary care of congenital and acquired heart disease in children of all ages and also, increasingly, in adolescents and adults. Thanks to constantly improving treatment that also covers the most complex heart defects, more and more children with heart disease reach adulthood today. This group of patients poses new challenges, not only to pediatric cardiologists, but increasingly to specialists in other fields such as intensive medicine, cardiac surgery, internal medical cardiology, and general medicine. These special problems have led to the development of a new subspecialty called "Grown-Up Congenital Heart Disease" (GUCH).

Heart defects and residual defects following procedures can now often be treated definitively with catheterization and interventional techniques. Until recently, surgery was the only treatment option for many of these defects. In addition, hybrid operations, combining surgery with catheterization in a single procedure (such as an intervention during an operation on the heart-lung machine), have led to completely new options. All these advances make it increasingly difficult for practicing physicians as well as specialists from related fields to keep up with developments, especially if they do not deal with the specific issues of pediatric cardiology on a daily basis or are just beginning training in pediatric cardiology.

The first German edition was developed on the basis of various scripts and teaching material that we created during our training or—later on—when training our junior (and senior) colleagues, students, and nurses. It is evident that a textbook created by only two authors cannot provide the complete scientific expert knowledge of this fascinating specialty. Based on the daily challenges of our practical work we were able nevertheless to combine the appropriate scientific background with all practically relevant aspects and answer all the necessary questions for clinical patient care.

We would like to give special thanks to all those who have supported us during the preparation of the initial German edition and subsequent English edition of our textbook. First of all to our families, who accepted and tolerated the additional workload and encouraged us to continue; then the team at Georg Thieme Verlag, notably Dr. Christian Urbanowicz and the editor Tom Böttcher for their support with the German edition; and finally to Ms. Angelika-Marie Findgott and Ms. Joanne Stead of Thieme Publishers for their editorial support on the English edition, our translator Ms. Melanie Nassar for the excellent translation and, more importantly, to the Editorial and Production staff for their never-ending patience awaiting our input during the final corrections. In addition, we would like to express our sincere thanks to Occlutech GmbH, Jena, Germany, for their financial support of the translation process that made this English edition possible.

Last but not least we offer special thanks to our clinical and scientific mentors and teachers, who have translated their passion for this field into our daily clinical practice. Their spirit and passion, together with the challenge of training young colleagues, their questions, the overcoming of difficulties in understanding, and their constant urge to learn and understand led to the development of this textbook.

We hope that this textbook may provide adequate information for daily practice to those who treat patients with congenital heart disease and for those who want to learn. We would be happy for any feedback and look forward to improving the next edition based on your input.

Nikolaus A. Haas, MD
Ulrich Kleideiter, MD

Abbreviations

ACT	activated clotting time
ACC	American College of Cardiology
ACE	angiotensin converting enzyme
ADH	antidiuretic hormone
AHA	American Heart Association
AICD	automatic implant cardioverter/ defibrillator
ALT	alanine transaminase
ANA	antinuclear antibody
ANP	atrial natriuretic peptide
Ao	aorta
AP	anteroposterior, alkaline phosphatase
ASD	atrial septal defect
AST	aspartate aminotransferase
AT	antithrombin
ATP	adenosine triphosphate
AV	atrioventricular, arteriovenous
AVNRT	atrioventricular nodal re-entrant tachycardia
AVRC	arrhythmogenic right ventricular cardiomyopathy
AVRT	atrioventricular re-entrant tachycardia with accessory pathway
AVSD	atrioventricular septal defect
BE	base excess
BNP	B-type (brain) natriuretic peptide
BSA	body surface area
c-ANCA	(cytoplasmic)-antineutrophil cytoplasmic antibody
CAT	chaotic atrial tachycardia
cc	congenitally corrected
CDG	congenital disorder of glycosylation
CK-MB	creatine kinase, isozyme MB
CNP	C-type natriuretic peptide
CRP	C-reactive protein
CT	computed tomography
CVC	central venous catheter
CVP	central venous pressure
CW	continuous wave
d-	dextro
DCM	dilated cardiomyopathy
DILV	double inlet left ventricle
DIRV	double inlet right ventricle
DORV	double outlet right ventricle
EAT	ectopic atrial tachycardia
EBV	Epstein–Barr virus
ECMO	extracorporeal membrane oxygenation
EF	ejection fraction
EFE	endocardial fibroelastosis
EPE	electrophysiological examination
ESR	erythrocyte sedimentation rate
FFP	fresh frozen plasma
FS	fractional shortening
GT	glutamyl transferase
HCM	hypertrophic cardiomyopathy
HDL	high density lipoprotein
HHV	human herpesvirus
HLHS	hypoplastic left heart syndrome
HOCM	hypertrophic obstructive cardiomyopathy
IART	atrial flutter and intra-atrial re-entrant tachycardia
ICD	implantable converter defibrillator / intracardiac defibrillator
ICS	intercostal space
ICU	intensive care unit
INR	international normalized ratio
JET	junctional ectopic tachycardia
LA	left atrium
LAD	left anterior descending (artery, branch)
LAH	left anterior hemiblock
LBBB	left bundle branch block
LCA	left coronary artery
LDH	lactate dehydrogenase
LPH	Left posterior hemiblock
LSVC	left superior vena cava
LV	left ventricle
MAPCAs	major aortopulmonary collateral arteries
MAT	multifocal atrial tachycardia
MCL	mid-clavicular line
MHC	major histocompatibility complex
MIBI	methoxyisobutylisonitrile
MMR	measles, mumps, rubella
MRI	magnetic resonance imaging
MRSA	methicillin resistant Staphylococcus aureus
MVV	maximum voluntary ventilation
NASPE	North American Society of Pacing and Electrophysiology
NCC	noncompaction cardiomyopathy

NSAID	nonsteroidal anti-inflammatory drug
NYHA	New York Heart Association
PA	posteroanterior; pulmonary artery; pulmonary atresia
PA/IVS	pulmonary atresia with intact ventricular septum
PAP	pulmonary arterial pressure
PAPVC	partial anomalous pulmonary venous connection
PA-VSD	pulmonary atresia with ventricular septal defect
PCR	polymerase chain reaction
PEEP	positive end expiratory pressure
PFO	patent foramen ovale
PiCCO	pulse contour cardiac output
PJRT	permanent junctional reciprocating tachycardia
PMI	point of maximum impulse
POTS	postural orthostatic tachycardia syndrome
PTCA	percutaneous transluminal coronary angioplasty
PTT	partial thromboplastin time
RA	right atrium
RAAS	renin–angiotensin–aldosterone system
RBBB	right bundle branch block
RCA	right coronary artery
RCM	restrictive cardiomyopathy
RCX	ramus circumflexus of the left coronary artery
RI	resistance index
RSV	respiratory syncytial virus
RV	right ventricle
SA	sinoatrial
SAM	systolic anterior movement
SGA	small for gestational age
SIRS	systemic inflammatory response syndrome
SLE	systemic lupus arteriosus
SVES	supraventricular extrasystole
SVT	supraventricular tachycardia
TCPC	total cavopulmonary connection
TEE	transesophageal echocardiography
TGA	transposition of the great arteries
TSH	thyroid stimulating hormone
VACTERL	vertebral, anal, cardiac, tracheo-esophageal, esophageal, renal and radial, and limb defects
VSD	ventricular septal defect
VT	ventricular tachycardia
WPW	Wolff–Parkinson–White

List of Videos

Part I

Basics and Diagnostics

1 Clinical History and Examination in Pediatric Cardiology

1.1 Basics

Every pediatric cardiology evaluation starts with a thorough medical history and clinical examination. Because of the increasing number of technical diagnostic procedures available, there is a tendency to place less importance on medical history and examination. However, a comprehensive medical history and clinical examination are essential for determining potential differential diagnoses and arranging for further examinations using technical procedures.

1.2 Medical History

In pediatric cardiology, the medical history consists of current complaints and of gestational and perinatal history, family medical history, and the child's physical development. Of course it must also include any current medication.

1.2.1 Gestational History

The gestational history includes the following specific questions:

- Were there any indications of a congenital heart defect in the fetal ultrasound examinations? A large percentage of congenital heart defects can now be diagnosed prenatally using fetal echocardiography.
- Were any chromosome anomalies or genetic diseases suspected or diagnosed prenatally?
  A number of genetic syndromes are associated with congenital heart defects (Chapter 23.1). Some of the most important are:
  - Trisomy 21 (atrioventricular [AV] canal defect, ventricular septal defect [VSD], tetralogy of Fallot)
  - Trisomy 13 (VSD)
  - Trisomy 18 (VSD)
  - VACTERL association (VSD)
  - Microdeletion 22q11 (conotruncal heart defects such as tetralogy of Fallot, pulmonary atresia, truncus arteriosus communis)
  - Noonan syndrome (pulmonary stenosis, hypertrophic cardiomyopathy)
  - Turner syndrome (coarctation of the aorta, aortic stenosis, cardiomyopathy)
  - Williams–Beuren syndrome (supravalvular aortic stenosis, peripheral pulmonary stenosis, coarctation of the aorta)
  - Marfan syndrome (aortic root dilatation, aortic insufficiency, mitral valve prolapse, mitral valve insufficiency)
- Did the mother take any medication or drugs or drink alcohol during pregnancy?
  Many medications are considered to be teratogenic. Taking any of the following products during pregnancy has been associated with congenital heart defects:
  - Phenytoin (pulmonary stenosis, aortic stenosis, coarctation of the aorta, patent ductus arteriosus [PDA])
  - Valproate (ASD, VSD, aortic stenosis, pulmonary atresia with intact ventricular septum, coarctation of the aorta)
  - Lithium (Ebstein anomaly)
  - Retinoic acid (conotruncal heart defects such as tetralogy of Fallot, truncus arteriosus communis)
  - Amphetamines (VSD, PDA, ASD, transposition of the great arteries [TGA])
  - Progesterone/estrogen (VSD, TGA, tetralogy of Fallot)
  - Alcohol (VSD, PDA, ASD, tetralogy of Fallot)
- Did or does the mother have diabetes mellitus or gestational diabetes mellitus?
  If the mother has diabetes mellitus, the child is at an increased risk of hypertrophic cardiomyopathy (reversible), TGA, VSD, and coarctation of the aorta.
- Does the mother have systemic lupus erythematosus (SLE)?
  If the mother has SLE, the child has an increased risk of developing a congenital AV block. The transplacental transmission of maternal antibodies can destroy the child's cardiac conduction system. Sometimes SLE has not yet been detected in the mother and is not diagnosed until an AV block is found in the child.
- Did the mother contract a viral infection during pregnancy?
  A maternal infection with rubella in the first trimester can lead to peripheral pulmonary stenosis, PDA, and/or VSD.
  Infections with cytomegalovirus, herpes simplex, or Coxsackie B virus are considered to be potentially teratogenic. In late pregnancy, viral infections can cause congenital myocarditis.

1.2.2 Perinatal History

The perinatal history must include the following:

- Birth weight, gestational age?
  The birth weight is the basis for monitoring progress. A low birth weight ("small for gestational age" [SGA]) can be an indication of an intrauterine infection.
  Neonates of mothers with diabetes mellitus are typically abnormally large and heavy.
  Neonates with TGA also frequently have a relatively high birth weight, but the cause for this is unclear.

Table 1.1 Risk of repetition of heart defects if a sibling is affected (from Nora JJ, Nora AH 1978)

Heart defect	Risk of repetition
VSD	3%
PDA	3%
ASD	2.5%
Tetralogy of Fallot	2.5%
Pulmonary stenosis	2%
Coarctation of the aorta	2%
Aortic stenosis	2%
TGA	1.5%
AV canal	2%
Endocardial fibroelastosis	4%
Tricuspid atresia	1%
Ebstein anomaly	1%
Truncus arteriosus communis	1%
Pulmonary atresia	1%
Hypoplastic left heart syndrome	1%

- Assessment of postnatal adaptation (Apgar score, pH)
  Cyanotic heart defects are a risk factor for perinatal asphyxia.
- If cyanosis occurred, was there improvement after oxygen was administered?
  Hyperoxia test—an increase in pulse oximetry oxygen saturation after the administration of oxygen is more indicative of a pulmonary problem than of a cardiac problem.
- Was a heart murmur found soon after birth?
  Cardiac defects that lead to obstruction (e.g., aortic stenosis, pulmonary stenosis) generally cause a heart murmur at an early stage. On the other hand, a murmur from a shunt defect (VSD, PDA) can usually not be heard until the pulmonary vascular resistance is lowered when the flow in the shunt increases.

1.2.3 Family History

The family history can determine whether there is a familial disposition for cardiac disease.

- Have there been any congenital heart defects among close relatives?
  Around 1% of all neonates have a congenital heart defect. The risk is greater if there are close relatives with a congenital heart defect. In general, the risk is about 3% if a sibling has had a congenital heart defect. However, this risk varies depending on the kind of heart defect (▸ Table 1.1). If the mother had a congenital heart defect, the risk is greater than if the father was affected (▸ Table 1.2).

Table 1.2 Child's risk of certain heart defects if a parent is affected by this defect (from Nora JJ, Nora AH 1978)

Heart defect	Mother affected	Father affected
Aortic stenosis	13–18%	3%
ASD	4–4.5%	1.5%
AV canal	14%	1%
Coarctation of the aorta	4%	2%
PDA	3.5–4%	2%
Pulmonary stenosis	4–6.5%	2%
Tetralogy of Fallot	6–10%	1.5%
VSD	6%	2%

- Are there any genetic diseases associated with a heart defect or arrhythmia in the family?
  The most common genetic diseases associated with heart defects have already been listed above (e.g., Marfan syndrome). Examples of familial arrhythmia are long QT syndrome, Brugada syndrome, or familial atrial fibrillation.
- Have there been frequent deaths or syncopes of unknown origin in the family?
  If the family history yields any such information, a differential diagnosis of ventricular arrhythmia, long QT syndrome, Brugada syndrome, and hypertrophic cardiomyopathy must be considered.
- Has any family member had a heart attack at a young age?
  In this case, possible coronary anomalies and risk factors for coronary heart disease such as hereditary thrombophilia or hypertension must be explored.

1.2.4 Development of the Child

In this part of the medical history, specific questions are asked about symptoms that could indicate heart failure or cyanosis.

▸ **Weight gain.** Insufficient weight gain is a typical sign of heart failure. Weight gain is generally more affected than growth in length in children with heart failure.

▸ **Feeding behavior.** Feeding difficulties may indicate heart failure, especially when associated with rapid fatigue or sweating when feeding.

▸ **Physical performance in comparison with age group.** Reduced exercise capacity can be a sign of heart failure and a symptom of all relevant cardiac diseases—for example, shunt defects, cyanotic heart disease, relevant valve obstruction, valve insufficiency, or severe arrhythmia.

In neonates and infants, physical capacity is best evaluated by observing feeding.

▶ **Tachypnea, dyspnea.** Tachypnea and/or dyspnea are typical signs of heart failure. The symptoms generally increase under stress.

▶ **Frequent respiratory infections.** Heart defects with a relevant left-to-right shunt and excessive blood flow to the lungs (e.g., a large VSD or AV canal) are predisposing factors for pulmonary infections. Chronic respiratory problems should alert to the possibility of vascular rings that compress the trachea (e.g., a dual aortic arch or right aortic arch with a left ductus/ligamentum).

▶ **Edema.** Edema is a typical sign of heart failure. In neonates and infants, the first edema seen is generally eyelid edema.

1.2.5 Current Symptoms

The symptoms listed below are frequently the reason for consulting a pediatric cardiologist. The detailed differential diagnoses of the symptoms are presented in Chapters 11 to 15.

▶ **Chest pain.** Most instances of chest pain in childhood and adolescence are not related to cardiac disease. The most frequent causes are costochondritis, muscle problems, respiratory diseases, or trauma. Gastroesophageal reflux or gastritis can also lead to chest pain.

Cardiac diseases that can cause chest pain include mainly myocarditis and pericarditis; other possibilities are relevant aortic stenosis, hypertrophic obstructive cardiomyopathy, pulmonary hypertension, mitral valve prolapse, myocarditis, or pericarditis.

▶ **Syncopes.** When syncopes occur under stress and/or are associated with chest pain, a cardiac cause must be ruled out. Possible cardiac causes are arrhythmia (e.g., in the context of long QT syndrome), relevant aortic stenosis, or hypertrophic obstructive cardiomyopathy. Furthermore, congenital or already surgically treated heart defects in patients with syncopes must always alert to the possibility of a cardiac cause. The most important differential diagnoses are vasovagal syncopes and cerebral seizures.

▶ **Palpitations.** Palpitations can be caused by paroxysmal or permanent tachycardia or extrasystoles. A mitral valve prolapse or hyperthyroidism should be ruled out.

▶ **Cyanosis.** Parents are often concerned about cyanosis in young infants. If only the hands and feet are affected, it is generally a harmless peripheral cyanosis. However, cyanosis that occurs in mucosa and fingernail beds is indicative of central cyanosis. The time when the cyanosis first occurred needs to be clarified (at birth, a few days after birth), whether it is continuous or paroxysmal, and whether it increases under stress (e.g., during feeding). In addition to cyanotic heart defects, "breath-holding spells" should be considered, in which infants hold their breath, especially after exertion, and become cyanotic.

1.3 Clinical Examination

The clinical pediatric cardiology examination includes taking vital signs (pulse, respiratory rate, oxygen saturation, blood pressure) and inspection, palpation, and auscultation.

1.3.1 Inspection

The first step of the clinical examination is inspection. The examiner can get a first impression of the child while taking the medical history. The inspection should focus on the following aspects.

▶ **Nutritional condition.** Heart defects that are associated with a large left-to-right shunt, pulmonary edema, or reduced ventricular function can lead to slow weight gain. Cardiac related failure to thrive is an indication for anti-congestive therapy (digoxin, diuretics, ACE inhibitors, possibly beta blockers) and for caloric supplementation if needed.

▶ **Extracardiac malformations.** Extracardiac malformations occur in around 20% of all children with congenital heart defects. They frequently occur in combination with syndromal diseases. The most common syndromal diseases associated with a heart defect are presented in Chapter 23.

▶ **Skin color.** If the hemoglobin level is normal, cyanosis will be noted if oxygen saturation is below 85%. Peripheral cyanosis and central cyanosis must be distinguished. In *central cyanosis*, arterial oxygen saturation is reduced. Correspondingly, the mucosa, tongue, and fingernail beds are cyanotic. In *peripheral cyanosis*, however, arterial oxygen saturation is normal. In this case, the cyanosis is caused by increased oxygen depletion at the periphery—for example, resulting from vasoconstriction due to cold or reduced cardiac output (heart failure). Isolated perioral cyanosis is observed especially in neonates and infants with pale skin and usually has no pathological significance.

Pronounced *pallor* can be a sign of vasoconstriction, when associated with heart failure or shock, for example.

▶ **Clubbing.** Curvature of the nails and clubbed fingernails and toenails are typical signs of chronic cyanosis. Today they are seen almost only in adult patients with an Eisenmenger reaction.

► **Edema.** In neonates and infants, edema occurs primarily around the eyelids and flanks. Pretibial edema and edema at the dorsum of the foot usually do not occur until children are older.

► **Sweating.** Children with heart failure experience cold sweats due to activation of the sympathetic nervous system. The forehead is especially affected in children.

► **Thorax.** When evaluating the thorax, *thorax malformations* should be noted. A funnel chest (pectus excavatum) and a pigeon chest (pectus carinatum) occurs frequently with Marfan syndrome. *Scoliosis* can be the result of a thoracotomy. A bulging chest (*voussure*) occurs in association with cardiomegaly. *Hyperactive precordium* is characteristic for volume overload (especially associated with a pronounced left-to-right shunt or severe valve insufficiency).

► **Respiration.** *Tachypnea* can be characteristic not only of parenchymal lung disease, but is also a classic sign of a shunt defect with pulmonary hypertension, pulmonary edema, or metabolic acidosis. Tachypnea is often associated with subcostal, intercostal, or substernal retractions that indicate reduced pulmonary compliance. A Harrison groove (groove along the lower border of the thorax at the insertion of the diaphragm) indicates chronic reduction of pulmonary compliance or chronic dyspnea.

Orthopnea is a sign of reduced left ventricular function or increased pulmonary venous pressure.

► **Jugular veins.** The jugular veins should not be visible in a half-sitting position at a 45° angle. Visible filling and pulsation of the jugular veins are signs of increased venous pressure (heart failure).

1.3.2 Palpation

Palpation includes palpation of pulses, the precordium, and the abdomen.

► **Pulses.** The pulses should always be palpated on all four limbs. In neonates and infants, it is useful to palpate the pulse on the fontanelle as well. The quality (strong, weak, absent) of each pulse should be evaluated.

A *weak pulse* on all limbs is found in conjunction with a severe reduction of the left ventricular ejection fraction (e.g., critical aortic stenosis, hypoplastic left heart syndrome) or in manifest heart failure.

Strong pulses in the upper limbs and weakened or absent pulses in the lower limbs are a classical sign of coarctation of the aorta or an interrupted aortic arch.

A *water hammer pulse* (bounding, rapidly increasing pulse; *pulsus celer et altus*) is characteristic of aortic leak (run-off) and is typically found with severe aortic insufficiency, a relevant PDA, an aortopulmonary window, or an AV fistula.

Pulsus paradoxus describes an inspiratory drop in blood pressure amplitude by more than 10 mmHg. A pulsus paradoxus can occur with pericardial tamponade, constrictive pericarditis, relevant pleural effusion, or respiratory problems (e.g., asthma).

► **Precordium.** The *apex beat* can normally be palpated in the left midclavicular line (MCL) in the 4th/5th intercostal space (ICS). When associated with left ventricular volume overload (e.g., left-to-right shunt, aortic or mitral regurgitation), it is displaced to the left side and when associated with dextrocardia, to the right.

A *thrill* is a palpable vibration caused by turbulent flow. The location of the thrill varies depending on the heart defect—upper left sternal border (e.g., pulmonary stenosis), upper right sternal border (e.g., aortic stenosis), lower left sternal border (VSD), suprasternal (e.g., aortic stenosis, pulmonary stenosis), or base of the heart (e.g., left ventricular obstruction). A continuous thrill at the upper left sternal border may occur rarely with a large PDA.

Note

A thrill felt in patients with pulmonary or aortic stenosis indicates a relevant obstruction.

► **Abdomen.** If the liver is palpated on the right side it is in the normal visceral location; if palpated on the left there is situs inversus, and a liver palpated in the middle indicates situs ambiguus or heterotaxy. In infants and young children, the liver can generally be palpated about 2 cm below the costal arch, in older children approximately 1 cm below the costal arch. An enlarged liver is a sign of elevated central venous pressure and venous congestion. Hepatomegaly is thus a classic sign of heart failure. Pulsation during the liver palpation is a sign of elevated right atrial pressure, usually accompanied by relevant tricuspid regurgitation.

Splenomegaly in young children is usually not a sign of elevated central venous pressure or venous congestion. In children, splenomegaly more often occurs with an infection.

1.3.3 Blood Pressure Measurement

Every pediatric cardiology examination should include noninvasive measurement of blood pressure. The blood pressure should be measured on both the upper and lower limbs so that coarctation of the aorta or interrupted aortic arch is not overlooked. For screening, it is generally sufficient to measure the blood pressure on the right arm and one of the legs. The right arm is preferable because if there is coarctation of the aorta, the left subclavian artery may be involved in the stenosis. Blood pressure is frequently measured on all four limbs. The advantage is that a pressure gradient can be measured even if there is a rare aberrant origin of the right subclavian artery, the last aortic arch vessel distal to the left subclavian artery (as arteria lusoria) associated with coarctation of the aorta. If the blood pressure of the right arm were compared only with that of the legs, no gradient could be determined, because the right arm is also supplied by a vessel (arteria lusoria) that arises distal to the stenosis.

It is important that the blood pressure cuff has the proper width, which should be about two-thirds of the upper arm. A cuff that is too narrow yields a false high blood pressure; a cuff that is too wide gives a false low value.

The systolic pressure measured on the legs is generally 5 to 10 mmHg higher than that measured on the arms. Systolic blood pressure measured on the arms that is more than 10 mmHg higher than on the legs is a sign of coarctation of the aorta.

1.3.4 Auscultation

Auscultation of the heart includes an evaluation of the heart sounds and the exclusion or evaluation of heart murmurs in the different phases of the cardiac cycle. Auscultation is performed in a sitting and lying position and includes not only the precordium and thorax, but the neck and back as well. An aortic coarctation murmur can often be heard best in the interscapular region. The membrane and the bell of the stethoscope are both used for auscultation. High-frequency sounds are best heard with the membrane and low-frequency sounds with the bell.

The auscultation finding includes a description of the heart sounds and for heart murmurs includes intensity, timing within the cardiac cycle, tone quality, localization, and radiation if present.

Heart Sounds

► **First heart sound.** The first heart sound (S_1) is low frequency and sounds dull. It coincides with the closure of the tricuspid and mitral valves, thus marking the start of the systole. Generally, the first heart sound is heard as a single sound in auscultation, as both AV valves close nearly simultaneously. A split first heart sound may occur in a right bundle branch block or Ebstein anomaly where there is delayed closure of the tricuspid valve. As a differential diagnosis, a split first heart sound must be distinguished from a systolic ejection click associated with stenosis of the aortic or a pulmonary valve.

The first heart sound becomes louder with high cardiac output and softer with low output.

► **Second heart sound.** The second heart sound (S_2) has a higher frequency than the first heart sound. Two components can generally be heard—the aortic sound and the pulmonary valve sound (A_2 and P_2). The second heart sound can be best heard at the upper left sternal border. The aortic valve generally closes before the pulmonary valve, so the aortic click occurs before the pulmonary click. The respiration-related split of the second heart sound is significant. During inspiration, venous return to the right heart is increased. This prolongs the systole of the right ventricle. Splitting of the second heart sound increases correspondingly during inspiration. This is reversed during expiration, with reduced splitting of the second heart sound during expiration.

Wide splitting of the second heart sound occurs when right ventricular ejection lasts longer than usual or left ventricular ejection is shortened. This is also known as fixed or respiration-independent splitting of the second heart sound. The most important example of fixed splitting of the second heart sound is right ventricular volume overload due to an atrial septal defect.

Narrow splitting of the second heart sound occurs when the pulmonary valve closes earlier than normal or when aortic valve closure is delayed. Possible causes are pulmonary hypertension or an aortic stenosis.

A single, second heart sound occurs when only one semilunar valve is present (aortic or pulmonary atresia, truncus arteriosus communis) or the pulmonary valve click cannot be heard (in TGA, for example, pulmonary valve click cannot be appreciated in auscultation due to its relatively posterior position).

A paradoxical split of the second heart sound occurs when the pulmonary valve closes before the aortic valve, that is, if the systole of the left ventricle is delayed (e.g., severe aortic stenosis, left bundle branch block).

The intensity of the second heart sound depends primarily on the pressure with which the semilunar valves close. The most common cause of a loud second heart sound is pulmonary hypertension. The second heart sound is also louder when the aorta is in a relatively anterior position, for example, in TGA, tetralogy of Fallot, or pulmonary atresia.

► **Third heart sound.** The third heart sound (S_3) is a low-frequency sound that can be best heard over the cardiac apex. It is produced during the rapid filling phase of the ventricles in the early diastole. A third heart sound is normal in childhood and adolescence, but due its low frequency, it is not often heard. A loud third heart sound is abnormal and occurs when the ventricles are dilated and ventricular compliance is reduced (e.g., associated with manifest heart failure or volume overload). In this case, the sound heard in auscultation has a gallop rhythm like the word "Ken-tuc-ky" (Kentucky gallop). The third syllable of this sequence represents the third heart sound.

► **Fourth heart sound.** The fourth heart sound (S_4) is a low-frequency sound that can be best heard over the apex of the heart. It is most likely produced by increased atrial contraction during the late diastole. A fourth heart sound heard in auscultation is always pathological. It occurs with decreased ventricular compliance when increased atrial contraction is needed to fill the ventricle (e.g., heart failure, ventricular hypertrophy). The gallop rhythm that arises has a cadence like "Ten-nes-see," where the first syllable of the sequence represents the fourth heart sound.

▶ **Summation gallop.** A summation gallop is a quadruple rhythm that occurs when both third and fourth heart sounds can be heard.

▶ **Ejection click.** An ejection click is a short, high-frequency, sometimes metallic systolic sound. It is caused by the opening of an abnormal semilunar valve. An ejection click therefore occurs primarily in association with a valvular aortic or pulmonary stenosis. The click of an aortic stenosis or bicuspid aortic valve can be best heard over the cardiac apex, that of a pulmonary stenosis over the left sternal border.

Clicks occur less frequently in association with dilatation of the aorta or pulmonary artery (aortic or pulmonary artery dilatation click).

▶ **Mid-systolic click.** A mid-systolic click occurs with a mitral valve prolapse.

▶ **Mitral opening sound.** A mitral opening sound (MOS) is a high-frequency diastolic sound associated with a mitral stenosis. The earlier the MOS is auscultated, the more severe the stenosis is.

1.3.5 Cardiac Murmurs

Cardiac murmurs are graded according to timing in the cardiac cycle, intensity, frequency, tone quality, point of maximum intensity, and sound radiation. They represent turbulent blood flow (see Chapter 11).

Types of Cardiac Murmurs

We distinguish between innocent, functional, and organic cardiac murmurs:

Table 1.3 Innocent cardiac murmurs (from Hofbeck M, Apitz C 2007)

Cardiac murmur	Age peak	Point of maximum intensity	Timing in cardiac cycle, character	Remarks
Still murmur	Toddlers	Left 3rd–5th ICS parasternal	Systolic, musical tone	The sound is typically loudest when the patient is lying, becoming softer after standing. Possibly arises from vibrations of tendon fibers in the left ventricle or from vibrations of the normal pulmonary valve flap
Turbulence at the bifurcation of the pulmonary artery	Neonates, young infants	Left and right 2nd ICS parasternal, extending to the back	Systolic, harsh	In fetuses, the stem of the pulmonary artery is large, but the branches of the pulmonary arteries are slender, as they receive very little intrauterine blood flow. After the closure of the ductus, the entire cardiac output suddenly flows through the relatively hypoplastic branches of the pulmonary arteries
Pulmonary artery turbulence	Toddlers, school-age children, adolescents	Left 2nd ICS parasternal	Systolic, harsh	
Supraclavicular arterial murmur (carotid bruit)	School-age children, adolescents	Left 2nd ICS parasternal	Systolic, harsh	
Venous hum	Toddlers	Supraclavicular, more pronounced on the right, extending in an infraclavicular direction	Continuous systolic-diastolic sound (louder diastolic segment), soft humming tone	Venous turbulence that typically disappears when the head is turned

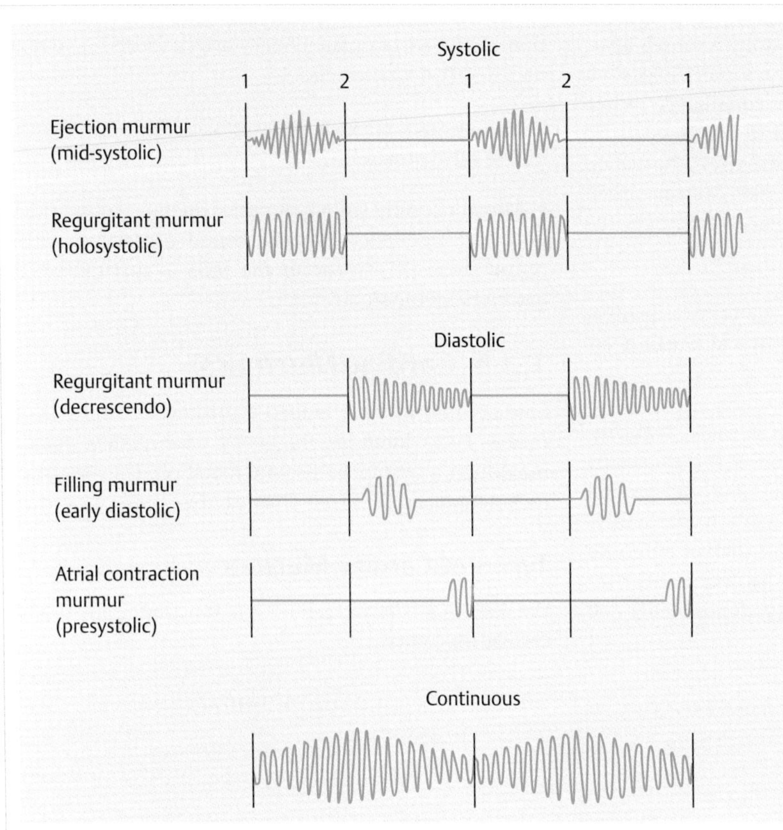

Fig. 1.1 Classification of cardiac murmurs and typical auscultation findings in the phonocardiogram.[1]

Innocent cardiac murmurs occur in children with no cardiac disease without any pathological anomaly of the cardiovascular system being found. They are almost never louder than 3/6 and are considered harmless. The most important innocent cardiac murmurs are listed in ▶ Table 1.3.

Functional cardiac murmurs are flow phenomena that occur when elevated cardiac output flows through the valves at an increased flow velocity. The most common causes in childhood are fever, anemia, or hyperthyroidism.

Organic cardiac murmurs are caused by a pathological change in the cardiovascular system. This may be stenosis of a valve or vessel, valve regurgitation, or a pathological shunt.

Intensity

Cardiac murmurs are graded on a 6-point scale depending on intensity:

- 1/6: faint murmur barely audible over breathing
- 2/6: soft, readily audible murmur
- 3/6: moderately loud murmur not associated with a thrill
- 4/6: loud murmur with a thrill
- 5/6: loud murmur audible through the palpating finger
- 6/6: loud murmur audible without a stethoscope

Frequency

The frequency of a murmur depends on the pressure gradient that causes the turbulent blood flow. The greater the pressure gradient, the higher the frequency of the murmur will be.

Accordingly, the murmurs from aortic or mitral regurgitation with their high gradients have the highest frequencies. A mitral stenosis on the other hand causes a low-frequency murmur because the gradient between the left atrium and left ventricle associated with a mitral stenosis is only about 5 to 15 mmHg.

Timing

Depending on when the murmur occurs during the cardiac cycle, we distinguish between systolic, diastolic, and continuous (systolic-diastolic) cardiac murmurs (▶ Fig. 1.1).

Systolic Cardiac Murmurs

Systolic cardiac murmurs occur during systole, that is, they can be heard between the first and second heart sounds. A distinction is made between systolic ejection and systolic regurgitant murmurs.

▶ **Systolic ejection murmurs.** Organic ejection murmurs arise from obstructions between the ventricles and the major vessels. The maximum intensity of the murmur is mid-systolic when the blood flow through the obstruction is greatest. It starts after the first heart sound and ends before the second heart sound. Ejection murmurs are also described as spindle-shaped, crescendo-decrescendo, or mid-systolic murmurs.

► **Systolic regurgitant murmurs.** Systolic regurgitant murmurs arise as a result of AV valve insufficiency when blood flows back into the atrium during the systole. Systolic murmurs caused by a VSD are also considered regurgitant murmurs, although the term "regurgitation" is actually not pathophysiologically correct in this case.

Regurgitant murmurs begin with the first heart sound and are plateau-shaped and holosystolic.

Diastolic Cardiac Murmurs

The diastolic cardiac murmurs are classified as diastolic regurgitant murmurs, diastolic filling murmurs, or atrial contraction murmurs.

Note

Diastolic heart murmurs are always pathological.

► **Diastolic regurgitant murmurs.** Diastolic regurgitant murmurs are caused by insufficiency of the semilunar valves. They begin with the second heart sound, decrease in intensity (decrescendo), and last almost until the first heart sound. Due to the larger gradient, an aortic regurgitant murmur is generally louder and has a higher frequency than a pulmonary regurgitant murmur.

► **Diastolic filling murmurs.** Diastolic filling murmurs are caused when increased blood volume (e.g., as a result of volume load from a shunt defect) flows through an AV valve. This usually involves a relative AV valve stenosis. "True" AV valve stenosis is less frequent. Due to the low gradient between atrium and ventricle during diastole,

Location	Systolic	Diastolic	Systolic/diastolic
(1) 2nd right ICS	Aortic stenosis	Aortic insufficiency	Aortic stenosis + insufficiency
(2) 2nd left ICS	Pulmonary stenosis	Pulmonary insufficiency	Pulmonary stenosis + insufficiency, patent ductus arteriosus
(3) 3rd–4th left ICS	Ventricular septal defect		Ventricular septal defect + aortic insufficiency, coronary aneurysm
(4) Apex	Mitral insufficiency	Mitral stenosis	Mitral insufficiency + stenosis
(4) Back	Coarctation of the aorta		

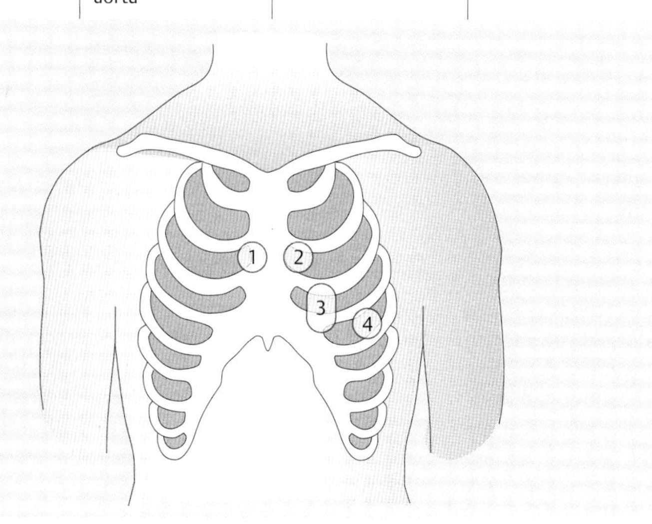

Fig. 1.2 Typical auscultation locations for important cardiac defects.[14]

Table 1.4 Typical auscultation and other indicative findings of common congenital heart defects in older children (from Hofbeck M and Apitz C 2007)

Diagnosis	Heart murmur	Point of maximum intensity/ radiation	Remarks
Small VSD	Grade 2/6–3/6 high-frequency systolic murmur	Left 3rd–4th ICS parasternal	Asymptomatic children ("much ado about nothing")
Moderate VSD without pulmonary hypertension	Harsh, grade 3/6–4/6 systolic murmur	Left 3rd–4th ICS parasternal	Possibly mild signs of heart failure, normal or slightly increased pulmonary vascular markings
Large VSD with pulmonary hypertension	Grade 1/6–3/6 systolic murmur, pronounced 2nd heart sound	Left 3rd ICS parasternal	Usually clear signs of heart failure, increased pulmonary vascular markings and cardiomegaly in chest X-ray
Large AVSD	Grade 2/6–3/6 systolic murmur, pronounced 2nd heart sound	Left 3rd ICS parasternal	Left heart axis in ECG, association with trisomy 21
Small PDA	Grade 2/6–3/6 systolic murmur	Left 2nd ICS parasternal	Frequent in premature infants
Moderate PDA	Grade 2/6–4/6 systolic-diastolic machinery murmur	Left 2nd ICS parasternal	Strong pulse, frequent in premature infants, increased pulmonary vascular markings in chest X-ray (DD: AV fistula)
ASD with relevant left-to-right shunt	Grade 2/6–3/6 systolic ejection murmur (relative pulmonary stenosis murmur), fixed split 2nd heart sound	Left 2nd ICS parasternal	Usually asymptomatic, possible frequent respiratory infections
Pulmonary stenosis	Harsh grade 2/6–4/6 systolic ejection murmur, possibly ejection click with valvular stenosis	Left 2nd ICS parasternal, radiation to the back	Usually asymptomatic
Aortic stenosis	Harsh grade 2/6–5/6 systolic ejection murmur, possibly ejection click with valvular stenosis	Right 2nd ICS parasternal, radiation to carotids	Usually asymptomatic, chest pain or syncopes under stress if stenosis is pronounced
Aortic insufficiency	High-frequency, grade 2/6–3/6 diastolic murmur	Left 3rd–4th ICS	Strong pulses, often associated with aortic stenosis
Coarctation of the aorta	Grade 1/6–3/6 systolic ejection murmur	Interscapular	Blood pressure difference between upper and lower limbs
Tetralogy of Fallot	Grade 2/6–3/6 systolic ejection murmur	Left 2nd–3rd ICS parasternal, radiation to the back	Reduced pulmonary vascular marking and normal-sized heart in chest X-ray

AVSD = atrioventricular septum defect.

these murmurs have a low frequency and are rather soft. They occur primarily during early diastole.

▶ **Atrial contraction murmurs.** Atrial contraction murmurs occur in association with AV valve stenosis. When there is an AV valve stenosis, increased atrial contraction means that maximum flow velocity for ventricular filling is not reached until late diastole. Atrial contraction murmurs are therefore not heard until late diastole or during presystole. Because of the low gradient between atrium and ventricle in diastole, these murmurs have a low frequency and are soft-pitched. They are relatively rare in childhood.

Continuous Cardiac Murmurs

Continuous heart murmurs can be heard during both systole and diastole. They usually reach maximum intensity around the second heart sound and are also described as a machinery murmur. Pathological continuous heart murmurs are caused by a short circuit when there is a pronounced difference in pressure between the vessels, both systolic and diastolic. Important examples of this are patent ductus arteriosus (PDA) and an aortopulmonary window, but also include a ruptured aneurysm of the Valsalva sinus, coronary fistulas, or AV fistulas.

One example of a harmless innocent continuous heart murmur is “venous hum.”

► **Tone quality.** Ejection murmurs and the typical VSD murmur are frequently described as harsh. Regurgitant murmurs through AV valves are typically soft-pitched, flowing, blowing, or gurgling. A diastolic murmur from an AV valve stenosis has a rumbling quality. The innocent Still murmur has a musical quality and sounds like the vibration of a string instrument.

► **Location and transmission.** The typical locations of heart murmurs are summarized in ► Fig. 1.2 and ► Table 1.4.

1.3.6 Extracardiac Murmurs

Pericardial friction rub occurs when inflamed visceral and parietal pericardial surfaces rub together—for example, associated with pericarditis or after surgery involving opening the pericardial space. If there is relevant pericardial effusion, the two surfaces of the pericardium cannot rub together and the murmur is not present. Pericardial friction rub can be best heard during inspiration and when the patient is sitting and leaning forward. The murmur can be heard during systole and diastole and often has several components. It has a grating quality and sounds near, sometimes reminiscent of walking in snow or the squeaking of leather shoes.

2 Electrocardiography

2.1 Basics

The "ECG" is one of the basic diagnostic tests in pediatric cardiology. The standard electrocardiogram (ECG) in childhood includes 12 leads:

- Bipolar limb leads (Einthoven triangle) (I, II, III)
- Unipolar limb leads (Goldberger augmented leads) (aVR, aVL, aVF)
- Precordial leads (Wilson) (V_1 to V_6; ▶ Fig. 2.1). In pediatric cardiology, the Wilson leads V_1 to V_6 are often complemented by the right precordial leads V_3R and V_4R that can contribute additional information for diagnosing hypertrophy:
  - V_1: right sternal border in the 4th intercostal space (ICS)
  - V_2: left sternal border in the 4th ICS
  - V_3: midway between V_2 and V_4
  - V_4: left mid-clavicular line (MCL) in the 5th ICS
  - V_5: left anterior axillary line in the 5th ICS
  - V_6: left mid-axillary line in the 5th ICS

The additional right precordial leads are designated with an "R." They correspond with the location of the left precordial leads on the right side of the thorax (i.e., V_4R: right MCL in the 5th ICS).

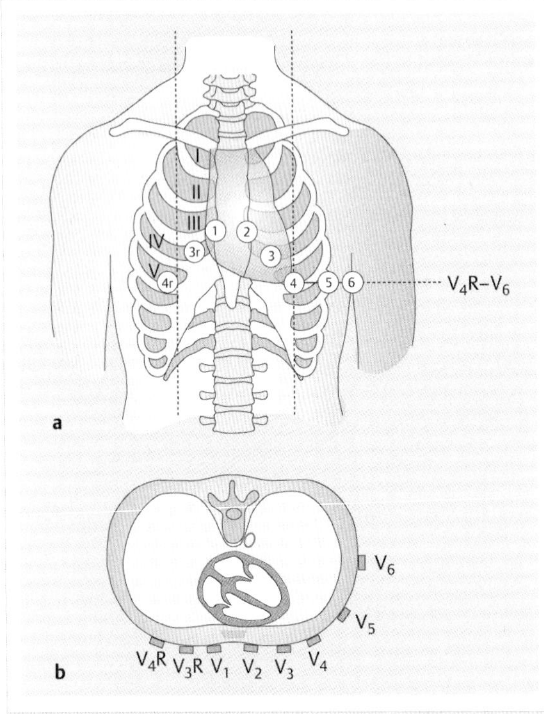

Fig. 2.1 Locations of the Wilson leads on the thorax wall.

Leads I, aVL, and V_4 to V_6 (left precordial leads) normally represent the left ventricle; while leads V_1 to V_3 and the right ventricular Wilson leads V_3R and V_4R (right precordial leads) represent the right ventricle.

The standard paper feed speed when recording is 50 mm/s. For recording over a long period, the feed speed can be reduced to 25 mm/s ("rhythm strips"). In the English-speaking world, a paper feed speed of 25 mm/s is routinely used.

Generally, the amplitude on the paper is set so that 1 cm of paper is equivalent to 1 mV. For very high amplitudes (e.g., with ventricular hypertrophy) amplification can be modified so that an amplitude of 0.5 cm is equivalent to 1 mV.

2.2 Special Features of the Pediatric ECG

Compared with an adult ECG, an ECG in childhood has the following special features (▶ Fig. 2.2):

- Higher heart rate
- Shorter conduction intervals (PQ interval, QRS duration, QT interval)
- Right ventricular dominance:
  - Axis deviation of the QRS complex to the right
  - High R wave in the right precordial leads (V_4R, V_3R, V_1, V_2, aVR)
  - Deep S wave in the left precordial leads (V_5, V_6, I)
- Negative T wave in V_1. Immediately after birth, the T waves are positive in all precordial leads in the first 4 to 8 days of life. After this, negative T waves are found in children in the right precordial leads (V_4R to V_1) and positive T waves in the left precordial leads. This pattern persists into adolescence before only positive T waves can be found in the precordial leads in adults.

Since the right ventricular muscle mass increases primarily in the last weeks of gestation, right ventricular dominance is less pronounced in premature infants. In addition, the amplitudes of the QRS complex and T wave are lower.

A *bundle branch block* features an M-shaped QRS complex. The second notch of the R wave is then designated R′ or r′, a second S notch is S′ or s′ by analogy. A capital or lower-case letter is used depending on the amplitude of the respective notch. A large notch is given a capital letter and a small notch, a lower-case letter.

An entirely *negative QRS complex* is described as QS. Examples are shown in ▶ Fig. 2.3.

ECG findings associated with some congenital heart defects are listed in ▶ Table 2.1.

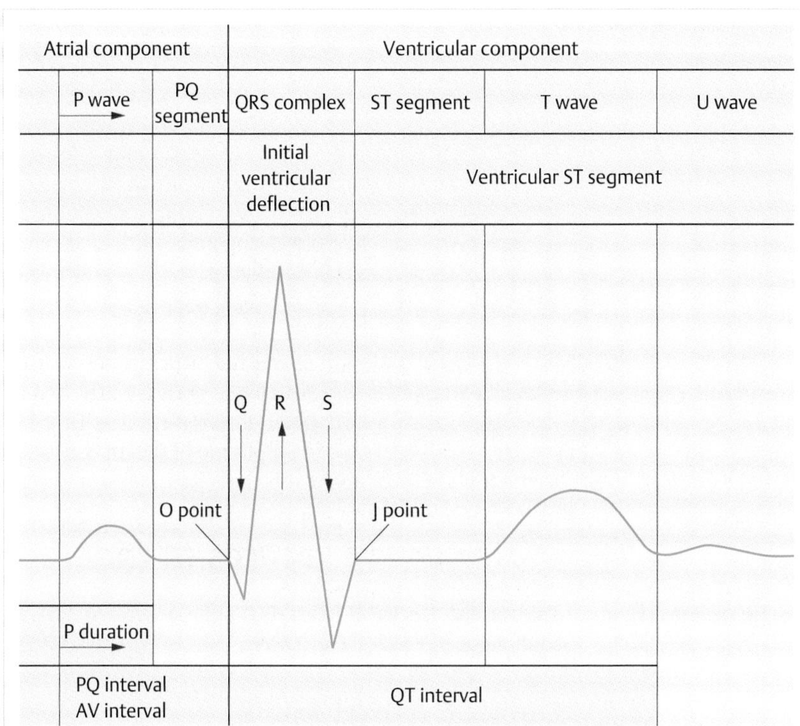

Fig. 2.2 Designation of waves, notches, and intervals in an ECG.

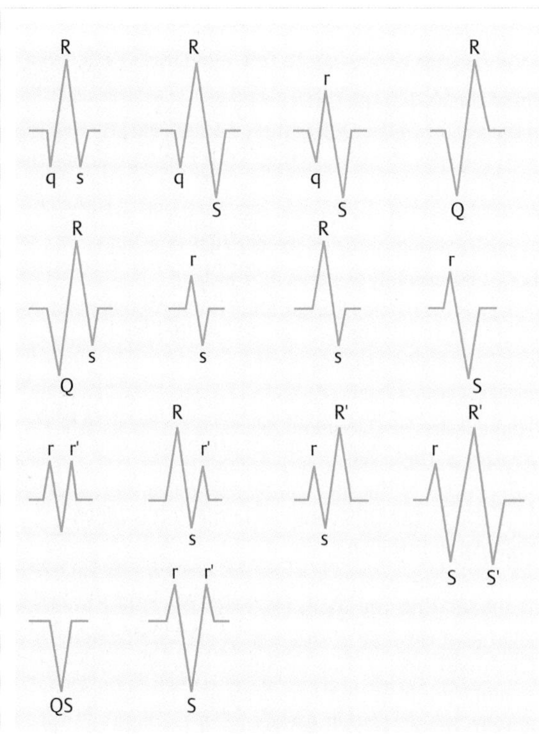

Fig. 2.3 Nomenclature of various QRS complexes depending on the amplitudes.[15]

2.3 Evaluation

The routine evaluation of an ECG should include the following points:

- Heart rhythm (e.g., sinus rhythm, ectopic atrial rhythm, escape rhythm)
- Heart rate
- Cardiac axis or QRS axis, T axis
- Conduction intervals: PQ, QRS, QT, and QTc
- Evaluation of the P wave: amplitude, duration, shape
- Evaluation of the QRS complex: amplitude, duration, shape, evaluation of the R/S ratio in the precordial leads
- Evaluation of the ST segment: take-off and course in relation to the PQ segment
- Evaluation of the T wave: amplitude, duration, direction of deflection in comparison with the QRS complex (concordant, discordant)
- Possibly evidence and evaluation of a U wave
- Evidence or exclusion of extrasystoles
- Overall assessment: Is the ECG consistent with a heart defect? Are there changes from the previous ECG?

2.3.1 Cardiac Rhythm

In an anatomically normal heart, the electrical impulse spreads from the sinus node in the upper right atrium to the lower left towards the AV node. This results in a P wave vector between 0° and 90°. Correspondingly, the P wave is positive in leads I and aVF. If the P wave has a

Table 2.1 Indicative ECG findings for some congenital heart defects

Heart defect	Indicative findings
Atrioventricular septal defect ("AV canal")	Left axis deviation, possibly AV block I°
Atrial septal defect, ostium secundum (ASD II)	Incomplete right bundle branch block of the volume overload type (rsR′)
Atrial septal defect, ostium primum (ASD I)	Left axis deviation (minimal variant of an AV canal)
Bland–White–Garland syndrome (abnormal origin of the left coronary artery from the pulmonary)	Anterolateral myocardial infarction (I, aVL, V_5, V_6)
Tricuspid atresia	Left axis deviation
Congenitally corrected transposition of the great arteries	Q waves in V_1, no Q waves in the left precordial leads V_5 and V_6, frequently AV block I–III, sometimes accessory pathways with pre-excitation and supraventricular tachycardia
Single ventricle	Monomorphic QRS complexes in all precordial leads, unusual Q waves
Mitral valve prolapse	Usually unremarkable ECG, sometimes abnormal repolarization in II, III, aVF: non-specific ST segment changes, conspicuous T waves, T wave inversion, etc.

different axis, there is usually an ectopic pacemaker in the atrial region.

Normally, every P wave is followed by a QRS complex. Otherwise there is an AV block or an escape rhythm or re-entrant tachycardia. If the P waves are missing and the QRS complexes are narrow, there is usually a junctional escape rhythm located around the AV node. Less frequently there may be a ventricular escape rhythm with wide ventricular complexes.

2.3.2 Heart Rate

The heart rate at rest is age dependent. The younger the child is, the higher the normal heart rate is:

- Neonates: 90 to 160/min
- 1 to 5 years: 70 to 150/min
- 6 to 10 years: 60 to 140/min
- 10 to 15 years: 60 to 130/min
- Over 15 years: 60 to 100/min

The heart rate is generally determined using an ECG ruler. Alternatively, it can be calculated using the R-R interval:

$$\text{Heart rate} = \frac{60}{\text{R-R interval}}$$

At a paper feed speed of 50 mm/s, 1 cm on the strip is equivalent to 0.2 s.

2.3.3 Determining the Cardiac Axis or the Axes of the QRS Complex and T Wave

The axis of the QRS complex corresponds with the spread of intraventricular excitation and is age dependent. Compared with older children and adults, neonates have a deviation of the electrical cardiac axis to the right. By age 3 years, the electrical heart axis approaches the normal adult value of + 50° (▶ Fig. 2.4).

Cardiac Electrical Axis

The axis of the QRS vector can be determined using the Cabrera circle on the basis of the limb leads (▶ Fig. 2.5).

The direction of deflection of the limb leads can be best pictured using ▶ Fig. 2.6.

The following considerations are useful when determining the axis of the QRS complex:

- If the vector of the QRS complex points exactly to a lead axis, the QRS complex in the ECG is completely positive in this lead.
- If the vector of the QRS complex points in the exact opposite direction of a lead, the QRS complex in the ECG is completely negative in this lead.
- If the vector of the QRS complex is exactly perpendicular to a lead, the QRS complex in the ECG is equally positive and negative in this lead.
- If the vector of the QRS complex deviates less than 90° from a lead, the QRS complex in the ECG is mostly positive in this lead.
- If the vector of the QRS complex deviates more than 90° from a lead, the QRS complex in the ECG is mostly negative in this lead.

This means that the main vector of the QRS complex is located near the lead with the greatest R deflection.

The main vector can be more precisely defined by observing the lead that is exactly at a right angle to the lead with the greatest R deflection. If the QRS complex is predominantly positive in this lead, the QRS vector deviates somewhat towards this lead. If it is mainly negative, it deviates in the opposite direction (▶ Fig. 2.7).

The vectors of the P and T waves can be determined in the same way.

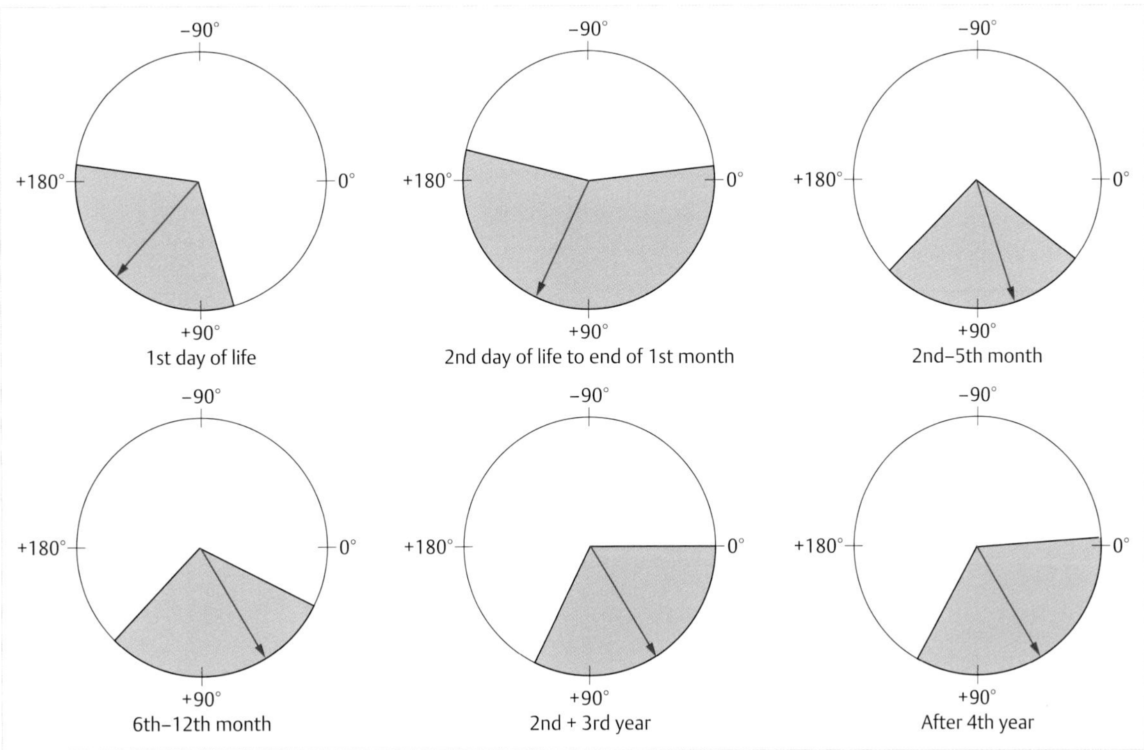

Fig. 2.4 Normal ranges of the electrical heart axis in the different age groups (from Ziegler 1951).[114]

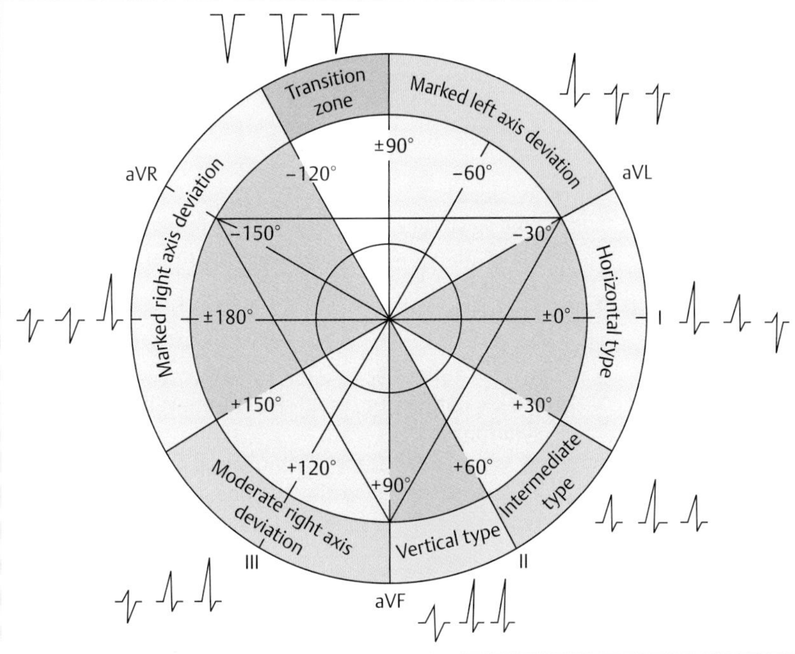

Fig. 2.5 Cabrera circle for determining the electrical axis. In most cases in clinical practice, it suffices to indicate the type of the heart's electrical axis. Typical ECG patterns of the various electrical axis types.[15]

Aside from the electrical axes described above, there are two others in which the QRS vector cannot be determined using the criteria listed. In these electrical axes, the main vector is not in the vertical plane that is measured with the limb leads, but in the horizontal plane. In the sagittal axis (also known as SI, SII, SIII type) the QRS complexes in all limb leads are approximately equally positive and negative.

In the SI-QIII type there is a conspicuously pronounced Q wave in lead III and a conspicuously deep S wave in lead I.

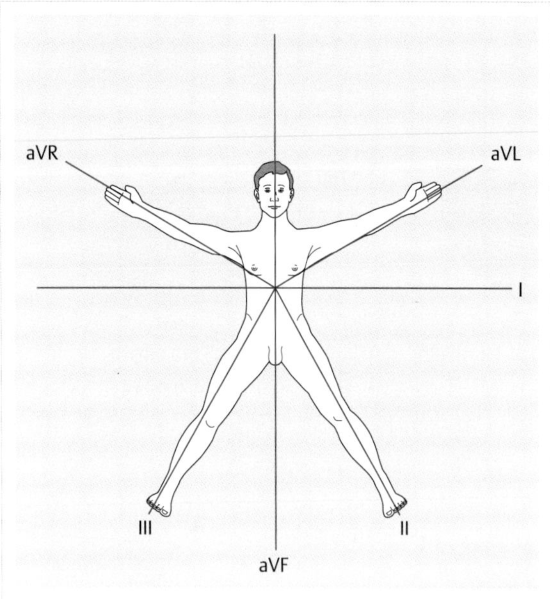

Fig. 2.6 Main deflections of the limb leads.

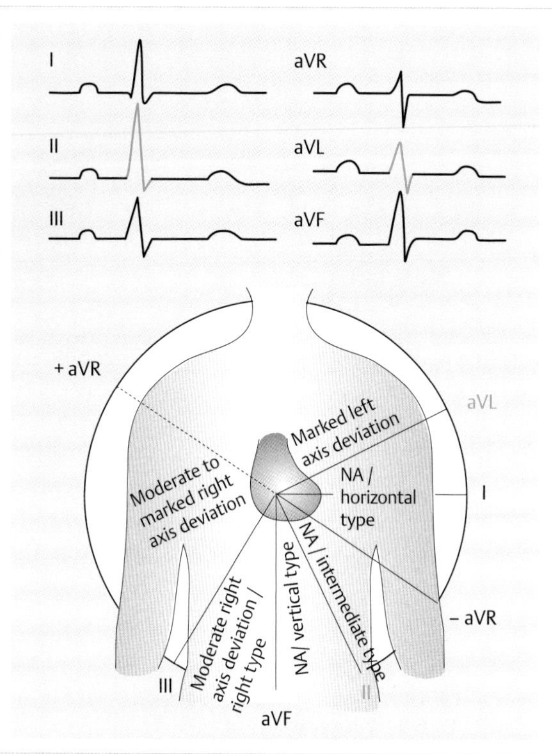

Fig. 2.7 Example for determining the heart's electrical axis. The QRS vector with the largest deflection is in lead II at about 60°. Lead aVL is perpendicular to lead II. The QRS complex is mainly positive in lead aVL. The QRS vector therefore deviates somewhat towards aVL. The angle of the QRS vector is thus around 50° (normal axis).[38] NA = Normal axis

These axis types occur with right heart stress, unusual thorax configurations, or can be constitutional with no pathological significance.

A deviation from the normal QRS axis for the child's age occurs in the following situations:

- Deviation of the QRS vector to the right: right heart hypertrophy
- Deviation of the QRS vector to the left: left heart hypertrophy (left heart hypertrophy is less sensitive to detection in an ECG than right heart hypertrophy)

In addition, left axis deviation is almost pathognomonic with atrioventricular septal defects (AV canal, AVSD) or tricuspid atresia.

A left axis deviation can also be a sign of a left anterior hemiblock. In this event, S waves can be detected up to lead V_6.

T Vector

The vector of the T wave is normally located in the vicinity of the QRS vector. An axis of the T wave that deviates from the QRS axis by more than 60° (up to 90°) is pathological and can be a sign of hypertrophy, myocardial dysfunction, ischemia, or inflammatory heart disease. The direction of deflection of the T waves in the ECG then differs from the associated QRS complex. This is called negative T wave discordance or strain pattern.

2.3.4 Conduction Intervals

► **PQ interval.** The PQ interval corresponds with the AV conduction time and is independent of age or heart rate. Causes of a prolonged PQ interval are:

- AV block I
- high vagal tone, pronounced sinus bradycardia
- Medication (digoxin, beta blockers, antiarrhythmic agents such as verapamil)
- hypokalemia

Causes of a shortened PQ interval are:

- Pre-excitation (e.g., Wolff–Parkinson–White [WPW] syndrome)
- AV ventricular escape rhythm (atrial excitation via an ectopic focus near the AV node; the P waves are typically negative in leads II and III)

► **QRS duration.** The QRS complex represents the spread of excitation to the ventricles. The duration of the QRS complex increases with age. If there is an intraventricular conduction abnormality, the QRS complex is deformed and the QRS duration is prolonged.

Possible causes of a widened QRS complex:

- Bundle branch blocks
- Pre-excitation (e.g., WPW syndrome)
- Pronounced hyperkalemia

Ventricular extrasystoles, a ventricular rhythm, or a pacemaker with ventricular stimulation can also widen the QRS complex.

► **QT interval.** The QT interval depends mainly on the heart rate. To evaluate the QT interval independently of the heart rate, the corrected QT interval is calculated (QTc) using the Bazett formula:

$$QT_C = \frac{\text{QT interval}}{\sqrt{\text{R-R interval}}}$$

The QTc interval should not exceed 0.44 s. A QTc interval up to 0.49 s can only be considered normal in children under 6 months of age. The QT interval can be most reliably determined in lead II.

A prolonged QTc interval is caused by:

- Long QT syndrome (Chapter 18.23)
- Hypocalcemia, hypokalemia
- Inflammatory heart disease
- Myocardial disease
- Traumatic brain injury
- Medication (e.g., antiarrhythmic agents of classes IA, IC, and III, antidepressants, antihistamines)
- Bundle branch blocks (in these cases, lengthening of the QT interval is a result of the widened QRS complex)

A shortened QT interval is caused by:

- Short QT syndrome (Chapter 18.24)
- Digoxin
- Hypercalcemia, hyperkalemia

2.3.5 Evaluation of the P Wave

The P wave represents the spread of excitation to the atria. Since the right atrium is normally reached first in a normal sinus rhythm, the initial segment of the P wave represents excitation in the right atrium and the terminal segment represents excitation in the left atrium.

An amplitude of the P wave greater than 3 mm indicates right atrial overload ("P dextrocardiale" or "P pulmonale").

If the P wave in an infant is wider than 0.07 s or wider than 0.09 s in older children, it is an indication of left atrial overload ("P sinistrocardiale" or "P mitrale"). The P wave frequently has two peaks in leads I and II in these cases.

2.3.6 Evaluation of the QRS Complex

The QRS complex represents the spread of ventricular excitation. The Q wave reflects the spread of excitation in the ventricular septum of the morphological left ventricle and can thus provide an indication of the position of the ventricles. Q waves can normally be seen in the left precordial leads V_5 and V_6. If there are no Q waves in these leads and they are found in the right precordial leads (V_1, V_2) instead, it is an indication of ventricular inversion, in which the morphological left ventricle is located on the right and the morphological right ventricle on the left.

Abnormally deep Q waves are considered to be a sign of hypertrophy resulting from volume overload. Deep, wide Q waves occur in myocardial infarctions. The duration of a Q wave should not exceed 0.03 s.

The amplitude of the QRS complex and especially the ratio of the R wave to the S wave in a lead (R/S ratio) are significant for diagnosing hypertrophy.

High R waves in a lead indicate hypertrophy in the ventricle represented by this lead. The opposite leads are a mirror image with deep S waves (► Fig. 2.8).

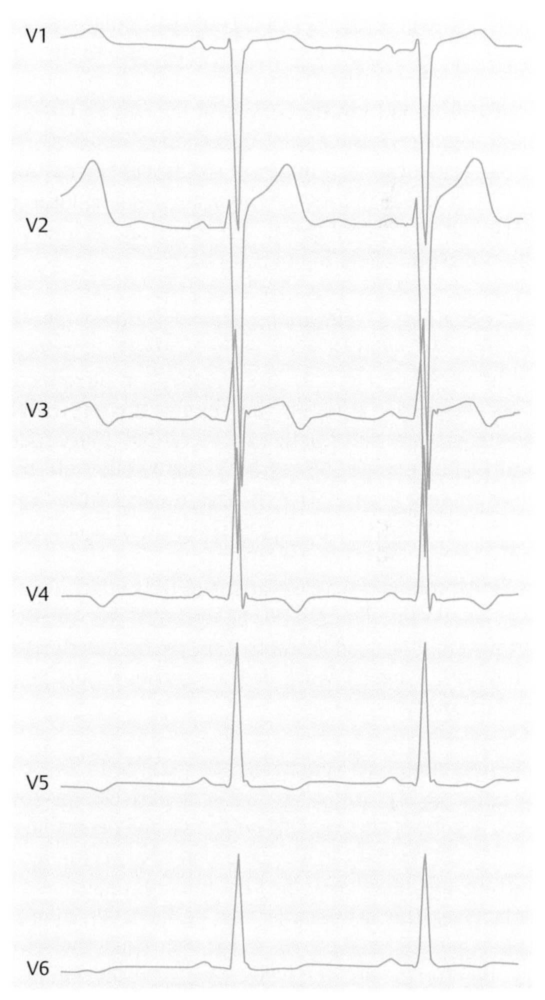

Fig. 2.8 Example of signs of left ventricular hypertrophy in the ECG associated with valvular aortic stenosis. High R waves in the left precordial leads mirror deep S waves in the right precordial leads. There is also a slight strain pattern in the left ventricular leads.

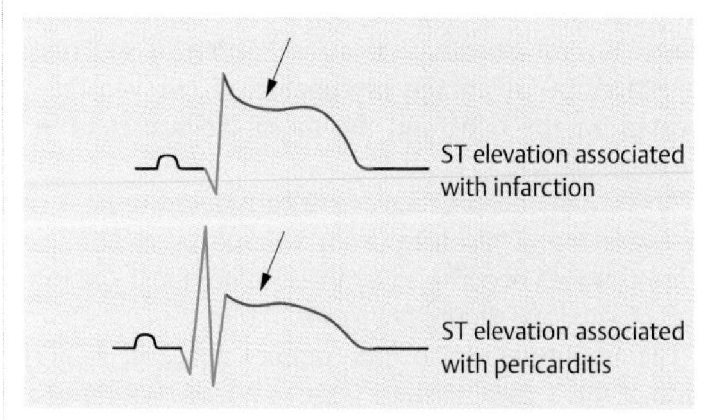

Fig. 2.9 Morphology of ST elevations in myocardial infarction and pericarditis.[38]

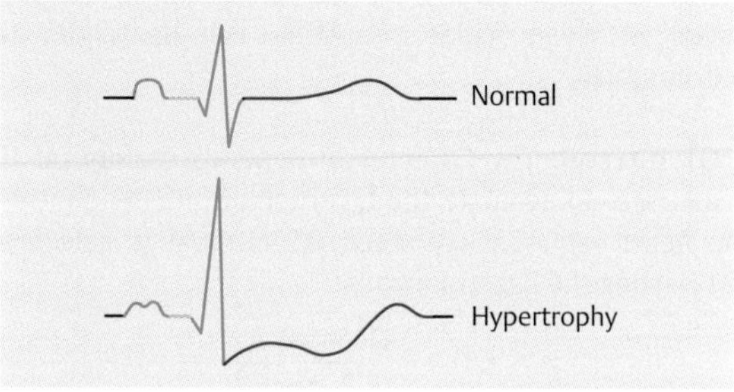

Fig. 2.10 Typical pattern of the ST segment in ventricular hypertrophy ("strain pattern").[38]

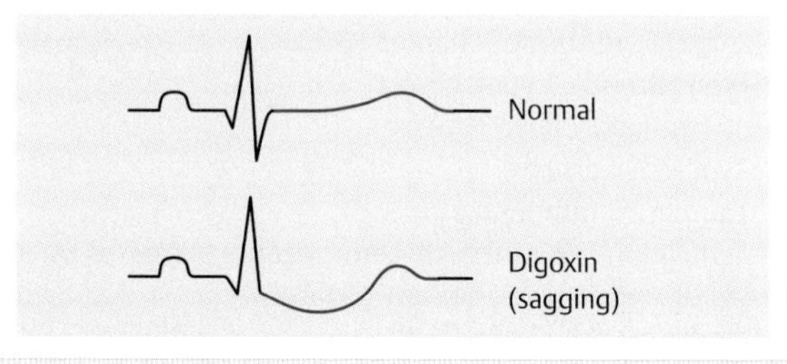

Fig. 2.11 Typical pattern of a sagging ST depression associated with digoxin medication.[38]

2.3.7 Evaluation of the ST Segment

The ST segment indicates the start of ventricular repolarization. Its normal course is along the isoelectric line (reference point is the PQ segment).

The transition from the S wave of the QRS complex to the ST segment is the J point. Elevation or depression of the ST segment up to 1 mm may still be considered normal. ST segment depressions indicate a subendocardial injury, and ST segment elevation a subepicardial injury or myocardial infarction (injury potential).

► **ST elevation.** ST elevations and ST segment take-off from the descending R wave occur primarily in myocardial infarction (► Fig. 2.9). The changes can be detected in the respective leads of the supply territory of the affected coronary artery. In a subepicardial injury (pericarditis), the elevated ST segment usually takes off from the ascending S wave. The changes in pericarditis cannot be allocated to the supply territory of a coronary artery.

Mildly pronounced ST elevations in the mid-precordial leads or the inferior leads II, III, and aVF are usually a harmless finding in adolescents. They are frequently associated with a high T wave and are attributed to "early repolarization."

► **ST depression.** ST depression may occur with endocardial ischemia (e.g., with severe aortic stenosis). In this case, the ST segments are generally horizontal and descending.

An ST depression can also be a sign of hypertrophy. In this case, the direction of the ST segment is opposite (discordant) to the main deflection of the QRS complex ("strain pattern"; ► Fig. 2.10). In left ventricular hypertrophy, the corresponding changes are typically found in leads I, aVL, V_5, and V_6; in right ventricular hypertrophy in leads V_1 and V_2.

Sagging ST depressions occur typically when digoxin is taken (► Fig. 2.11). Descending ST depressions and preterminal negative T waves in leads II, III, and aVF are typical findings of a mitral valve prolapse.

In addition, abnormal repolarization occurs with bundle branch blocks and pre-excitation syndromes. In these cases, the ST segments are not useful for making a diagnosis.

Evaluation of the T Wave

The amplitude of the T wave is usually at least one-sixth to a maximum of one-third of the preceding R wave. The T wave in the limb leads is generally concordant with the respective QRS complex. This means that in a positive QRS complex, the associated T wave is also positive. The opposite applies to negative QRS complexes, which are normally followed by a negative T wave in the corresponding lead. *Discordant negative T waves* occur, for example, after pericarditis or as a sign of myocardial hypertrophy associated with a "strain pattern" (► Fig. 2.10).

High T waves occur with high vagotonus (e.g., in physically fit adolescents), with sinus bradycardia, or with hyperkalemia (peaked, sharp T wave).

T wave alternans (alternation between positive and negative T waves in one lead) is typical of long QT syndrome.

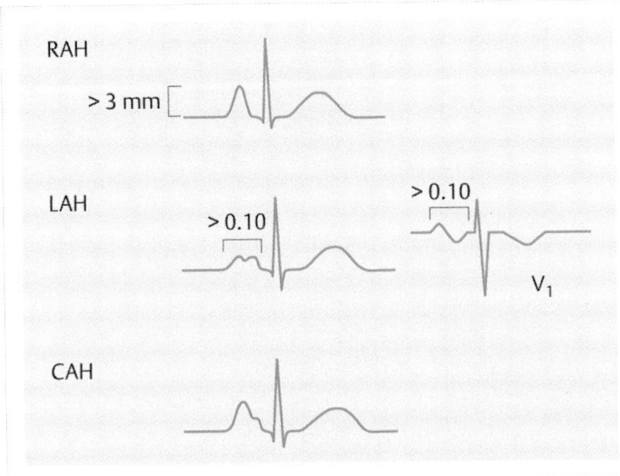

Fig. 2.12 Typical ECG changes in right atrial hypertrophy (RAH), left atrial hypertrophy (LAH), and combined hypertrophy (CAH).[29]

> **Note**
>
> Negative T waves in V_1 are normal after the fourth to eighth day of life until adolescence. QRS complexes and T waves are usually concordant in the limb leads (I, II, III, aVL, aVR, aVF).

Evaluation of the U Wave

A U wave cannot always be detected. It possibly corresponds with repolarization in the Purkinje system. Unlike the other waves and notches, the U wave is located in the diastole of the cardiac cycle. The polarity of the U wave generally corresponds with that of the T wave.

Abnormally high U waves are found in:

- hypokalemia
- left ventricular hypertrophy (the higher the R amplitude, the more positive or negative the U wave is)

Abnormally configured U waves are also frequently found in long QT syndrome.

2.3.8 Criteria for Hypertrophy in an ECG

Atrial Hypertrophy

Changes in the amplitude and duration of P waves are indications of atrial hypertrophy (▸ Fig. 2.12).

A P wave over 3 mm high ("P pulmonale"; usually in lead II or the right precordial leads V_1/V_2) is a sign of *right atrial hypertrophy*.

A P wave duration of more than 0.1 s, or more than 0.08 s in children under 1 year old, is a sign of *left atrial hypertrophy*. The P wave in these cases frequently has double peaks or is biphasic in lead V_1.

In *biatrial hypertrophy* there is a combination of an excessively high and widened P wave.

Ventricular Hypertrophy

Typical changes can occur in the ECG due to ventricular hypertrophy. The leads in which the changes can be detected indicate whether there is right ventricular hypertrophy, left ventricular hypertrophy, or combined hypertrophy. Typical changes that indicate ventricular hypertrophy are (▸ Fig. 2.13):

- deviations from the QRS axis,
- increase in QRS amplitude and R/S ratio,
- evidence of abnormal Q waves,
- changes in the repolarization phase ("strain pattern," ST depression),
- increase in the QRS interval (intraventricular conduction disorder).

▸ **Right ventricular hypertrophy.** There are somewhat different signs in the ECG for hypertrophy involving pressure and volume overload.

Signs of a right ventricular pressure overload hypertrophy (e.g., associated with severe pulmonary stenosis) are:

- cardiac axis deviation (QRS vector) to the right
- high, narrow R waves in the right precordial leads (V_1/V_2); the height of the R waves frequently correlates well with right ventricular pressure overload
- ST depression and negative T waves in the right precordial leads

Signs of right ventricular *volume overload* (e.g., hemodynamically relevant ASD) are:

- slight cardiac axis deviation (QRS vector) to the right
- borderline wide or slightly widened QRS complex with fragmentation of the QRS, complex as in an incomplete right bundle branch block (typical configuration: rsR′ or rR′s, i.e., R′ > r)
- amplitude of the R waves usually less pronounced than in systolic overload
- ST depression and negative T waves in the right precordial leads

▸ **Left ventricular hypertrophy.** Compared with the criteria for right ventricular hypertrophy, the sensitivity with respect to left ventricular hypertrophy is clearly lower in the ECG.

Signs of left ventricular *pressure overload hypertrophy* are:

- cardiac axis deviation to the left (not always present)
- high R waves in the left precordial leads (V_5/V_6)
- ST depression and negative T waves in the left precordial leads
- deep S waves in the right precordial leads (V_1/V_2)

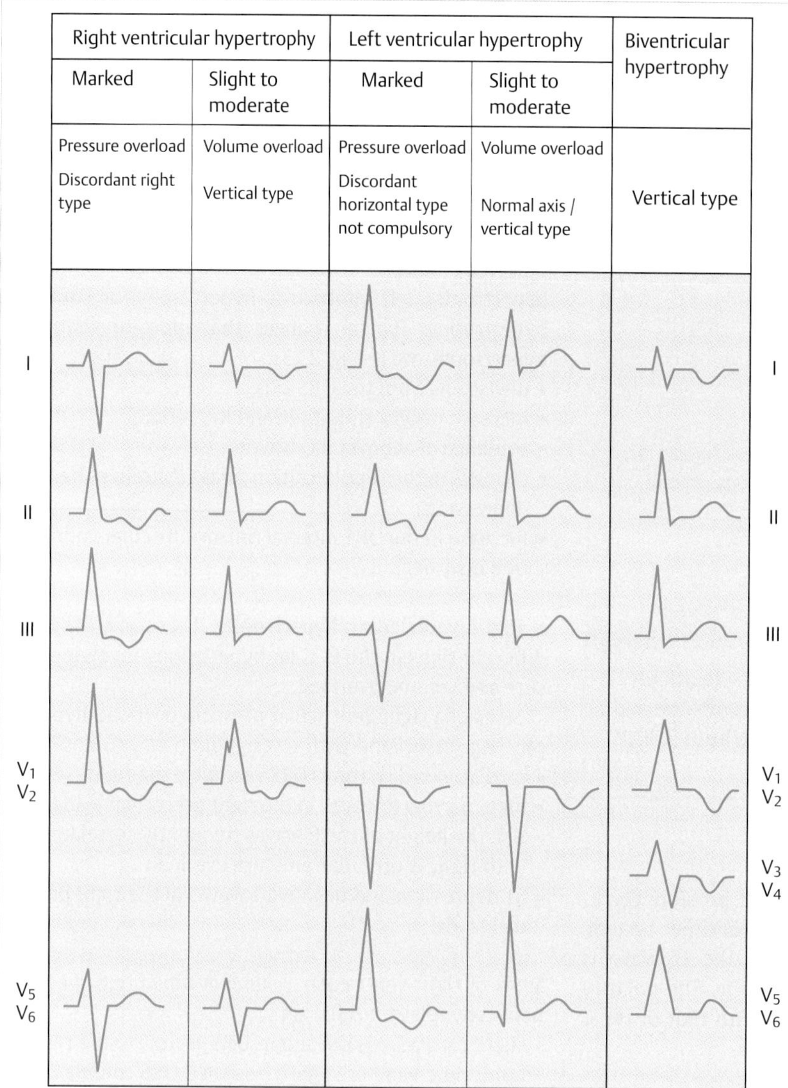

Fig. 2.13 Summary of the typical ECG changes associated with right and left ventricular pressure or volume overload and biventricular hypertrophy.[15]

Signs of left ventricular *volume overload hypertrophy* are:

- deep S waves in the right precordial leads
- pronounced Q waves in the left precordial leads
- slightly elevated R waves (possible slight fragmentation) in the left precordial leads

▶ **Biventricular hypertrophy.** In biventricular hypertrophy there are simultaneous signs of left and right ventricular hypertrophy. There is typically a relatively uniform picture in the precordial leads from V_1 to V_6 in the sense of a continuous rS or RS configuration of the QRS complex.

3 Echocardiography

3.1 Transthoracic Echocardiography

3.1.1 Basics

Two-dimensional (2D) echocardiography is the most important noninvasive imaging procedure in pediatric cardiology. It provides cross-sectional images of the heart and great vessels. The examination is performed using standard cross-sectional planes.

In routine diagnostics, 2D echocardiography is supplemented by examinations using M-mode, Doppler, and color Doppler imaging techniques. In some cases, three-dimensional (3D) echocardiography and tissue Doppler examinations can provide additional information.

M-mode Echocardiography

M-mode echocardiography is a one-dimensional technique (▸ Fig. 3.1). M-mode is used to observe a small segment of the heart over a certain period. The advantage of this method is its good temporal resolution. The method is used in particular for time-dependent visualization of moving structures (e.g., cardiac valves) and for measuring size (e.g., systolic and diastolic diameter of the ventricles).

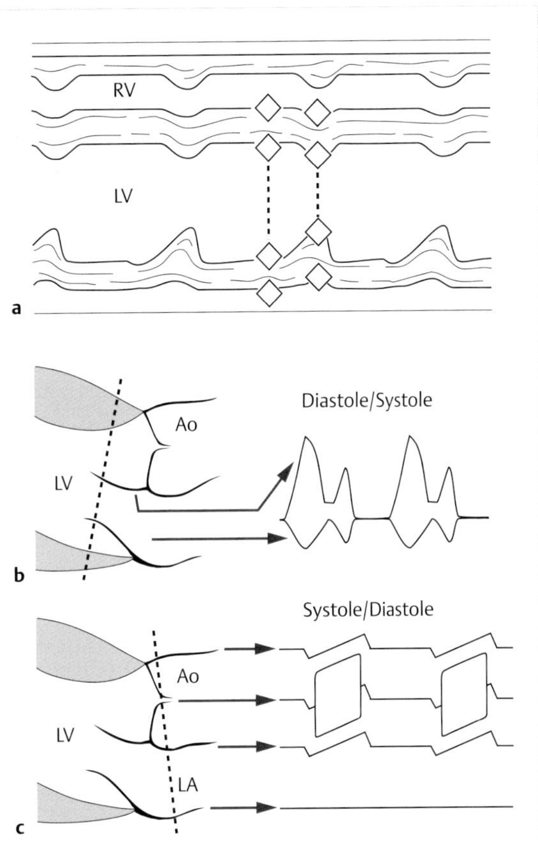

Fig. 3.1 M-mode in the left parasternal longitudinal axis.[26] **a** Most common uses of M-mode. In the left parasternal axis, M-mode is used at the ventricular level to determine the size of the right ventricle (RV), the interventricular septum (IVS), the left ventricle (LV), and the left ventricular posterior wall (LVPW) in diastole and systole. In addition, the systolic and end-diastolic diameter of the left ventricle can be used to calculate fractional shortening. Maximum diameter of the left ventricle occurs during diastolic filling. It contracts during the systole. The IVS and the LVPW normally move closer during the systole. **b** When the ultrasound beam is directed through the mitral valve, the M-shaped opening pattern of the anterior mitral valve leaflet and the mirror-image W-shaped pattern of the posterior mitral valve leaflet can be visualized during diastole. **c** When the beam is directed toward the aortic valve, the parallelogram-shaped opening pattern in systole is visualized. The mid-echo of the closed aortic valve can be seen during diastole.

Doppler Echocardiography

Doppler echocardiography utilizes the Doppler effect. Moving an ultrasound transducer closer to or further from the receiver results in a frequency shift of the ultrasound waves. The Doppler effect can be used to measure the direction and velocity of the acoustic source. An example from everyday life is that a pedestrian can distinguish whether an ambulance with a siren is approaching (increasing pitch of the siren) or moving away (decreasing pitch). The pedestrian can also estimate whether the ambulance is approaching or moving away rapidly or slowly (extent of the increase or decrease in pitch).

Doppler echocardiography utilizes the frequency shift that occurs when ultrasound waves are reflected off moving blood cells, allowing the velocity and direction of blood flow to be determined (▸ Table 3.1 and ▸ Table 3.2). However, measurement is reliable only if the flow direction is nearly parallel to the ultrasound beam, in other words moving directly toward or away from the ultrasound beam. The procedure therefore depends on the angle of the beam.

The most common procedures in echocardiography are pulsed wave (PW) Doppler, continuous wave (CW) Doppler, and color Doppler.

▸ **Pulsed wave Doppler.** In this method, the transducer emits and receives ultrasound waves in rapid succession. The next pulse is not sent until the previous one is received. This procedure enables flow velocities to be measured in a certain sample volume. In practice, this means that the region along the ultrasound beam where flow velocity is to be measured can be set. For example, when the ultrasound beam is directed across the right ventricular outflow tract, the pulmonary valve, and the main pulmonary artery, one can choose whether to

Table 3.1 Standard Doppler echocardiography measurements (from Lai WW et al. 2006)[83]

Anatomical structure	Measurements
Tricuspid valve	E wave and A wave velocity, mean pressure gradient, IVRT, velocity of the regurgitation flow if there is tricuspid valve insufficiency
Right ventricular outflow tract	Peak gradient, mean pressure gradient
Pulmonary valve	Peak gradient, mean pressure gradient, velocity of the regurgitation flow if there is pulmonary valve insufficiency
Pulmonary artery branches	Peak gradient, mean pressure gradient
Mitral valve	E wave and A wave velocity, mean pressure gradient, IVRT, pressure half time (PHT) if there is a mitral valve stenosis
Left ventricular outflow tract	Peak gradient, mean pressure gradient
Aortic valve	Peak gradient, mean pressure gradient
Aortic arch, aortic isthmus	Peak gradient, mean pressure gradient

IVRT, isovolumetric relaxation time

Table 3.2 Normal flow velocities in children measured using Doppler echocardiography (from Goldberg SJ et al. 1985)[12]

Structure	Mean (m/s)	Normal range (m/s)
Aorta	1.5	1.2–1.8
Mitral valve inflow	1.0	0.8–1.3
Tricuspid valve inflow	0.6	0.5–0.8
Pulmonary artery	0.9	0.7–1.1

measure blood flow velocity in the infundibulum, across the pulmonary valve, or in the main pulmonary artery.

However, the disadvantage of this method is that it cannot be used to measure high flow velocities. Blood flow moving toward the transducer is normally displayed above the zero line and blood flow moving away from the transducer is displayed below the zero line. However, if a certain maximum velocity is exceeded (Nyquist limit), aliasing occurs, meaning that the curve generated by the blood flow on the monitor is cut off and displayed on the other side of the zero line. Neither flow direction nor velocity can then be reliably assessed.

► **Continuous wave Doppler.** In this Doppler method, continuous ultrasound waves are emitted and received. The disadvantage is that it is impossible to distinguish at which location of the beam certain Doppler signals are generated. It is thus not possible to determine precisely where along the ultrasound beam the flow velocities occur. In the above example, the maximum flow velocity in the right ventricular outflow tract through the pulmonary valve and in the pulmonary artery can be determined, but not the precise location. The advantage is that very high flow velocities can be measured using CW Doppler. Aliasing practically never occurs.

► **Color Doppler.** Blood flow in the heart and great vessels can be displayed well using color Doppler. Blood flow directed toward the transducer is generally displayed in red; blood flow in the opposite direction appears blue. Turbulent blood flow is green or a mosaic of colors. Since the color Doppler is based on a PW Doppler technique, color reversal (aliasing) occurs when a certain velocity is exceeded.

► **3D echocardiography.** Modern equipment makes it possible to produce a three-dimensional image. These techniques have not yet become common in routine diagnostics. They are sometimes used to obtain a detailed image of cardiac valves or to determine the volume of the heart chambers.

► **Tissue Doppler.** Tissue Doppler imaging is a method for assessing tissue movement, which is relatively slow compared with blood flow. Special velocity and amplitude filters are required for this. Tissue movements primarily involve myocardial motion. In clinical practice, tissue Doppler imaging is most frequently used to evaluate diastolic function (see Chapter 3.1.2).

Regional myocardial deformation can be quantified using "strain" and "strain rate." The significance of these relatively new parameters is currently being investigated in many clinical trials.

3.1.2 Standard Examination and Standard Planes

The various standard planes are presented below. In addition to 2D echocardiography, the relevant Doppler and M-mode measurements that can be made in the respective planes are explained.

Overview of the standard planes (► Table 3.3):

Table 3.3 Standard echocardiographic measurements of cardiovascular structures (from Lai WW et al. 2006)[83]

Anatomical structure	Measurement timepoint	Suitable standard views
Tricuspid valve annulus	Diastole	Apical four-chamber view
Mitral valve annulus	Diastole	Apical four-chamber view, left parasternal long axis
Diameter of the left atrium	Diastole	Left parasternal long axis
Pulmonary valve annulus	Systole	Left parasternal long axis, tilted left parasternal long axis
Main pulmonary artery	Systole	Left parasternal short axis, tilted left parasternal short axis
Pulmonary artery branches	Systole	Left parasternal short axis, tilted left parasternal long axis
Aortic valve annulus	Systole	Left parasternal long axis
Aortic root	Systole	Left parasternal long axis
Ascending aorta	Systole	Left parasternal long axis
Transverse aortic arch	Systole	Suprasternal view (long axis)
Aortic isthmus	Systole	Suprasternal view (long axis)

- Apical planes:
  - Four-chamber view
  - Five-chamber view
  - Two-chamber or three-chamber view
- Parasternal planes:
  - Left parasternal longitudinal views (long axis)
  - Left parasternal transverse views (short axis)
- Subcostal planes
  - Subcostal longitudinal views
  - Subcostal transverse views
- Suprasternal planes:
  - Suprasternal longitudinal view
  - Suprasternal transverse view
- Abdominal planes

The transducer positions for the various planes are depicted in ▶ Fig. 3.2.

The examination is generally performed in the supine position on neonates and infants and is best performed in the left lateral position on older children to prevent artifacts from air in the lungs.

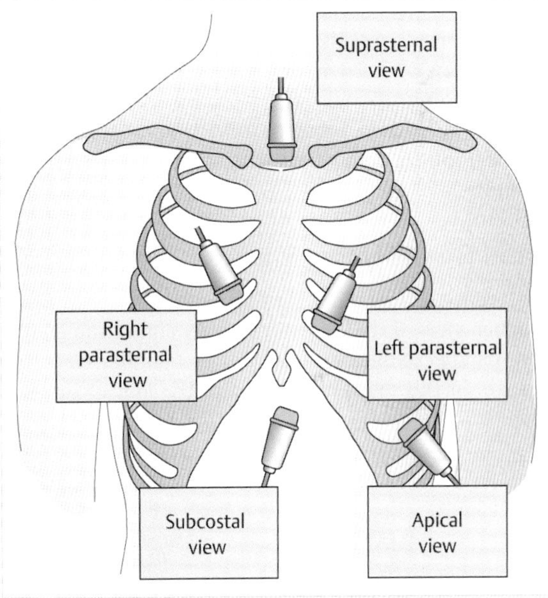

Fig. 3.2 Positions of the transducer in standard echocardiography planes.[18]

Apical Planes

For apical planes, the transducer is placed near the cardiac apex. The transducer marking points to the patient's left side, so the patient's right side is displayed on the left of the monitor.

Apical Four-Chamber View

▶ **2D echocardiography.** The apical four-chamber view should be used first as it enables an initial assessment of the size and function of ventricles and atria to be made. Moreover, a muscular ventricular septal defect (VSD) can be visualized very well in this plane.

The apical four-chamber view is set so that all four cardiac chambers can be seen. It is necessary to invert the image on the monitor. In this "anatomically correct" display (surgical view), the atria are displayed at the top of the monitor and the ventricles at the bottom. The ventricular septum should be as vertical as possible in the apical four-chamber view. The right ventricle can be readily recognized by the tricuspid valve that is somewhat closer to the apex than the mitral valve. In addition, there is a thick muscular band (moderator band) at the right ventricular apex that cannot be detected in the left ventricle.

▶ **Doppler.** The apical four-chamber view displays the diastolic inflow through the mitral and tricuspid valves into the left and right ventricles using Doppler and color Doppler techniques.

In the PW Doppler profile, the typical M-shaped configuration of diastolic inflow is seen. The two peaks of the "M" are designated E wave and A wave. The E wave represents "early" diastolic filling and the A wave represents "atrial" contraction flow. AV valve stenosis can be quantified by determining the mean pressure gradient through the valve. This is done by tracing the contour of the M-shaped Doppler signal. Modern echocardiography equipment then calculates the mean pressure gradient using the area under the curve.

AV valve insufficiency can be seen in the color Doppler. In these cases, regurgitation through the affected valve into the atrium is seen during diastole. In the color Doppler, the regurgitation jet is blue. Using the Bernoulli equation, the maximum velocity of the regurgitation jet is used to estimate the gradient across the valve and thus the pressure in the affected chamber. If the maximum velocity of regurgitation is 3 m/s, for example, the pressure difference across the valve according to the Bernoulli equation ($4 \times V_2$) is 36 mmHg. If it is then assumed that the pressure in the right atrium, which is equivalent to the central venous pressure (CVP), is approximately 4 mmHg, the right ventricular pressure must be around 40 mmHg.

Apical Five-Chamber View

▶ **2D echocardiography.** Starting with the apical four-chamber view, if the acoustic beam is aimed somewhat more parallel to the sternum, the five-chamber view can be seen. In this view, in addition to the four chambers, the left ventricular outflow tract, the aortic valve, and the ascending aorta as "fifth chamber" can be seen.

In this plane, any obstruction of the function of the aortic valve and the left ventricular outflow tract can be assessed. Ectasia of the ascending aorta can also be visualized well in this plane.

▶ **Doppler.** Since the flow in the left ventricular outflow tract and across the aortic valve is almost parallel to the acoustic beam in this plane, it is particularly suitable for quantifying aortic valve stenosis and obstructions of the left ventricular outflow tract. In Doppler ultrasonography, aortic valve insufficiency is seen as regurgitation during the diastole.

Apical Four-Chamber View (posterior angulation)

▶ **2D echocardiography.** Starting from the four-chamber view, tilting the transducer further backward (steeper) brings an additional structure into view, the coronary sinus (▶ Fig. 3.3), which receives venous blood from the coronary vessels, proceeds along the lower wall of the left atrium, and empties into the right atrium. The left atrium can be clearly distinguished from the right atrium by the coronary sinus. A dilated coronary sinus is a sign of a left persistent superior vena cava, which frequently empties into the coronary sinus.

Apical Two-Chamber or Three-Chamber View

▶ **2D echocardiography.** Rotating the transducer 90° clockwise from the four-chamber view position yields the two-chamber view (▶ Fig. 3.4). This view shows the left

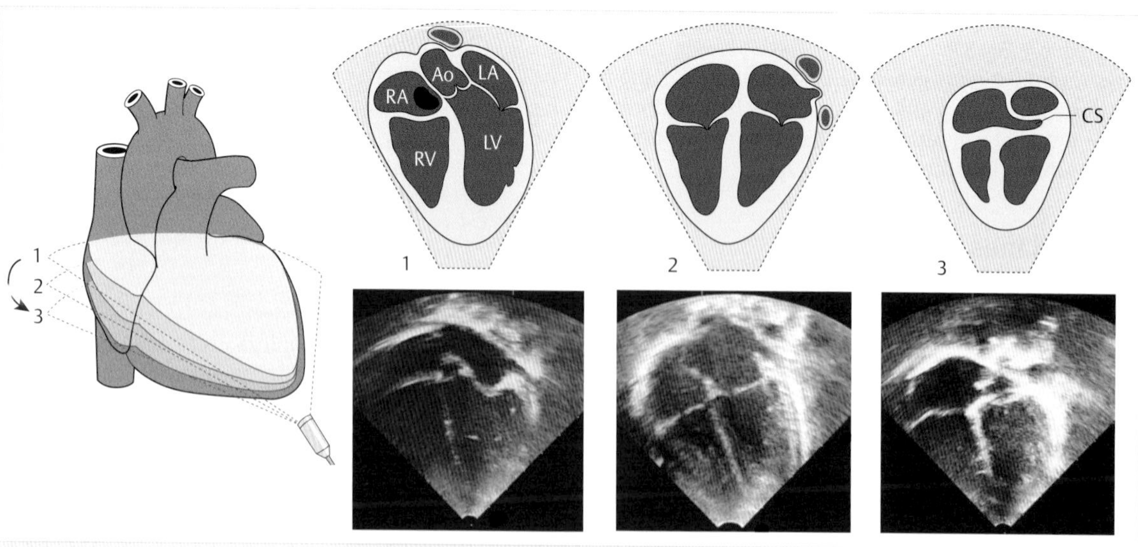

Fig. 3.3 Standard sections of the apical four-chamber view and five-chamber view (inverted).
RA, right atrium; LA, left atrium; RV, right ventricle; LV, left ventricle; Ao, aorta; CS, coronary sinus.

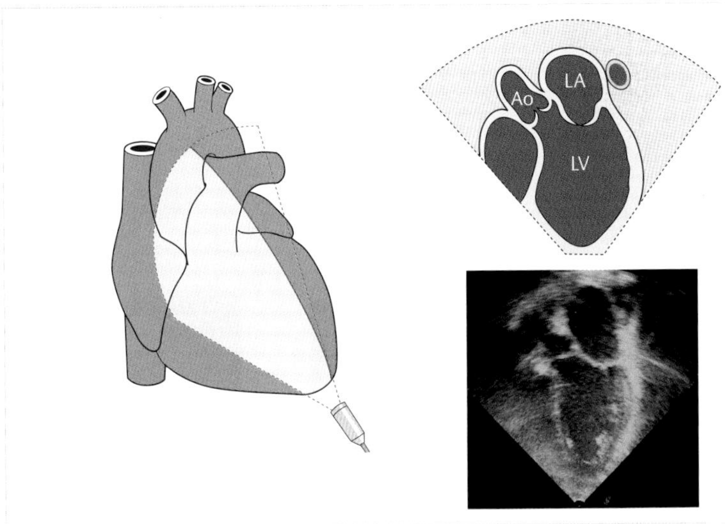

Fig. 3.4 The apical two-chamber view. LA, left atrium; LV, left ventricle; Ao, aorta.

ventricle, the left atrium, and the aorta. If the aortic valve and the ascending aorta are also included, it is called the apical three-chamber view.

▸ **Doppler.** In this position, color Doppler ultrasound can be used to visualize mitral and aortic valve insufficiency. Flow velocity over the mitral valve, the left ventricular outflow tract, and the aortic valve can also be determined.

Left Parasternal Planes

Left Parasternal Long Axis

▸ **2D echocardiography.** The left parasternal long axis runs parallel to the ventricular septum. The marking on the transducer points approximately to the patient's right shoulder. The right ventricle is located immediately below the transducer, followed by the interventricular septum, the left ventricle, and the left ventricular posterior wall. In this plane, the junction of the interventricular septum and the anterior wall of the aorta and ascending aorta can also be seen. The aortic valve is readily visible and its function can be evaluated.

The left atrium is located behind the ascending aorta. The anterior leaflet of the mitral valve is contiguous with the aorta with no myocardial tissue separating them. This is called "aortomitral continuity," a characteristic feature of the left ventricle. The anatomy and function of the mitral valve can also be readily evaluated in this position.

In addition, any movement of the septum or regional dyskinesia should be noted. Dilatation in the ascending aorta that can occur with aortic ectasia (e.g., associated with Marfan syndrome) must be excluded. Malalignment VSD with an overriding vessel (e.g., in tetralogy of Fallot or truncus arteriosus communis) can be readily visualized in the 2D view of this plane.

▸ **Doppler.** Insufficiency of the aortic and mitral valves can be visualized using color Doppler. In this setting, perimembranous and sometimes muscular VSD can be visualized using color Doppler.

▸ **M-mode.** The left parasternal long axis is the standard plane for many M-mode measurements. The interventricular septum and the left ventricular posterior wall appear nearly perpendicular in this plane. Positioning the beam of the M-mode through both ventricles allows the thickness of the interventricular septum, the size of the left ventricle, and the dimensions of the left ventricular posterior wall in systole and diastole to be reliably determined (see ▸ Fig. 3.1). Fractional shortening can be calculated as an indication of left ventricular function (Chapter 3.1.3).

By positioning the beam of the M-mode to include the distal ends of the mitral leaflets, the M-shaped motion of the anterior mitral leaflet and the mirror-image motion of the posterior leaflet can be seen. If there is an obstruction in the left ventricular outflow tract, the anterior mitral leaflet is "drawn into" the left ventricular outflow tract during systole. In the M-mode, this phenomenon can be seen as "systolic anterior movement" (SAM phenomenon). In a mitral valve prolapse, "sagging" of one or both mitral leaflets is observed during systole.

When the beam of the M-mode is positioned further in the cranial direction, the ascending aorta, aortic valve, and left atrium can be visualized together. The ratio of the size of the ascending aorta and the left atrium is normally about 1:1. If there is relevant patent ductus arteriosus (PDA), the size of the atrium increases disproportionately and the ratio of ascending aorta to the atrium increases to 1:1.3 to 1.5 or more. The measurements are made in the end systole when the left atrium has reached its maximum size.

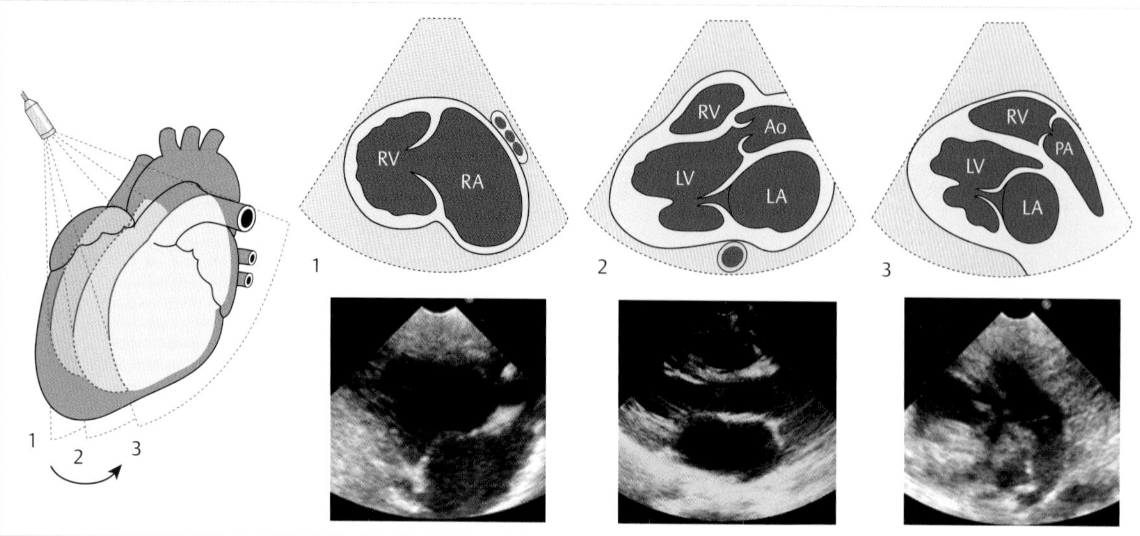

Fig. 3.5 The left parasternal long axes. RA, right atrium; LA, left atrium; RV, right ventricle; LV, left ventricle; Ao, aorta; PA, pulmonary artery.

The aortic valve opening can also be visualized in the left parasternal long axis. In M-mode, the opened aortic valve looks like a parallelogram. When the valve is closed, the mid-echo normally runs midway between the anterior and posterior wall of the aorta. If the aortic valve is bicuspid, the mid-echo is eccentric.

Left Parasternal Long Axis (rotate left)

► **2D echocardiography.** Starting from the left parasternal long axis, tilting the transducer slightly to the left toward the patient's left shoulder brings the right ventricular outflow tract, the pulmonary valve, and the main pulmonary artery into view. This view is suitable for evaluating an infundibular stenosis of the outflow tract, for example, and for visualizing the pulmonary valve and the main pulmonary artery.

► **Doppler.** Using the Doppler technique, flow velocities and thus the gradients in the right ventricular outflow tract, across the pulmonary valve, and in the main pulmonary artery can be measured. Pulmonary insufficiency can be visualized using color Doppler.

Left Parasternal Long Axis (rotate right)

► **2D echocardiography.** Starting from the left parasternal long axis, tilting the transducer slightly to the right toward the patient's right hip brings the right atrium, tricuspid valve, and right ventricle into view (► Fig. 3.5). This view is well suited for evaluating the tricuspid valve.
► **Doppler.** Using color Doppler, tricuspid insufficiency can be reliably assessed in this position. The right ventricular pressure can be estimated using the velocity of the regurgitation jet and the Bernoulli equation.

Left Parasternal Short Axis (at the level of the aortic valve)

► **2D echocardiography.** For this position, the transducer is rotated about 90° clockwise from the left parasternal axis. At the center of the image is the cross-section of the aortic valve with its three cusps, similar to a Mercedes star. By moving the transducer slightly, it is usually possible to visualize the origins of the coronary arteries from the left and right coronary sinus. Behind the aortic valve is the left atrium, which is separated from the right atrium by the atrial septum. The right atrium opens into the right ventricle through the tricuspid valve. Part of the pulmonary valve can be seen to the left of the aortic valve. The pulmonary valve annulus can be reliably measured in this position. The right ventricular outflow tract is visualized directly below the valve. Infundibular stenosis can be readily detected here. Distal to the pulmonary valve are the main pulmonary artery and the Y-shaped bifurcation into its two main branches. Ostial stenosis of the pulmonary arteries can be readily visualized in this view.

► **Doppler.** Using color Doppler, pulmonary insufficiency can be detected in this view. In addition, obstructions or stenosis of the right ventricular outflow tract, the pulmonary valve, or the origins of the pulmonary arteries are seen as flow turbulence.

A shunt in the region of the atrial septum can sometimes be visualized in this view using color Doppler. The parasternal short axis is also suitable for screening for a PDA. A PDA with a left-to-right shunt leads to diastolic flow in the main pulmonary artery moving toward the pulmonary valve.

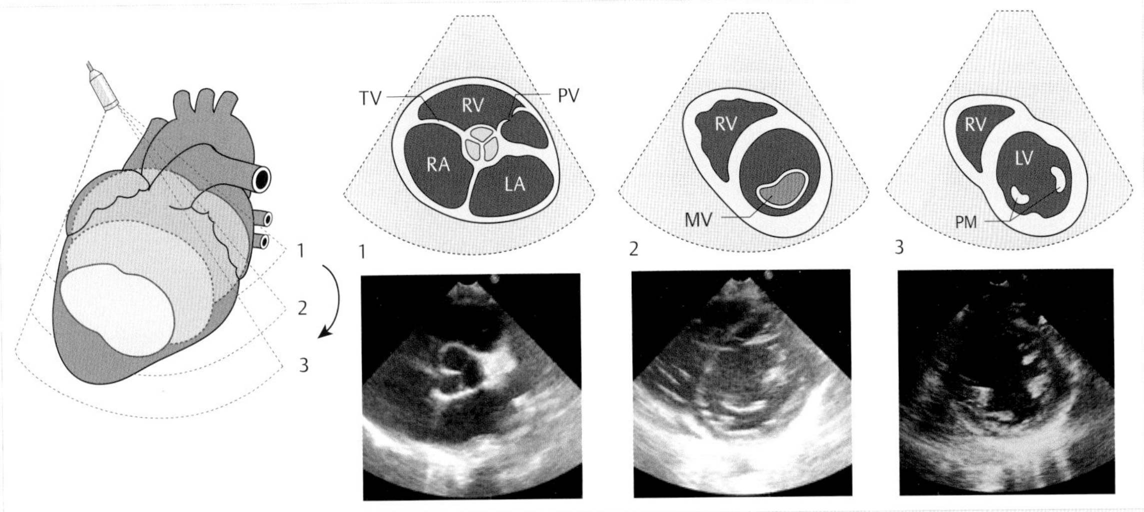

Fig. 3.6 The left parasternal short axes. RA, right atrium; LA, left atrium; RV, right ventricle; LV, left ventricle; PV, pulmonary valve; TV, tricuspid valve; MV, mitral valve; PM, papillary muscle insertions.

Left Parasternal Short Axis (at the level of the mitral valve)

▸ **2D echocardiography.** When the transducer is moved further in a caudal direction, a cross-section of the left ventricle is reached where the mitral valve can be visualized particularly well. The characteristic fish-mouth opening motion of the mitral valve can be seen and anomalies of the mitral valve (e.g., cleft) can be reliably assessed. The muscular segment of the ventricular septum is also imaged, meaning that a muscular VSD can be detected in this plane. Inlet VSDs are located relatively far back and can extend up to the level of the AV valve.

▸ **Doppler.** Mitral valve insufficiency is readily visible in color Doppler. The muscular ventricular septum and the inlet septum should be checked for defects.

Left Parasternal Short Axis (at the level of the papillary muscles)

▸ **2D echocardiography.** When the transducer is aimed still further in a caudal direction, the papillary muscle insertions can be seen (▸ Fig. 3.6). They are located at around the 5 and 7 o'clock positions. The left ventricle appears nearly perfectly round. The apical segment of the interventricular septum can be readily assessed in this view.

▸ **Doppler.** Using color Doppler, apical muscular VSDs are visible in this plane.

Subcostal Planes

The subcostal planes are usually the most difficult for beginners to evaluate, but they provide a large amount of information and an almost complete impression of cardiac anatomy, especially in neonates and young infants, for whom the acoustic window is especially suitable for these planes. The acoustic conditions for subcostal planes deteriorate increasingly in older children and adults.

In order to more easily understand the complex spatial relationships, it is necessary to invert the image on the monitor so that it is "anatomically correct." The segments of the heart that are located closer to the feet are displayed at the bottom of the monitor in the inverted image. It appears as if the patient were standing and facing the examiner.

Subcostal View (long axes)

In this view, the transducer is held so the marking points to the left. The transducer is "aimed" toward the sternum, keeping it as flat as possible. This allows the structures located at the front of the heart to be imaged—the right atrium and the right ventricular inflow and outflow tract including the pulmonary valve (▸ Fig. 3.7).

Tilting the transducer further in a dorsal direction yields a subcostal five-chamber view of a sort. It includes the right atrium with the openings of the vena cava, part of the right ventricle, and the aorta arising from the left ventricle.

If the transducer is panned even further in a dorsal direction, the subcostal four-chamber view can be seen. Both atria and both ventricles are displayed. The atrial septum is almost perpendicular, so an ASD or patent foramen ovale can be readily visualized.

▸ **Doppler.** In Doppler ultrasound scanning of the long subcostal axes, the flow in the right ventricular outflow tract and across the pulmonary valve and—when panning

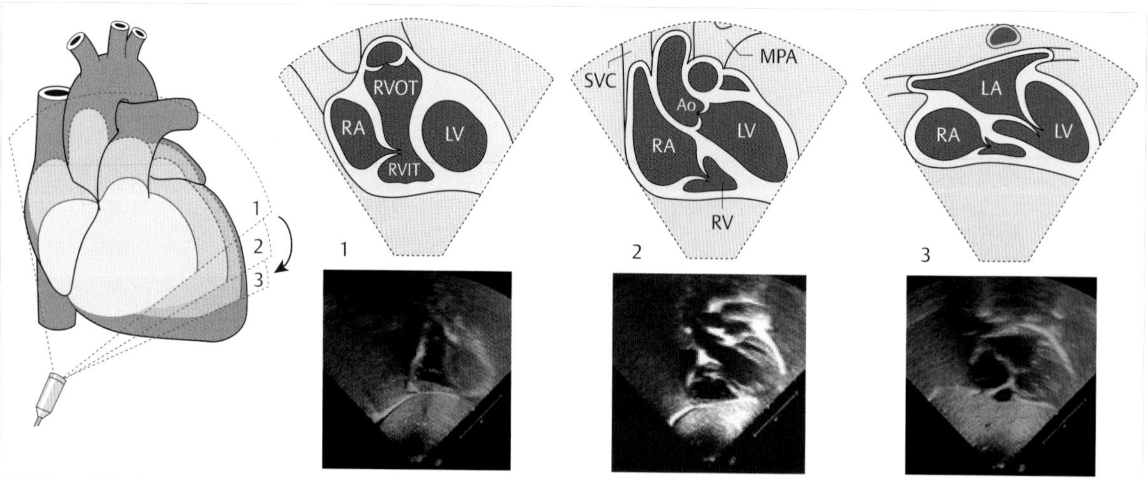

Fig. 3.7 Subcostal long axes (inverted image). RA, right atrium; LA, left atrium; RV, right ventricle; LV, left ventricle; Ao, aorta; MPA, main pulmonary artery; SVC, superior vena cava; RVOT, right ventricular outflow tract; RVIT, right ventricular inflow tract.

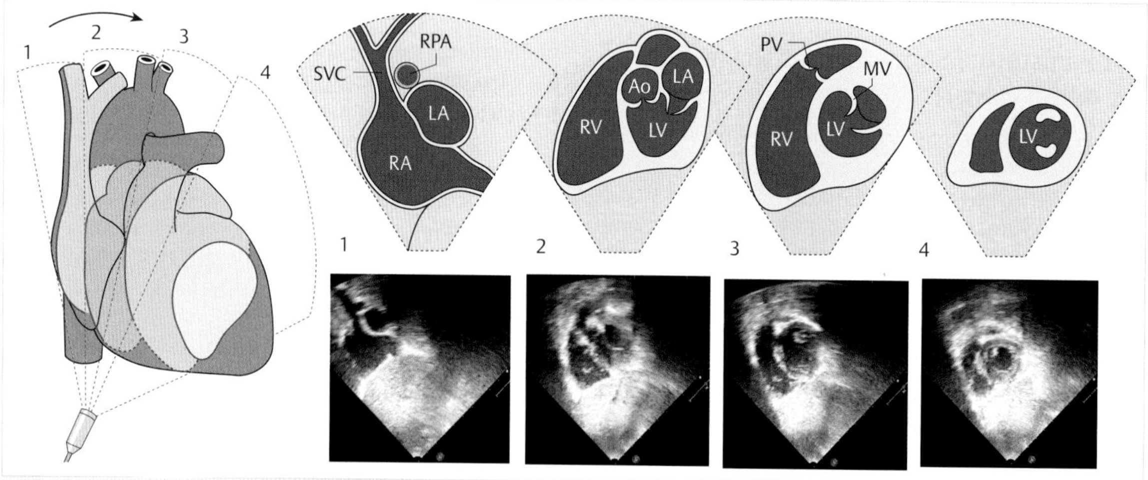

Fig. 3.8 Subcostal short axes (inverted view). RA, right atrium; LA, left atrium; RV, right ventricle; LV, left ventricle; Ao, aorta; PV, pulmonary valve; MV, mitral valve; SVC, superior vena cava; RPA, right pulmonary artery.

in a dorsal direction—the flow in the left ventricular outflow tract and the aortic valve can be imaged particularly well. Tilting even further in a dorsal direction displays the flow of the vena cava. In addition, the subcostal four-chamber view is particularly suited for detecting a shunt at the atrial level using color Doppler.

Subcostal View (short axes)

▸ **2D echocardiography.** Starting from the subcostal long axes, the transducer is rotated 90° clockwise for these planes. The marking on the transducer is pointed downward. In general, this examination begins at the right and images the right atrium so that the junctions of both venae cavae are visualized (bicaval view). The left atrium can be seen at the left of the right atrium. In this view, the entire atrial septum can be readily evaluated (▸ Fig. 3.8).

Later in the course of this examination, the transducer is pointed more and more to the left so that the basal segments of both ventricles with the AV valves and the aortic valve come into view.

When the transducer is panned further to the left, the right ventricle with the right ventricular outflow tract and the pulmonary valve are visualized. In this illustration, the right ventricle and its outflow tract partly encircle the left ventricle.

When the transducer is moved further to the left, the apical segments of both ventricles are reached.

▸ **Doppler.** The subcostal short axes are particularly suited for Doppler ultrasound measurement of flow

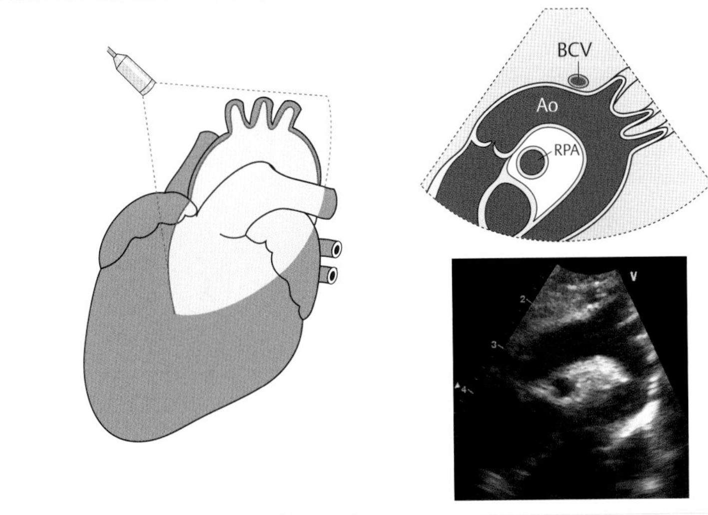

Fig. 3.9 Suprasternal view (long axis). Ao, aorta; RPA, right pulmonary artery; BCV, brachiocephalic vein.

velocity in the right ventricular outflow tract and across the pulmonary valve. In the bicaval view, the blood flow in the superior and inferior venae cavae can also be visualized. This is especially important after a superior cavopulmonary shunt procedure or for Fontan patients. Using color Doppler, a shunt in the atrial septum can also be detected.

Suprasternal Views

The suprasternal planes generally come at the end of the examination because they are the most uncomfortable for the patient. For this examination, the patient is requested to hyperextend his or her neck so that the transducer can be positioned in the suprasternal notch. It may be helpful to place padding under the shoulders of neonates or young infants. The patient's head should be turned as far to the left as possible. For the long axes, the marking on the transducer is pointed approximately toward the patient's left ear and for the short axis toward the left shoulder.

Suprasternal View (long axis)

▶ **2D echocardiography.** In this plane, the entire aortic arch including the aortic isthmus is visualized (▶ Fig. 3.9). The aortic arch looks like the knob of a walking stick. The brachiocephalic trunk, the left common carotid artery, and the left subclavian artery originate from the aortic arch. The aortic isthmus can be seen distal to the left subclavian artery. In this position, a cross-section of the right pulmonary artery can be seen behind the aorta and a cross-section of the brachiocephalic vein in front of the brachiocephalic trunk. In neonates and young infants, a similar view can be obtained by positioning the transducer in the parasternal second right intercostal space owing to the good acoustic window caused by the still large thymus.

▶ **Doppler.** The aortic isthmus can be especially well identified in the suprasternal long axis using color Doppler ultrasound. Accelerated blood flow and saw-tooth appearance of the flow curve in the Doppler are the typical findings of coarctation of the aorta. The aortic valve can sometimes also be easily examined by Doppler ultrasound in the suprasternal view.

Suprasternal View (short axis)

▶ **2D echocardiography.** The left atrium with the junctions of the pulmonary veins can often be best visualized in the suprasternal short axis. The left atrium with the pulmonary veins has been described as a crab, a turtle, or a bearskin. The pulmonary veins correspond to the animal's legs in this image. Above the left atrium is a longitudinal section of the right pulmonary artery; above that is a cross-section of the aorta (▶ Fig. 3.10). Optimally, the brachiocephalic vein with its junction to the superior vena cava will also be visualized above the aorta.

▶ **Doppler.** In color Doppler ultrasound scanning, the junction of the pulmonary veins with the left atrium can be visualized. Blood flow from left and right and from above and below can be visualized in color. The color jets of the four pulmonary veins frequently intersect in the center of the left atrium.

Abdominal Planes

Echocardiography is supplemented by the examination of the abdomen. The positions of the inferior vena cava, the aorta, and the large abdominal organs (liver, stomach, and spleen) are of particular interest. In situs solitus, the liver is located on the right and the spleen and stomach on the left. In heterotaxy syndromes, which are nearly always associated with cardiac anomalies, the liver may be located in the middle and the spleen can be entirely absent.

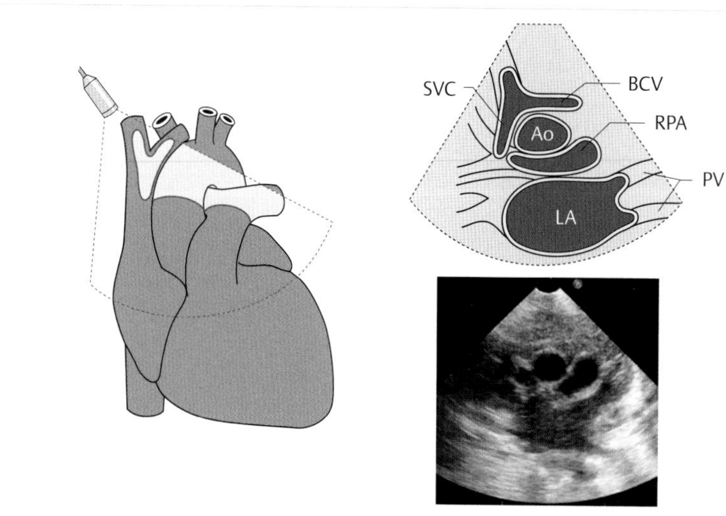

Fig. 3.10 Suprasternal view (short axis). SVC, superior vena cava; BCV, brachiocephalic vein; Ao, aorta; LA, left atrium; RPA, right pulmonary artery; PV, pulmonary veins.

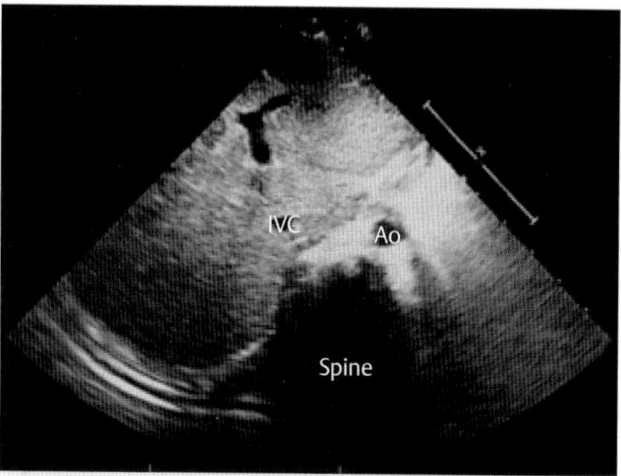

Fig. 3.11 Abdominal cross-section including the inferior vena cava (IVC) at the right of the spinal column and the abdominal aorta (Ao) at the left of the spine.

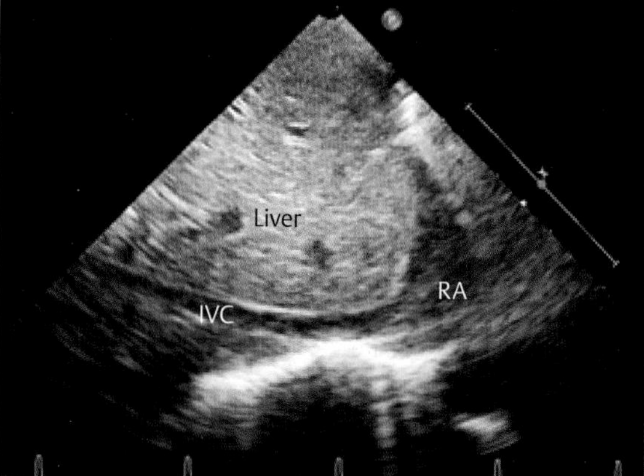

Fig. 3.12 Abdominal longitudinal section through the inferior vena cava (IVC) with the junction of the vena cava with the right atrium (RA).

▸ **2D echocardiography.** The cross-section shows that the aorta is normally at the left and the inferior vena cava at the right of the spinal column (▸ Fig. 3.11).

In the longitudinal section, the inferior vena cava and the junction to the right atrium can be visualized (▸ Fig. 3.12). Dilatation of the inferior vena cava may be a sign of right heart insufficiency.

When the transducer is rotated slightly to the left, a longitudinal section of the abdominal aorta where the celiac trunk and the superior mesenteric artery branch off can be seen (▸ Fig. 3.13).

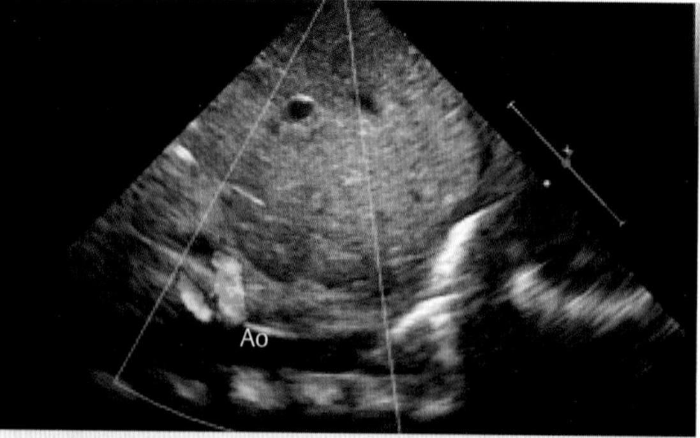

Fig. 3.13 Abdominal longitudinal section through the abdominal aorta (Ao).

▸ **Doppler.** Blood flow in the celiac trunk is routinely determined by Doppler ultrasonography. A weakened flow signal can be a sign of coarctation of the aorta. Diastolic flow approaching zero or even negative (diastolic run-off) can occur if there is a relevant shunt of the great vessels, for example. The clinically most significant example is a PDA.

3.1.3 Quantitative Analyses

Systolic Function

Fractional Shortening

The systolic function of the left ventricle can be easily described using fractional shortening. Fractional shortening (*FS*) is calculated from the end diastolic diameter (*LVEDd*) and the end-systolic diameter (*LVEDs*) of the left ventricle:

$$FS(\%) = \frac{LVEDd - LVEDs}{LVEDd \times 100}$$

Both diameters are easiest to determine in the parasternal long axis in M-mode just below the mitral valve—or alternatively in the parasternal short axis.

Note

The normal value for fractional shortening is between 28% and 44% (mean 36%).

Fractional shortening is *reduced* when ventricular function is impaired. It is *elevated* as a compensation mechanism if there is volume or pressure overload of the ventricle (e.g., VSD, mitral valve insufficiency, aortic stenosis, hypertrophic obstructive cardiomyopathy).

If the motion of the ventricular septum is flattened or paradoxical (e.g., associated with right ventricular dilatation), the quotient *FS* only poorly represents ventricular function. The values for *FS* are then too low. If there is a regional contraction disorder, *FS* naturally does not reflect the function of the entire ventricle.

Fractional shortening of the right ventricle can be determined by analogy with the procedure described above.

Ejection Fraction

To calculate the ejection fraction (*EF*), the volume of the left ventricle, assumed to be approximately the diameter raised to the third power, is used instead of the diameter:

$$EF(\%) = \frac{LVEDd^3 - LVEDs^3}{LVEDd^3 \times 100}$$

Note

The normal value of the ejection fraction is between 56% and 78% (mean 66%).

Using this procedure, however, ventricular volume is determined using only a diameter measured in the short axis. This is not mathematically correct, and the resulting values can be considered only an approximation.

Modern echocardiography devices have the option of determining ventricular volume more precisely. In one of the most frequently used methods (Simpson's slice summation method), the end-systolic and end-diastolic contours of the ventricle are traced with the cursor. The system software then calculates the volume and the *EF*.

Diastolic Function

The diastolic function involves a complex interplay of different factors. The diastole is composed of several phases:

- Isovolumetric relaxation
- Rapid ventricular filling
- Passive ventricular filling
- Atrial contraction

Diastolic function is more difficult to evaluate using echocardiography than systolic function. Suitable parameters have been found to be the Doppler profile of the inflow through the AV valves, left ventricular filling index (*E*/*E′*), and the isovolumetric relaxation time (*IVRT*) in particular.

Doppler Profile Across the AV Valves

The Doppler profile across the AV valves is M-shaped (▶ Fig. 3.14) and consists of the maximum velocity during passive filling into the ventricle (E wave) and during atrial contraction (A wave). The E wave is normally greater than the A wave. The normal E/A ratio of the mitral valve inflow with respect to the maximum flow velocity of the respective wave is 1.2 ± 0.3 for children under the age of 1 year and 1.9 ± 0.5 for children over age 1 year (Reynolds 2002).[31]

If relaxation is abnormal, the filling profile through the AV valves is changed. The maximum velocity of the E wave decreases, while the velocity of the A wave increases. If restriction is pronounced, the E wave is excessively increased and the A wave velocity decreases. However, there may also be a completely normal filling profile between the two stages despite relevant abnormal relaxation. This is called pseudonormalization.

A color Doppler examination of the mitral valve annulus can be useful for distinguishing between the two stages (▶ Fig. 3.14). The E wave is usually more pronounced in a color Doppler. If there is abnormal diastolic function, the E wave across the mitral valve annulus is also less pronounced than the A wave—this also applies to the phase of pseudonormalization of the mitral valve inflow profile.

Left Ventricular Filling Index

The ratio of the early diastolic E wave of the blood flow through the mitral valve (E wave) to the early diastolic E′ wave of the tissue Doppler in the mitral valve annulus (E′ wave) has proved to be an easily determined parameter for diastolic function. Each maximum flow velocity is measured and a ratio is formed (*E/E'*). This ratio correlates with the pressure in the left atrium or with the left ventricular end-diastolic pressure (LVEDP) and thus with the preload of the left ventricle.

Note

A normal E/E' ratio is below 8. A ratio of 8 to 15 is borderline, and a ratio over 15 is definitely elevated.

Isovolumetric Relaxation Time

The isovolumetric relaxation time (IVRT) is the period between the closure of the aortic valve and the diastolic inflow through the mitral valve. It is determined by placing the region of interest of the PW Doppler in the region of the left ventricular outflow tract near the anterior mitral valve leaflet (▶ Fig. 3.15). In this way, the left ventricular outflow up to the closure of the aortic valve and the transmitral inflow can both be visualized. The IVRT is the time between the end of left ventricular outflow and the start of transmitral inflow.

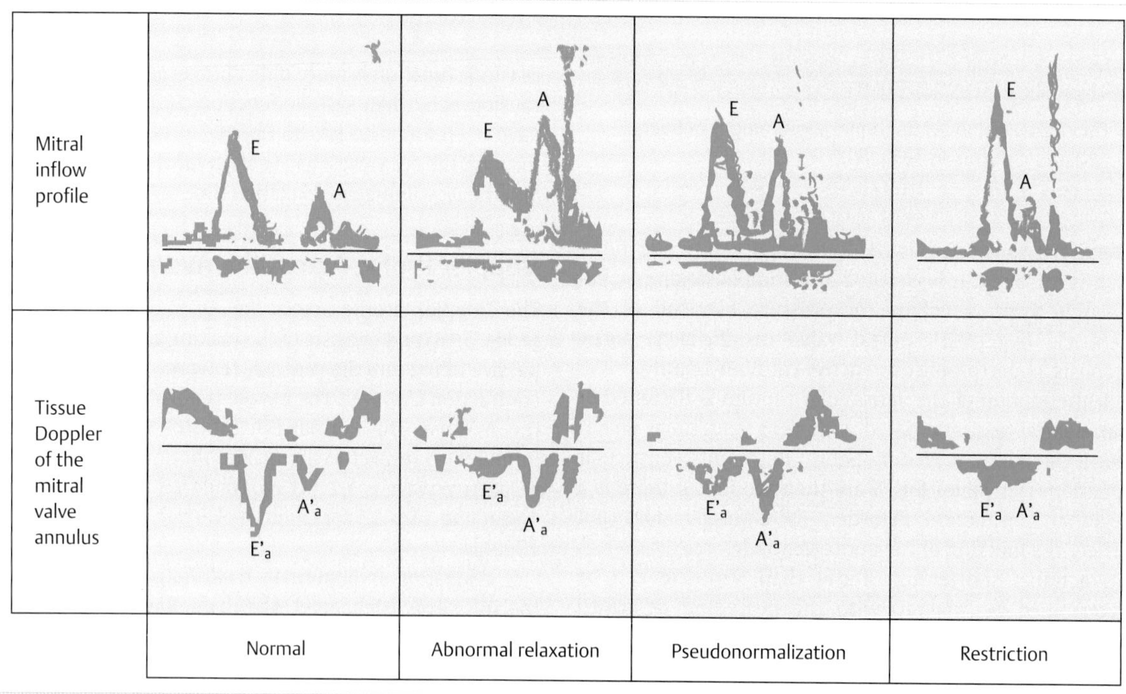

Fig. 3.14 Overview of the typical profiles for classifying diastolic function using the mitral inflow profile and tissue Doppler of the mitral valve annulus.[113]

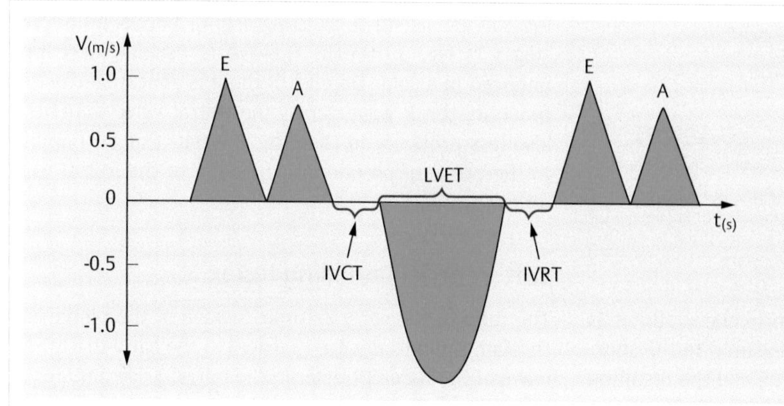

Fig. 3.15 Determining the IVRT using Doppler echocardiography.[43]

Note

The IVRT is normally 30 to 50 ms in children.[115] It is prolonged if there is abnormal relaxation and shortened with pronounced restriction.

Pressure Gradients

When fluid flows through a tube, flow is accelerated where the tube is narrowed. The more pronounced the narrowing, the faster the fluid flows at this location. The extent of the stenosis (i.e., the pressure gradient) can be determined based on the flow velocity. This principle applies the simplified Bernoulli equation:

$$\Delta p(\text{mmHg}) = 4 \times v^2(\text{m/s})$$

The pressure gradient (Δp) at a stenosis (measured in mmHg) is equal to four times the square of the flow velocity (measured in m/s) at the stenosis. For example, if a maximum velocity of 4 m/s is measured at a pulmonary stenosis, the gradient through the stenosis is approximately. 64 mmHg.

Note

The simplified Bernoulli equation can be applied only to short segments of stenosis.

If the flow velocity is already increased before the stenosis, the flow acceleration before the stenosis must be taken into consideration and included in the Bernoulli equation. In practice, this plays a role in coarctation of the aorta, when the flow is already accelerated in the aortic arch before the stenosis. Another example is a valvular aortic stenosis downstream from a subvalvular stenosis. In cases such as this, the following equation applies:

$$\Delta p(\text{mmHg}) = 4 \times (V_2{}^2(\text{m/s}) - V_1{}^2(\text{m/s}))$$

where V_1 is the velocity before the stenosis and V_2 is the velocity in the stenosis.

The acoustic beam should be as near to parallel to the flow direction as possible in all Doppler measurements. In practice, it is useful to aim the beam at a stenosis using various acoustic angles. The highest velocity measured is then used to calculate the gradient.

The systolic gradient measured using the Bernoulli equation is frequently higher than that measured in the catheterization laboratory using the pressure pull-back curve. This is partly because the instant gradient, that is the maximum gradient, is calculated using Doppler and the Bernoulli equation, while in the catheterization laboratory the "peak-to-peak" gradient is measured. The measurements from the heart catheterization laboratory therefore usually correlate better with the mean pressure gradients. Among other things, the integral of the area below the Doppler curve must be calculated for this. In practice, this means that the flow curve must be traced with the cursor, from which the software of the echocardiography device calculates the mean pressure gradient.

Intracardiac and Intravascular Pressures

Using the simplified Bernoulli equation, the pressures in the cardiac chambers and pulmonary flow path can also be estimated. The most important example from clinical practice is determining right ventricular pressure.

► **Right ventricular pressure associated with tricuspid valve insufficiency.** In tricuspid valve insufficiency, the gradient between the right atrium and ventricle can be calculated using the Bernoulli equation based on the regurgitation velocity of the blood during systole. If the pressure in the right atrium (which is equivalent to the central venous pressure) is added to this gradient, the result is the right ventricular systolic pressure. For example, if the velocity measured through an insufficient tricuspid valve is 3 m/s, a gradient of 36 mmHg is calculated between the right atrium and ventricle using the Bernoulli equation. If we assume a pressure of 5 to 10 mmHg in the right atrium, the right ventricular pressure is 41 to 46 mmHg.

► **Right ventricular pressure associated with VSD.** By analogy with this method, the right ventricular pressure across a VSD can also be estimated. The pressure in the left ventricle is approximately equivalent to the systemic blood pressure. If the gradient determined across the VSD is subtracted from the actual blood pressure, the result is the right ventricular pressure. The prerequisite for this is, of course, that the systolic pressure in the left ventricle is approximately equal to the systemic pressure. A relevant aortic stenosis or coarctation of the aorta must be ruled out. For example, the systolic blood pressure is 120 mmHg. A flow velocity of 5 m/s is measured across a small VSD. This is equivalent to a gradient of 100 mmHg, so the systolic pressure in the right ventricle in this example is approximately 20 mmHg.

Using the same principle, in a patent ductus, the pressure in the pulmonary artery can also be estimated taking the systemic blood pressure into consideration.

3.2 Transesophageal Echocardiography

In transesophageal echocardiography (TEE), an ultrasound probe is advanced through the esophagus similarly to an endoscopic procedure. Since the heart, or more precisely the left atrium, is located directly in front of the esophagus, an echocardiographic examination of the heart can be made using this technique with no artifacts from bones or lungs. The disadvantage of this method is that children tolerate the examination only under deep sedation and it can sometimes be performed on infants only under general anesthesia.

In children, TEE is primarily used intraoperatively to monitor surgical correction of heart defects, as the esophageal access does not obstruct the surgeon. Another typical indication is the interventional closure of an atrial or ventricular septal defect by catheterization. Using TEE, the exact size of the defect can be measured and later the correct position of the closure system can be checked.

TEE often provides considerably better options for visualizing cardiac structures in adolescents and adults, in whom the acoustic window for transthoracic echocardiography is poorer. The atria, the interatrial septum, and the aortic and mitral valves can be visualized especially well using TEE. The interventricular septum and the ascending aorta can also be readily assessed. Because they are positioned further away from the probe, however, the pulmonary and tricuspid valves are only conditionally suitable for assessment using TEE.

Typical indications for TEE are to search for atrial thrombi, visualize the connections of the pulmonary veins, exclude or detect endocarditis vegetation at the mitral and aortic valve, detect a patent foramen ovale or atrial septal defect, and for postoperative monitoring in the intensive care unit.

3.3 Fetal Echocardiography

Fetal echocardiography is performed by prenatal diagnosticians and pediatric cardiologists. The reliability of the examination—as is the case for most other examinations—depends to a great extent on the experience and qualification of the examiner. Therefore, only an initial cursory overview of fetal echocardiography is given here.

The best time to make a fetal echocardiogram is in the 20th to 22nd week of gestation. Cardiac abnormalities can generally be reliably diagnosed or ruled out at this point and there is also still enough time to initiate other diagnostic or therapeutic measures.

In exceptional cases, fetal echocardiography can also be performed as early as the 12th to 15th week of gestation. Sometimes a transvaginal examination is performed at such an early stage of pregnancy. In this case, however, a follow-up examination should always be performed at a later stage.

Typical indications for fetal echocardiography are:

- Familial disposition for congenital heart defects
- Conspicuities detected in the fetus that are frequently associated with cardiac anomalies (e.g., esophageal atresia, hiatus hernia, situs inversus or ambiguus, omphalocele, hydronephrosis, limb deformities, CNS abnormalities, persistent left superior vena cava, single umbilical artery, ductus venosus agenesis)
- Proven chromosome anomaly in the fetus
- Increased fetal nuchal translucency thickness
- Nonimmune fetal hydrops, nuchal edema, hygroma colli
- Fetal arrhythmia
- Maternal diseases or infections associated with an increased risk of congenital heart defect (e.g., diabetes mellitus, phenylketonuria, collagenosis, TORCH infections)
- Maternal medication associated with an increased risk of congenital heart defect (e.g., anticonvulsants, lithium, alcohol, vitamin A), or drug consumption
- High doses of ionizing radiation during pregnancy

4 Chest X-ray

4.1 Basics

Despite the availability of modern imaging methods, the chest X-ray remains an essential component of diagnostic measures in pediatric cardiology. An X-ray image provides information on the size and shape of the heart, enlargement of any parts of the heart, the position of the heart in the thorax, lung perfusion, lung parenchyma, abdominal situs, and any bone anomalies that may be associated with heart defects.

Routine projections in childhood are anterior–posterior (AP) or posterior–anterior (PA) and lateral images. In neonates and infants, the AP projection is preferred; a PA projection is preferred for older children as it is for adults.

4.2 Heart Size

As a rule of thumb, the transverse diameter of the heart is half that of the thorax. The size of the heart can be more correctly described using the cardiothoracic ratio, which is calculated by dividing the greatest transverse diameter of the heart by the greatest inner diameter of the thorax (▶ Fig. 4.1). A cardiothoracic ratio of over 0.5 is a sign of cardiomegaly except in neonates.

4.3 Heart Shape

A diagram of the structures normally forming the borders of the heart is shown in ▶ Fig. 4.2. In AP projection, the right border of the heart is formed by the superior vena cava and right atrium. On the left side, the cardiac silhouette is bordered from top to bottom by the aortic knob, the pulmonary artery, and the left ventricle in AP projection. In a neonate, the left border of the heart may still be formed by the right ventricle, but at a later age this is pathological.

In the lateral projection, the right ventricle is located directly behind the sternum. The posterior border is formed by the left atrium at the top and the left ventricle at the bottom. The left ventricle and inferior vena cava overlap just above the diaphragm (▶ Fig. 4.2).

In *neonates* the cardiac silhouette is frequently concealed by the presence of a still large thymus. The thymus is located in the anterior and superior mediastinum and often appears as an unusually wide base of the heart. In addition, the heart is wide at the diaphragm in neonates. The thorax of the neonate appears broader and deeper. The ribs are horizontal. Only as the heart continues to grow does it assume the typical, almost vertical position in adults. The contours of the cardiac silhouette are then better defined. In neonates, the cardiac silhouette appears more rounded. Since the right ventricle in neonates still forms the left border of the heart, the apex appears to be higher. A cardiothoracic ratio of over 0.5 can still be normal in neonates and young infants.

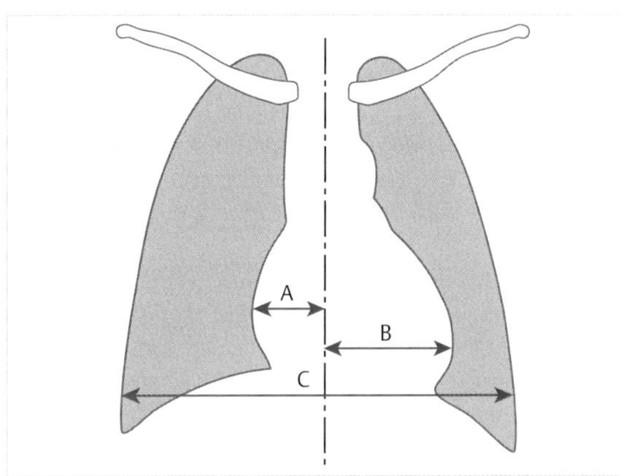

Fig. 4.1 Determining the cardiothoracic ratio in a PA image. Cardiothoracic ratio = (A + B)/C

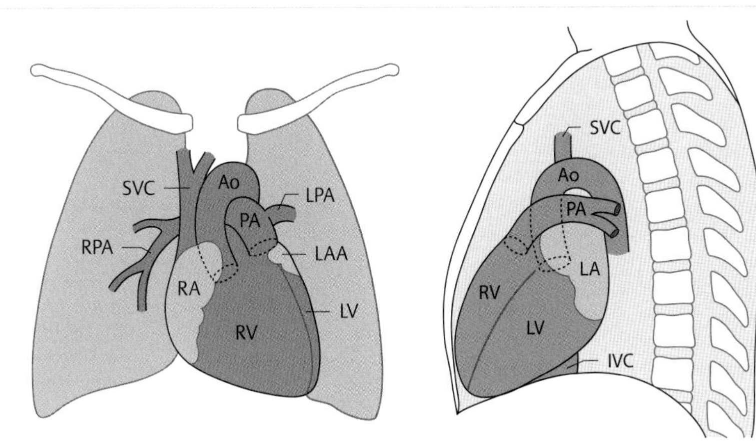

Fig. 4.2 Normal cardiac silhouette in PA and lateral projections.[29] RA, right atrium; RV, right ventricle; LA, left atrium; LV, left ventricle; Ao, aorta; PA, main pulmonary artery; RPA, right pulmonary artery; LPA, left pulmonary artery; SVC, superior vena cava; IVC, inferior vena cava; LAA, left atrial appendage.

4.4 Assessment of Atria, Ventricles, and Great Vessels

Enlarged atria and ventricles have different effects on the shape of the heart. Changes in heart shape therefore provide information on enlargement of certain parts of the cardiac. However, most cardiac defects involve not only one atrium or one ventricle, but generally a combination.

▶ **Enlargement of the left atrium.** The left atrium is directly adjacent to the tracheal bifurcation. An enlarged left atrium therefore increases the angle of the bifurcation (▶ Fig. 4.3) and typically displaces the main bronchus upward. In addition, in AP projection, an enlarged left atrium can appear as a dense shadow in the cardiac silhouette. The left atrial appendage can also form the left border of the heart. The bulge in the posterior superior cardiac silhouette is prominent in the lateral projection.

▶ **Enlargement of the left ventricle.** Since the left ventricle normally forms the left border of the heart, the left border is more prominent if it is enlarged. In addition, the cardiac apex is displaced downward. The cardiac apex appears to "dip" into the diaphragm.

In the lateral projection, the posterior inferior border of the cardiac silhouette is displaced further in a posterior and inferior direction. The lower border of the heart (formed by the left ventricle) and the inferior vena cava do not intersect until below the diaphragm. (▶ Fig. 4.4)

▶ **Enlargement of the right atrium.** When the right atrium is dilated, the lower right edge of the cardiac silhouette becomes more prominent (▶ Fig. 4.5). In the lateral projection, the inferior retrocardiac space is not constricted unless the right atrium is massively enlarged.

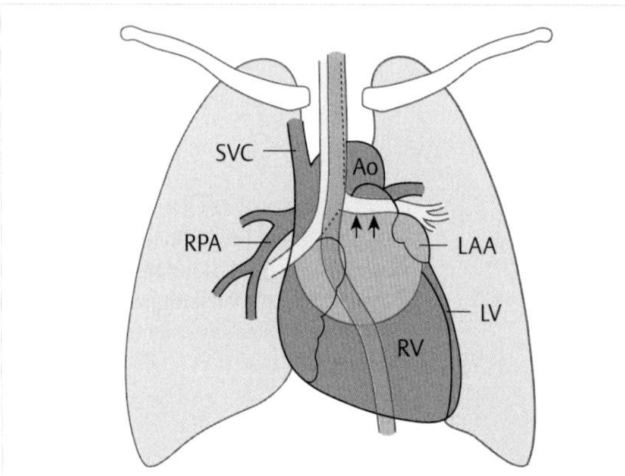

Fig. 4.3 Typical radiological findings associated with an enlarged left atrium in the PA projection. The left main bronchus is elevated and the angle of the tracheal bifurcation is increased.[29] SVC, superior vena cava; RPA, right pulmonary artery; Ao, aorta; LAA, left atrial appendage; LV, left ventricle; RV, right ventricle

▶ **Enlargement of the right ventricle.** The cardiac apex is elevated when the right ventricle is enlarged. An enlarged right ventricle can also displace the left ventricle to the left and the right atrium to the right, widening the cardiac silhouette. The right ventricle does not normally form the right border, but if it is greatly enlarged, the right ventricle may form the right border.

Right ventricular enlargement is often best detected in the lateral projection, in which the retrosternal space is constricted (▶ Fig. 4.6).

▶ **Dilatation of the pulmonary artery.** Dilatation of the pulmonary artery results in a prominent pulmonary artery segment in the X-ray (▶ Fig. 4.7). It may be a sign of poststenotic dilatation of a pulmonary artery stenosis, increased blood flow associated with a shunt defect, or elevated pulmonary artery pressure.

▶ **"Absent" pulmonary artery segment.** Hypoplasia or even atresia of the pulmonary artery leads to a concavity

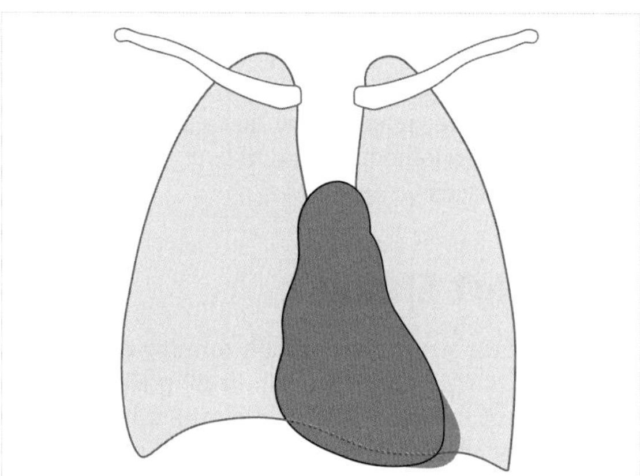

Fig. 4.4 Typical radiological findings associated with an enlarged left ventricle in the PA projection.[26]

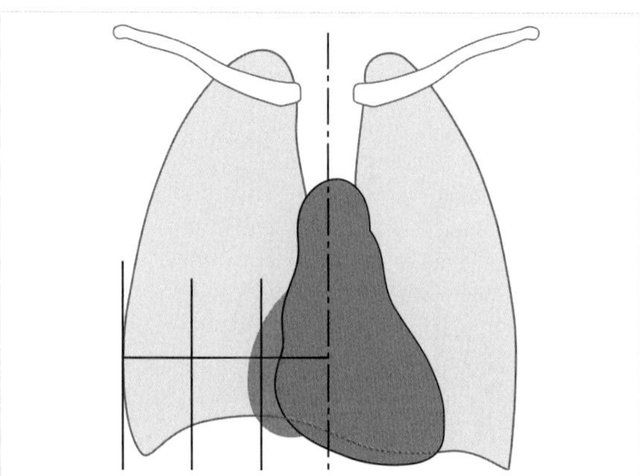

Fig. 4.5 Typical radiological findings associated with an enlarged right atrium in the PA projection.[26]

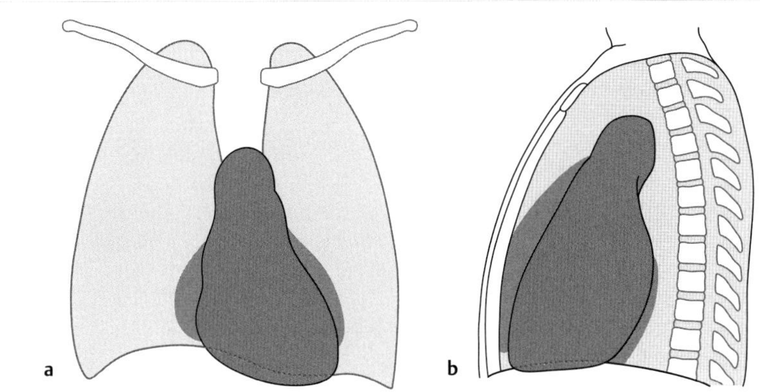

Fig. 4.6 Typical finding associated with an enlarged right ventricle in the PA (**a**) and lateral (**b**) projections.[26]

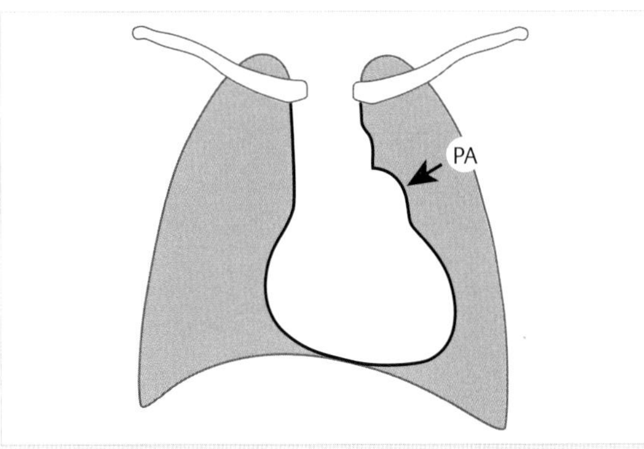

Fig. 4.7 Prominent pulmonary artery segment (arrow) in the PA projection.[29]

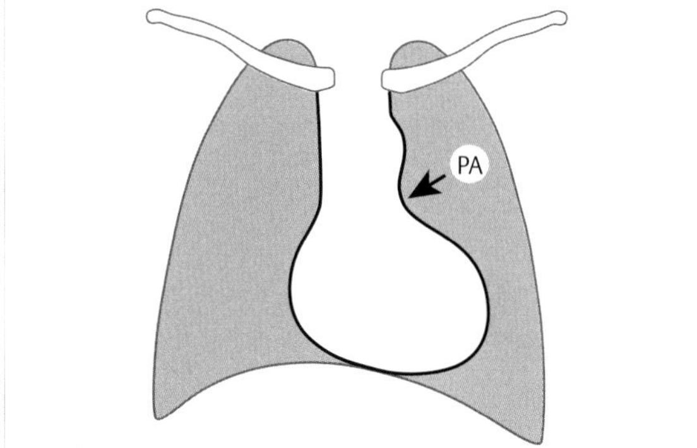

Fig. 4.8 "Absent" pulmonary artery segment (arrow) in the PA projection.[29]

of the pulmonary artery. This is termed an "absent" pulmonary artery segment (▸ Fig. 4.8). The cardiac waist is then prominent. This configuration of the cardiac silhouette is also described as "boot shaped."

▸ **Dilatation of the ascending aorta and aortic arch.** The ascending aorta does not usually form the right border. It does not cross the superior vena cava. If the ascending aorta is dilated it can form the right border, or the entire aortic arch may be widened (▸ Fig. 4.9). The cause may be aortic insufficiency (volume overload from regurgitant blood flow), poststenotic dilatation of the ascending aorta associated with an aortic stenosis, or a shunt defect that results in increased perfusion of the aorta.

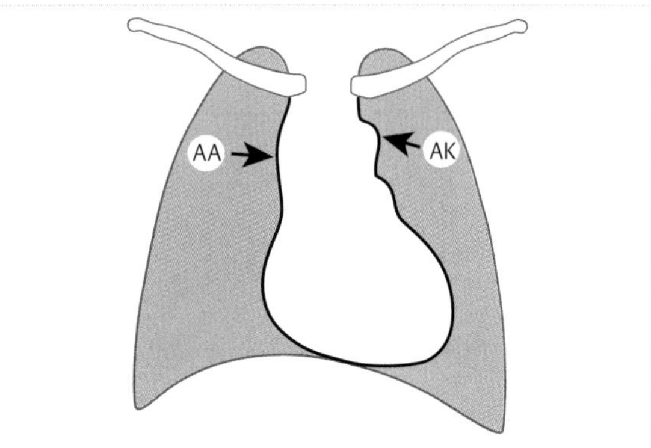

Fig. 4.9 Dilatation of the entire aortic arch in the PA projection.[29] AA, ascending aorta; AK, aortic knob.

▸ **Left and right aortic arch.** Normally, a *left aortic arch* crosses the left main bronchus and proceeds downward at the left of the spinal column. The course of the aorta along the left edge of the spinal column can generally be followed on the X-ray image. In addition, with a left aortic arch, the esophagus and trachea are displaced slightly to the right of the midline.

If a *right aortic arch* descends on the right, the aortic silhouette is detected at the right of the spinal column. A right aortic arch also forms the right border. The trachea and esophagus are typically displaced to the left.

A right aortic arch is frequently found with tetralogy of Fallot, pulmonary artery atresia with ventricular septal defect (VSD), or with a truncus arteriosus communis. In particular if none of these congenital heart defects is

Table 4.1 Characteristic radiological findings associated with some congenital heart defects

Heart defect	Characteristic radiological finding	Diagram
Dextro-transposition of the great arteries (d-TGA)	"Egg on side" appearance. Elevated cardiac apex, narrow annulus	
Tetralogy of Fallot, pulmonary atresia with ventricular septal defect	"Boot-shaped" heart. Elevated cardiac apex, prominent cardiac waist	
Total anomalous pulmonary venous connection, supracardiac type	"Snowman" or "figure 8." The upper segment of the 8 or snowman is formed by a dilated vertical vein on the left, through which the common pulmonary venous sinus drains into the brachiocephalic vein. The lower part of the figure is caused by an enlarged cardiac silhouette.	
Coarctation of the aorta in older children	Rib notching. Defects at the lower edge of the ribs from collateral blood flow through the intercostal arteries	
Ebstein anomaly	"Globe-shaped" silhouette with a narrow waist. The enlarged right atrium usually extends the cardiac silhouette to the right.	

present, a pulmonary annulus must always be considered if there is a right aortic arch (Chapter 15.26).

▸ **Congenital heart defects.** Characteristic radiological findings associated with some congenital heart defects are summarized in ▸ Table 4.1.

4.5 Pulmonary Vascular Markings

The pulmonary vessels normally taper down continuously starting at the hilum. Usually no pulmonary vessels can be seen in the outer one-third of the lung fields and in the apical segments in an X-ray photo. Pathological lung perfusion (increased pulmonary circulation associated with shunt defects, reduced pulmonary perfusion, pulmonary hypertension, venous pulmonary congestion) can be detected in an X-ray image based on changes in the pulmonary vessels.

▸ **Increased lung perfusion.** Lung perfusion is increased in heart defects involving a left-to-right shunt (e.g., relevant VSD, patent ductus arteriosus [PDA], partial anomalous pulmonary venous connection, ASD). Typical radiological signs of increased lung perfusion are dilated pulmonary vessels that can be followed up to the lateral one-third of the lung fields. In addition, pulmonary vessels can be seen in the apical segments of the lungs. The central pulmonary vessels are dilated. Excessive blood flow to the lungs is characteristically associated with a diameter of right pulmonary artery in the hilum greater than the inner diameter of the trachea.

► **Reduced lung perfusion.** Reduced lung perfusion may occur with tetralogy of Fallot or extremely severe pulmonary stenosis or atresia. The pulmonary vascular markings are then reduced; the lung fields are extremely radiotranslucent. Unilaterally reduced lung perfusion can occur if there is a relevant stenosis of the left or right pulmonary artery.

► **Pulmonary venous congestion.** Obstruction of the pulmonary venous return leads to congestion in the dilated pulmonary veins; however, this is rather rare in children. It can be caused by left heart failure, mitral valve stenosis, or total anomalous pulmonary venous connection with obstruction of the pulmonary vein. Interstitial edema occurs, appearing as a network of streaky pulmonary markings on an X-ray image. Kerley B lines are horizontal densities that can be most readily identified in the costophrenic angles. They are a sign of interstitial edema in the interlobular septa. Alveolar edema leads to diffuse opacification of the cardiac silhouette.

► **Pulmonary hypertension.** Pulmonary hypertension leads to increasing constriction of the peripheral pulmonary arteries and an increase in pulmonary vascular resistance, while the central pulmonary arteries are enlarged. The X-ray image features abrupt changes in the caliber of pulmonary arteries and discontinuity. While there is opacification in the pulmonary hili, the peripheral lung segments are conspicuously radiolucent. The discrepancy in size of the peripheral and central pulmonary arteries is called pruning (► Fig. 4.10).

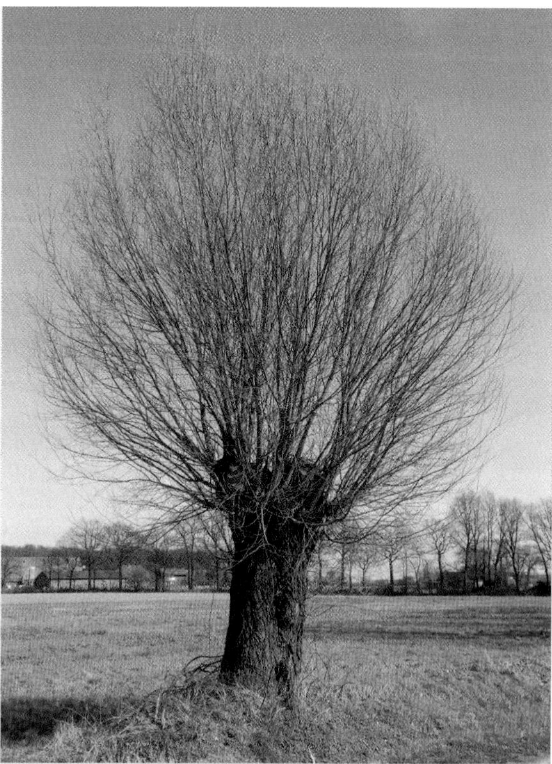

Fig. 4.10 Pruned tree with a large trunk and slender branches.

4.6 Abdominal Situs

In situs solitus (normal situs), the heart and stomach are located on the left side and the liver is on the right side below the cervical pleura. In situs inversus totalis, the stomach and heart are on the right and the liver on the left side.

In heterotaxy syndromes (Chapter 15.34) the stomach and heart may be located on different sides. This may also be associated with situs ambiguous with the liver in the middle and malrotation of the gastrointestinal tract. Heterotaxy syndromes are almost always associated with complex cyanotic heart defects.

4.7 Bony Structures of the Chest

The most common bone anomalies include scoliosis, which is found rather frequently in patients who have had heart surgery (e.g., after a left lateral thoracotomy). Anomalies of the vertebrae also occur with syndromes associated with cardiac anomalies. Examples of this are a VACTERL association or Alagille syndrome, which is frequently associated with butterfly vertebrae.

Rib notching is a typical finding in older children with untreated coarctation of the aorta. The recesses or notches that occur at the lower edge of the ribs are the result of collateral blood flow through the intercostal arteries that causes a large increase in their diameter. These changes are seen only rarely today because aortic coarctation is generally diagnosed and surgically corrected before notching occurs.

5 Cardiac Magnetic Resonance Imaging and Computed Tomography

5.1 Cardiac Magnetic Resonance Imaging

5.1.1 Basics

Magnetic resonance imaging (MRI) is a modern, noninvasive technique for obtaining cross-sectional images that is also very valuable for diagnosing congenital heart defects.

▸ **Advantages and disadvantages.** One major advantage of the method is that it does not require the use of ionizing radiation or iodinated contrast medium. The disadvantage is the long time needed for the examination, which may be over an hour for typical pediatric cardiology problems. Anesthesia is therefore generally needed for uncooperative younger children. Since many images must be made using the breath-hold technique, endotracheal anesthesia is usually the method of choice for uncooperative patients.

▸ **Functional principle.** The principle of MRI can be briefly summarized as follows. The protons in the nucleus of an atom have intrinsic angular momentum (spin) that gives the nuclei a magnetic moment. Due to the strong magnetic field of the MRI, the nuclei are aligned in a certain direction. Radio waves are used to deflect the nuclei from their normal alignment. The nuclei begin to wobble. After the radio waves are switched off, the nuclei return to the aligned positions. The atomic nuclei display different behavior depending on their surroundings. In this process, they emit weak magnetic signals that can be measured by the MRI unit, from which cross-sectional images can be made.

Rapidly switching the magnetic field on and off generates electromagnetic fields that pull on the coils of the MRI unit and cause the typical thumping sound during the examination.

Gadolinium (Gd), a paramagnetic substance, is used as a contrast medium for a cardiac MRI. Gadolinium is toxic and must be bound in a stable chelate molecule (e.g., in the form of Gd-DTPA).

Frequently, 3D datasets are made that can later be reconstructed in various ways.

▸ **Imaging process.** MRI examinations were originally performed using primarily spin-echo sequences. Now considerably faster sequences are commonly used. More technical details are available in the specific literature.

▸ **Contraindications.** Due to the very strong magnetic field, patients must remove all metal items (watch, wallet, piercings, etc.) before an MRI scan. The magnetic strips on chip cards will also be permanently erased by the magnetic field. Patients with ferromagnetic implants (cardiac pacemakers, AICDs, cochlear implants), or large tattoos (metallic dyes) can generally undergo an MRI scan only if special measures are taken. There is a relative contraindication for this examination for such patients. However, occlusion systems implanted in a catheter-based procedure such as ASD occluders or coils and artificial heart valves are usually not a problem. The wire cerclage used after a sternotomy also poses no problem, but the metallic parts can cause artifacts in the surrounding area.

▸ **Indications.** MRI is particularly suited for displaying non-bony structures such as soft tissue, brain, internal organs, and cartilage. Only lung tissue and bones are difficult to assess. The disadvantages compared with cardiac catheterization are mainly that the pressures in the heart chambers and great vessels cannot be measured directly and that no intervention is possible.

Cardiac MRI is especially useful for the following examinations:

- Determining cardiac anatomy (in addition to the other imaging methods)
- Assessing global and regional cardiac function
- Volumetric analysis of the different cardiac chambers
- Measuring and analyzing blood flow (e.g., determining systemic and pulmonary blood flow)
- Quantifying shunts
- Characterizing tissue (e.g., more precise classification of a cardiac tumor)
- Assessing myocardial perfusion
- Assessing myocardial vitality (using the delayed enhancement technique)
- Visualizing the great vessels using MR angiography

The most frequent clinical questions for cardiac MRI in childhood are listed in ▸ Table 5.1.

▸ **Cardiac anatomy.** The examination process is based on standard planes, similar to echocardiography, which can, however, be freely varied depending on the clinical question. The individual sections can be selected in all spatial planes. Examples of the most common standard sections are presented in ▸ Fig. 5.1.

▸ **Global and regional myocardial function.** Global and regional myocardial function is generally displayed using cine sequences. These sequences, which are usually executed as breath-hold, ECG-triggered images, yield a kind of short film of several cardiac cycles.

Table 5.1 Typical clinical questions and indications for an MRI in childhood

Heart defect/disease	Clinical question
ASD	• Exclusion or detection of an anomalous pulmonary venous connection (esp. with sinus venosus defects) • Quantification of the shunt
Partial anomalous pulmonary venous connection	• Visualization of the anomalous connection • Quantification of the shunt
VSD	• Quantification of the shunt • Location of the defect
PDA	• Quantification of the shunt
Coarctation of the aorta	• Detailed visualization of the entire aorta including the head/neck vessels and renal arteries (incl. 3D reconstruction of the vessels) • Detection or exclusion of collateral vessels • Evaluation of left ventricular function and size
Aortic aneurysm	• Follow-up (especially in adolescents and adults when echocardiography is limited by a poor acoustic window) • Exclusion of an aortic dissection
Vascular rings	• Detailed visualization of the vascular ring and spatial relationship with the trachea and bronchi (incl. 3D-reconstruction of the vascular ring)
Tetralogy of Fallot	Preoperative: • Clarification of pulmonary blood supply (pulmonary arteries, aortopulmonary collaterals, PDA) • Visualization of coronary arteries (exclusion of a coronary artery transecting the right ventricular outflow tract) Postoperative: • Assessment of pulmonary insufficiency • Determination of right ventricular function and precise quantification of right ventricular dilatation • Exclusion or assessment of an aneurysm of the right ventricular outflow tract • Assessment of left ventricular function • Exclusion or visualization of peripheral pulmonary stenoses
TGA	Postoperative after atrial switch operation (Mustard/Senning procedure): • Assessment of the size and function of the right (systemic) ventricle • Exclusion of systemic and pulmonary venous inflow stenoses • Exclusion of a baffle leak • Assessment of tricuspid insufficiency (systemic AV valve) Postoperative after switch operation: • Exclusion or assessment of supravalvular pulmonary stenoses as a result of the switch procedure and dilatation of the aortic root • Assessment of the coronary arteries and their branches
Fontan patients	Before Fontan completion: • Visualization of systemic and pulmonary veins • Visualization of the branches of the pulmonary artery • Exclusion of an aortic arch obstruction • Assessment of semilunar and AV valve function • Assessment of system ventricular function • Exclusion of collateral vessels After Fontan completion: • Exclusion of stenoses in the region of the cavopulmonary anastomoses • Exclusion of thrombi in the Fontan tunnel • Exclusion or visualization of fenestration or leakage in the Fontan tunnel • Assessment of the function and size of the systemic ventricle • Assessment of the AV and semilunar valves • Visualization of the aorta to exclude stenosis or aneurysm • Exclusion of collaterals
Anomalous coronary artery	• Visualization of origin and course of the coronary arteries • Assessment of myocardial perfusion and vitality
Kawasaki syndrome	• Detection and follow-up of aneurysms of the coronary arteries and other vessels

Continued

Table 5.1 continued

Heart defect/disease	Clinical question
Hypertrophic cardiomyopathy	• Distribution pattern of myocardial hypertrophy • Assessment of left ventricular function • Assessment of obstruction of the left ventricular outflow tract
Arrhythmogenic right ventricular cardiomyopathy	• Detection of fatty and connective tissue dysplasia in the right ventricle (esp. lateral wall and outflow tract affected)
Restrictive cardiomyopathy	• If a secondary cardiomyopathy is suspected, changed contrast medium and signal behavior associated with amyloidosis, sarcoidosis, hemochromatosis
Myocarditis	• Quantification of ventricular function • "Delayed enhancement" after application of contrast medium (nonspecific)
Cardiac tumors	• Differentiation based on contrast medium and signal behavior • Precise determination of size and location

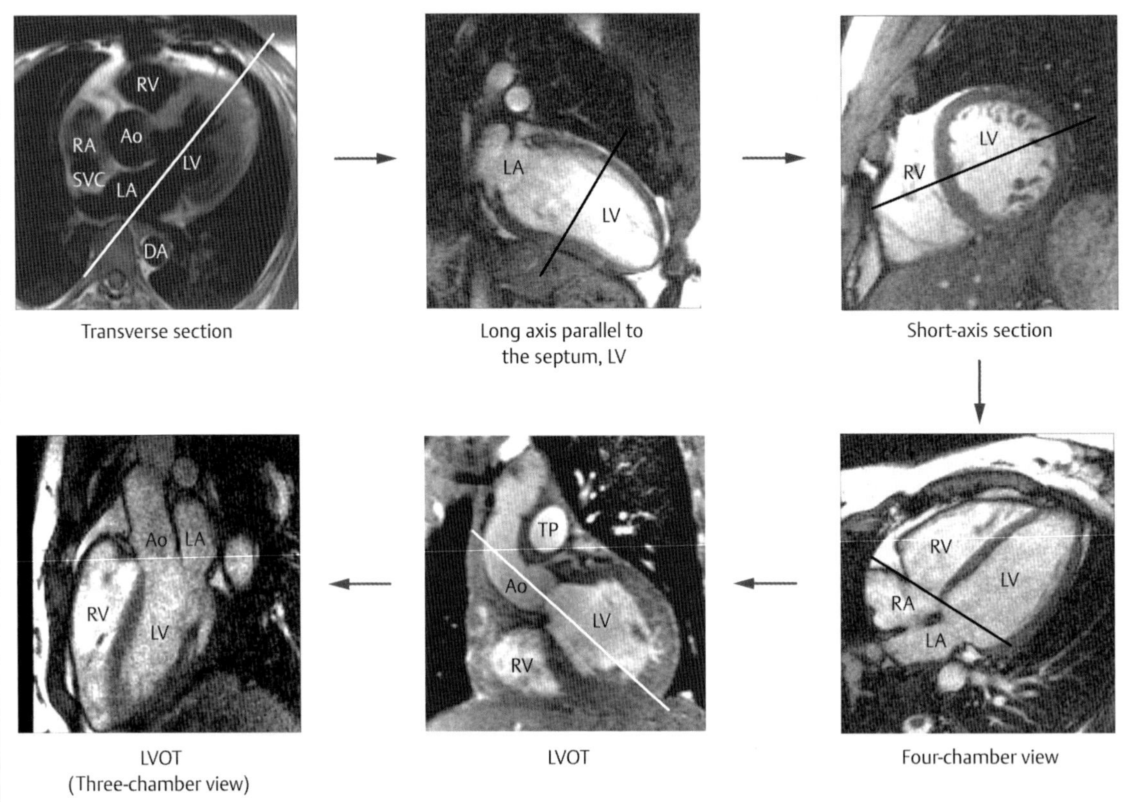

Fig. 5.1 Angulation of standard sections. The plane for each subsequent angulation is marked.[5] In cardiac diagnostics, various standard planes are used for imaging procedures. Examples of a few important standard sections that form the basis of an MRI scan are shown here. They are a starting point for the further course of the examination depending on the clinical question.
The standard sections are obtained by determining the angulation for the subsequent plane from an already existing plane. Starting with the transverse section, the next section is positioned, as marked, through the left atrium and ventricle. This plane is equivalent to a longitudinal section through the left ventricle and left atrium (long axis parallel to the septum). Setting the next angulation perpendicular to the long axis of the ventricle results in a short axis section through the left and the right ventricle. Setting the next plane through the middle of the two ventricles results in the typical four-chamber view. The next two angulations are used for the specific display of the left ventricular outflow tract.
LA, left atrium; LV, left ventricle; LVOT, left ventricular outflow tract; RA, right atrium; RV, right ventricle; Ao, ascending aorta; DA, descending aorta; TP, truncus pulmonalis; SVC, superior vena cava.

▶ **Volumetric analysis.** A complete series of short-axis slices from the base of the heart to the apex is used to quantify the volume of the ventricles. Ventricular volume is calculated using the planimetric data of ventricular surface areas combined with slice thickness and spacing (single-plane Simpson formula). Stroke volume, ejection fraction, and cardiac output are calculated using the ventricular volume measurements.

▶ **Measurement and analysis of blood flow.** Vascular blood flow is usually determined using phase contrast flow measurement. Similar to the method used in Doppler ultrasound, the approximate estimated flow velocity must be set to achieve the best possible results. Flow is optimally measured in a direction orthogonal to the respective blood vessel.

▶ **Quantifying shunts.** An intracardiac shunt is easy to quantify using the ratio of pulmonary blood flow (Q_p) to systemic blood flow (Q_s). To do this, flow is measured in the pulmonary artery and aorta and the ratio is calculated (Q_p/Q_s). As in cardiac catheterization, a ratio of more than 1 is a sign of a left-to-right shunt and a ratio less than 1 indicates a right-to-left shunt. If the ratio of Q_p/Q_s is 1, there is no shunt.

▶ **Myocardial perfusion.** Contrast medium (normally Gd-DTPA) can be administered to assess myocardial perfusion. Depending on how the contrast medium travels in the heart, myocardial perfusion can be assessed both visually-qualitatively and quantitatively.

▶ **Myocardial vitality.** The vitality of myocardial tissue can be assessed using the delayed enhancement technique. After intravenous administration of contrast medium, delayed images are made in which the nonviable myocardial tissue shows contrast medium enhancement. This technique is used to visualize myocardial scars after infarctions or from coronary artery stenosis as well as after myocyte damage due to other causes (myocarditis, cardiomyopathy). Even compared with the gold standard diagnostic measure for vitality, the PET scan, the sensitivity and specificity for detecting nonviable myocardial tissue using this method are very high.

▶ **MR angiography.** In MR angiography, the thoracic vessels can be readily visualized after contrast medium is administered. These images are generally made while the breath is held. Modern devices generate a complete 3D dataset within 30 seconds. Indications for an MR angiography are primarily stenoses in the thoracic aorta (e.g., coarctation), peripheral pulmonary stenoses, and anomalous pulmonary venous connections.

5.2 Cardiac Computed Tomography

Computed tomography (CT) uses X-rays to make cross-sectional images of the body. The advantages of CT are the brief examination time and very good spatial resolution. Unlike MRI, the lung parenchyma can also be readily evaluated in a CT scan. After application of an iodinated contrast medium, a CT angiography can also be made.

In pediatric cardiology, however, routine CT is of limited value because it involves considerable exposure to radiation and provides little information about function. Modern dual source CT scanners may be used more frequently due to a substantial reduction in radiation exposure. In addition, contrast in soft tissues is relatively low compared with MRI.

Cardiac CT scans are primarily made in pediatric cardiology when cross-sectional images are needed and cardiac MRI is not possible—for example, in patients with a pacemaker or an AICD or if metal implants such as coils or the like would result in strong artifacts in the region to be assessed.

6 Nuclear Medicine in Pediatric Cardiology

6.1 Basics

In nuclear medical examinations, radionuclides are introduced into human metabolism. Radionuclides are nucleotides that emit radioactive energy and undergo spontaneous transformation to nuclei of another element. Radionuclides are also called tracers. The radiation they emit can be measured using special detectors. This yields images of the tracer uptake in various regions of the heart.

The two nuclear medicine techniques primarily used in cardiology are:

- SPECT (single photon emission computed tomography), used in myocardial perfusion imaging
- PET (positron emission tomography), gold standard for assessing myocardial vitality

6.2 Myocardial Perfusion Imaging

For myocardial perfusion imaging, a tracer is injected intravenously. This tracer accumulates in perfused areas of the myocardium, while nonperfused areas show no uptake. This allows perfusion of the myocardium to be visualized. Myocardial perfusion imaging is indicated primarily for assessing and visualizing the extent of myocardial ischemia.

The tracers usually used are thallium-201 chloride or technetium-99 m methoxyisobutylisonitrile (MIBI). Thallium-201 chloride is a potassium analog that, like potassium, enters cardiomyocytes via the Na,K-ATPase proportional to regional blood flow. After a delay, thallium-201 chloride is then cleared out of the system. The tracer is washed out more slowly in poorly perfused areas. However, due to the exposure to radiation, which is almost double that of technetium-99 m MIBI, thallium-201 chloride should not be used in children.

Technetium-99 m MIBI is a lipophilic substance that diffuses into cardiomyocytes through the cell membrane, but it does not accumulate in the affected area of the heart if perfusion is insufficient. Unlike thallium-201 chloride, the examination using technetium-99 m MIBI is not based on washout, but on measuring tracer uptake.

However, since even severe coronary stenoses allow sufficient perfusion of the heart at rest (coronary reserve), the scan is performed both at rest and after exercise. A bicycle ergometer or medication (e.g., dobutamine or adenosine) can be used for exercise testing.

6.3 Positron Emission Tomography

Positron emission tomography (PET) measures glucose metabolism. A PET scan is currently the gold standard for diagnosing myocardial vitality. 18-Fluorodeoxyglucose (^{18}F-FDG) is used as a tracer. ^{18}F-FDG is transported into the cells like glucose and phosphorylated. However, since glucose uptake in cardiomyocytes must be stimulated by insulin, glucose must be given orally or insulin administered in addition to the tracer.

^{18}F-FDG accumulates in vital myocytes, but there is no ^{18}F-FDG uptake in "dead," irreversibly damaged tissue.

By combining this vitality diagnostic test with a method of measuring perfusion, it is possible to differentiate whether or not nonperfused myocardial tissue is still vital. Nonperfused or poorly perfused myocardial tissue that is still vital leads to a discrepancy between perfusion and vitality diagnostics (perfusion-metabolism mismatch). In this case, the patient would benefit from revascularization (e.g., bypass). If, however, perfusion is reduced and no vitality is detected (perfusion-metabolism match), patients do not benefit from revascularization.

Myocardial perfusion is determined either by myocardial SPECT imaging or again by PET scan, but using a different tracer, most often ^{13}N-ammonia.

7 Pediatric Exercise Testing

7.1 Exercise Test

7.1.1 Indications and Contraindications

▶ **Indications.** Exercise tests in childhood are used primarily for detecting and evaluating cardiac arrhythmia and myocardial ischemia as well as for objectifying physical capacity. Blood pressure behavior can be assessed by simultaneously measuring blood pressure. Another aim of exercise testing is to investigate stress-related symptoms (e.g., shortness of breath) and verify the effectiveness of treatment for certain diseases (hypertension, arrhythmia, abnormal circulatory regulation). For some clinical questions, it can also be useful to monitor oxygen saturation by pulse oximetry.

Specific clinical questions for exercise testing for a few selected diseases are listed in ▶ Table 7.1.

Table 7.1 Typical indications for exercise testing in childhood and adolescence

Disease	Question/findings
Aortic stenosis	Detection of subendocardial ischemia (ST depression), occurrence of arrhythmia during exercise Caution: The gradient of an aortic stenosis increases during exercise, thus potentially insufficient increase in blood pressure
Coarctation	Increase of the arterial hypertension during exercise, increase of the gradient during exercise
Arterial hypertension	Blood pressure behavior during exercise, check of effective medication
Extrasystoles	Rule of thumb for structurally unremarkable hearts—harmless extrasystoles disappear during exercise, malignant extrasystoles increase during exercise. Cardiomyopathies (hypertrophic cardiomyopathy, right ventricular arrhythmogenic cardiomyopathy) or catecholamine-induced ventricular tachycardia, for example, must then be excluded
AV block	Determination of maximum achievable heart rate. AV blocks resulting from high vagal tone disappear during exercise
Long QT syndrome	In long QT syndrome, a prolonged QTc interval is observed during exercise. T wave changes and ventricular extrasystoles should also be noted Caution: Tachycardia can be induced by exercise
WPW syndrome	The disappearance of the delta wave during exercise is a sign of a relatively long refractory period of the accessory pathway (favorable prognosis)
Fontan patients	Assessment of physical capacity. An increase in cyanosis during exercise is a sign of venovenous collaterals or a right-to-left shunt through an atrial tunnel window, tunnel leak, or the like
After coronary artery surgery (arterial switch operation, Ross procedure, ascending aortic replacement, correction of Bland–White–Garland syndrome), after Kawasaki syndrome	Evidence of myocardial ischemia (ST depression, AV block, ventricular extrasystoles) should be particularly noted
Syncopes	Exclusion of arrhythmia; possible sudden drop in blood pressure associated with cardioinhibitory syncopes
Reduced physical capacity	Objective assessment of capacity, exclusion of underlying causes
Pacemaker	Monitoring rate adaptation (R function) of the pacemaker, which should lead to an adequate increase in the heart rate during exercise

► **Contraindications.** Absolute contraindications for exercise testing are:
- Acute myocardial infarction or unstable angina pectoris
- Decompensated heart failure
- Acute inflammatory heart disease
- Acute lung embolism
- Congestive lung disease
- High-grade aortic stenosis (subvalvular, valvular, supravalvular), aortic coarctation, aortic arch interruption
- Significant hypertrophic obstructive cardiomyopathy (HOCM)
- Uncontrolled symptomatic arrhythmia
- Aortic dissection/aneurysm

Special caution is required if there are pre-existing cardiac arrhythmias, arterial or pulmonary hypertension, or certain heart defects. Particular caution is recommended especially for mild to moderate forms of aortic stenosis, aortic coarctation, HOCM, or other stenosis of the left ventricular outflow tract where exercise testing is not entirely contraindicated, as the gradient can increase considerably during exercise.

7.1.2 Procedure

Exercise testing is usually performed on a treadmill or bicycle ergometer. The treadmill more closely approaches naturally induced stress. However, because of the many possible movement artifacts using the treadmill ergometer, a bicycle ergometer is usually the preferred method for children, and is possible for children over the age of 5 who are at least 110 cm tall. However, especially in younger children, rapid fatigue of the thigh muscles in bicycle exercise testing means that maximum workload is not achieved.

► **Preparation.** Complete emergency equipment including a defibrillator and oxygen supply must be present at all times. The limb leads of the ECG are attached to the torso to reduce movement artifacts. Precordial leads must be used to detect ischemic changes. The total duration of exercise is usually under 15 minutes. The patients should not have fasted longer than 3 to 4 hours prior to the test.

► **Exercise protocol.** Maximum cardiac workload is assumed when the maximum heart rate is reached.
- Bicycle ergometer: maximum heart rate = 200 – age (years)
- Treadmill ergometer: maximum heart rate = 220 – age (years)

The exercise test is begun after a warm-up period according to a step or ramp protocol. In the step protocol, the workload remains the same for 2 to 3 minutes and is then gradually increased. In the ramp protocol, the workload is increased continuously. The exercise test is followed by a recovery period. As a rule of thumb, healthy boys achieve an average maximum workload of 3 to 3.5 W/kg, healthy girls an average of around 2.5 to 3 W/kg.

Note

In childhood, arrhythmia during exercise testing often does not occur until the recovery period or increases in this phase.

Below are some examples of test protocols for bicycle and treadmill exercise testing as recommended by the German Society of Pediatric Cardiology (step protocols).
- Bicycle ergometer:
  - Warm-up period: 2 min freewheel
  - Exercise period: start with 0.5 W/kg; increase by 0.5 W/kg every 2 min
  - Recovery period: 2 min freewheel

During all phases, a regular pedal rate of approximately 50 to 60/min should be maintained.
- Treadmill ergometer
  - Resting period: 90 s
  - Exercise period: start with 2.5 km/h and a 0% incline, increase speed in increments of 0.5 km/h and incline by 3% (up to max. 21%) every 1.5 min
  - Recovery period: 2 km/h at a 0% incline.

► **Termination criteria.** The test is terminated at the latest when the maximum workload is reached (maximum heart rate, see above). The following are additional criteria for termination:
- Absolute criteria for termination:
  - Signs of cardiac ischemia (ST segment changes ±3 mm in the ECG
  - Ventricular tachycardia longer than 30 s
  - Subjective fatigue and complaints (dizziness, ataxia, dyspnea)
  - Severe angina pectoris
  - Failure of monitoring equipment
- Relative criteria for termination:
  - Signs of hypoperfusion (cyanosis)
  - Progressive drop in heart rate and/or blood pressure
  - Increase of systolic blood pressure over 220 mmHg and/or diastolic pressure over 110 mmHg
  - More than 10 mmHg drop in blood pressure without signs of myocardial ischemia
  - Occurrence of conduction disturbances (AV block II° or III°, bundle branch block)
  - Supraventricular tachycardia
  - Complex arrhythmia longer than 30 s
  - Bradyarrhythmia
  - Increasing angina pectoris

7.1.3 Evaluation

The evaluation report should include the following information:

- Patient's cooperation
- Duration of exercise, maximum workload, and assessment of maximum workload
- Reasons for terminating exercise
- Heart rate and blood pressure at rest and under maximum workload
- Heart rhythm during exercise (occurrence of extrasystoles, salvos, etc. during exercise or in the recovery period)
- Evaluation of signs of ischemia
- Symptoms occurring during exercise

► **Heart rate.** The heart rate increases with increasing workload during the test. The maximum achievable heart rate is estimated using the previously mentioned formulas. Fit athletes have a lower resting heart rate. Patients who take beta blockers also have a lower resting heart rate, but unlike trained athletes, the maximum heart rate of these patients is not reached.

An inadequate increase or abnormal behavior of the heart rate can be an expression of chronotropic incompetence in patients with a sick sinus syndrome (e.g., after Fontan procedure or atrial switch operation). An abrupt increase in the heart rate is more likely a sign of ectopic focus or re-entrant tachycardia than of sinus tachycardia. However, re-entrant tachycardia can very rarely be triggered by an exercise test.

Adequate increase in the heart rate can be tested by an exercise ECG in patients with a rate-responsive pacemaker (R function) who show an increase in heart rate during exercise.

► **Blood pressure.** In childhood and adolescence, the systolic pressure during exercise does not usually exceed 200 mmHg (150 mmHg in young children). The systolic blood pressure should rise by at least 25% during exercise.

Stress-dependent hypertension may reflect developing hypertension. An excessive rise in blood pressure measured on the arms is typically found in patients with aortic coarctation (sometimes even after correction), and also in patients with renal artery stenosis, essential hypertension, or vasculitis.

An insufficient rise in the blood pressure is found in patients with stenosis of the left ventricular outflow tract (aortic stenosis, hypertrophic cardiomyopathy), severe aortic or pulmonary insufficiency, pulmonary hypertension, cardiomyopathy, and coronary anomalies. The exercise test must be terminated immediately if there is an abrupt drop in blood pressure. A sudden, dramatic drop in blood pressure can occur in patients with cardio-inhibitory syncopes.

► **ECG.** As the heart rate increases, PQ and QT intervals decrease, but the QTc time remains unchanged. Arrhythmias that originate from ectopic foci that can be suppressed under exercise are usually benign in a structurally unremarkable heart.

Note

If the frequency or the incidence of arrhythmia increases during exercise, underlying heart disease must be ruled out, in particular myocardial ischemia, myocarditis, cardiomyopathy, prolonged QT syndrome, and catecholamine-sensitive ventricular tachycardia.

The exercise ECG is also used to differentiate *AV blocks*. An AV block as a result of a high vagal tone (e.g., in trained athletes) disappears during exercise. AV blocks due to AV nodal disease can develop into a more severe blockage during exercise.

In patients with *long QT syndromes*, the physiological shortening of the QT interval as the heart rate increases does not usually take place. In addition, T wave changes may occur.

Note

In long QT syndrome, physical stress can trigger ventricular tachycardia up to Torsades de pointes tachycardia.

In patients with a *WPW syndrome*, the disappearance of the delta wave during exercise is a favorable sign. It is believed that in these patients, the refractory period of the accessory pathway is relatively long, so that the accessory pathway no longer communicates when the heart rate increases, thus lowering the risk of ventricular fibrillation as a result of an unchecked conduction of atrial fibrillation to the ventricles.

Exercise ECG is used in children less commonly than in adults for investigating *myocardial ischemia*. However, an ST elevation or depression of more than 2 to 3 mm is pathological in children. The ST segment is typically horizontal if ischemia is present. In addition, T wave inversion frequently occurs. Causes of myocardial ischemia can be congenital or acquired coronary anomalies (e.g., stenosis after coronary transfer during a switch operation for TGA or as a result of Kawasaki syndrome). However, an increased oxygen demand of the myocardium—associated with aortic stenosis or hypertrophic cardiomyopathy, for example—can cause myocardial ischemia.

7.2 Spiroergometry

In spiroergometric testing, exercise is supplemented by parameters that measure respiration and energy

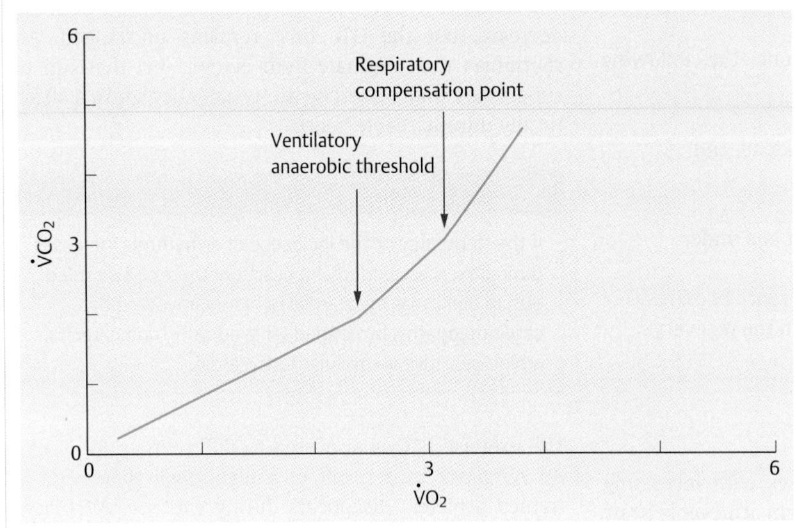

Fig. 7.1 Ventilatory anaerobic threshold.

metabolism in addition to assessing the cardiovascular system. In principle, the same conditions as for exercise testing apply, including exercise protocols with identical contraindications and termination criteria.

Muscle work requires energy. The body consumes oxygen (aerobic conditions) to generate this energy from fats and carbohydrates. If an oxygen deficit exists (anaerobic conditions), energy can still be taken from carbohydrates. However, this method of utilizing energy is substantially less efficient—under aerobic conditions one molecule of glucose yields 37 molecules of ATP and under anaerobic conditions only 3. Furthermore, lactate is produced as a result of anaerobic energy generation. Lactate leads to metabolic acidosis and inhibits energy metabolism. Metabolic acidosis is buffered and compensated by bicarbonate. When lactate is buffered, CO_2 is produced and exhaled through the lungs. Energy supply to the body and the removal of metabolic end-products are therefore directly linked to the cardiovascular system.

7.2.1 Parameters

In spiroergometry, in addition to the ECG and blood pressure, the oxygen and carbon dioxide content in exhaled air is measured using a mask or a mouthpiece with a nose clip, and the tidal volume and the expiratory minute volume are recorded. In addition to end-expiratory (end-tidal) partial pressures for oxygen and carbon dioxide, oxygen consumption and carbon dioxide production are determined. Furthermore, capillary and arterial blood gas analyses are made during the examination.

▸ **Respiratory rate (RR).** As exercise progresses, the respiratory rate increases slowly and steadily. With more intensive exercise, the respiratory rate increases more rapidly and can reach three times the baseline rate under maximum workload.

▸ **Tidal volume (V_T).** The tidal volume increases relatively quickly as exercise increases and reaches a plateau about three times the baseline value at a relative early stage of exercise.

▸ **Ventilatory anaerobic threshold (A_T).** The ventilatory threshold describes the range of workload at which a relative oxygen deficit leads to anaerobic metabolism. Increased lactate production is then found in the blood gas analysis. Furthermore, due to the buffering process, carbon dioxide accumulates and is exhaled through an increased respiratory drive. However, lactate buffering does not increase oxygen consumption. When plotting carbon dioxide production against oxygen consumption, a sudden, disproportionate increase in carbon dioxide production occurs at the ventilatory anaerobic threshold —a kink in the graph. An additional kink appears when excessive carbon dioxide increases the respiratory drive and hyperventilation occurs. This second kink on the graph is the "respiratory compensation point" (▸ Fig. 7.1).

▸ **Maximum oxygen consumption ($V'O_2$ max).** Oxygen consumption is calculated from the inspiratory and expiratory volume as well as from the mean inspiratory and expiratory oxygen concentration.

Below the anaerobic threshold, oxygen consumption increases nearly linearly as the workload increases. At a certain workload, a plateau is reached that is referred to as maximum oxygen consumption. This describes the highest possible oxygen consumption that cannot be increased even if the workload is increased.

Note

Maximum oxygen consumption is considered to be the best parameter for assessing fitness or cardiovascular capacity.

In children, however, maximal oxygen consumption is not usually reached during exercise testing on the bicycle ergometer. In these cases, the peak oxygen consumption (peak $V''O_2$) is used. This is the highest value reached in an average period of 30 s. Until puberty, the rule of thumb is that 40 ± 7 mL/kg/min is assumed to be the standard value for peak oxygen consumption.

► **Oxygen pulse ($V'O_2$/heart rate).** The oxygen pulse indicates how much oxygen is transported per heartbeat. Usually the oxygen pulse during exercises increases continuously, eventually reaching a plateau, which is usually reached at maximum workload. A high oxygen pulse indicates good physical capacity, a low one indicates poor capacity.

► **Respiratory equivalent for oxygen ($V'E/V'O_2$).** The respiratory equivalent for oxygen is an indicator for the efficiency of respiration. It describes the minute ventilation needed to take in 1 liter of oxygen. This parameter has no dimension. The normal range at the anaerobic threshold is around 25 to 30. The larger the respiratory equivalent, the poorer capacity is. A pathologically high respiratory equivalent may also be a sign of ventilation-perfusion mismatch.

► **Respiratory equivalent for carbon dioxide ($V'E/V'CO_2$).** By analogy with the respiratory equivalent for oxygen, the respiratory equivalent for carbon dioxide describes the minute ventilation needed to exhale 1 liter of carbon dioxide. The normal value at the anaerobic threshold is around 25 to 30.

► **Respiratory quotient (CO_2 production/O_2 consumption).** The respiratory quotient gives information about the main source of energy. A respiratory quotient of 1 indicates carbohydrate metabolism. The respiratory quotient for fatty acid metabolism is 0.71. At rest, about 40% of the muscle's energy demand is covered by carbohydrates and about 60% by fats. This yields a respiratory quotient of around 0.8. During exercise, energy demand is increasingly covered by carbohydrates. However, an individual in good physical condition metabolizes an increased amount of fat during exercise as well. The respiratory quotient allows an estimate to be made of the proportion of energy generated from carbohydrates or fats during exercise.

An increase in the respiratory quotient to greater than 1 indicates full metabolic workload. Exhalation of carbon dioxide is greater than oxygen intake. This ratio arises because lactate is buffered during metabolic acidosis and carbon dioxide thus accumulates and must be exhaled.

► **Carbon dioxide production ($V'CO_2$).** Production of carbon dioxide initially increases linearly as the workload is increased. At the transition between aerobic and anaerobic energy production, carbon dioxide production increases disproportionately. This increase can be explained by the fact that buffering the lactate that is produced leads to the accumulation of carbon dioxide that must then be exhaled. This disproportionately steep increase in the production of carbon dioxide is used to determine the ventilatory anaerobic threshold (see above).

► **Respiratory threshold (maximum voluntary ventilation, MVV).** The respiratory threshold describes the maximum amount of air that can be inhaled and exhaled by a patient within 1 minute. The respiratory threshold can be estimated using the FEV_1 (forced expiratory volume in the first second of expiration) determined by spirometry ($FEV_1 \times 40 = MVV$). The respiratory threshold can generally not be reached under spiroergometry exercise (except by very well trained athletes). Reaching the

Panel 1	Panel 2	Panel 3
Minute volume vs. Workload	Heart rate and oxygen pulse vs. Workload	Oxygen consumption and carbon dioxide production vs. Workload
Panel 4	**Panel 5**	**Panel 6**
Minute volume vs. Carbon dioxide production	Carbon dioxide production and heart rate vs. Oxygen consumption	Ventilatory equivalent for oxygen and carbon dioxide vs. Workload
Panel 7	**Panel 8**	**Panel 9**
Tidal volume vs. Ventilatory equivalent	Respiratory quotient vs. Workload	End-expiratory oxygen and carbon dioxide partial pressure vs. Workload

Fig. 7.2 Nine-panel plot proposed by Wasserman. Panels 2, 3, 5, and 8 marked in red concern mainly parameters of cardiac capacity. The blue panels 1, 4, and 7 describe primarily the respiratory mechanism. Gas exchange is best assessed using panels 6 and 9 (in green).[116]

respiratory threshold during exercise is a sign of impaired pulmonary capacity.

▸ **End expiratory oxygen and carbon dioxide partial pressure** ($PETO_2$, $PETCO_2$). At rest, the arterial and end expiratory values measured for oxygen and carbon dioxide are almost identical in a healthy person. The occurrence of a relevant difference between arterial and end expiratory carbon dioxide values during exercise indicates a ventilation–perfusion mismatch. This means that carbon dioxide cannot be completely exhaled and accumulates in the blood. The same is true for right-to-left shunt defects, where venous blood rich in carbon dioxide bypasses the lung. In such cases, the amount of carbon dioxide in the exhaled air is low compared with the amount of carbon dioxide in the blood.

▸ **Lactate.** The anaerobic threshold is considered as safely reached when the lactate level exceeds 4 mmol/L. After a short period, lactate is buffered away by bicarbonate, which leads to a drop in the standard bicarbonate.

7.2.2 Evaluation

The nine-panel plot proposed by Wasserman (Wasserman et al. 2005)[116] is usually used to evaluate the results of spiroergometric testing. With the appropriate software, this plot is created and printed out by modern equipment immediately after the test (▸ Fig. 7.2).

The assessment of the test includes statements on the maximum workload based on the maximum or peak oxygen consumption, the anaerobic threshold, the respiratory mechanism, and on gas exchange in addition to pulse and blood pressure behavior and the ECG during exercise and in the recovery period (▸ Fig. 7.3).

7.3 Six-Minute Walk Test

For patients who cannot be subjected to the high stress of exercise or spiroergometric testing (e.g., patients with uncorrected cyanotic heart defects or pulmonary hypertension), the six-minute walk test can be used to assess physical capacity.

In this test, after resting, the patient is asked to walk for six minutes on level ground at a pace chosen by him or her that seems to be just barely tolerable. The distance covered is measured and used to evaluate capacity. The patient's ECG and oxygen saturation are monitored during the test. Respiratory rate and blood pressure are measured before and after exercise. The same termination criteria used in the other exercise tests apply.

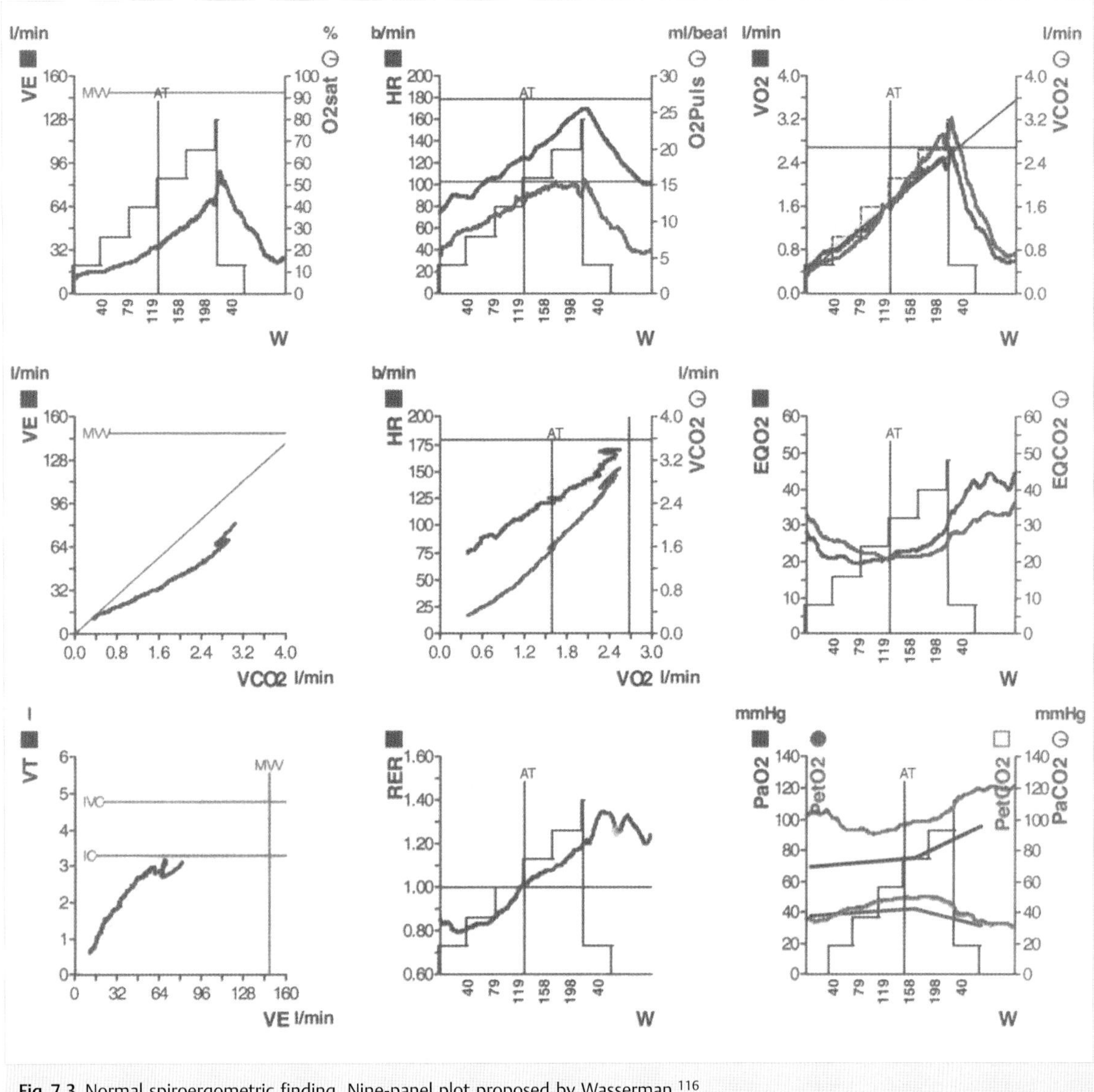

Fig. 7.3 Normal spiroergometric finding. Nine-panel plot proposed by Wasserman.[116]

8 Cardiac Catheterization

8.1 Basics

Today, only very few purely diagnostic cardiac catheterizations are performed, as the anatomical situation for most heart defects can be visualized very precisely using echocardiography or magnetic resonance tomography, which is used especially in larger patients and adults.

Nevertheless, diagnostic cardiac catheterizations are occasionally needed for specific clinical questions such as for exact blood pressure measurements and the calculation of blood flow resistance, to quantify shunts, or in those cases where findings from noninvasive diagnostics were unclear or contradictory. Pressure values, oxygen content in the individual cardiac chambers or segments of blood vessels, and additional indicator methods, if needed, are used to assess the hemodynamic situation (e.g., calculating cardiac output or identifying shunts).

Another indication not to be underestimated is the surgeon's desire and need to obtain additional morphological information preoperatively so that the surgery can proceed more quickly and more safely. Furthermore, there are a number of patients in whom an accurate diagnosis is possible only by cardiac catheterization; for example, if the diagnostic window is insufficient for echocardiography and MRI cannot be performed due to a pacemaker.

The special features of diagnostic cardiac catheterizations for some typical cardiac defects are discussed below.

8.2 Vascular Access Routes

Normally, most cardiac catheterization examinations in children as well as adults are performed via vascular access routes in the groin (femoral artery and vein; ▸ Fig. 8.1). The vessel is punctured using the Seldinger technique and the sheath is inserted over a guidewire. These sheaths consist of a hemostatic valve (rubber plug) through which the actual catheters can be inserted, and a side port through which the sheath can be flushed with saline solution, for example, and blood samples can be drawn. Standard sheaths are available in various sizes with an inner lumen from 4 F to 16 F (1 F = ⅓ mm).

Other access routes may become necessary because of vascular occlusions (▸ Fig. 8.1). Commonly used access routes in this event are the brachial or axillary vessels, the jugular vein, the carotid artery, and the subclavian vein. Access via the umbilical vessels is also possible in neonates—for a Rashkind procedure or treatment of a critical aortic stenosis, for example.

The transhepatic access is very rarely used, but is a safe access should the peripheral venous accesses be completely occluded. A percutaneous puncture of the hepatic vein is made under sonographic or fluoroscopic guidance and the sheath then advanced into the right atrium.

8.3 The Catheter Examination

The cardiac catheter examination procedure should be standardized to allow a precise hemodynamic examination with valid results. To ensure this, the following steps are helpful.

▸ **Documentation of the baseline condition.** This includes documentation and monitoring of the vital signs, including pulse, ECG, transcutaneous O_2 saturation, and noninvasive blood pressure.

▸ **Initial adequate stable hemodynamic situation.** The patient should be calm and at rest and have no significant episodes of excitation. In most modern centers, the examination is performed even in small children under deep conscious sedation and with spontaneous breathing. General anesthesia is not routinely needed. A blood gas analysis should be performed to document adequate ventilation.

▸ **Measuring blood pressure and shunt fraction.** These steps should best be taken initially, before the contrast

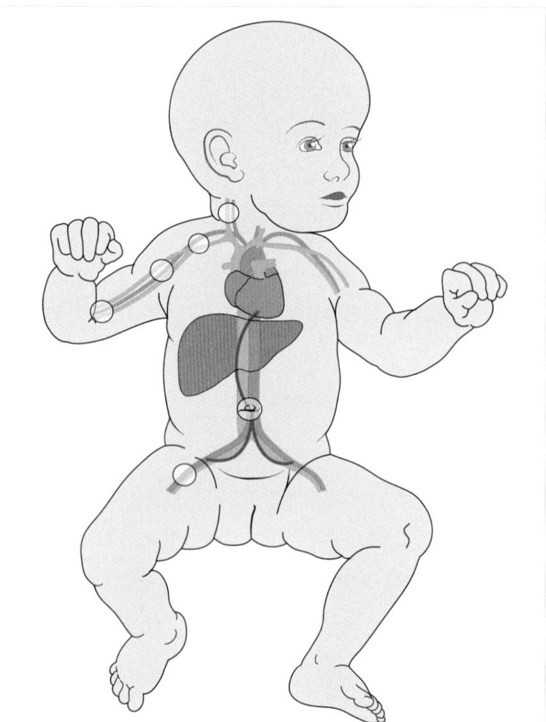

Fig. 8.1 Typical vascular access routes for cardiac catheterization in children: femoral artery and vein, brachial artery and vein, axillary artery and vein, carotid artery, jugular vein, umbilical artery and vein, and subclavian vein.

medium is administered, as the contrast medium can lead to volume load that may result in false high blood pressure readings (e.g., high end-diastolic pressures). The pressure curves are recorded at defined positions of the heart. In addition, pressure curves are recorded along the course of blood vessels or anatomical structures (pull-back pressure curves). The first blood gas analysis should be made in room air or at FiO_2 of less than 0.3. Depending on the results of these baseline recordings, a subsequent analysis can be made later with increased oxygen supply, for example, to test the responsiveness of the pulmonary vascular system.

► **Angiographies.** After the hemodynamic situation has been determined, the vascular segments or cardiac chambers to be examined are visualized by the use of angiography. A sufficient amount of contrast medium is injected via the cardiac catheter using a high-pressure injection pump and the images are recorded continuously on film or in digital form.

► **Interventions.** If an intervention is performed, the major and important steps of the procedure should also be documented (e.g., balloon inflation for valve stenosis or stent placement in a stenotic segment of a vessel). In addition, the result of the intervention and any complications that may have occurred (e.g., development of a new valvular insufficiency or contrast media extravasation) must be documented.

► **Final documentation.** After the catheterization is completed, the patient's condition must be assessed and documented before he or she is transferred to the ward for further monitoring and care. In addition to vital signs, this also includes checking the vascular status and the perfusion of the limb where the puncture was made.

8.4 Various Catheters

An important part of the careful planning of a cardiac catheterization involves the precise selection of the examination catheters to be used. A variety of different catheters are available for the different stages of the examination and for accessing the various cardiac chambers and vascular segments.

► **Flexible balloon catheter.** These catheters have a small balloon at the tip that can be filled with air or carbon dioxide (► Fig. 8.2). This balloon allows the tip of the catheter to float with or be carried by the bloodstream. Typical uses for these catheters include, for example, entry to the pulmonary artery from the right atrium and ventricle, or for an antegrade access to the aorta from the left ventricle (► Fig. 8.3 and ► Fig. 8.4). Balloon catheters are very soft and flexible, but they can be temporarily stiffened and shaped with a guidewire and be moved along the wire into certain vascular segments or even against the bloodstream. Balloon catheters can have open or closed tips and are suitable for precise blood pressure readings (including pulmonary capillary occlusion pressure, wedge pressure), for angiography, or to determine the cardiac output by thermodilution (Swan-Ganz catheter).

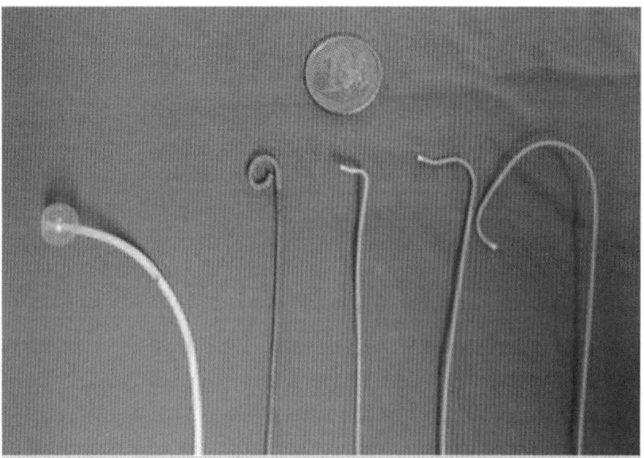

Fig. 8.2 Various cardiac catheters. From left to right: balloon catheter, pigtail catheter, special coronary catheters.

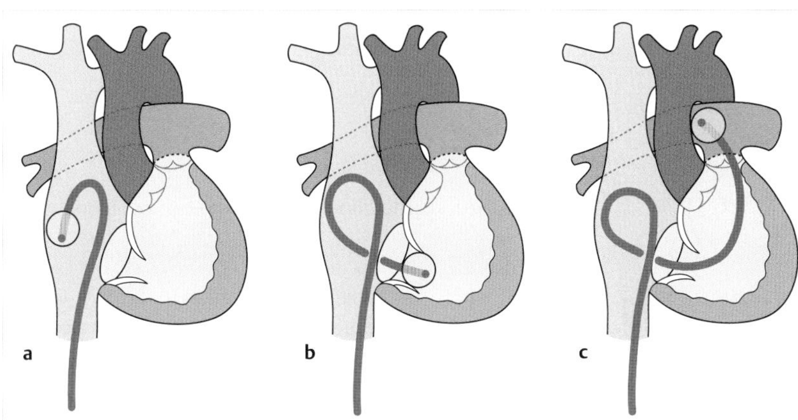

Fig. 8.3 Flow-directed placement of a balloon catheter from the right atrium into the pulmonary artery. **a** The balloon catheter is inserted via the inferior vena cava into the right atrium and then inflated. **b** The inflated balloon is carried by the bloodstream through the tricuspid valve into the right ventricle. **c** The inflated balloon is then carried by the bloodstream through the pulmonary valve and into the pulmonary artery in the direction of normal blood flow.

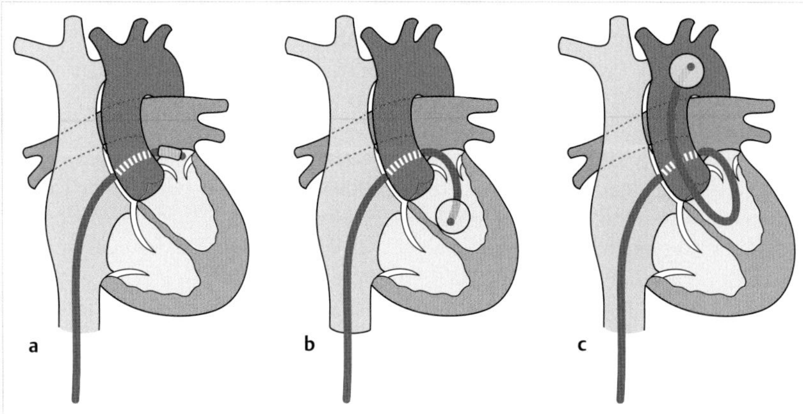

Fig. 8.4 Flow-directed placement of a balloon catheter from the left ventricle to the aorta. **a** The deflated balloon catheter is advanced through the inferior vena cava to the right atrium. It is then advanced further into the left atrium through a hole in the atrium (patent foramen ovale or atrial septal defect). **b** The balloon is inflated in the left atrium and carried by the bloodstream through the mitral valve into the left ventricle. **c** From the left ventricle, the catheter follows the bloodstream through the aortic valve into the ascending aorta.

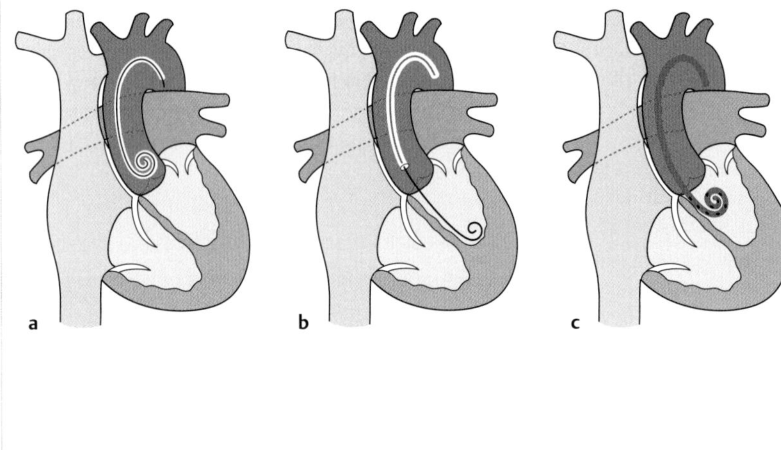

Fig. 8.5 Passage of a pigtail catheter through the aortic valve with a wire into the left ventricle. **a** Retrograde advancement of the pigtail catheter through an arterial access into the ascending aorta. A wire is then pushed through the catheter. This straightens the pigtail-shaped distal end of the catheter; the catheter is lengthened. **b** Now the thin, soft end of the wire is advanced carefully until it passes the aortic valve in a retrograde direction. **c** The wire serves as a guide over which the pigtail catheter can be advanced into the left ventricle. Finally, the wire is retracted and the pigtail catheter remains in the left ventricle.

► **Preshaped plastic catheters.** These are predominantly catheters with an open tip and with a predefined typical shape that also gives them their individual names. Typical examples are the pigtail catheter, the right and left coronary catheter, or the multipurpose catheter (► Fig. 8.2). Some of them have only one hole at the tip, but many catheters have several side holes at the end through which contrast medium can be injected using a high-pressure pump. Their predefined shape can be changed or temporarily modified by guidewires (► Fig. 8.5 and ► Fig. 8.6). Since these catheters are more rigid than balloon catheters, they can be used to examine difficult-to-reach segments of the heart or blood vessels. However, the risk of injury is higher when using these catheters. Guidewires with soft, flexible ends are therefore often used for exact positioning.

8.5 Hemodynamic Monitoring

Hemodynamic monitoring is an essential component of cardiac catheterizations in childhood and for congenital heart defects. The blood pressure in the individual segments of the heart or blood vessel is transmitted through the hollow catheter via the continuous blood or fluid column to a pressure sensor and then on to the measuring system for analysis. The typical pull-back pressure curves are recorded when the catheter is moved through segments of the heart and blood vessels.

In addition, the catheters can be used to take a blood sample at individual segments of the heart or blood vessels for determining hemoglobin and oxygen concentrations. The cardiac output and shunt fraction can be determined from these values (see Chapter 8.5.2 and Chapter 8.5.3).

8.5.1 Pressure Curves

A standard examination includes measuring blood pressure in all segments of the heart and blood vessels that are probed and documenting pressure curves across valves when the catheter is withdrawn through valves, septa, or stenotic segments. Since there is usually a certain amount of variation from breathing, at least 10 pressure curves should be recorded, the mean values calculated, and artifacts eliminated.

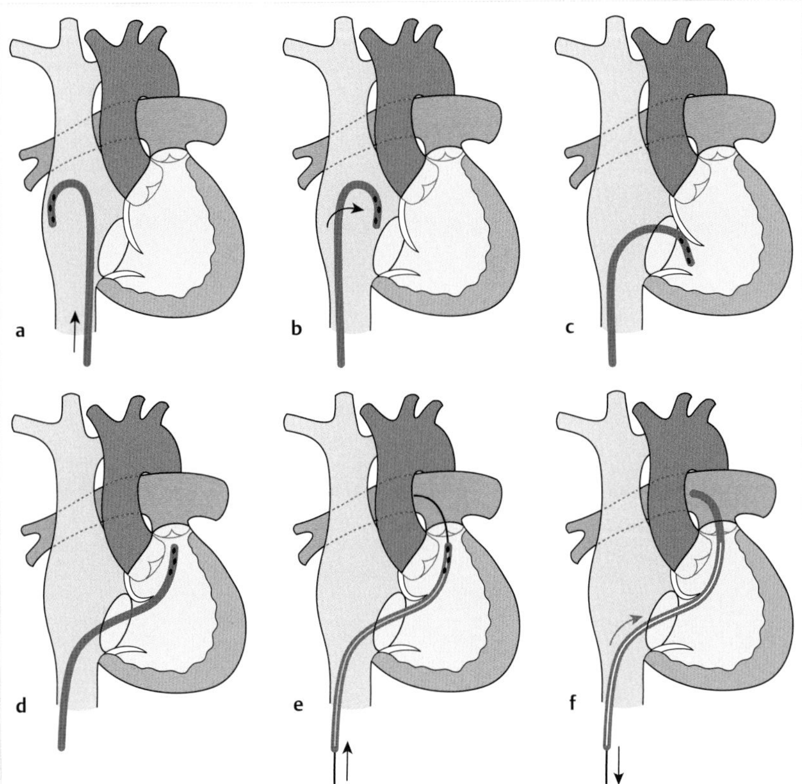

Fig. 8.6 Passage of a preshaped multipurpose catheter with a wire from the right atrium into the pulmonary artery. The multipurpose catheter is advanced through the inferior vena cava into the right atrium (**a**). The tip of the catheter is rotated and pushed (**b**) to direct it through the tricuspid valve (**c**) so that the distal end of the catheter is located below the pulmonary valve (**d**). A thin wire is now advanced through the multipurpose catheter; it passes through the pulmonary valve and reaches the pulmonary artery (**e**). This wire now serves as the guidewire for advancing the multipurpose catheter into the pulmonary artery. Finally, the wire is retracted (**f**).

► **Atrial pressure curves.** These curves consist mainly of an A wave and V wave, corresponding to the atrial contraction (A wave) and atrial filling (V wave). The V wave is caused by an increase in pressure in the atrium from the venous backflow or from atrial filling after closure of the AV valve. In the right atrium, the A wave is usually larger than the V wave; vice versa in the left atrium. The pressure in the left atrium is normally higher than in the right atrium. However, if there is a large atrial septal defect, the pressure between the two atria is generally equalized. In addition to pressure curves, the mean pressure is also important (► Fig. 8.7 and ► Fig. 8.8).

► **Wedge pressure (pulmonary capillary occlusion pressure).** This pressure is measured by advancing an open-tip balloon catheter into the pulmonary artery in the flow direction and inflating the balloon at the distal end of the artery. This prevents transmission of pressure from the pulmonary artery via the bloodstream. The pressure measured in this way corresponds with the pressure of the vascular segment located behind the catheter in the flow direction, namely the pulmonary tissue, the pulmonary vein, or the left atrium (► Fig. 8.9). The E wave and A wave of the left atrium can also be seen here. If there is no stenosis in the pulmonary veins, the wedge pressure is equivalent to that in the left atrium (principle of communicating tubes). However, if there is a stenosis in the pulmonary vein, the wedge pressure is higher than the pressure in the left atrium.

► **Ventricular pressure curves.** During ventricular systole, the ventricular pressure increases rapidly until it exceeds the diastolic pressure of the downstream vessel and the ventricle ejects blood. This is followed by a definite plateau, during which blood continues to flow into the vessel. Diastole then leads to a relaxation of the ventricle; the pressure approaches 0 mmHg, and now additional blood flows in from the atrium. After the end of diastole, there is an isovolumetric contraction of the ventricle before a new ejection phase starts (► Fig. 8.10 and ► Fig. 8.11). This dip in the ascending segment of the ventricular pressure curve corresponds with the end-diastolic pressure. No mean pressure is calculated for the ventricle, as diastole is always 0 mmHg (exceptions are cardiomyopathy or tamponade, for example). The end-diastolic pressure of a ventricle is normally equivalent to the mean pressure of the upstream atrium. If this is not the case, there is a stenosis of the mitral or tricuspid valve.

► **Vascular pressure curves.** The typical systolic–diastolic blood pressure curves that arise from vascular wall tone, systole, vascular resistance, and Windkessel function (► Fig. 8.12) are documented in blood vessels. The normal arterial blood pressure varies depending on age

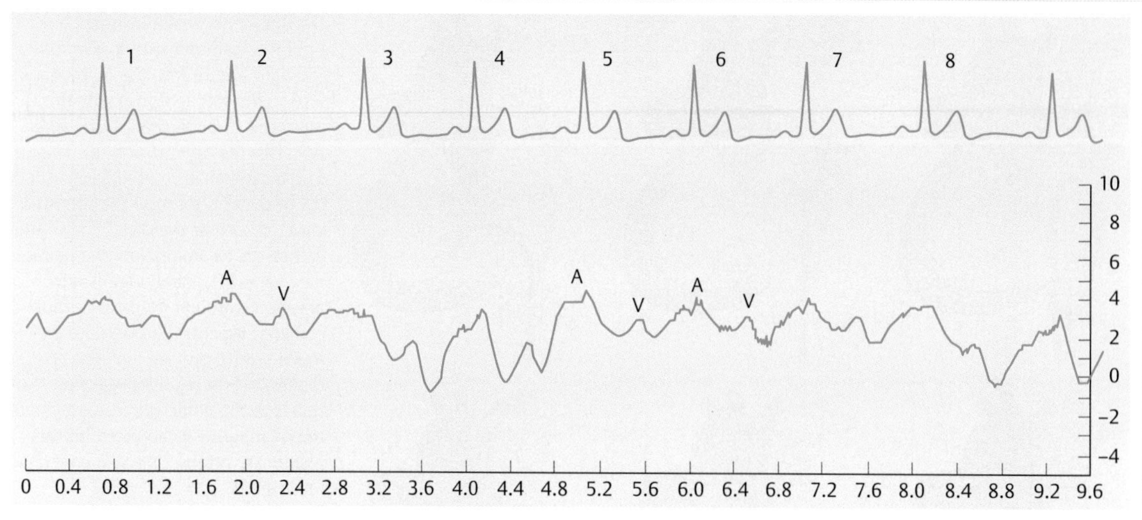

Fig. 8.7 Typical pressure curve from the right atrium.

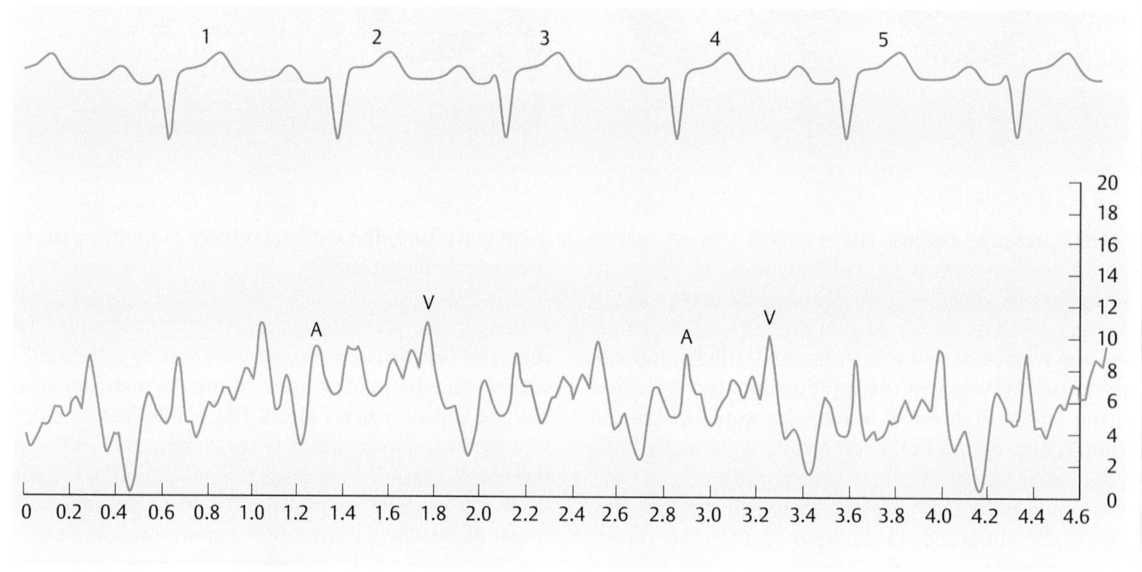

Fig. 8.8 Typical pressure curve from the left atrium.

and weight. The blood pressure in the pulmonary artery is identical for all age and weight groups with the exception of the period immediately after birth, when there is physiological pulmonary hypertension.

Systolic and diastolic pressures are elevated in a rigid vessel (e.g., due to atherosclerosis, scarring). If the volume of blood is large and the Windkessel function is absent (e. g., due to aortic insufficiency, patent ductus arteriosus [PDA]), the result is very high amplitude with low diastole (pulsus celer et altus). If the valve does not close, the diastolic pressure is usually considerably lower or is only 0 to 1 mmHg (e.g., pulmonary insufficiency) and may appear similar to a ventricular pressure curve.

► **Pull-back curves.** For pull-back curves, blood pressure is measured continuously while the catheter is simultaneously pulled back through a segment of the heart or blood vessel. This allows the blood pressure curve in front of and behind an anatomical structure (e.g., valve) or stenosis to be determined (► Fig. 8.13, ► Fig. 8.14, ► Fig. 8.15, ► Fig. 8.16). A pull-back pressure curve can be used to prove or rule out a pressure gradient.

The systolic and the middle pressure gradient can be measured in vessels with pressure differences. In valve stenosis the systolic pressure difference is usually measured between the ventricle systole and the systolic blood pressure of the downstream blood vessel.

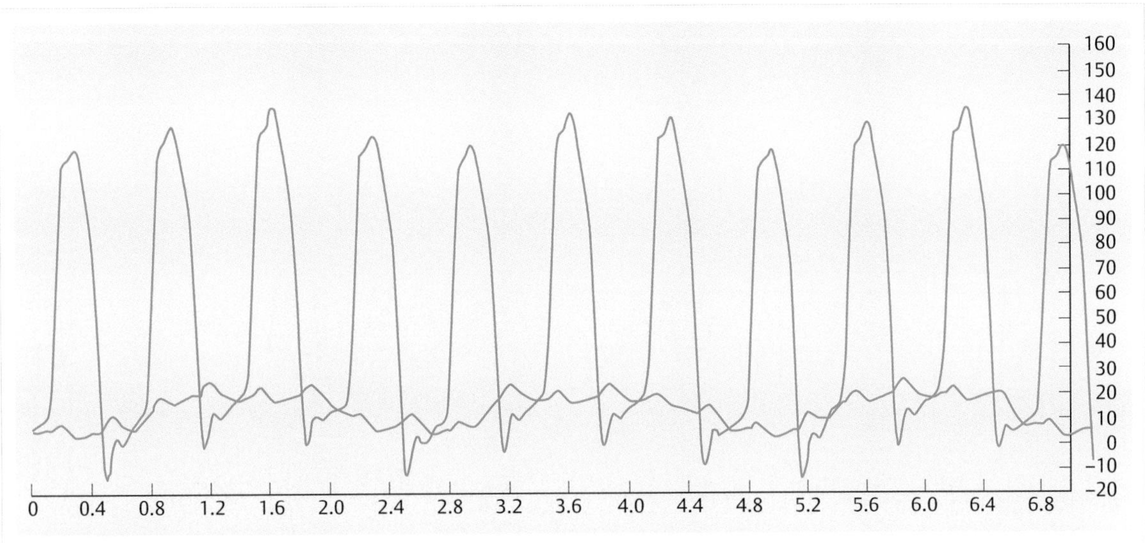

Fig. 8.9 Typical pressure curve of wedge pressure after the balloon is inflated in the pulmonary artery. Simultaneous measurement of wedge pressure and pressure in the left ventricle.

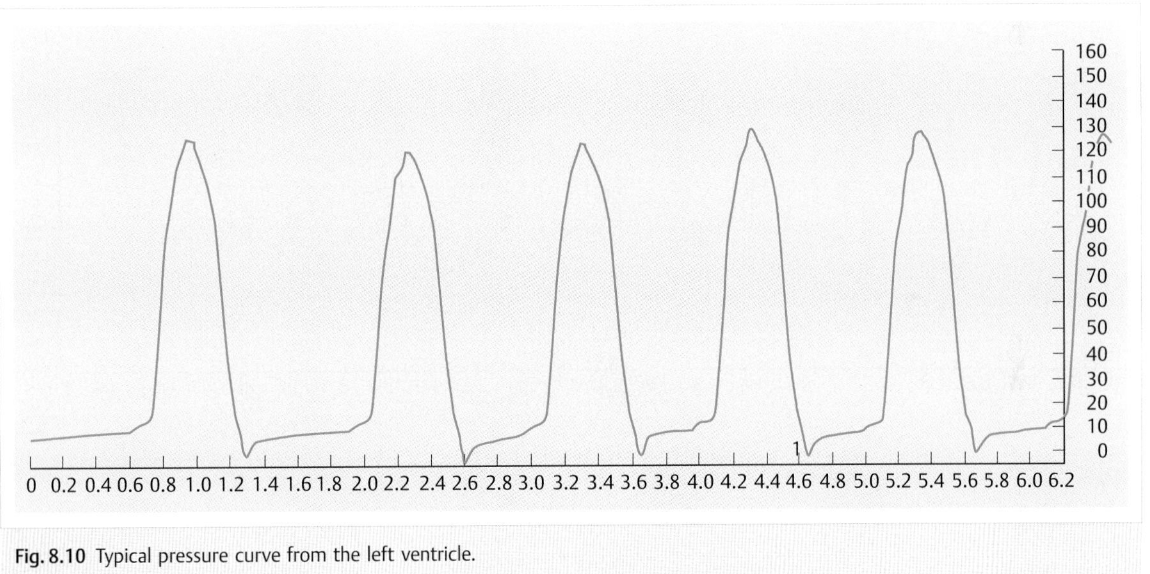

Fig. 8.10 Typical pressure curve from the left ventricle.

▸ **Simultaneous measurements.** In simultaneous measurements, pressures are recorded at the same time in different segments of the heart and vessels (▸ Fig. 8.17 and ▸ Fig. 8.18). Simultaneous measurements are used in particular when a pull-back pressure curve is technically impossible or extremely difficult (e.g., mitral stenosis—wedge pressure or pressure in the left atrium and end-diastolic pressure in the left ventricle), or when a direct comparison between different vessels and heart segments is important (e.g., pulmonary pressure and aortic pressure for testing pulmonary vascular response).(▸ Fig. 8.18. Normal reference values for pressures and saturation in an adult with a healthy heart are shown in ▸ Fig. 8.19)

8.5.2 Determining Blood Flow and Cardiac Output

Determining cardiac output is an integral part of cardiac catheterization and reliable, reproducible methods for measuring it are indispensable. Although cardiac output is affected to a certain extent by respiratory variability and also by the cardiac cycle, these minimal factors can be ignored and cardiac output is determined as the flow per time unit. There are two methods for determining cardiac output: the direct Fick principle, and the indicator dilution method. Both methods measure the pulmonary blood flow, which can be considered the equivalent of

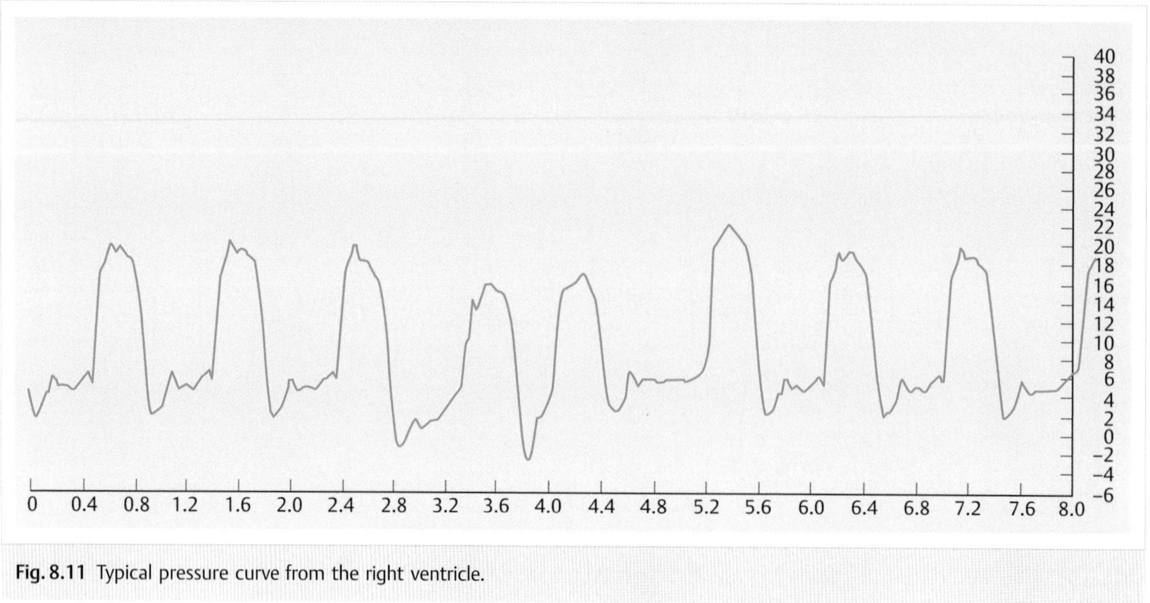

Fig. 8.11 Typical pressure curve from the right ventricle.

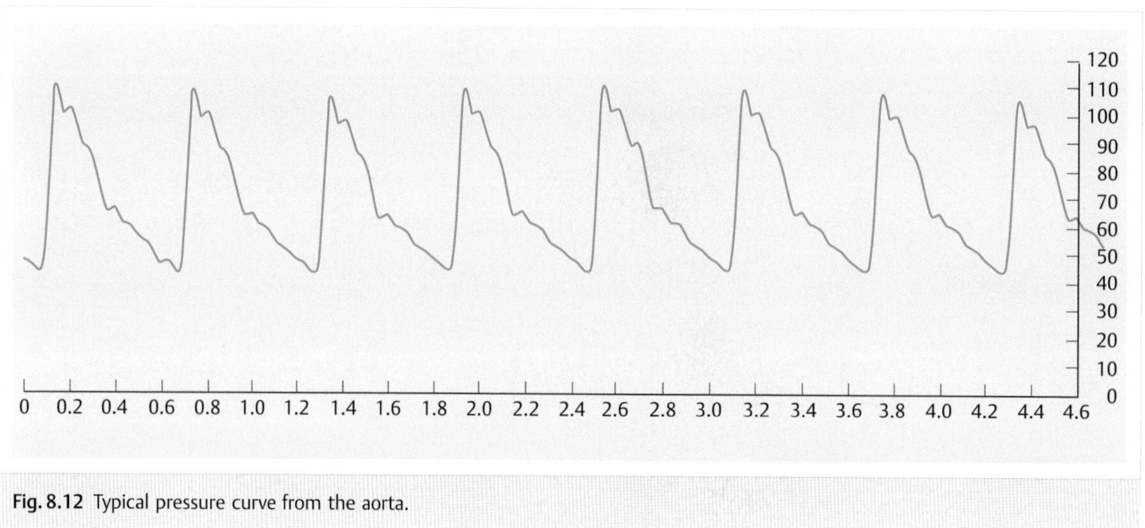

Fig. 8.12 Typical pressure curve from the aorta.

systemic blood flow if there are no intrapulmonary or intracardiac shunts. The small additional flow from the bronchial arteries is negligible.

The flow through a specific vascular bed can generally be measured using an indicator over a unit of time if the original and final concentrations are known.

$$\text{Flow(Q)} = \frac{\text{Change in indicator quantity}}{\text{Mean difference in concentration (inflow – outflow)}}$$

The more of the added indicator that is removed from the blood or diluted per time unit, the higher the blood flow is. For accurate determination, the indicator must have been mixed thoroughly with the blood and there may no undetected inflow or outflow of the indicator. Usually the cardiac output in humans is approximately. 3.5 L/min per m^2 body surface (± 0.7).

Direct Fick Principle

► **Pulmonary blood flow (Q_P).** The indicator for calculating cardiac output with this method is oxygen. Oxygen is consumed by the lungs during inspiration (this is the measurement profile, equivalent to pulmonary blood flow). A portion of the oxygen that was taken in through inspiration is supplied to the venous blood of the lungs. This process is called oxygen intake or oxygen

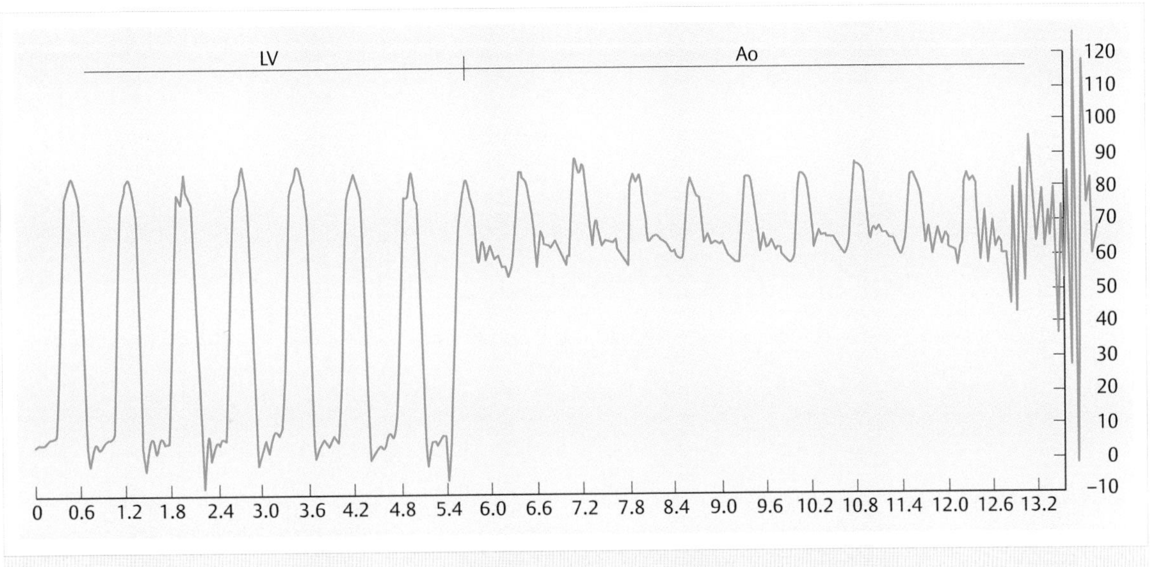

Fig. 8.13 Typical pull-back pressure curve from the left ventricle to the aorta. LV, left ventricle; Ao, aorta.

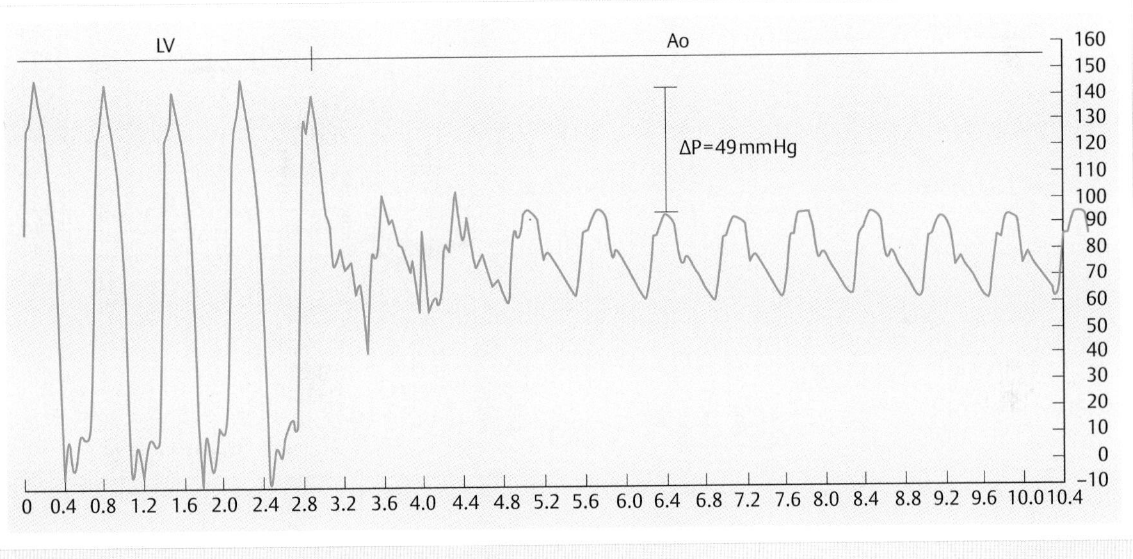

Fig. 8.14 Typical pull-back pressure curve with aortic stenosis. LV, left ventricle; Ao, aorta.

consumption ($V \cdot O_2$). The oxygen content in the venous blood is called mixed venous oxygen content (MVO_2), expressed in milliliters O_2/100 mL blood. The higher oxygen content in the pulmonary veins after passing through the lungs is called PVO_2. It is also expressed in milliliters O_2/100 mL blood. This makes it clear that every 100 mL blood that flows through the lungs takes in the difference in the amount of oxygen between PVO_2 and MVO_2 while passing through the lungs. This amount is usually is around 25 to 50 mL per liter. If the amount of oxygen consumed by the lungs during inspiration is known ($V \cdot O_2$), the pulmonary blood flow (Q_P) can be calculated.

$$Q_P(L/min/m^2) = \frac{V \cdot O_2(mL/min)}{PVO_2 - MVO_2/100\ mL\ blood} \times 10$$

The 100 mL is multiplied by 10 to convert it to one liter so the cardiac output can be expressed in L/min.

▸ **Systemic blood flow (Q_S).** Since the two blood flows are connected in a series, the pulmonary blood flow, Q_P, is equal to the systemic blood flow, Q_S. If no systemic venous oxygen is added and no oxygen is removed, the pulmonary venous oxygen content (PVO_2) is equal to the arterial oxygen content (SAO_2). (This should not be confused with

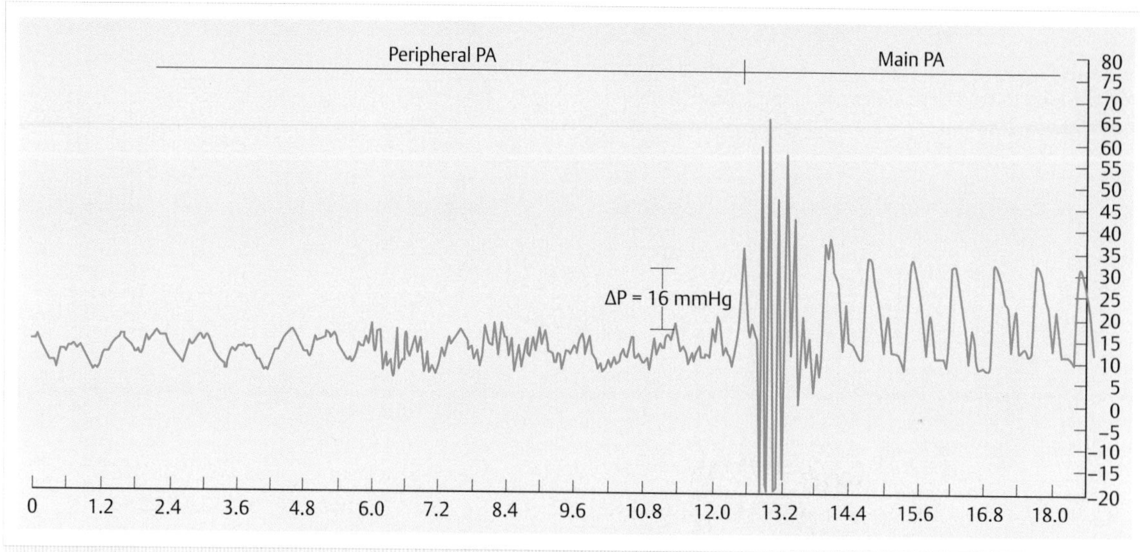

Fig. 8.15 Typical pull-back pressure curve with peripheral pulmonary stenosis. PA, pulmonary artery.

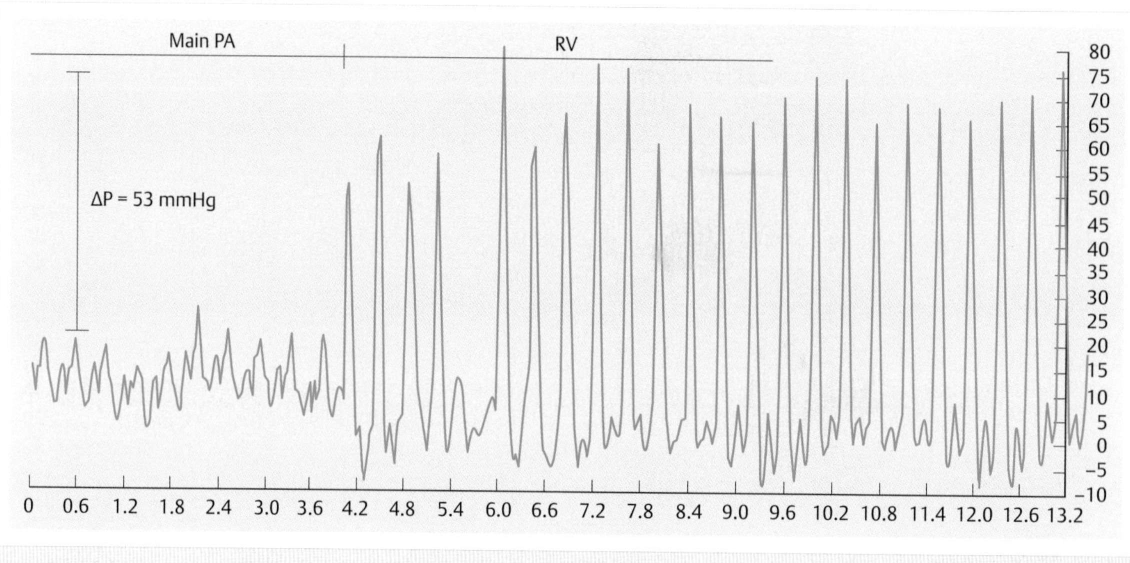

Fig. 8.16 Typical pull-back pressure curve with pulmonary valve stenosis. Main PA, main pulmonary artery; RV, right ventricle.

oxygen saturation, SaO_2.) Hence the following formula is valid for calculating the systemic blood flow, Q_S:

$$Q_S(\text{L/min/m}^2) = \frac{V \cdot O_2(\text{mL/min})}{SAO_2\text{–}MVO_2/100\text{ mL blood}} \times 10$$

▸ **Oxygen consumption ($V \cdot O_2$).** It is technically difficult, however, to calculate oxygen consumption ($V \cdot O_2$). Formerly, rebreathing bags were used for this purpose. Other methods use measurement instruments in ventilators but require intubation and anesthesia. In routine practice, standard tables are used that show oxygen consumption ($V \cdot O_2$) in relation to height and weight. In adults, oxygen consumption is usually around 200 to 250 mL/min. The formula below can also be used to estimate oxygen consumption:

$$\text{Oxygen consumption } (V \cdot O_2) = \text{BSA } (\text{m}^2) \times 150 \text{ mL/min}$$

where BSA is the body surface area.

▸ **Mixed venous oxygen content (MVO_2).** Another problem is measuring the mixed venous oxygen content (MVO_2). By definition, the oxygen content in the pulmonary artery is referred to as mixed venous oxygen

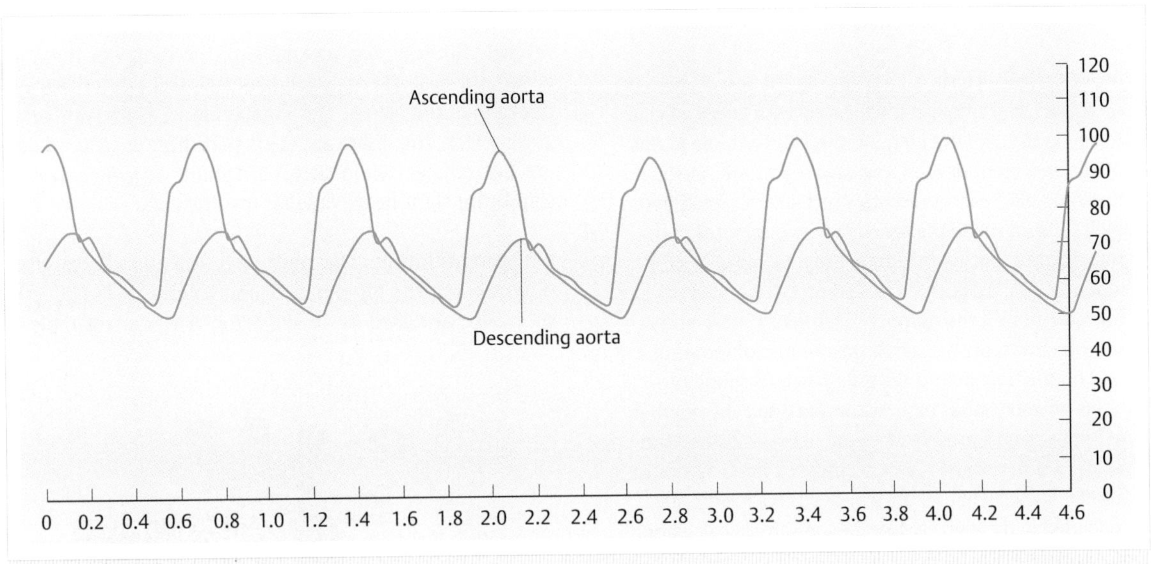

Fig. 8.17 Typical pressure curve associated with aortic coarctation. Simultaneous pressure measurement of the ascending and descending aorta.

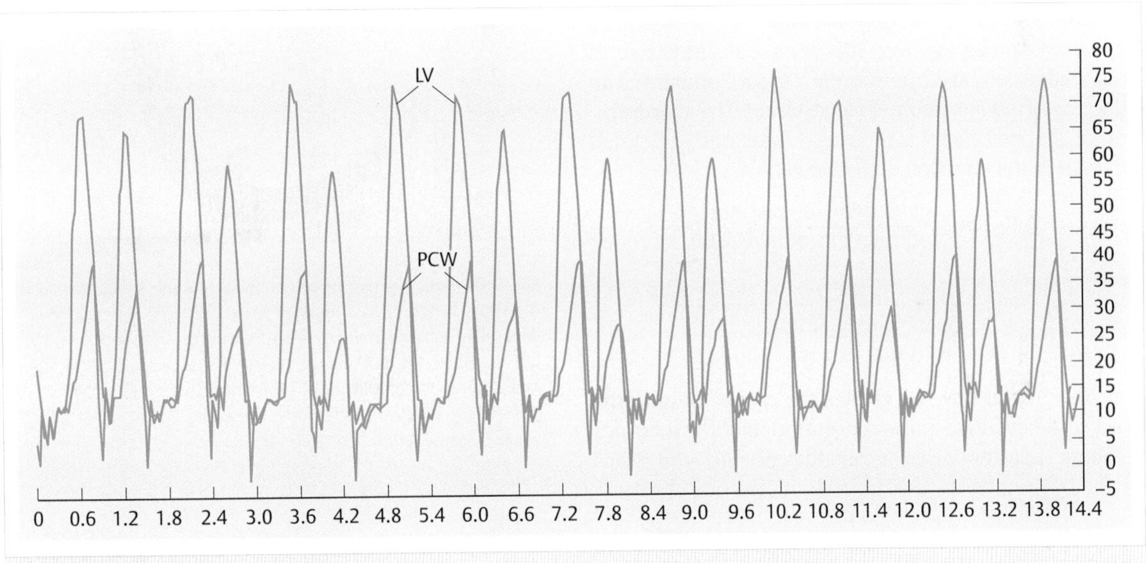

Fig. 8.18 Typical pressure curve associated with severe mitral insufficiency. Simultaneous pressure measurement in the left ventricle (LV) and pulmonary capillary wedge pressure (PCW).

content (MVO_2). To measure it, the pulmonary artery must be probed with a catheter and blood taken there. Using the oxygen content in other large veins close to the heart, such as the superior vena cava ($SVCO_2$) or the inferior vena cava ($IVCO_2$) involves errors, because different blood streams from different tributary areas have different saturations. However, the oxygen content of the superior vena cava often corresponds to the mixed venous oxygen content. Therefore some centers use this oxygen content as MVO_2. The following formula is commonly used to calculate the mixed venous oxygen content:

$$MVO_2 = \frac{3 \times SVCO_2 + 1 \times IVCO_2}{4}$$

Excursus

In 2006, Driscoll gave a simplified illustration of the Fick principle using a freight train loaded with lumps of coal traveling through the lungs. In this example, the lumps of coal represent oxygen, the train represents the blood flow, and each car represents a certain amount of hemoglobin. To calculate the speed (cars per minute) of the train (cardiac output in L/min), the total number of lumps of coal that can be loaded on the train per minute (oxygen intake), the number of lumps a car can carry (oxygen transport capacity), the number of lumps of coal on the train before the train passes through the lungs (mixed venous oxygen content), and the number of lumps of coal present after the train has passed the lungs (arterial oxygen content) must be known. It must also be known whether any lumps of coal have been unloaded in the lungs themselves. A sample calculation is shown in ▶ Fig. 8.20.

Indicator Dilution Methods

▶ **Classic indicator dilution methods.** These methods have been known for over 100 years and are based, as described above, on administering a known amount of an indicator as a bolus into the bloodstream. The concentration of the indicator C over time is measured at defined intervals in the direction of the blood flow.

$$Q\ (\text{L/min}) = \frac{\text{Quantity of indicator}}{C\ (\text{mg/L}) \times t\ (\text{min}) \times 60}$$

or

$$\frac{\text{Quantity of indicator}}{C\ (\text{mg/L}) \times t\ (\text{s})}$$

It is only logical that the greater the cardiac output, the quicker the decrease in the concentration of the indicator is. Some indicators used are methylene blue and Evans blue (both historic) as well as indocyanine green and recently lithium. The advantage of the indicator methods is the speed of the measurement, the semi-automatic generation of the values, and independence from ventilation parameters. The disadvantage is that these measurements are not reliable when there is a shunt or when there is significant right heart valvular insufficiency.

▶ **Thermodilution.** This method is also an indicator dilution method. The temperature and volume of the injected substance are used as an indicator. A classic example of

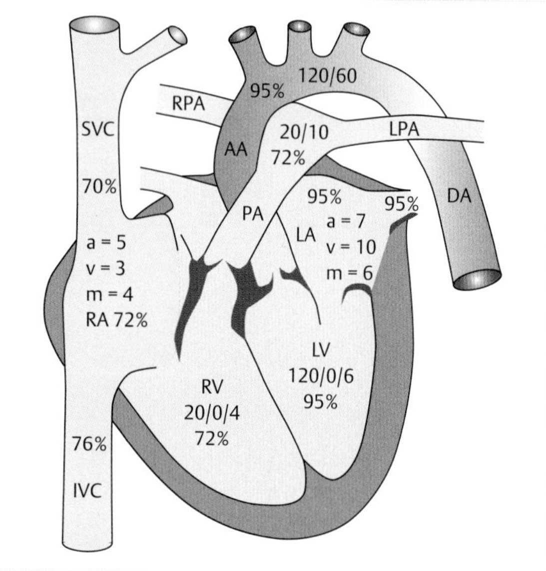

Fig. 8.19 Typical pressure and saturation levels in an adult with a healthy heart.[37] SVC, superior vena cava; IVC, inferior vena cava; RA, right atrium; LA, left atrium; RV, right ventricle; LV, left ventricle; PA, pulmonary artery; AA, ascending aorta; DA, descending aorta; RPA, right pulmonary artery; LPA, left pulmonary artery; a, atrial wave pressure; v, ventricular filling wave pressure; m, mean pressure.

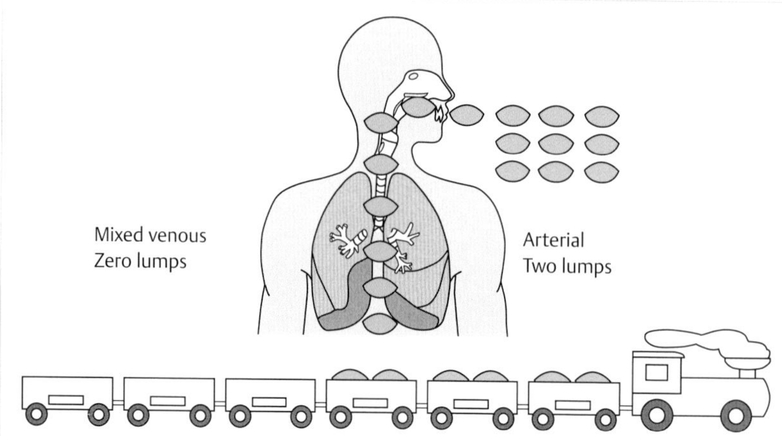

Fig. 8.20 Schematic representation of the Fick principle (from Driscoll 2006). Ten lumps of coal are loaded onto the train per minute (coal consumption = oxygen consumption). Two lumps of coal are loaded onto each car (coal-carrying capacity = oxygen-carrying capacity). Before passing through the lungs, the individual cars held no lumps of coal (mixed venous oxygen content); after passing through the lungs, they had 2 lumps (arterial oxygen content). The train is thus driving at a speed of 5 cars per minute (cardiac output in L/min).

this method is the Swan-Ganz catheter used routinely worldwide. A well-defined amount of a cold substance (5 or 10 mL NaCl 0.9% or glucose 5%, temp. 4°C) is injected through the catheter as a quick bolus into the right atrium and the temperature profile in the pulmonary artery is measured over time. The cardiac output is calculated as follows:

$$Q = \text{CO (cardiac output)} = \frac{(\text{Tb} - \text{Ti}) \times V \times 60 \times 1.08 \times 0.825}{\text{D6(t)dt}}$$

In this formula, "D6(t)dt" represents the area under the curve of the temperature change over time and Tb is body temperature. Ti is the temperature of the injected material. V stands for the volume of the injected material, and multiplying by 60 converts from seconds to minutes. 1.08 is the correction factor of the heat coefficient and 0.825 is the correction factor for the loss of heat at the moment of injection.

This formula is usually generated automatically by the computer. Here again, cardiac output is high when a large, rapid change in temperature is registered which subsides again just as quickly. When the change in temperature is slow and changes only slightly, cardiac output is low.

8.5.3 Shunt Calculations

The most common method for measuring shunts is oximetry. In this method, the oxygen content of a blood sample taken from a certain segment of the heart or blood vessel is measured. The oxygen content in a segment of a vessel is almost never constant—variations of about 1% to 5% are common. Applying the Fick principle, the values for the mixed venous (MVO_2), pulmonary venous (PVO_2), pulmonary arterial (PAO_2), and the systemic arterial oxygen (SAO_2) content are used to calculate the shunt volume using the following equations:

$$\text{Blood flow Q (L/min/m}^2) = \frac{\text{Oxygen consumption } V \cdot O_2 \text{ (mL/min)}}{\text{Arteriovenous difference (mL } O_2\text{/L blood)}}$$

$$\text{Pulmonary blood flow} = \frac{\text{Oxygen consumption}}{PVO_2 - PAO_2\text{/mL } O_2\text{/L blood}}$$

$$\text{Systemic blood flow} = \frac{\text{Oxygen consumption}}{SAO_2 - MVO_2\text{/mL } O_2\text{/L blood}}$$

$$\text{Effective pulmonary blood flow} = \frac{\text{Oxygen consumption}}{PVO_2 - MVO_2\text{/mL } O_2\text{/L blood}}$$

The effective lung flow, Qe_P, is equivalent to the venous blood—the unoxygenated blood that flows back to the heart—which absorbs oxygen while passing through the lungs. If there is no circulatory shunt, all three blood flow volumes are identical, that is $Q_P = Q_S = Qe_P$. In a left-to-right shunt, Q_S is equal to Qe_P, but Q_P is elevated. In a right-to-left shunt, Q_P is equal to Qe_P but Q_S is elevated.

In practice, oxygen saturation is generally measured instead of oxygen content. However, to obtain accurate values, the oxygen content should actually be used instead of saturation. The oxygen content includes saturation, that is the amount of oxygen bound to hemoglobin, as well as physically diluted oxygen. As 1 g hemoglobin (Hb) can bind 1.34 mL oxygen, therefore:

$$\text{Oxygen content (mL/L)} = \text{Oxygen saturation (\%)} \times \text{Hb (g/dL)} \times 1.34 \times 10$$

The hemoglobin concentration is again converted to g/L by multiplying by 10. The oxygen content can be ignored in a spontaneously breathing patient in room air or FiO_2 below 0.3. In this case, determining the oxygen saturation is sufficient for the calculations. If the patient is ventilated or given oxygen, oxygen content should be taken into consideration to yield a more accurate calculation.

▸ **Right-to-left shunt (R-L shunt).** The right-to-left shunt is marked by low saturation. The cause can be prepulmonary (e.g., tetralogy of Fallot), intrapulmonary (venous malformations) or postpulmonary (unroofed coronary sinus). The greater the degree of undersaturation, the larger the right-to-left shunt is. The volume of the shunt is calculated as follows:

$$Q_S \text{ (L/min)} = Q_{eP} \text{ (L/min)} + \text{R-L shunt,}$$

that is:

$$\text{R-L shunt} = Q_S \text{ (L/min)} - Q_{eP} \text{ (L/min)}$$

▸ **Left-to-right shunt (L-R shunt).** In a left-to-right shunt, additional blood which is rich in oxygen reaches the pulmonary circulation and saturation increases (e.g., in cases of ASD, VSD, PDA). The larger the shunt, the greater the saturation (or increase in saturation) in the pulmonary artery is. Therefore, an exact calculation of the left-to-right shunt can be made in the same way:

$$Q_P \text{ (L/min)} = Q_{eP} \text{ (L/min)} + \text{L-R shunt,}$$

that is:

$$\text{L-R shunt} = Q_P \text{ (L/min)} - Q_{eP} \text{ (L/min)}$$

This additional shunt quantity is usually given as a percentage of the systemic shunt, thus for a left-to-right shunt:

$$\text{\% shunt} = \frac{Q_P \text{ (L/min)} - Q_{eP} \text{ (L/min)}}{Q_P \text{ (L/min)}} \times 100$$

8.5.4 Flow Conditions

In pediatric cardiology, the absolute values can be calculated using numerous programs in the cardiac catheterization laboratory; however, these values are of minor significance in clinical practice. The relative flow conditions can be determined based on normal cardiac output (whatever that may mean). For a left-to-right shunt, the additional amount of blood that passes through the lung compared with systemic cardiac output is measured. This is indicated as the extent of recirculation, for example, 2:1 or 3:1. For a right-to-left shunt, the amount that pulmonary blood flow is reduced compared with the systemic blood flow is indicated, for example, 0.7:1. It is advantageous that these calculations can be made without elaborate measurements of oxygen consumption or oxygen content.

To calculate the ratio between the pulmonary blood flow (Q_P) and systemic blood flow (Q_S) the ratio of Q_P and Q_S must be calculated:

$$\text{Flow ratio} = \frac{Q_P}{Q_S}$$

If we now substitute the above equations for Q_P and Q_S, we obtain:

$$\text{Flow ratio } Q_P/Q_S \text{ (L/min)} = \frac{SAO_2 - MVO_2}{PVO_2 - PAO_2}$$

Most heart defects can be adequately described in this way; the shunt fraction is therefore usually expressed as Q_P/Q_S. A shunt fraction of more than 1.5:1 is an indication for surgery.

However, for more accurate flow and resistance calculations of pulmonary vascular resistance associated with long-term shunt defects and pulmonary hypertension, the calculations must be made using oxygen content (Chapter 21).

8.5.5 Resistance Calculations

Vascular resistances can be calculated from the pressure and flow values previously measured, generated and determined. For this, according to Ohm's law:

$$\text{Resistance (mmHg/L/min)} = \frac{\text{Mean pressure loss (mmHg)}}{\text{Blood flow (L/min)}}$$

In this context, the *systemic* vascular resistance (R_S) can be calculated based on the mean arterial pressure (MAP), central venous pressure (CVP), and systemic blood flow (Q_S):

$$\text{Systemic vascular resistance } R_S \text{ (mmHg/L/min)} = \frac{\text{MAD} - \text{CVP (mmHg)}}{Q_S \text{ (L/min)}}$$

By analogy, the ***pulmonary*** vascular resistance (R_P) can be determined based on pulmonary artery pressure (PAP), pulmonary venous pressure (PVP), and pulmonary blood flow (Q_P). Instead of PVP, the wedge pressure (PCW) or the left atrial pressure (LAP) can also be used.

$$\text{Pulmonary vascular resistance } R_P \text{ (mmHg/L/min)} = \frac{\text{PAP} - \text{PVP (mmHg)}}{Q_P \text{ (L/min)}}$$

The resistance is indicated in mmHg/L/min. This unit is also known as the Wood unit. In children, resistance is usually related to the body surface by multiplying it by the body surface area (Wood units × m^2). The pulmonary vascular resistance is approximately one-tenth of systemic vascular resistance.

As in the shunt calculations, the resistance values are often expressed as relative resistance, viz. the ratio of pulmonary resistance, R_P, to systemic resistance, R_S. The normal pulmonary vascular resistance is at most 0.2 of systemic vascular resistance ($R_P/R_S = 0.2:1$). To calculate the relative resistance, the ratio of R_P and R_S is determined:

$$\text{Relative resistance} = \frac{R_P}{R_S}$$

If we now substitute the above equations for R_P and R_S, we obtain:

$$\text{Relative resistance } R_P/R_S = \frac{\text{PAP} - \text{LAP}}{\text{MAD} - \text{CVP}} \times \frac{Q_S}{Q_P}$$

The wedge pressure can also be used instead of the LAP in this formula.

8.5.6 Indications for Cardiac Catheterization

▶ Table 8.1 lists the most common heart defects with the possible indications for cardiac catheterization. In most cases, however, primarily in neonates and infants, therapy can be started before diagnostic cardiac catheterization. The indication should always be made in close consultation with the surgeon before a scheduled operation.

Table 8.1 Diagnostic cardiac catheterization to evaluate the most frequent cardiac defects

Cardiac defect	Diagnostic question
Atrial septal defect (ASD)	Pulmonary arterial pressure, shunt fraction, exclusion of an anomalous pulmonary vein connection
Sinus venosus defect	Pulmonary arterial pressure, shunt fraction, exclusion of an anomalous pulmonary vein connection
Ventricular septal defect (VSD)	Pulmonary arterial pressure, shunt fraction
Atrioventricular septal defect	Pulmonary arterial pressure, shunt fraction, AV valve insufficiency, accompanying dysplasias
Patent ductus arteriosus	Pulmonary arterial pressure
Anomalous pulmonary venous connection	Shunt fraction, pulmonary arterial pressure
Vena cava anomaly	Preoperative clarification of the anatomy
Tetralogy of Fallot	Anatomy of the coronaries, diameter of the pulmonary valve annulus and pulmonary arteries, Nakata and McGoon index, anatomy of the right ventricular outflow tract
Pulmonary atresia without VSD	Myocardial sinusoid, pulmonary vascular bed
Pulmonary atresia with VSD	Pulmonary vessels, major aorto-pulmonary collateral arteries
Double-outlet right ventricle	Coronary anomaly
Transposition of the great vessels	Coronary anatomy
Transposition after switch operation	Coronary stenosis
Transposition of the great arteries after Mustard/Senning procedure	Hemodynamics, pulmonary arterial pressure, stenosis in the atrial region or of the veins
Bland–White–Garland syndrome	Detection or exclusion of coronary anomalies
Mitral stenosis	Pulmonary arterial pressure, cardiac output, stress test
Mitral insufficiency	Pulmonary arterial pressure, hemodynamics
Aortic stenosis	Pressure gradient, possibly coronaries
Aortic insufficiency	Function of the left ventricle, possibly coronaries
Pulmonary stenosis	Pressure gradient, peripheral vascular anatomy
Pulmonary insufficiency	Function of the right ventricle, peripheral pulmonary vessels
Aortic coarctation	Aortic arch anatomy, pressure gradient
Univentricular heart, congenital	Very rare, unclear anatomy
Univentricular heart, before upper cavopulmonary anastomosis	Pulmonary vascular anatomy, pulmonary arterial pressure
Univentricular heart, after upper cavopulmonary anastomosis	Pulmonary vascular anatomy, fistula
Univentricular heart, after Fontan completion	Pressure ratios, fistula, vascular anatomy (stenosis)
Coronary heart disease in adults, e.g., over age 40	Anatomy/pathology of the coronaries
Kawasaki syndrome	Anatomy of the coronaries, status of the other vessels
Williams–Beuren syndrome	Pulmonary vessels, arterial vessels
Trisomy 21	Pulmonary hypertension
Alagille syndrome	Pulmonary perfusion
Myocarditis, cardiomyopathy	Cardiac output, pulmonary arterial pressure, biopsy
Heart transplantation	Cardiac output, coronaries, biopsy

9 Electrophysiology Studies

9.1 Basics

An electrophysiological examination study (EPS) is an invasive procedure in which intracardiac potentials are recorded using catheter electrodes. The electrodes are inserted into the heart using the Seldinger technique, similar to cardiac catheterization. EPS makes it possible to obtain detailed images of the spread of electrical excitation in the heart and to measure conduction and refraction times precisely. In addition, by inducing arrhythmia during the examination, the underlying pathological mechanism of the rhythm disorder (e.g., an accessory conduction pathway) can be determined.

In addition to a purely diagnostic purpose, it is also possible to destroy or modify the morphological correlate of a rhythm disorder using an ablation catheter and thus effectively treat the arrhythmia.

9.2 Indication

The indication for an EPS must be made on a case-by-case basis. Among other things, it depends on the underlying arrhythmia, the age of the child, the symptoms, the treatment options, and any potential underlying structural heart disease.

In childhood, an EPS is most frequently performed to investigate supraventricular tachycardia—usually with the option of catheter ablation. Other indications are cardiovascular arrest of unclear cause or syncopes for which no conclusive explanation could be found using non-invasive diagnostic tests.

Note

When determining the indication for EPS in childhood, it must be taken into consideration that in children weighing less than 15 kg, the rate of complications of the examination and ablation is considerably higher than for larger children.

9.3 Procedure

The examination is generally performed under deep sedation in children, but longer procedures when ablation is planned are usually performed under general anesthesia. After consulting with the electrophysiologists who will perform the examination, anti-arrhythmic agents should be discontinued five half-lives before the examination if clinically tolerable.

During the examination, electrode catheters are inserted into the femoral vein after it is punctured using the Seldinger technique. It may be difficult to probe the coronary venous sinus, which is particularly necessary to investigate supraventricular tachycardia (see Chapter 9.3.1), via an inguinal access, so that an access from above may have to be selected (left basilic vein, right internal jugular vein, or left subclavian vein). If the left ventricle or the area of the mitral valve annulus need to be examined more closely (e.g., for left accessory pathways), the femoral artery is also punctured and the catheter is advanced by retrograde insertion into the left ventricle. For an examination of the left atrium—if the foramen ovale is closed and there is no atrial septal defect—the atrial septum must be punctured in order to access the left atrium from the right atrium (transseptal puncture).

The catheter electrodes are generally positioned under fluoroscopy guidance. Multipolar catheters are used. The electrodes at the tips of the catheters are spaced at 2 to 5 mm.

9.3.1 Catheter Positions

For an EPS, four standard electrode positions are usually used (▶ Fig. 9.1):

- High right atrium (HRA)
- Bundle of His (HB)
- Right ventricular apex (RVA)
- Coronary sinus (CS)

▶ **High right atrium (HRA).** Positioning the electrode catheter at the junction between the superior vena cava and the right atrium allows potentials from the area of the sinus node to be measured. Sometimes the catheter is also advanced into the right atrial appendage. The HRA potential is the earliest potential recorded in the intracardiac lead. The right atrium can also be stimulated via the catheter.

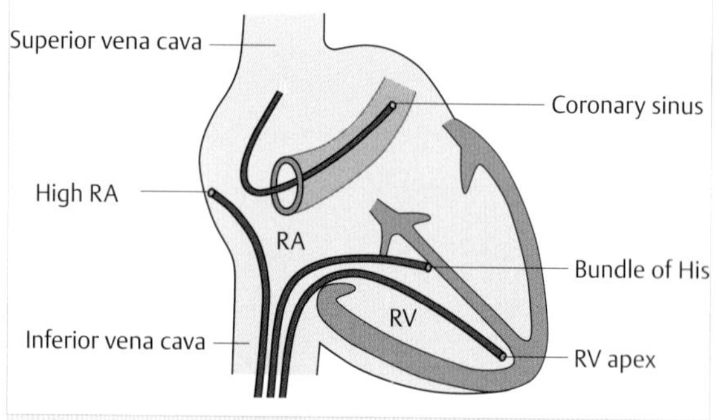

Fig. 9.1 Positions of electrode catheters.[39]

► **Bundle of His (HB).** In order to position the catheter in the region of the bundle of His, it is first advanced into the right ventricle. Then it is withdrawn toward the right atrium until an atrial signal appears in addition to the ventricular signal. After rotating the catheter slightly in a dorsal direction, the His potential appears between the atrial and the ventricular signal.

The bundle of His ECG is important for investigating atrioventricular (AV) conduction disorders and diagnosing arrhythmia. Signals that appear before the bundle of His potential have a supraventricular origin. Signals recorded after the bundle of His potential stem from the ventricle.

► **Right ventricular apex (RVA).** The right ventricular catheter is generally positioned in the right ventricular apex, less frequently in the right ventricular outflow tract to answer a specific clinical question.

► **Coronary venous sinus (CS).** The coronary sinus catheter records signals from the left atrium as well as from the left ventricle. A coronary sinus catheter is used primarily to evaluate supraventricular tachycardias—especially if an accessory pathway is suspected.

9.3.2 Evaluation of an Intracardiac ECG

► **Atrial signals.** Normally, the first signal of the intracardiac ECG that appears is the signal from the HRA catheter positioned near the sinus node (► Fig. 9.2). This is followed by the signal from the lower right atrium recorded from the bundle of His catheter. The last atrial signal is the left lateral atrial signal recorded from the coronary venous sinus. If there are ectopic atrial foci or supraventricular tachycardias, the order of the signals changes depending on the origin of the arrhythmia and speed of excitation.

► **AV and His transition.** The AV transition is determined on the basis of the AH interval. The AH interval extends from the start of atrial depolarization (A) to the start of the His bundle potential (H). The AH interval in children is normally 50 to 120 ms (► Table 9.1).

In the His–Purkinje system, transition is reflected by the HV interval recorded from the His bundle catheter. The normal values for children are 25 to 50 ms (► Table 9.1). A shortened HV interval can occur with accessory conduction pathways, for example.

► **Ventricular signals.** The spread of excitation to the ventricles is described based on three catheter locations:

- Right ventricular apex (RVA catheter)
- Right ventricular inflow tract (ventricular signal of the His bundle catheter)
- Left ventricular base (ventricular signal of the coronary sinus catheter)

Generally, the signal of the RVA catheter is the first potential to appear shortly after the appearance of the QRS complex in the ECG. A right bundle branch block can delay the RVA signal. If there are accessory conduction pathways, the first signal to appear may be the ventricular potential from the His bundle catheter or

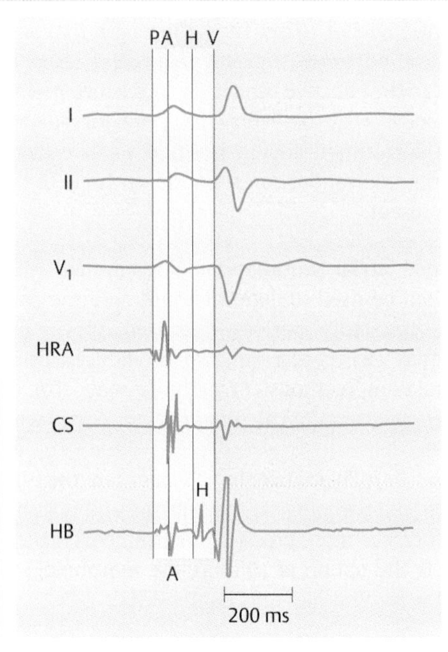

PA: Interval from the start of the P wave in the surface ECG to the start of atrial depolarization (A) in the His bundle electrogram

AH: Interval from the start of atrial depolarization (A) to the start of the His potential (H)

HV: Interval from the start of the His potential (H) until the earliest ventricular excitation in a surface or intracardiac ECG

Fig. 9.2 Simultaneous recording of a superficial ECG (I, II, V_1) and an intracardiac ECG (HRA, CS, HB).[39]

Table 9.1 Normal values of the most important electrophysiological parameters in childhood (from Pass RH and Walsh EP 2001)

Parameter	Normal value
AH interval	50–120 ms
HV interval	25–50 ms
RVA activation	5–35 ms
Corrected sinus node recovery period	< 275 ms
Sinus node recovery period in percent	< 166%
Wenckebach point	< 380 ms
Sinoatrial transition period	< 200 ms
Atrial effective refractory period	170–250 ms
AV node effective refractory period	220–350 ms
Ventricular effective refractory period	200–300 ms

the coronary sinus catheter, depending on the location of the pathway.

► **Sinus node function.** Sinus node function is generally assessed by means of the sinus node recovery period. To measure this, the right atrium is stimulated by the HRA catheter for 30 to 60 s at a rate higher than the patient's resting rate. When the stimulation is abruptly ended, there is a brief pause before the sinus node itself jumps into action again as a pacemaker. An excessively long pause is a sign of sinus node dysfunction. The sinus node recovery period is usually indicated as the corrected sinus node recovery period. To determine this, the normal interval between two normal sinus beats at rest is subtracted from the interval between the last stimulus and the first sinus node activity.

Alternately, the sinus node recovery period can also be indicated as a percentage of the normal interval between two sinus beats at rest.

► **AV node function.** AV node function is assessed using the *Wenckebach point.* When the Wenckebach point is exceeded, not every atrial action is transmitted to the ventricle. The Wenckebach point is determined by first stimulating the atrium at a fixed frequency and then reducing the time between two stimuli in 10-ms increments, that is, continuously increasing the stimulation rate. Normally, the interval between two stimuli before Wenckebach symptoms occur should be less than 380 ms in adolescents and adults, equivalent to a frequency of over 185/min.

The *effective refractory period* of the AV node is determined by first conducting basis stimulation in the atrium, usually with eight stimuli. The stimulation is applied at a rate somewhat exceeding the patient's own rate and ensures "electrophysiological stability." Subsequently, an extra stimulus is coupled 10 ms prematurely. This extra stimulus is delivered progressively earlier in 10-ms increments. Due to the decremental (delayed) conduction of the AV node, the interval between atrial stimulation and ventricular response (AH interval) is increasingly lengthened. When the coupling interval is sufficiently short, conduction in the AV node ceases. This interval between the last stimulus conducted and the first stimulus that is not conducted is described as the effective refractory period of the AV node. In children, it is between 220 and 350 ms.

The effective refractory period of the atrial myocardium can be determined by analogy.

► **Dual AV node physiology.** Different AH conduction periods may be noted using programmed atrial stimulation. The different conduction periods are signs of two or more AV node pathways with varying refractory periods (dual AV nodes).

A patient with a dual AV node is predisposed to AV nodal re-entrant tachycardia. By definition, a dual AV node is present if a "jump" can be detected in the intracardiac ECG. An AH interval (or VA interval) that increases by more than 50 ms after the extra stimulus is shortened by 10 ms is proof of a dual AV node.

► **Ventricular effective refractory period.** The ventricular effective refractory period is determined in a manner similar to the effective refractory period of the atrial myocardium and the AV node. Using the RVA catheter, several (usually eight) ventricular stimuli are first delivered at a base cycle length before shortening the cycle length in increments of 10 ms. The cycle length that is so short that it can no longer trigger a ventricular response is equivalent to the effective ventricular refractory period. In addition, measuring the ventricular refractory period with ventricular stimuli should be used to investigate whether retrograde conduction from the ventricle to the atria is also present.

► **Programmed atrial stimulation.** Programmed atrial stimulation can be used to determine not only the conduction and refractory periods discussed above, but supraventricular tachycardia can also be induced using special stimulation methods. Arrhythmia may also be triggered by pharmaceutical provocation (e.g., with orciprenaline).

When supraventricular arrhythmia is induced, the type of arrhythmia, the pathological mechanism, and possibly how to end it can be more precisely determined. Furthermore, there is the option of ablating the morphological correlate of the arrhythmia (see Chapter 9.3.3).

▸ **Programmed ventricular stimulation.** Different sites of the ventricles can be stimulated. Stimulation is routinely delivered to the apex of the right ventricle, but it can also be delivered in the right ventricular outflow tract or in the left ventricle if needed. In addition to determining the ventricular refractory period described above and investigating retrograde conduction from the ventricles to the atria, an attempt can be made to induce ventricular arrhythmia using stimuli with different cycle lengths, possibly at different locations. The origin of spontaneous ventricular arrhythmia can be detected in this way and it may also be possible to ablate the morphological correlate of the arrhythmia.

▸ **Pace mapping.** The principle of pace mapping is to use atrial or ventricular stimulation to find the location at which the rhythm induced by stimulation has the same morphology as spontaneously occurring tachycardia. A 12-channel ECG that was recorded during spontaneous tachycardia must be available in order to compare the induced rhythm and spontaneous tachycardia.

▸ **Catheter mapping.** In catheter mapping, an intracardiac ECG is recorded to see where the earliest excitation during tachycardia occurs, for which it must be possible to induce tachycardia using EPE. Computer-assisted navigation systems and visual methods (e.g., LocaLisa, CARTO map) are usually used for precise mapping. These methods reduce fluoroscopy time and increase patient safety.

9.3.3 Ablation Treatment

In principle, it is possible to ablate the arrhythmogenic substrate of a rhythm disorder by interventional catheterization. Two methods are available in clinical practice:

- Radiofrequency ablation
- Cryoablation

Table 9.2 Overview of catheter ablation of certain rhythm disorders in childhood

Arrhythmia	Treatment principle	Comment
Ectopic atrial tachycardia (EAT)	Ablation of the ectopic atrial focus	Recurrence rate 20–30%
Multifocal atrial tachycardia (MAT)	Ablation of the ectopic atrial foci	More difficult procedure with lower chances of success than EAT due to multiple foci
Typical atrial flutter	Typical atrial flutter is caused by counterclockwise rotation of excitation around the tricuspid valve. The treatment principle is to interrupt the re-entrant circuit by creating a linear lesion between the tricuspid valve and the inferior vena cava (cavotricuspid isthmus) using radiofrequency or cryoablation	If complete interruption is achieved at the cavotricuspid isthmus, the recurrence rate is below 10%
Intra-atrial re-entrant tachycardia (IART) following atrial surgery (e.g., Mustard/Senning atrial switch procedure, Fontan procedure or other surgical scars at atrial level)	Re-entrant circuits are caused by scars, patches, AV valve annulus, etc. The treatment principle is to interrupt the circular excitation by creating a linear lesion using radiofrequency or cryoablation.	Visualizing the complex excitation sequences and performing ablation using modern mapping methods improves the chances of success
Accessory conduction pathways	Estimation of the location of the accessory pathway using surface ECG, precise mapping during EPE, ablation of the accessory pathway	
AV nodal re-entrant tachycardia	Tachycardia caused by dual AV node physiology with one rapid and one slower pathway. Treatment consists of modulating the slower conduction pathway	Modulating the slow pathway involves a lower risk of inducing an AV block than modulating the fast pathway. Unlike ablation, after modulating a pathway, dual conduction properties of the AV node can still be detected. However, the risk of a recurrence is not greater than after ablation, so modulation is generally the preferred method for children.
Ventricular tachycardia	The ectopic focus can be ablated	The chances of success depend on the location of the ectopic focus and absence or presence of a structural heart defect, among other things

► **Radiofrequency ablation.** Radiofrequency ablation is the older of the two methods. After the arrhythmogenic substrate is located, high-frequency current is emitted from the tip of the ablation catheter. Heat develops in the cardiac tissue, inducing coagulation necrosis that obliterates the arrhythmogenic substrate.

► **Cryoablation.** Cryoablation is a newer method, in which tissue is necrotized by applying extreme cold. The advantage of this method is that it allows a kind of "trial ablation." The effect of ablation can be predicted in this trial before irreversible cryoablation at a temperature of –75 to –80°C is carried out. This method reduces the risk of an iatrogenic AV block, but the recurrence rate appears to be somewhat higher.

► **Complications.** The most important complication of ablation or modulation of accessory conduction pathways or of dual AV nodal conduction is inducing an AV block. General risks of the examination are myocardial perforation (pericardial tamponade), thromboembolic events, and inducing life-threatening arrhythmia.

The indications and prospects for success of catheter ablation for different cardiac rhythm disorders are discussed in the respective chapters. ► Table 9.2 shows a brief overview.

Part II

Leading Symptoms

10 Cyanosis

10.1 Definition

Cyanosis is a bluish discoloration of the skin and mucous membranes. It occurs when the hemoglobin is not adequately saturated with oxygen. Cyanosis becomes clinically visible when the amount of unsaturated hemoglobin in the veins of the skin exceeds 4 to 5 g per 100 mL of blood.

The extent of cyanosis correlates with the *absolute* amount of unsaturated (reduced) hemoglobin. Cyanosis may therefore not be visible in anemia (low hemoglobin content in blood), although oxygen saturation is low. However, cyanosis quickly becomes apparent even in patients with polyglobulia (high hemoglobin content in blood) who have relatively low undersaturation with oxygen.

10.2 Classification

A differentiation is made between central and peripheral cyanosis.

▶ **Central cyanosis.** Central cyanosis stems from low arterial oxygen saturation. It is caused by intracardiac right-to-left shunts, by insufficient oxygenation of the blood in the lungs, or rarely by reduced oxygen-binding capacity of hemoglobin (e.g., associated with methemoglobinemia).

▶ **Peripheral cyanosis.** Peripheral cyanosis stems from increased oxygen extraction from the blood when arterial oxygen saturation is normal. In most cases, it is caused by a large reduction of cardiac output due to heart failure. The skin is noticeably cool in this case.

One cause of localized peripheral cyanosis is reduced local perfusion or obstructed venous blood flow, for example, due to a thrombosis, venous congestion, or impaired peripheral blood flow. Increased vasoconstriction due to cold also leads to increased oxygen extraction (blue lips from the cold).

10.3 Diagnostic Measures

▶ **Symptoms.** The leading symptom is the bluish discoloration of the skin and mucosa, which is best seen at the fingernails, lips, ear lobes, and oral mucous membranes. Clinically, a distinction is made between central and peripheral cyanosis:

- In *central cyanosis*, the tongue is cyanotic and the mucosae are a deep red. The skin is warm.
- In *peripheral cyanosis*, the tongue is not cyanotic. In peripheral cyanosis resulting from reduced cardiac output, the skin is cool.
- Impaired venous outflow (thrombosis or venous congestion) leads to swelling proximal to the congestion.

▶ **Oxygen saturation.** In *central cyanosis*, arterial oxygen saturation is reduced. In *peripheral cyanosis*, arterial oxygen saturation is normal, but because of increased oxygen extraction in the periphery, mixed venous oxygen saturation is reduced.

▶ **Hyperoxia test.** The hyperoxia test is used to distinguish between cardiac or pulmonary cyanosis. The cyanotic patient is given 100% oxygen to breathe for a few minutes. If there is a pulmonary cause, the cyanosis disappears or is considerably reduced and there is a relevant increase in oxygen saturation. If there is a cardiac cause, oxygen saturation remains unchanged because the cardiac right-to-left shunt is not overcome by applying oxygen.

▶ **Echocardiography.** Cyanotic heart defects can generally be reliably diagnosed by echocardiography. Echocardiography is therefore indispensable in patients with cyanosis.

▶ **Differential diagnoses.** The most common cyanotic heart defects are:

- Transposition of the great arteries
- Fallot group:
  - Tetralogy of Fallot
  - Pulmonary atresia with ventricular septal defect
  - Pulmonary atresia with intact ventricular septum
  - "Double-outlet right ventricle"
- Univentricular heart:
  - Tricuspid atresia
  - Single ventricle
  - Hypoplastic left heart syndrome
- Ebstein anomaly
- Total anomalous pulmonary venous connection
- Truncus arteriosus communis

The most common differential diagnoses for cyanosis are summarized in ▶ Table 10.1.

Note

Investigation of perioral cyanosis or acrocyanosis is one of the most frequent reasons for presenting a child to a pediatric cardiology practice or clinic. If reduced cardiac output (heart failure, shock) can be ruled out, it is almost always a harmless phenomenon. In these cases oxygen extraction is increased, which probably occurs due to a slow blood flow in the capillary bed in conjunction with vasoconstriction or temporary hypotension. Perioral cyanosis is particularly noticeable in children with light skin.

Table 10.1 Frequent causes of cyanosis in childhood

Central cyanosis
Reduced alveolar ventilation: • Apnea (premature birth, asphyxia, seizures, CNS damage) • Inadequate respiratory drive (Pickwick syndrome) • Airway obstruction (choanal atresia, tracheal stenosis, Pierre Robin sequence, bronchial asthma, croup, aspiration of a foreign body) • Parenchymal lung disease (pneumonia, acute respiratory syndrome, meconium aspiration, lung deformities) • Restrictive lung diseases (pneumothorax, pleural effusions, diaphragmatic hernia, severe thorax deformity) • Ventilation–perfusion mismatch • Weakness of the respiratory muscles and respiratory regulation disorders (myopathies, Ondine syndrome
Right-to-left shunts: • Right-to-left intracardiac shunts (cyanotic heart defect) • Intrapulmonary shunts • Pulmonary hypertension resulting in a right-to-left shunt (persistent pulmonary hypertension in the neonate, Eisenmenger syndrome)
Peripheral cyanosis
• Shock, sepsis • Heart failure • Hypothermia • Isolated perioral cyanosis and acrocyanosis • Low cardiac output
Methemoglobinemia
• Congenital methemoglobinemia • Toxins (e.g., nitrates, nitrites, amines)

10.4 Complications

Over a long period, chronic cyanosis can lead to typical complications.

▶ **Polyglobulia.** The low arterial oxygen content stimulates the bone marrow to produce more red blood cells by releasing more erythropoietin in the kidneys. This increases the oxygen-binding capacity of the blood so that more oxygen is bound in the lungs and made available to the body. However, if the hematocrit exceeds a level of about 65%, the viscosity of the blood increases markedly. This has an unfavorable effect on peripheral blood flow. Due to increased erythropoiesis, cyanotic patients have a higher demand for iron. If they become anemic, microcythemia develops, which also has an unfavorable effect on the rheological properties of the blood. Many patients with chronic cyanosis therefore benefit from iron substitution.

Note

A normal and age-appropriate hemoglobin level constitutes relative anemia in a cyanotic patient.

▶ **Clubbing (drumstick fingers and watch-glass nails).** Chronic central cyanosis leads to characteristic trophic changes in distal phalanxes of the fingers and toes and the fingernails and toenails. The distal phalanxes of the fingers and toes are widened like a drumstick and thickened; the fingernails have a convex shape (▶ Fig. 10.1).

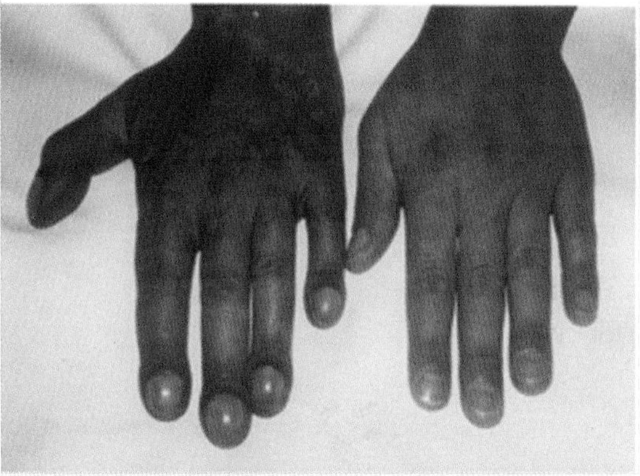

Fig. 10.1 Clubbing (drumstick fingers and watch-glass nails) associated with chronic cyanosis (left) compared with a normal finding (right).

▶ **Tendency to bleed.** Chronic cyanotic patients frequently have an increased tendency to bleed. Thrombocytopenia and platelet aggregation disorders are often found; occasionally the levels of fibrinogen or coagulation factors V and VIII are reduced.

▶ **Brain abscesses.** Chronic cyanotic patients tend to develop brain abscesses. The reduced viscosity of the blood may possibly lead to micro-infarctions with secondary bacterial colonization. Bacterial colonization is probably promoted by the fact that venous blood passes to the brain through an intracardiac right-to-left shunt without being filtered in the pulmonary capillary bed.

Note

In cyanotic patients, the constellation of "fever, headache, and focal neurological symptoms" should always suggest the possibility of a brain abscess. Sinovenous thromboses are also found more frequently in cyanotic patients.

► **Hyperuricemia.** As a result of the increased cell turnover in polycythemia, patients with chronic cyanosis frequently develop hyperuricemia or gout.

11 Cardiac Murmurs

A murmur can often be the most significant leading symptom of a congenital or acquired heart defect, but cardiac murmurs are also a harmless phenomenon in around half of all children.

11.1 Classification

Cardiac murmurs are classified as organic, functional, and innocent murmurs. The majority of murmurs auscultated in children are harmless functional or innocent heart murmurs. However, when investigating a murmur, an organic cause must be reliably excluded.

▸ **Organic murmurs.** Organic heart murmurs are caused by congenital or acquired heart defects such as valvular stenosis or insufficiency or may be the result of pathological shunts. They are thus always pathological.

▸ **Functional murmurs.** Functional heart murmurs are caused by extracardiac diseases that result in a change in blood flow or viscosity. These flow phenomena may be a result of fever, severe anemia, or hyperthyroidism, for example.

▸ **Innocent murmurs.** Innocent heart murmurs are harmless, physiological acoustic phenomena that often occur in childhood (especially in young children) and are not pathological. The most important innocent heart murmurs are listed in ▸ Table 1.1 and ▸ Fig. 11.1.

11.2 Special Features of Heart Murmurs in Neonates and Young Infants

While innocent and functional murmurs are the most frequent in older children, organic murmurs indicating a congenital heart defect are found more often in neonates and young infants. Neonates or young infants in whom a murmur is detected should therefore be examined promptly by a pediatric cardiologist.

▸ **Additional symptoms.** Additional symptoms aside from the murmur are particularly significant for the differential diagnosis.

The leading symptom of defects with reduced pulmonary perfusion, a right-to-left shunt, or parallel circulation of both systems is *cyanosis.*

Excessive pulmonary blood flow (e.g., as a result of a large left-to-right shunt) or severe left heart obstruction lead to *heart failure* (leading symptoms: tachypnea, tachycardia, hepatomegaly, pallor, failure to thrive, feeding problems, increased sweating).

▸ **Typical auscultation findings.** ▸ Table 11.2 and ▸ Table 11.3 list typical findings of heart defects that can cause a heart murmur and other symptoms in neonates and young infants. Because of the significance for the differential diagnosis, congenital heart defects are categorized

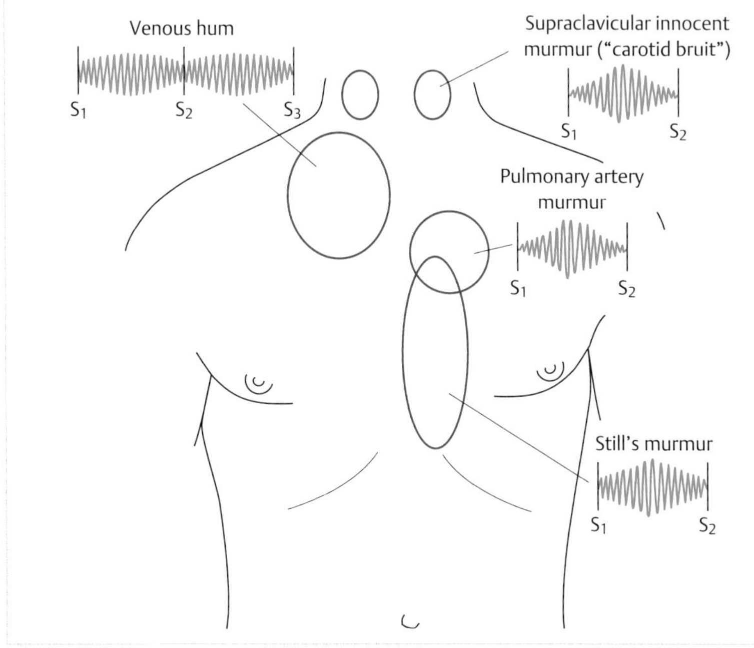

Fig. 11.1 Location and characteristics of the most common innocent heart murmurs (from Driscoll DJ 2006).

Table 11.1 Questions that should be asked when investigating a heart murmur

Question	Significance
Family history	
Are there any family members with a congenital heart defect?	Increased risk of repetition
Gestational and perinatal history	
Were there any infections during pregnancy (e.g., rubella)?	Increased risk for a congenital heart defect (e.g., pulmonary stenosis, PDA)
Did the mother take any medication or consume excessive alcohol during pregnancy?	Increased risk for a congenital heart defect (e.g., Ebstein anomaly if lithium was taken)
Did the mother have poorly controlled (gestational) diabetes during pregnancy?	Increased risk for a congenital heart defect (hypertrophic obstructive cardiomyopathy, VSD, TGA, etc.)
Was it a premature birth?	Increased risk for PDA
Personal history	
Signs of failure to thrive, feeding problems, increased sweating, tachypnea, reduced physical capacity, or pallor?	Signs of heart failure (e.g., associated with relevant shunt defects such as a large VSD or left heart obstruction)
Is cyanosis present?	Defects with right-to-left shunts or relevant reduction of lung perfusion or parallel circulation of the two systems; examples: pulmonary atresia, tetralogy of Fallot, tricuspid atresia, TGA
Are there frequent respiratory infections?	Sign of a defect with increased lung perfusion (ASD, VSD, PDA)
Does the patient have syncopes or presyncopes (esp. associated with exertion)?	Typical signs of left heart obstruction (e.g., aortic stenosis, hypertrophic obstructive cardiomyopathy) in older children or adolescents

as those associated with cyanosis and those in which heart failure is the leading symptom.

The characteristic findings of the most common heart defects on auscultation and other indicative findings in older children are summarized in ▶ Table 11.2 and ▶ Table 11.3 .

▶ **Heart defects with no indicative auscultation finding.** It should be noted that some congenital heart defects do not cause a murmur in the first few days of life when pulmonary resistance is still high. For example, a ventricular septal defect (VSD) does not cause a murmur until there is a pressure gradient between the two ventricles after pulmonary vascular resistance drops and a relevant shunt develops.

Other examples of severe congenital heart defects that do not necessarily have an indicative auscultation finding are an isolated d-TGA (dextro-transposition of the great arteries) with no other accompanying heart defects or a hypoplastic left heart syndrome. A typical heart murmur may also be absent in the presence of severe heart failure. In these cases, cardiac output is no longer sufficient to generate a heart murmur.

Generally, only a systolic bruit is associated with patent ductus arteriosus (PDA) in neonates. The typical, continuous, machine-like systolic-diastolic heart murmur (to-and-fro murmur) does not develop until after pulmonary vascular pressure drops, when both systolic and diastolic pressures in the aorta are greater than the pressure in the pulmonary artery.

Note

Organic heart murmurs are more common in neonates and young infants, while functional and innocent heart murmurs are more frequently found in older children. However, even severe heart defects can be present in neonates without an indicative heart murmur.

11.3 Diagnostic Measures

▶ **Medical history.** The most important points of the medical history when investigating a heart murmur are listed in ▶ Table 11.1.

▶ **Inspection and palpation.** Clinical signs of heart failure (tachypnea, hepatomegaly, pallor, etc.) should be noted as well as signs and symptoms of syndromes. The most common syndromes associated with congenital

Table 11.2 Typical auscultation findings and other indicative findings in neonates and young infants with the most frequent cyanotic heart defects

Diagnosis	Heart murmur	Point of maximum intensity / radiation	Other indicative findings
d-TGA simplex	No indicative heart murmur, possibly 1/6–2/6 systolic bruit	Parasternal 2nd left intercostal space (ICS)	Normal heart size, narrow upper mediastinum in X-ray (egg on its side)
Critical pulmonary stenosis	2/6–3/6 systolic bruit	Parasternal 2nd left ICS, radiation to the back	Usually decreased pulmonary vascular markings
Pulmonary atresia with/without VSD	2/6–3/6 systolic bruit	Parasternal 2nd left ICS	Decreased pulmonary vascular markings
Tetralogy of Fallot	2/6–3/6 systolic bruit	Parasternal 2nd left ICS, radiation to the back	Decreased pulmonary vascular markings, cyanotic spells usually only after early infancy
Total anomalous pulmonary venous connection	1/6–2/6 systolic bruit or no indicative heart murmur	Parasternal 2nd left ICS	Pronounced signs of heart failure; without obstruction of the pulmonary veins there is only slight cyanosis with clearly increased pulmonary vascular markings and cardiomegaly; with obstruction of the pulmonary veins there is pulmonary congestion and cyanosis
Truncus arteriosus communis	2/6–3/6 systolic bruit, additional (soft) diastolic bruit with truncus valve insufficiency	Parasternal 3rd left ICS	Heart failure, usually only slight cyanosis due to pulmonary recirculation

heart defects include trisomy 21, 13, and 18 and the Ullrich–Turner syndrome (leading symptom: edema on the backs of the hands and feet in female neonates) or Noonan syndrome.

In order to exclude aortic coarctation, the pulses should be palpated on the lower limbs and blood pressures measured in the upper and lower halves of the body in all children who present with a heart murmur. It is also advisable to measure oxygen saturation by pulse oximetry to avoid overlooking discrete cyanosis.

During palpation, any thrills in the thorax should be noted, which define a heart murmur with an intensity of ≥ 4/6.

▸ **Auscultation.** Auscultation of the heart is described in detail in Chapter 1.3.4. The assessment of the heart sounds provides important information on the differential diagnosis of a heart murmur. For example, a conspicuously loud, pronounced second heart sound is a sign of pulmonary hypertension. A respiration-related variable split second heart sound is physiological in children. Fixed splitting of the second heart sound occurs when the pulmonary valve always closes after the aortic valve due to pulmonary volume overload (e.g., in a large atrial septal defect [ASD]).

Typical auscultation findings are listed in ▸ Table 11.2 and ▸ Table 11.3.

Note

Innocent or functional heart murmurs are almost never louder than 3/6. If a thrill can be palpated, the heart murmur is pathological. Diastolic heart murmurs are always pathological.

▸ **Phonocardiogram.** Until just a few years ago, a phonocardiogram was generally recorded to document the heart murmur, which aided in reliably assigning the murmurs to the phases of the cardiac cycle. As echocardiography becomes more important, however, the phonocardiogram is used only rarely in routine examinations.

▸ **ECG.** Some ECG findings can be indicative of a certain heart defect. The most important example is a marked left axis deviation associated with an atrioventricular septal defect (AVSD). Tricuspid atresia must be considered as a differential diagnosis if a marked left axis deviation is found.

Table 11.3 Typical auscultation findings and other indicative findings in neonates and young infants with congenital heart defects leading to heart failure

Diagnosis	Heart murmur	Point of maximum intensity/ radiation	Other indicative findings
Hypoplastic left heart syndrome/ critical aortic stenosis	Possibly 1/6–3/6 systolic bruit	Parasternal 2nd/3rd left and/or right intercostal space (ICS)	Cardiomegaly, lung congestion in X-ray, sepsislike symptoms, weak pulses
Critical aortic coarctation / interrupted aortic arch	1/6–2/6 systolic bruit	Parasternal 2nd left ICS	Weakened pulses in the lower limbs, heart failure if decompensation develops
Tricuspid atresia	2/6–3/6 systolic bruit	Parasternal 3rd left ICS (for VSD) Parasternal 2nd left ICS (for pulmonary stenosis)	Slight cyanosis, excessive pulmonary blood flow, cardiomegaly, marked left axis deviation in ECG
Large VSD	1/6–3/6 systolic bruit, pronounced 2nd heart sound with pulmonary hypertension	Parasternal 3rd left ICS	Heart failure with a drop in pulmonary resistance
Complete AVSD	2/6–3/6 systolic bruit, pronounced 2nd heart sound	Parasternal 3rd left ICS	Marked left axis deviation in ECG, association with trisomy 21
Large PDA	2/6–4/6 systolic bruit, generally no typical systolic–diastolic machine sound in neonates	Parasternal 2nd left ICS	Water hammer pulse, frequently excessive pulmonary blood flow in premature infants
Truncus arteriosus communis	2/6–3/6 systolic bruit, additional (soft) diastolic bruit with truncus valve insufficiency	Parasternal 3rd left ICS	Excessive pulmonary blood flow, slight cyanosis
Total anomalous pulmonary venous connection	1/6–2/6 systolic bruit or no indicative heart murmur	Parasternal 2nd left ICS	Without obstruction of the pulmonary veins there is only slight cyanosis and clearly increased pulmonary vascular markings and cardiomegaly; with obstruction of the pulmonary veins there is pulmonary congestion and cyanosis
Ebstein anomaly / severe tricuspid insufficiency	3/6–4/6 systolic bruit	Parasternal 3rd/4th left ICS	Cyanosis, decreased lung perfusion, marked hepatomegaly

► **Chest X-ray.** X-rays are used primarily to assess global heart size, dilatation of specific cardiac chambers or vessels, and pulmonary vascular markings, and can be helpful for a differential diagnosis. Especially if there are complex defects that are sometimes associated with an abnormal visceral situs, the position of the gastric air bubble should be noted.

► **Echocardiography.** Echocardiography is the diagnostic method of choice for investigating a heart murmur. A congenital or acquired heart defect can almost always be diagnosed or excluded by echocardiography by an experienced examiner.

12 Chest Pain

12.1 Basics

▶ **Epidemiology.** Patients who present with chest pain are more often children and adolescents between the ages of 12 and 14 years. Boys and girls are equally affected. Since chest pain in adults is a typical symptom of serious diseases (myocardial infarction, pulmonary embolism, etc.), chest pain in children is often perceived to be just as threatening, thus giving rise to anxiety. However, chest pain in children and adolescents only rarely has a cardiac cause.

▶ **Etiology.** Most chest pain in childhood and adolescence is idiopathic. If any cause is found, it is usually a musculoskeletal or pulmonary disease. At most, only 1% to 3% of cases have cardiac causes. Psychogenic chest pain is more common in children over age 12 than in younger children.

Chest pains can also stem from the esophagus, stomach, or gall bladder. The most common causes of chest pain in childhood and adolescence are listed in ▶ Table 12.1.

Cardiac causes of chest pain in children and adolescents are rare. However, an underlying cardiac disease is more probable if there are other cardiac symptoms such as syncopes or palpitations in addition to chest pain.

The most important cardiac causes of chest pain in childhood and adolescence are listed in ▶ Table 12.2.

12.2 Diagnostic Procedures

▶ **Medical history.** The medical history frequently provides clues for the cause of the chest pain. The following points should be clarified when taking the medical history:

- When did the pain first occur?
- Onset of pain (acute or gradual onset?)
- How can the pain be described (e.g., burning, pressing, dull)?
- What is the exact location of the pain?
- Does physical exertion increase the pain?
- Does it get better at rest?
- Was there any recent trauma or muscle strain?
- Risk factors for thromboembolism (e.g., recent operation or cardiac catheterization, thrombophilia, thrombosis, oral contraceptives, air travel, obesity)
- Psychosocial stress factors (e.g., problems at school, serious illness or death in the family, depression)
- Associated symptoms (e.g., palpitations, dizziness, syncopes, nausea, vomiting, dyspnea, fever, cough, swollen joints)
- Underlying diseases: sickle cell anemia, Kawasaki syndrome, Marfan syndrome, Turner syndrome, rheumatic diseases
- Drug and medication use (e.g., cocaine, nicotine, betamimetics)
- Family history: hypertrophic cardiomyopathy, connective tissue disorders (Marfan syndrome), or sudden cardiac death in the family

> **Note**
>
> In patients with chest pain, the following information in the medical history should be considered a warning sign for an underlying organic cause:
>
> - Sudden onset of severe pain and reduced general condition
> - Pain that increases during exertion or suggests myocardial ischemia
> - Associated cardiac symptoms such as palpitations, dizziness, or syncopes
> - Underlying diseases such as Marfan syndrome, Kawasaki syndrome, sickle cell anemia, thrombophilia, or rheumatic disease
> - Positive family history for cardiomyopathies, long QT syndrome, Marfan syndrome, or sudden deaths

▶ **Physical examination.** In the physical examination, the first step is to determine whether the patient is acutely ill and needs immediate treatment—for example, if he or she has pneumothorax or a dissected aortic aneurysm. However, in most cases, the patients who present with chest pain are not clinically impaired.

During inspection, any indication of an injury and conspicuous respiratory pattern or asymmetric chest movements should be noted. Indicative findings during auscultation of the lungs are weakened breath sounds on one side (pneumothorax, pleural effusions), fine moist rales (pneumonia), or expiratory obstruction (bronchial asthma).

Some examples of typical palpation findings are painful costochondral or costosternal junctions (costochondritis), muscle tension, or a painful epigastrium (gastritis).

In the auscultation of the chest, arrhythmia or tachycardia, a pathological murmur, and weakened heart sounds (pericardial effusion) or pericardial friction rub (pericardial effusion) should be noted.

▶ **ECG.** An ECG can sometimes yield indicative findings in patients with chest pain. The following findings should be noted in particular:

- Delta wave and shortened PQ interval: Wolff–Parkinson–White syndrome
- Signs of (left) ventricular hypertrophy: hypertrophic cardiomyopathy, severe aortic stenosis
- Prolonged QT interval: long QT syndrome

Table 12.1 The most common causes of chest pain in children and adolescents

Cause	Indicative findings
Musculoskeletal	
Excessive strain of the chest muscles (stiff muscles, e.g., from weight training or coughing), trauma, pulled muscle	Medical history, local palpation finding
Costochondritis	Reproducible tenderness at the costosternal or costochondral junctions of the ribs, usually on one side, increased by deep breathing or physical exertion, duration up to several months; harmless illness, generally no treatment needed
Tietze syndrome	Swelling at the costosternal junctions, usually affecting the upper ribs
Pulmonary	
Bronchial asthma	Dyspnea, retrosternal pain, auscultation, prolonged expiration, wheezing
Pneumonia	Cough, fever, respiration-related pain, auscultation, fine moist rales over the lungs, X-ray
Pleural effusion	Breathing-related pain (increase in pain on deep inspiration), effusion in ultrasound or X-ray
Pneumothorax	Sudden onset of pain, dyspnea, weakened breath sounds on one side
Pleurodynia	Chest pain after a virus infection, Coxsackie virus detected
Pulmonary embolism	Sudden onset of breathing-related pain, hypocapnia, tachycardia, coagulation disorder, thrombosis, fever
Aspiration of a foreign body	Medical history, sudden dyspnea and chest pain, possibly weakened breath sounds on one side, X-ray finding, bronchoscopy to confirm the diagnosis and remove the foreign body
Gastrointestinal	
Gastroesophageal reflux	Related to meals, coughing at night, possible failure to thrive, pH monitoring
Esophagitis	Retrosternal pain, difficulty swallowing, radiating to the back, endoscopy
Gastritis, ulcer	Epigastric pain, related to meals, endoscopy
Cholecystitis	Postprandial pain in the right upper abdomen and chest, ultrasound, evidence of gallstones
Pancreatitis	Upper abdominal pain, radiating to the chest, elevated serum lipase and amylase
Other causes	
Psychogenic	Stressful situation, family history of cardiac problems or chronic pain, girls more often affected, age over 12 years, psychological or psychiatric consultation
Sickle cell crisis	African origin, Hb electrophoresis
Herpes zoster	Stabbing pain, local blisters, previous chicken pox

- Diffuse ST segment and T wave anomalies: pericardial effusion
- Signs of infarction: Bland-White-Garland syndrome (deep Q in the anterolateral leads); rarely, signs of coronary stenoses following Kawasaki syndrome

▸ **Echocardiography.** In addition to ECG, echocardiography is one of the standard diagnostic measures in pediatric cardiology for patients with chest pain. It can be used to confirm a diagnosis or to rule out congenital or acquired cardiac diseases such as cardiomyopathies, valvular stenoses, pericardial effusions, and dilatations or aneurysms of the aorta. Furthermore, anomalies of the coronary arteries such as anomalous origins or aneurysms should be specifically looked for.

▸ **Chest X-ray.** The X-ray is primarily to exclude pulmonary diseases as the cause of chest pain (e.g., pneumothorax, pleural effusions, or pneumonia).

▸ **Exercise testing.** An exercise test can be useful if the chest pains occur during exercise. If there are indications of myocardial ischemia in the medical history, an exercise ECG may also provide additional information.

Table 12.2 Cardiac causes of chest pain in children and adolescents

Cardiac disease	Remark	Indicative clinical findings
Myocardial ischemia		
Severe aortic stenosis	Myocardial ischemia especially during exertion due to increased oxygen demand of the hypertrophic myocardium and elevated pressure in the left ventricle	Loud systolic bruit, PMI in the parasternal 2nd right ICS, radiating to the carotids, signs of left heart hypertrophy in the ECG, confirmed by echocardiography
Hypertrophic obstructive cardiomyopathy		Possible positive family history, possible signs of hypertrophy in the ECG, possibly systolic bruit, the murmur typically changes on inspiration and expiration, confirmed by echocardiography
Severe pulmonary stenosis	Considerably less frequent that aortic stenosis as the cause of myocardial ischemia	Loud systolic bruit, PMI in the parasternal 2nd left ICS, signs of right heart hypertrophy in the ECG, confirmed by echocardiography
Mitral valve prolapse	Correlation with chest pain is disputed, possibly ischemia of the papillary muscle	Mid-systolic click, sometimes systolic bruit, possibly T wave inversion in leads II, III, aVF, often asthenic habitus, possibly anomalies of the bony thorax, confirmed by echocardiography
Eisenmenger syndrome		Shunt defect, cyanosis, clubbed fingers, rounded nails, pronounced 2nd heart sound, signs of right heart hypertrophy in the ECG
Bland-White-Garland syndrome	Myocardial ischemia after the drop in pulmonary resistance, typically between the ages of 2 and 6 months	ECG: Q in I, aVL, V4–6 (anterolateral myocardial infarction), visualization of the coronary origins in echocardiography, if necessary coronary angiography
Rare aberrant origins of the coronary arteries (e.g., origin of the left coronary artery from the right sinus of Valsalva)	Compression of the affected coronary artery between the aorta and the pulmonary artery, myocardial ischemia especially during exertion	Visualization of the coronary origins in echocardiography, if necessary coronary angiography
Kawasaki syndrome	After coronary aneurysms, coronary stenoses can develop, the risk is greatest with very large aneurysms	Kawasaki syndrome in the patient history, evidence of myocardial ischemia in the ECG, confirmed by coronary angiography
Inflammatory heart disease		
Pericarditis	Usually infectious or immunological cause, also traumatic or from tumors	Sharply defined pain that increases when lying down and subsides when sitting up and leaning forward; possible pericardial friction rub, weakened heart sounds, ECG may have low voltage and ST segment changes, confirmed by echocardiography
Post-pericardiotomy syndrome	Immunologically caused pericardial effusion following open heart surgery	Findings similar to pericarditis, fever, pronounced discomfort
Myocarditis	Usually infectious	Often after previous viral infection, weakness, arrhythmia, enlarged heart with impaired function
Other causes		
Dissected aortic aneurysm	Especially feared in adolescent Marfan patients, less frequent than with Turner syndrome	Life-threatening emergency, intense chest pain, diagnosis by echocardiography, possibly chest CT or MRI scan

Table 12.2 continued

Cardiac disease	Remark	Indicative clinical findings
Arrhythmias	Palpitations are sometimes described by children as "heart pain." On the other hand, long lasting tachycardia in particular can lead to myocardial ischemia	Rapid heartbeat, palpitations, diagnosis confirmed by ECG, long-term ECG, or possibly event recorder
Cocaine consumption	Possible symptoms: chest pain (coronary vasoconstriction, increased myocardial oxygen consumption), pneumothorax, arrhythmia, hypertension	Medical history, drug screening

▶ **Laboratory.** If there are indications of myocardial ischemia, it may be useful, depending on the individual case, to determine the myocardial enzymes (esp. CK-MB test, troponin I). Elevated myocardial enzymes can also occur in myocarditis.

12.3 Therapy

In the many cases when no underlying organic cause is found, informing the patients and parents that a cardiac cause for the pain has been ruled out is helpful and reassuring in itself.

Otherwise the underlying diseases are treated. Musculoskeletal diseases can usually be treated by limiting physical activity and if necessary with a nonsteroidal anti-inflammatory drug. If esophagitis or gastritis is assumed to be the cause of the pain, prescribing an antacid can be useful, both as a diagnostic tool and for treatment. If there are signs of a chronic somatic disorder, the child should be evaluated by a pediatric psychiatrist.

12.4 Prognosis and Course

After organic causes have been excluded, the prognosis is generally very good. The pain is self-limiting in nearly all cases. If prolonged psychogenic chest pain is suspected, treatment by a pediatric psychiatrist should be initiated in an attempt to prevent the pain from becoming chronic. In the rare cases when an organic cause is found, the prognosis depends on the underlying disease.

13 Palpitations

13.1 Basics

▶ **Definition.** Palpitations are defined as the unpleasant awareness of your own heartbeat. Palpitations are often described by patients as pounding or skipping a beat. The heartbeat is perceived to be unpleasant when it is especially rapid or irregular or when individual heartbeats are unusually strong. However, individuals' awareness of their own heartbeat varies greatly.

▶ **Etiology.** Frequently, no organic cause for palpitations is found, but palpitations can be an indication of a relevant underlying rhythm disorder. Some of the cardiac diseases frequently associated with arrhythmias are:

- Status post correction of a congenital heart defect (especially after Fontan procedure or Mustard/Senning atrial baffle procedure)
- Hypertrophic obstructive cardiomyopathy
- Dilated cardiomyopathy
- Aortic stenosis
- Heart failure
- Cardiac tumor
- Myocarditis
- Mitral valve prolapse

In addition to cardiac causes of arrhythmia, numerous noncardiac causes can lead to palpitations, for example, hyperthyroidism or anemia. Other causes may be stimulants (caffeine, nicotine), drugs, or medication. Psychiatric disorders such as panic attacks or anxiety must also be ruled out. Palpitations can be physiological in association with exertion, agitation, or fever.

The most frequent causes of palpitations are listed in ▶ Table 13.1.

Note

The perception of palpitations alone provides little information on the type of underlying rhythm disorder. Palpitations may be physiological phenomena such as sinus tachycardia. On the other hand, even ventricular tachycardias can be completely asymptomatic.

If additional symptoms such as syncopes, dizziness, pallor, nausea, shortness of breath, or chest pain are present, an underlying organic cause is more likely.

Table 13.1 Frequent causes of palpitations

Physiological causes
• Physical or emotional stress, agitation
• Fever
Cardiac causes
• Extrasystoles (supraventricular, ventricular)
• Paroxysmal tachycardias such as AV nodal re-entrant tachycardia or AV re-entrant tachycardia (WPW syndrome)
• Other tachycardias (sinus tachycardia, postural tachycardia syndrome)
• Bradycardias (sinus node dysfunction, AV blocks)
• Atrial fibrillation (absolute arrhythmia)
Psychogenic causes and psychiatric disorders
• Anxiety, panic attacks
• Hyperventilation
Medication and drugs
• Stimulants: caffeine, nicotine, energy drinks
• Medication that can lead to tachycardia (catecholamines, betamimetics, theophylline, thyroid hormones, abrupt discontinuation of beta blockers)
• Medication that can lead to bradycardia (beta blockers, calcium antagonists)
• Potentially arrhythmogenic medication (antiarrhythmics, antidepressants)
Metabolic disorders
• Hyperthyroidism
• Hypoglycemia
Other causes
• Anemia
• Poor physical condition

13.2 Diagnostic Measures

▶ **Medical history.** In many cases, the medical history may provide clues. Supraventricular or ventricular extrasystoles are the most common reasons for consulting a pediatric cardiologist. In particular, patients experience the postextrasystolic compensatory pause as unpleasant ("my heart stops beating").

A sudden onset and abrupt end of the palpitations is a sign of paroxysmal supraventricular tachycardia such as AV nodal re-entrant tachycardia or a Wolf–Parkinson–White (WPW) syndrome. Children are often conspicuously pale or sweaty during the tachycardia.

Palpitations that occur during exertion may be normal in the sense of a sinus tachycardia (especially in children who are not physically fit). However, they must be distinguished from pathological exercise-related arrhythmias (e.g., as a result of a relevant aortic stenosis or hypertrophic obstructive cardiomyopathy).

Table 13.2 Characteristic findings from medical history and possible causes of palpitations

Characteristic finding	Possible causes
Isolated irregular pulse	Extrasystoles (supraventricular, ventricular)
Rapid, regular pulse	Sinus tachycardia, paroxysmal supraventricular tachycardia, atrial fibrillation, (slow) ventricular tachycardia, permanent junctional re-entrant tachycardia
Sudden onset and abrupt end of rapid heartbeat, possibly with pallor	AV nodal re-entrant tachycardia, WPW syndrome
Gradual onset and gradual end of rapid heartbeat	Sinus tachycardia
Slow, regular pulse	Sinus bradycardia, 2nd degree AV block Mobitz type II or 3rd degree AV block
Slow, irregular pulse	2nd degree AV block Mobitz type I (Wenckebach periodicity)
Completely irregular pulse	Absolute arrhythmia associated with atrial fibrillation, frequent extrasystoles (supraventricular, ventricular)
Rapid pulse, possibly with presyncopes after standing up or standing for a longer period	Postural tachycardia syndrome

Palpitations that occur when the patient stands up suddenly or after standing for a long period may be an indication of postural tachycardia syndrome.

When taking the family history, ask specifically about syncopes, sudden cardiac death, and arrhythmias. Use of medication, drugs, and stimulants including coffee and energy drinks should also be investigated.

Characteristic findings from the medical history and clinical findings of the most frequent causes of palpitations are summarized in ▶ Table 13.2.

▶ **Physical examination.** The physical examination is usually normal, but signs of hypothyroidism or hyperthyroidism should be noted. In the cardiac examination, particular attention should be paid to signs of a congenital or acquired heart defect (e.g., aortic stenosis, cardiomyopathies, mitral valve prolapse).

▶ **Laboratory.** If there are relevant clinical signs, anemia, electrolyte imbalances, hypoglycemia, and thyroid function disorders must be ruled out.

▶ **ECG.** If an ECG can be recorded during palpitations, it can provide clues for the diagnosis. But even the normal resting ECG can contribute important information on the origin of palpitations. Special attention should be given to AV blocks, a prolonged QTc interval (long QT syndrome), a delta wave (WPW syndrome), an atypical right bundle branch block with ST segment elevations in the right precordial leads (Brugada syndrome), an epsilon wave (right ventricular dysplasia), and signs of hypertrophy (e.g., hypertrophic cardiomyopathy).

▶ **Long-term ECG.** If palpitations occur frequently, the diagnosis can often be made using long-term ECG. The correlation of symptoms with the ECG findings should be noted.

▶ **Echocardiography.** Echocardiography is useful for ruling out structural heart disease.

▶ **Event recorder.** The event recorder can be used if the palpitations occur so rarely that it is unlikely that they will be "caught" in a long-term ECG.

▶ **Exercise ECG.** Exercise testing is useful for investigating palpitations that occur during exertion.

▶ **Electrophysiological examination.** An electrophysiological examination study (EPS) may be indicated if the medical history is typical for AV nodal re-entrant tachycardia or a WPW syndrome. An attempt can be made to ablate the anatomical correlate of tachycardia in the same session. An EPS can also be used to provoke supraventricular or ventricular tachycardia, the underlying causes of palpitations, using the relevant stimulation protocol.

13.3 Therapy

Many palpitations have no underlying disease (e.g., physiological sinus tachycardia during exertion) that needs to be treated. Isolated supraventricular and ventricular extrasystoles also do not generally require treatment. If they are felt to be extremely uncomfortable, medication can be helpful, for example, with a beta blocker. Otherwise substances that increase the frequency of extrasystoles should be avoided (coffee, energy drinks).

The therapy for arrhythmias is discussed in Chapter 18.

14 Syncope

14.1 Basics

▶ **Definition.** *Syncope* is the sudden, temporary loss of consciousness as a result of cerebral hypoperfusion associated with loss of muscular tone. Recovery is spontaneous. Unconsciousness usually lasts 30 to 60 seconds and up to 5 minutes at most.

There is no loss of consciousness in *presyncope*. Depending on the cause and duration, syncope may also be followed by cerebral seizures.

▶ **Epidemiology.** Around 15% of all children suffer at least one syncope episode in their life. The peak frequency is during adolescence. Syncope is rare in preschool children.

▶ **Etiology.** Syncope is most frequently (70%–80%) mediated neurally in children and adolescents. The term vasovagal syncope was previously used and the term neurocardiogenic syncope is sometimes used synonymously. Today, these types of syncope are described as vasodepressor, cardioinhibitory, or mixed, depending on the reaction pattern.

The most important causes and differential diagnoses of syncope are listed in ▶ Table 14.1 and ▶ Table 14.2.

The differential diagnoses listed in ▶ Table 14.2 must be distinguished from syncope. Breath-holding spells are frequent among toddlers, who may stop breathing until losing consciousness due to anger, fear, etc. Seizures, which should not be interpreted to be syncope, are also among the most frequent differential diagnoses.

14.2 Diagnostic Measures

▶ **Medical history.** The medical history is an important component of diagnosing syncope. In combination with the physical examination, it allows a majority of syncopes to be distinguished from differential diagnoses. The following points should be included in the medical history (▶ Table 14.3):

- Personal history:
  - Number and timing of the previous syncope episodes
  - Previous diseases (especially cardiac disease, epilepsy, migraines, diabetes mellitus, thyroid disease)
  - Possible pregnancy?
  - Medication history
  - Alcohol/drug consumption
  - Sleep habits
  - Fatigue, exhaustion, weight loss
  - Eating and drinking habits
  - Sports
- Family history:
  - Sudden deaths before age 30 years
  - Congenital heart defects or arrhythmias
  - Epilepsy or migraines
  - Syncope

Table 14.1 Causes of syncope

Neurally mediated syncope
• Reflex syncope (vasodepressor, cardioinhibitory, mixed)
• Postural tachycardia syndrome
• Dysautonomia (e.g., associated with neuropathies)
• Situational syncope (triggered by coughing, sneezing, pressing the carotid sinus, passing stools, pain)
Cardiac syncope
• Arrhythmias: ∘ Tachycardias: supraventricular tachycardia, atrial flutter/fibrillation, ventricular tachycardia, ventricular flutter/fibrillation (underlying diseases: long QT syndrome, short QT syndrome, Brugada syndrome, right ventricular dysplasia, myocarditis, catecholamine-induced ventricular tachycardia, right ventricular outflow tract tachycardia) ∘ Bradycardias: sinus bradycardia, sinus node dysfunction, AV block, pacemaker malfunction ∘ Asystole
• Cardiac obstructions: ∘ Outflow tract obstructions: aortic stenosis, hypertrophic obstructive cardiomyopathy ∘ Inflow tract obstructions: mitral stenosis, pericardial tamponade, constrictive pericarditis
• Myocardial dysfunction: dilative cardiomyopathy, hypertrophic cardiomyopathy, anomalous coronary arteries, myocardial ischemia
• Cyanotic spells associated with cyanotic defects (esp. tetralogy of Fallot)
• Pulmonary hypertension
• Mitral valve prolapse syndrome (very rare)

Table 14.2 Differential diagnoses of syncope

Neurological diseases
• Seizure
• Migraine ("confusional migraine")
• Intracranial pressure, tumors
• Cerebral hemorrhage, ischemia
• Encephalitis
Psychiatric disorders
• Panic attacks
• Conversion syndromes
• Hyperventilation
• Breath-holding spell
Metabolic diseases
• Hypoglycemia
• Electrolyte imbalances (incl. diabetes insipidus, inadequate ADH [antidiuretic hormone] secretion syndrome, adrenal insufficiency)
• Anorexia nervosa
• Toxins
• Anemia

- Situation before syncope:
  - Body position (sitting, lying, standing)
  - Physical exertion
  - Fear or scare, unexpected sound
  - Urination, bowel movement, coughing, pressing, swallowing
  - Turning the head, narrow collar
  - Meal
  - Full, overheated room
  - Menstruation
- Onset of the syncope:
  - Nausea, vomiting
  - Sweating
  - Dizziness
  - Blurred/double vision
  - Impaired speech
  - Impaired hearing
  - Palpitations, rapid heartbeat
  - Pain in the face or neck
  - Aura
  - Slumping, collapsing, falling down
- Description of the syncope:
  - Duration of unconsciousness
  - Skin color: pallor, cyanosis, flushed
  - Breathing: apnea, hyperventilation, stridor, snoring
  - Muscle tone: lax, heightened

Table 14.3 Frequent causes and differential diagnoses of syncope and indicative findings in the history

Cause	Indicative findings in the history
Neurally mediated syncope	• Prolonged standing • Prodromal stage (dizziness, sweating, spots before the eyes, nausea) • Loss of muscle tone, collapsing; convulsions are rare, but possible • Length of unconsciousness 0.5–5 min
Breath-holding spell	• Early childhood (toddlers) • Trigger: scare, anger, or fear • Often a short scream followed by apnea • Possible loss of consciousness, sometimes seizure
Cardiac syncope	• Sudden loss of consciousness without prodromes • Syncope during or shortly after physical exertion • Rapid heartbeat, chest pain • Positive family history of sudden cardiac death
Long QT syndrome (LQTS)	• LQTS 1: triggers are physical exertion, swimming • LQTS 2: triggers are acoustic signals, emotional stress • LQTS 3: triggers are resting, sleep • Jervell–Lange–Nielsen syndrome: inner ear hearing loss • Anderson or Timothy syndrome: musculoskeletal anomalies
Migraine	• Headache • Impaired vision • Nausea • Sometimes aura or confusion
Epilepsy	• Duration of unconsciousness usually longer than in neurally mediated syncope • Passing stool or urination • Biting the tongue • Postictal fatigue • Typical age of manifestation for various forms of epilepsy

  - Movements: myoclonic spasms, tonic–clonic movements, asymmetry
  - Gaze deviation
  - Biting the tongue, salivation, automatisms
- After the syncope:
  - Amnesia (antegrade, retrograde)
  - Injuries
  - Headache
  - Fatigue
  - Confusion
  - Speech disorders
  - Muscle pain
  - Chest pain
  - Palpitations, rapid heartbeat
  - Passing urine or stool

> **Note**
>
> Any of the following must be considered alarm signals as they may be indications of serious underlying diseases (from McLeod KA 2003):
> - Syncope during or shortly after physical exertion
> - Syncope that occurs while the patient is lying
> - Syncope that occurs after a noise, scare, in cold water, or after psychological stress
> - Positive family history for sudden heart death before age 30 years
> - Syncope lasting longer than 5 min

▸ **Physical examination.** The physical examination includes an assessment of the pulse, exclusion of a heart murmur, and a comprehensive evaluation of neurological status. In addition, the blood pressure should be measured when the patient has been lying down for at least 5 minutes and then shortly after standing up. A drop of at least 20 mmHg in systolic blood pressure is a sign of orthostatic hypotension.

▸ **ECG.** A resting ECG is one of the basic diagnostic measures for investigating syncope. Special attention should be given to arrhythmias, conduction disorders, signs of hypertrophy, signs of ischemia (e.g., Q notch), repolarization disorders, pre-excitation (delta wave), and the (corrected) QT interval. Furthermore, the ECG should be checked for an epsilon wave (right ventricular dysplasia), an atypical right bundle branch block configuration, and ST segment elevations in the right precordial leads (Brugada syndrome).

However, it should be taken into consideration that the ECG may not be sufficient to rule out a hypertrophic myocardiopathy. In addition, most coronary anomalies do not cause any typical changes in the ECG. If there is a borderline prolongation of the QTc interval and indications of a Brugada syndrome, an ECG of the siblings and parents may provide additional information. The ajmaline provocation test may show the typical ECG changes in patients with Brugada syndrome (Chapter 18.25).

> **Note**
>
> The basic diagnostic measures for investigating syncope include the medical history, the physical examination, and a resting ECG.

▸ **Echocardiography.** Echocardiography is indicated if the history or physical examination gives any evidence of a structural cardiac defect, but is not routinely needed after a syncope event. In addition to congenital heart defects (especially left heart obstructions), cardiomyopathies and inflammatory heart disease (myocarditis, Kawasaki syndrome) must be ruled out. In this examination, special attention should be paid to the origins and course of the coronary arteries to rule out anomalies.

▸ **24-hour Holter monitoring ECG..** If the history suggests rhythmogenic syncope or if the resting ECG is pathological, an attempt can be made to document the relevant arrhythmia using Holter monitoring, although the syncopes generally occur too infrequently to be recorded in a long-term ECG. In any case, when analyzing the long-term ECG, the correlation between the documented arrhythmias and the clinical symptoms should be considered. Otherwise there is the danger that actually harmless asymptomatic findings might be "overtreated."

▸ **Event recorder.** Event recorders are indicated in patients with frequent syncope events for which diagnostic measures have yielded no indicative findings. An external event recorder can be worn by a patient for several weeks. However, compliance generally decreases as the duration increases. If an event occurs, the ECG recording can be activated by the patient or another person. Depending on the programming, recording can also be triggered by bradycardia or tachycardia. After activation, the device saves a programmable interval before or after syncope.

In exceptional cases, it is even possible to implant an event recorder subcutaneously, similar to a pacemaker. This option is useful for patients who are severely impaired by syncopes that occur relatively rarely if other diagnostic methods do not provide any information on the cause of the syncopes.

▸ **Tilt table test.** The aim of a tilt table test is to reproduce and objectify the patient's symptoms through orthostatic stress. This should clarify whether the symptoms described by the patient are caused by neurocardiogenic syncope. A tilt table test is indicated for recurring syncopes for which other causes have been ruled out or for recurring syncopes with a high risk of injury. For patients with cardiac disease, the tilt table test is also used to clarify whether the syncopes are neurocardiogenic or caused by the cardiac disease itself. The tilt table test is generally not needed if the patient has the typical history and classic clinical symptoms of neurocardiogenic syncopes.

The reliability of tilt table test is limited. When establishing the indication, one should be aware that the test's sensitivity is relatively low. The test can also induce symptoms in patients who were previously asymptomatic.

Conducting the tilt table test: During the examination, the patient first lies on the table in horizontal position. An IV line is placed, an ECG is recorded continuously, and

Table 14.4 Pathological reaction types in the tilt table test (from Brignole M et al. 2004)[54]

Type of syncope	Pathological reaction type
Cardioinhibitory syncope:	
• Without asystole	• Drop in heart rate to below 40/min for more than 10 s • Without asystole lasting longer than 3 s
• With asystole	• Asystole lasting longer than 3 s
Vasodepressor syncope	• Drop in heart rate by less than 10% of maximum heart rate • Drop in blood pressure causes the syncope
Mixed syncope	• Drop in heart rate, but not below 40/min • With or without asystole for less than 3 s
Postural tachycardia syndrome	• Excessive increase in heart rate at the start of the tilting phase and during tilting by more than 30/min or to over 120/min • Usually only presyncope

the blood pressure is measured every 1 to 2 minutes. After several minutes in this position, the table is tilted, head-up, by 60 to 80°, with the patient's feet supported by a shelf. This position is maintained for 20 to 45 minutes or until symptoms occur. After a maximum of 45 minutes or when symptoms occur, the table is returned to the initial position. Most syncope events occur some 20 minutes after starting the test.

If the finding is negative, a repetition test with drug provocation (e.g., isoproterenol) may be recommended. However, this method is controversial, as the specificity of the test is reduced by provocation.

Evaluation of the tilt table test: The tilt table test is positive if clinically clear symptoms of presyncope or syncope can be provoked. The tilt table test is useful as a diagnostic tool if the patient's symptoms during the tilt table test correspond to the symptoms during previous syncopes. Asymptomatic fluctuations in blood pressure and pulse during the test are not relevant. ▶ Table 14.4 lists different reaction types depending on the behavior of blood pressure and pulse during the syncope.

▶ **Exercise testing.** An exercise test may be useful if there are unclear syncope events that occur during or after exertion. Prior to this, however, defects with a relevant left heart obstruction (e.g., aortic stenosis, hypertrophic obstructive cardiomyopathy) and a predisposition for ventricular tachycardias should be ruled out. The relevant precautionary measures (emergency medication, defibrillator) must be observed. Exercise testing can also help detect myocardial ischemia.

▶ **Electrophysiological examination study.** An EPS is rarely indicated for patients with structurally or functionally conspicuous hearts. But it can be useful if the initial examinations suggest a rhythmogenic cause of syncope in patients with cardiac disease, especially if they complain of palpitations or relevant arrhythmias (e.g., ventricular tachycardias) have already been detected. The EPS also includes atrial and ventricular stimulation to provoke the respective arrhythmias under controlled conditions.

Excursus: Neurally mediated syncope

Epidemiology

Neurally mediated syncope constitutes approximately 75% of all syncopes.

Pathogenesis

Neurally mediated syncope involves the reflex arc. All episodes are associated with the acute occurrence of pronounced vasodilatation with or without bradycardia or asystole. This leads to hypoperfusion of the brain and loss of consciousness.

The pathophysiological processes that lead to neurally mediated syncope are not fully understood. There is a complex underlying reflex pattern, the Bezold–Jarisch reflex. It is assumed that the blood pools in the lower half of the body when standing (venous pooling). The venous return to the heart is reduced. The circulatory system compensates for this initially by increasing inotropy in the heart and heart rate. Stimulating baroreceptors in the ventricular wall leads to transmission of the corresponding signals to the brain stem via vagal pathways. If these signals exceed a certain threshold (with great interindividual variance), reflex dilatation and bradycardia result. Similar reflex arcs can also be activated by anxiety, coughing, swallowing, urination, etc.

Symptoms

Prodromes such as weakness, fatigue, dizziness, nausea, yawning, cold sweats, blurred vision, or pallor are typical for neurocardiogenic syncope. Patients characteristically drop where they are standing when syncope occurs, but there can be dramatic falls. The duration of unconsciousness is rarely more than 60 s, extremely rarely more than 5 min. If syncope lasts longer, tonic–clonic spasms may occur in the limbs, which do not necessarily indicate epilepsy. Patients are generally quickly oriented again when they regain consciousness. Disorientation lasting more than 15 minutes indicates a cause other than syncope, but exhaustion, fatigue, and nausea may last for an even longer period.

Treatment

The first step in the treatment of neurocardiogenic syncope involves general measures, including:

- Avoiding triggers such as prolonged standing, loss of volume, crowded, warm environment
- Recognizing prodromal symptoms and developing strategies to avert impending syncope, for example, isometric exercise (crossing legs, clasping hands and pulling outwards, moving up and down on your toes, squatting)
- Endurance training
- Orthostatic training—patients can increase orthostatic tolerance by leaning with their back against the wall. After an initial duration of a few minutes, the period is increased to 30 minutes.
- Increased salt intake ("volume expansion").

If these general measures are unsuccessful, pharmacological approaches are available. However, it should be noted that there is little information on the pharmacological treatment of neurocardiogenic syncope. There are no generally valid recommendations for the various medications at this time.

The following methods are used in childhood and adolescence:

- *Beta blockers* block excessive activation of the sympathetic nervous system through the reflex arc, for example, metoprolol (0.5–1 mg/kg twice daily).
- *Mineralocorticoids* lead to an elevation of intravasal volume. Fludrocortisone is most frequently used. Dosage: e.g., oral administration of 0.1 mg twice daily.
- *Alpha-1 agonists* lead to vasoconstriction. Etilefrine was shown to be ineffective in trials, but midodrine appears to be effective. The disadvantage is that midodrine must be given in three single doses and the effective dose varies greatly from individual to individual. Dosage: e.g., oral administration of 2.5 mg three times a day.
- *Serotonin antagonists* are administered as there is evidence of central serotoninergic involvement in the genesis of syncope. An example is fluoxetine. Dosage: e.g., oral administration of 5 mg four times a day
- *Pacemaker:* The benefit of implanting a pacemaker for severe cardioinhibitory syncope associated with a marked drop in heart rate or even asystole is very controversial. Some problems with pacemaker therapy are, for example, that vasodilatation during syncope cannot be prevented by a pacemaker and that many patients do not develop bradycardia until after the drop in blood pressure.

Prognosis

The prognosis for neurocardiogenic syncope is very good. There is no increased mortality. In the great majority of cases in adolescent patients, syncope stops within a few years at the latest. It is absolutely necessary, however, to distinguish neurocardiogenic syncope from cardiac syncope, which has a high mortality if left untreated.

► **Laboratory.** Laboratory tests can be made to rule out anemia, hypoglycemia, electrolyte imbalances, and toxins. A pregnancy test may be carried out for women of childbearing age.

The reliability of laboratory tests is generally limited, however, by the fact that the blood samples are generally not taken immediately during the syncope. Acute hypoglycemia is therefore difficult to detect at a later time.

► **Supplementary diagnostic measures.** If there are indications of a neurological genesis, the diagnostic measures may be supplemented by pediatric neurology examinations such as an EEG and imaging modalities. If an underlying psychiatric disease is suspected, a psychiatric consultation is necessary.

Part III

Syndromes

15 Congenital Heart Defects

15.1 Atrial Septal Defects

15.1.1 Basics

Definition

An atrial septal defect (ASD) is a pathological connection between the left and the right atrium. The defect may be found at different sites on the atrial septum and leads to a left-to-right shunt at the atrial level with increased pulmonary blood flow. The most common type of ASD is the ostium secundum type (ASD II), which is found at the center of the atrial septum.

Epidemiology

ASDs constitute about 10% of all congenital heart defects. Women are affected around twice as often as men. A patent foramen ovale can be found in as many as one-third of all individuals.

Pathogenesis

During embryonic development, there is a wide opening between the two atria (ostium primum). This ostium primum increasingly narrows as the septum primum develops from a cranial direction. Before it fuses at the level of the atrioventricular (AV) valves, the upper portion of the septum primum tears, resulting in the ostium secundum. The septum secundum then grows in a caudal direction from the atrial roof to the right of the septum primum at the level of the AV valves. At the overlap with the ostium secundum, a crescent-shaped slit, the foramen ovale, forms between the septa. The foramen ovale functions as a check valve that opens when the pressure comes from the right and closes when the pressure comes from the left. The fusion of the septum primum with the septum secundum results in complete separation of the atria. A patent foramen ovale is the result of incomplete fusion. Inhibited development of the septum secundum leads to an ASD II.

Classification

Various types of ASD are differentiated according to their location in the atrial septum. (▸ Fig. 15.1):

- *Ostium secundum ASD* (ASD II; 70%): ASD II is the most common form. The defect is centrally located in the region of the foramen ovale and is surrounded on all sides by remnants of the atrial septum. ASD II is rarely associated with a partial anomalous pulmonary venous connection.
- *Ostium primum ASD* (ASD I; 20%): This defect is actually part of the AV canal (Chapter 15.3). The defect is located in the lower part of the atrium close to the AV valves and is almost always associated with an anomaly of the AV valves. Most common is a cleft in the anterior leaflet of the mitral valve that leads to mitral valve regurgitation.
- *Sinus venosus defect* (10%): Sinus venosus defects are located at the connection of the vena cava into the right atrium and are classified as upper or lower sinus venosus defects. They are usually associated with partial anomalous pulmonary venous connections.
  - *Superior sinus venosus defect*: An upper sinus venosus defect is located at the connection of the superior vena cava to the atrium. The actual atrial septum is intact, but the wall between some of the right pulmonary veins and the superior vena cava is missing, so that the pulmonary venous blood passes through the superior vena cava to the right atrium. The open connection between the two atria is located near the actual confluence of the pulmonary vein (▸ Fig. 15.2).
  - *Inferior sinus venosus defect (rare):* A lower sinus venosus defect is located where the inferior vena cava and the right inferior pulmonary vein connect to the atrium. This defect leads to a functional partial anomalous pulmonary venous connection.
- *Coronary sinus defect* (1%): This defect is the rarest form of ASD. In this form the coronary sinus connects not only to the right atrium but also to the left atrium. It is also called "unroofed coronary sinus" as the "roof" of the coronary sinus in the region of left atrium is

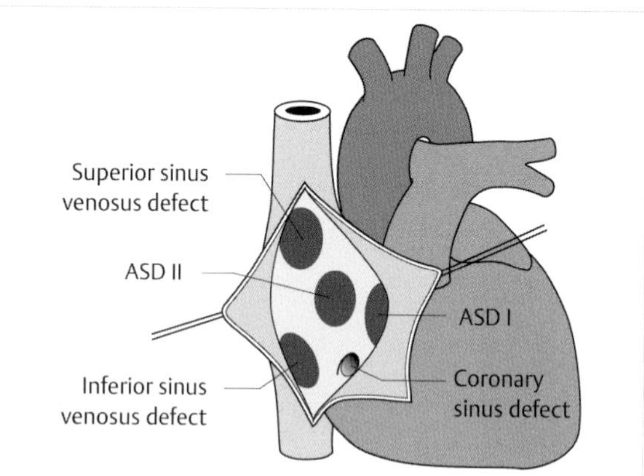

Fig. 15.1 Location of the atrial septum defects.
The right atrium is open with a view from the right atrium to the atrial septum. The typical ASD II is located at the center of the atrial septum. The ASD I is located in the lower part of the atrial septum in the immediate vicinity of the AV valves. The superior and inferior sinus venosus defects are located at the confluence of the superior and inferior vena cava in the right atrium. In the coronary sinus defect, left atrial blood reaches the right atrium through the unroofed coronary sinus in the left atrium.

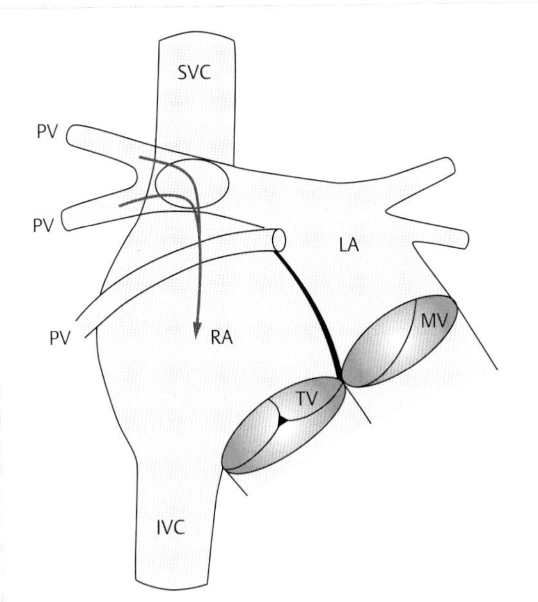

Fig. 15.2 Superior sinus venosus defect.[1]
In the upper sinus venosus defect, part of the wall between the right superior vena cava and the right upper pulmonary veins is missing, so that blood from the pulmonary veins reaches the right atrium. The connection between the two atria develops in the area where the right upper pulmonary veins normally connect to the left atrium.
SVC, superior vena cava; IVC, inferior vena cava; PV, pulmonary vein; RA, right atrium; LA, left atrium; TV, tricuspid valve; MV, mitral valve.

missing. This allows the blood from the left atrium to reach the coronary sinus and from there, the right atrium. As a result of the increased blood flow, the ostium of the coronary sinus is widened. The coronary sinus defect is almost always associated with a left persistent superior vena cava. It often occurs with a total anomalous pulmonary venous connection or heterotaxy syndromes.

- *Patent foramen ovale* (PFO): A PFO can be found in almost one-third of the population. It occurs when there is incomplete fusion of the ostium primum with the ostium secundum. There is no left-to-right shunt in a PFO. The foramen ovale may open like a valve when the pressure in the right atrium exceeds the pressure of the left atrium (e.g., during Valsalva maneuver, diving, or if there is pulmonary hypertension with high right atrial pressures). In this way venous thrombi from the right atrium can pass to the left atrium and cause systemic embolism (paradoxical embolism). The risk for this seems to be higher when the atrial septum in the oval fossa is widened by an aneurysm (atrial septum aneurysm). The relationship between PFO and migraine has also been discussed, although the exact pathological mechanism is still unclear.

Hemodynamics

There is a left-to-right shunt at the atrial level. The shunt direction is determined by the pressure difference in the atria, which in turn is dependent on the compliance of the ventricles and on the resistance in the pulmonary and the systemic circulatory system. The right ventricle normally has a better diastolic elasticity than the muscular left ventricle, so the pressure in the left atrium is higher than in the right atrium. This leads to a left-to-right shunt at atrial level left-to-right shunt with an increased volume overload in the right ventricle and pulmonary circulatory system.

After the drop in pulmonary vascular resistance beyond the neonatal period, the left-to-right shunt continues to increase. In a larger shunt there is a relative pulmonary stenosis (gradient usually 15–20 mmHg higher than the gradient across the aortic valves), because more blood passes through the pulmonary valve than the aortic valve. Likewise, tricuspid insufficiency can occur due to the volume-related dilatation of the right ventricle.

Associated Anomalies

ASDs occur in isolation or in combination with almost all congenital heart defects. Of particular importance are:

- Partial anomalous pulmonary venous connections: almost always present with sinus venosus defects, rarely with ASD II as well
- Persistent left superior vena cava
- Valvular or infundibular pulmonary stenosis
- Patent ductus arteriosus (PDA)
- Mitral valve anomalies—for example, cleft of the mitral valve associated with ASD I or a mitral valve prolapse associated with ASD II

Associated Syndromes

▸ **Lutembacher syndrome (extremely rare).** In Lutembacher syndrome there is a combination of an ASD II and an acquired or congenital mitral stenosis. Due to the mitral stenosis, the left-to-right shunt at the atrial level is more pronounced than with an isolated ASD.

▸ **Holt–Oram syndrome.** Holt–Oram syndrome is a combination of a heart defect (often an ASD) and a unilateral malformation of the forearm or hand (e.g., aplasia/hypoplasia of the radius or missing thumb).

15.1.2 Diagnostic Measures

Symptoms

Most children with an ASD are asymptomatic. Often the ASD is discovered as an incidental finding or the only symptom is a heart murmur. The symptoms depend on the size of the shunt. If there is a large shunt, the typical symptoms are:

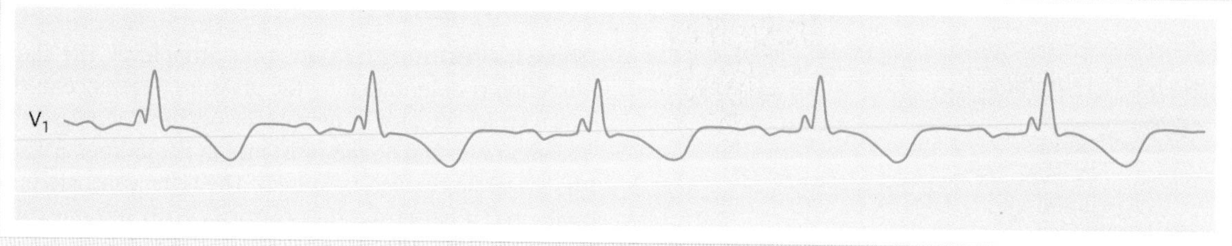

Fig. 15.3 Typical ECG associated with an ASD II. In a relevant ASD II there is typically an incomplete right bundle branch block with rsR′ configuration.

- Recurrent pulmonary infections (often the only symptom in childhood)
- slender body constitution and pale skin
- signs of congestive heart failure such as failure to thrive, poor feeding, and tachypnea or impaired physical capacity with dyspnea on exertion, which occur only if there is a large left-to-right shunt and are rare before the child reaches the toddler stage

Complications

Depending on the size of the shunt, in the long term, the increasing dilatation of the right atrium and ventricle leads to atrial arrhythmia, right ventricular failure, pulmonary congestion, and pulmonary hypertension. Paradoxical embolism may also occur.

Auscultation

The typical auscultation finding is fixed splitting of the second heart sound independent of respiration (not to be confused with the physiological respiratory-dependent split second heart sound) and a relative pulmonary stenosis murmur (2/6–3/6 systolic murmur with point of maximum impulse [PMI] in the 2nd–3rd left parasternal intercostal space [ICS]).

In a very large shunt there is also a rumbling, low-frequency diastolic bruit with PMI in the 4th left parasternal ICS as a sign of a relative tricuspid valve stenosis.

In an ASD I, there is often also a systolic mitral regurgitation murmur.

ECG

Typical ECG findings:

- Right axis deviation. However, in an ASD I there is typically a left axis deviation due to a shift in the conduction system.
- Incomplete right bundle branch block due to increased right ventricular volume (rSR′ configuration in V_1, ▶ Fig. 15.3). This finding should not be confused with the physiological Rsr′ configuration in V_1 in infancy.
- Signs of volume related hypertrophy of the right ventricle (slightly elevated R wave in the right precordial leads, deep and wide S wave in the left precordial leads), possibly abnormal repolarization in the right precordial leads (flattened T wave, T wave inversion, ST depression).
- AV block I (typical for ASD I, otherwise rare).
- An atrial rhythm with a P axis less than 30° is typical for a sinus venosus defect.
- Atrial arrhythmias such as atrial flutter or fibrillation may occur in adults.

Chest X-ray

Depending on the size of the shunt, there is moderate cardiomegaly, increased pulmonary vascular markings, a prominent right heart silhouette due to the enlarged right atrium, and a right ventricle that forms the left border of the heart with a rounded and elevated cardiac apex.

Echocardiography

Echocardiography is the diagnostic method of choice. Larger patients may require transesophageal echocardiography.

Echocardiography should be used to detect or exclude:

- Location and type of the atrial septal defect (▶ Fig. 15.4)
- Detection of a shunt using color Doppler
- Enlargement of the right atrium, right ventricle, and pulmonary artery
- Flattened or even paradoxical ventricular septal motion in M mode as a sign of volume overload. A paradoxical septal motion is evident when, during the systole, the ventricular septum moves away from the dorsal wall of the left ventricle and contracts in the direction of the right ventricle. The septum thus "helps" to empty the enlarged right ventricle
- Associated anomalies—for example, mitral valve cleft in ASD I, partial anomalous pulmonary venous connections in sinus venosus defects, or persistent left superior vena cava associated with a coronary sinus defect

Echocardiography should also be used:

- To visualize the distances of the defect borders to the adjacent structures (caudal: AV valves; cranial: superior vena cava; anterior: aorta; posterior: pulmonary vein).

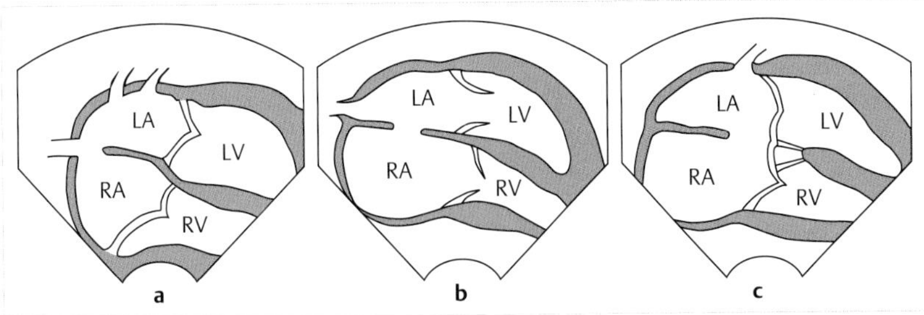

Fig. 15.4 Location of different ASDs in echocardiography in the subcostal longitudinal axis inverted view. **a** Superior sinus venosus defect. **b** ASD II. **c** ASD I.
LA, left atrium; LV, left ventricle; RA, right atrium; RV, right ventricle.[29]

It is especially important to visualize the spatial relationship of the defect borders to the adjacent structures for interventional closure.

- Caution: An superior sinus venosus defect can often be visualized only from the subcostal area. An indirect indication of a sinus venosus defect is a large right ventricle without any other obvious cause. If the right ventricle is enlarged, a partial anomalous pulmonary venous connection must also be considered as a differential diagnosis.

Cardiac Catheterization

Cardiac catheterization is not usually necessary for purely diagnostic reasons. When in doubt it is used to answer the following questions:

- To quantify shunts
- To exclude or detect associated anomalies (in particular anomalous pulmonary venous connections)
- To measure pressure in pulmonary circulation, possibly testing pulmonary vascular responsiveness

Cardiac catheterization is now performed almost only as interventional therapy for a typical ASD II.

MRI

In ambiguous cases (e.g., sinus venosus defect), an MRI scan can help locate the defect and detect or rule out associated anomalies. In addition, the shunt can be quantified.

15.1.3 Treatment

Conservative Treatment

Conservative treatment is rarely needed. Exceptional cases may need pharmacological treatment for heart failure.

Indications for ASD closure

- Any sign of right ventricular enlargement (dilatation of the right ventricle or paradoxical septal motion in echocardiography)
- Left-to-right shunt of more than 30% of the Q_P or Q_P: $Q_S > 1.5{:}1$
- Signs of congestive heart failure such as reduced capacity or delayed physical development
- Following a paradoxical embolism

An ASD is generally closed in preschool children between the ages of 3 and 5, earlier if it is symptomatic. In adults the closure can be performed electively after the diagnosis has been established.

► **Contraindication.** Closure of an ASD is contraindicated if pulmonary resistance is massively increased. Then a right-to-left shunt is necessary to make sure that there is sufficient cardiac output for systemic circulation. Due to the increased pulmonary resistance, sufficient blood cannot pass the lung to the left atrium. Filling the left atrium and the left ventricle is dependent on a right-to-left shunt across the ASD. Because of the right-to-left shunt, however, these patients are cyanotic.

Interventional Catheterization

Interventional catheterization is the method of choice for most cases of ASD II or patent foramen ovale. Usually, a double umbrella occluder system is implanted transvenously to close the defect. The residual atrial septum defects (ASD I, sinus venosus defects, coronary sinus defects) are not eligible for interventional catheter closure due to the lack of the border required for anchoring the double umbrella system.

Note

As a rule of thumb: If it has a sufficient rim area, an ASD II is suitable for an interventional catheterization closure when the maximal defect diameter (measured in mm) does not exceed the body weight (measured in kg). For example, most defects with a diameter up to 15 mm in a child weighing 15 kg can be closed by interventional catheterization (► Fig. 15.5).

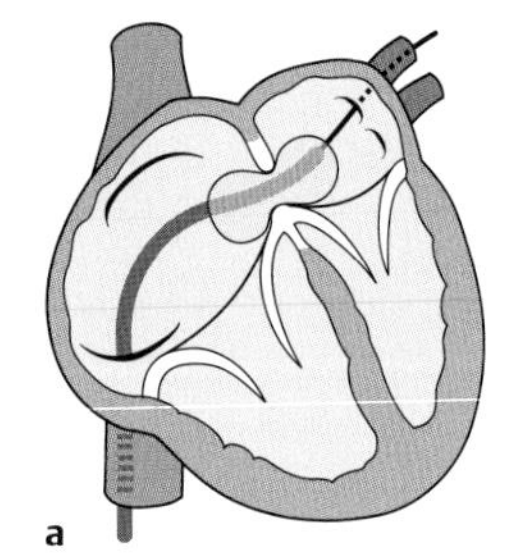

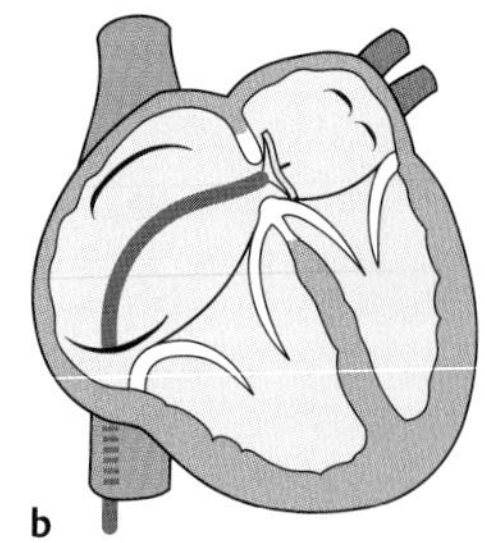

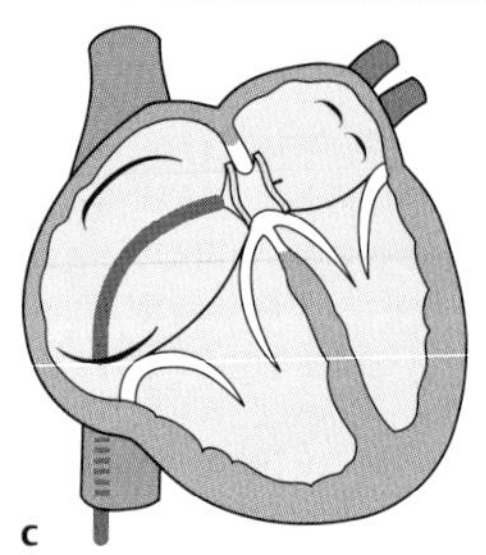

Fig. 15.5 Interventional catheter closure of an ASD II using a double umbrella occluder system. **a** First the size of the defect is measured with a balloon. **b** Then a catheter with a double umbrella is advanced through the defect into the left atrium. The left atrial part of the umbrella is unfolded and pulled up against the atrial septum. **c** Finally, the middle and the right atrial parts are unfolded before detaching the umbrella from the catheter.

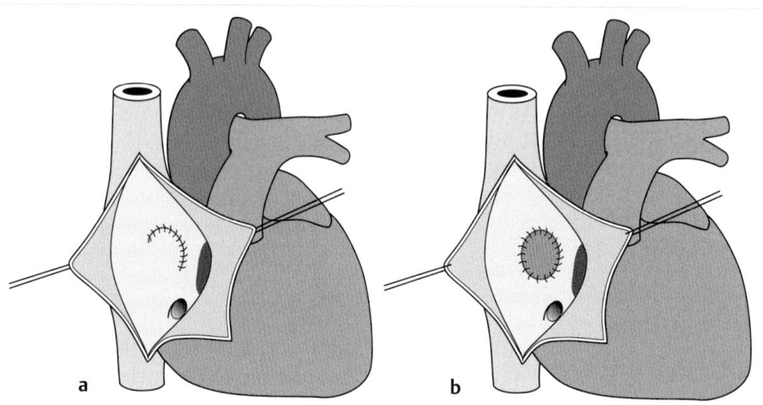

Fig. 15.6 Operative closure of an ASD. **a** Closure of an ASD with direct suture. **b** Closure of an ASD with a patch.

Surgery

If an interventional catheterization closure is not possible, the defect is closed by direct suturing or with a patch (mostly from autologous pericardium) under cardiopulmonary bypass (▶ Fig. 15.6). A median sternotomy is performed as an access route. Other cosmetically more favorable access routes are from anterolateral (right inframammary fold) or posterior access. Here, however, there is an increased risk of complications. In some centers the operation is also performed as a minimally invasive procedure.

15.1.4 Prognosis and Outcome

▶ **Long-term outcome.** Spontaneous closures of ASD II are common, in particular in small central defects of maximum 3 to 5 mm. Defects with a diameter of over 6 mm very rarely close spontaneously. Sinus venosus defects, ASD Is, and coronary sinus defects never close spontaneously.

The former average life expectancy without therapy was around 37 to 40 years. If the correction is performed before early adulthood, life expectancy is normal. If the correction is performed at a later time, statistical life expectancy is lower. Some of the reasons for this are arrhythmias and progressive pulmonary hypertension. Practically all patients with no contraindications benefit from an ASD closure even at a later stage.

The mortality rate of operative treatment or interventional catheterization in childhood is well below 1%; in uncomplicated cases in adulthood about 2%. Possible postoperative long-term effects are arrhythmias requiring treatment (e.g., sinus node dysfunction, atrial flutter/fibrillation), which in some cases may occur years after surgery.

There is a risk of paradoxical embolism if there are small defects that are not closed or a patent foramen ovale.

▶ **Outpatient follow-up.** Before correction, asymptomatic children need to be monitored only at longer intervals (e.g., annually). After surgery, they should first be monitored more frequently, then usually annually. Atrial arrhythmias should be observed.

Endocarditis prophylaxis is necessary in the first 6 months after interventional catheterization or operative closure with foreign material. If there are residual defects in the area of the foreign material, lifelong prophylaxis is required.

▶ **Physical capacity and lifestyle.** In an uncomplicated ASD and after a timely closure, physical capacity is normal.

► **Special aspects in adolescents and adults.** Clinical symptoms occur in patients if the defect was not corrected in time, usually as a result of a right heart failure, atrial arrhythmias (sick sinus syndrome, atrial flutter/fibrillation), pulmonary hypertension, or paradoxical embolism. Adults have a higher perioperative risk, especially if there is accompanying impaired (usually transient) left ventricular compliance. In adults, arrhythmias frequently persist despite successful correction.

15.2 Ventricular Septal Defects

15.2.1 Basics

Synonym: abnormal opening between the ventricles

Definition

A ventricular septal defect (VSD) is an interventricular connection. A VSD can occur in isolation or as an accompanying anomaly with complex heart defects.

Epidemiology

A VSD is the most common congenital heart defect, constituting up to 40% of all congenital heart defects. There is an accompanying anomaly in about half of these cases. Women are affected slightly more frequently than men.

Pathogenesis

A VSD is caused by a malformation of the interventricular septum during the first 7 weeks of gestation. The exact cause is usually unknown. A VSD can also occur in association with chromosome anomalies (e.g., trisomy 13, 18, 21) or other genetic diseases (e.g., Holt–Oram syndrome). Acquired VSDs following a cardiac contusion, a gunshot or knife wound, or myocardial infarction are rare.

Classification

The ventricular septum consists of the small high membranous septum and the larger muscular septum. The muscular septum has three segments:

- Inlet septum
- Trabecular septum
- Outlet septum (= infundibular septum, conus septum)

Various VSDs are described, depending on the location of the defect in the ventricular septum (► Fig. 15.7). However, the nomenclature is not uniform and is complicated by numerous terms that are sometimes used synonymously. The following classification has proven useful in practice.

► **Perimembranous VSD.** Synonyms: subaortic, infracristal, or membranous VSD. Perimembranous VSDs affect the membranous septum. They usually extend somewhat beyond the membranous septum into adjacent areas of the ventricular septum and are therefore termed perimembranous. They constitute approximately 70% of all VSDs.

The rare Gerbode defect is a special form of perimembranous VSD with a shunt between the left ventricle and right atrium (► Fig. 15.8). Such a shunt is possible because part of the membranous septum separates the left ventricle from the right atrium due to the difference in levels of the AV valves.

► **Muscular VSD.** Synonyms: trabecular, apical VSD. Muscular VSDs are in the trabecular segment of the muscular septum. These defects frequently occur in multiples (an extreme case is a Swiss cheese septum). With the improvement in diagnostic methods, the number of muscular VSDs detected, some of which are very small, has increased, but they frequently close spontaneously.

► **Infundibular VSD.** Synonyms: outlet, subpulmonary, supracristal, doubly-committed, subarterial VSD. In an infundibular VSD, there is a gap in the outlet septum below the aortic and pulmonary valves. There is a risk that the aortic valve cusp may prolapse into the VSD, leading to aortic insufficiency. In Western nations, the incidence of infundibular VSD is only 5 to 8%, but up to 30% in Asia.

► **Inlet VSD.** Synonym: AV canal type VSD. An inlet VSD is located in the inlet septum, that is, relatively posterior. It is limited from above by the tricuspid valve annulus. An inlet VSD occurs typically with an AV septal defect (AV canal), but can also occur in isolation. Inlet VSDs constitute 5 to 8% of all VSDs.

► **Malalignment VSD.** In a malalignment VSD there is an abnormal displacement of the outflow tract septum with the result that the semilunar valve overrides the VSD. Malalignment VSDs never occur in isolation, but are always associated with other cardiac anomalies. Typical examples are tetralogy of Fallot (aorta overrides the VSD) or truncus arteriosus (truncus valve overrides the VSD).

Hemodynamics

The hemodynamics in a VSD depends on the size of the VSD and the resistance in the systemic and pulmonary circulation. If the pressures are normal, the VSD leads to a left-to-right shunt at the ventricular level. This results in excessive pulmonary blood flow and volume overload in the left ventricle. The size of a VSD is often indicated in relation to the diameter of the aortic root:

- Small (restrictive) VSDs are less than 50% of the diameter of the aortic root.
- Mid-sized VSDs have 50 to 100% of the diameter of the aortic root.
- Large VSDs constitute more than 100% of the diameter of the aortic root.

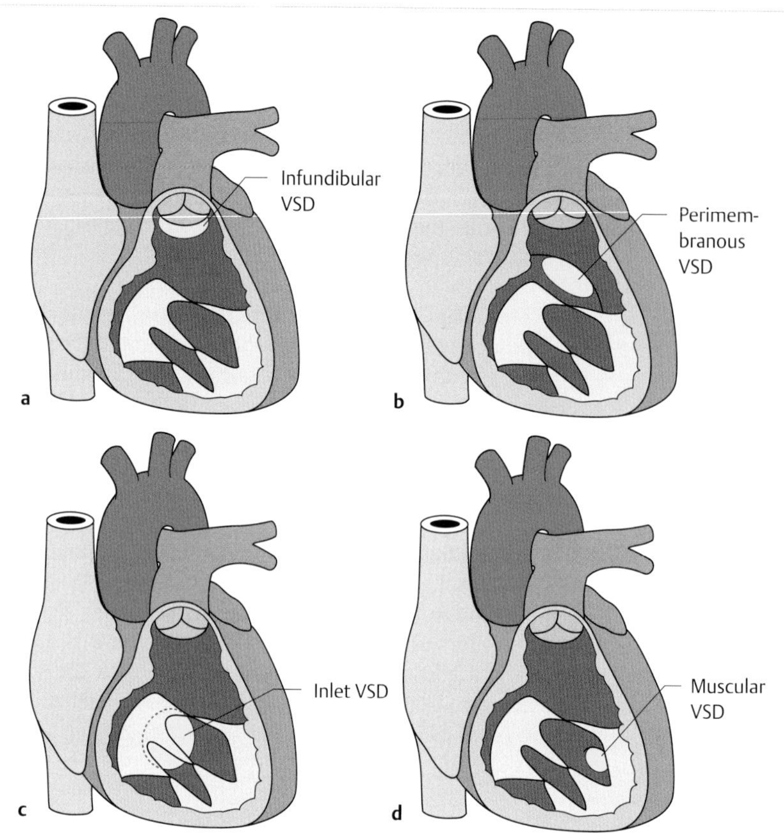

Fig. 15.7 Sites of the ventricular septal defects (VSDs). View of the different segments of the ventricular septum from the open right ventricle. **a** The infundibular VSD is located in the vicinity of the outlet septum directly below the pulmonary valve, but in close proximity to the aortic valve. **b** The perimembranous VSD is located in the membranous septum, but often extends into the adjacent segments of the septum. It is located below the aortic valve and in the vicinity of the septal leaflet of the tricuspid valve. **c** The typical inlet VSD is located relatively far to the posterior in the inlet septum and extends up to the tricuspid valve annulus. **d** Muscular VSDs are surrounded on all sides by the muscular septum. They sometimes occur in multiples.

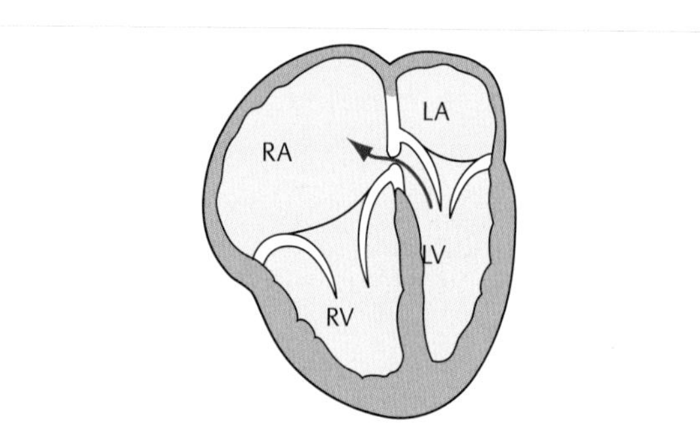

Fig. 15.8 Gerbode defect. The tricuspid valve is located further in an apical direction in the ventricle than the mitral valve. Part of the left ventricle thus borders the right atrium. A defect in this area that leads to a shunt from the left ventricle to the right atrium is called a Gerbode defect. LA, left atrium; LV, left ventricle; RA, right atrium; RV, right ventricle.

In mid-sized defects, the volume overload of the left ventricle is most significant; as the defect becomes larger, pressure overload of the pulmonary circulation and the right ventricle increase. If the diameter of the VSD exceeds 50 to 75% of the diameter of the aortic root, the pressure between the two ventricles is equalized (pressure-equalizing VSD). Then the shunt is determined only by pulmonary resistance, which increases steadily as a result of the volume overload of the pulmonary circulation. This ultimately results in the Eisenmenger reaction, which is a reversal of the shunt across the VSD. This results in a right-to-left shunt with cyanosis.

In VSDs near the aortic valve, the lack of resistance may cause the aortic valve leaflets to prolapse in the VSD, resulting in aortic insufficiency.

Associated Anomalies

VSDs often occur as an additional anomaly in almost all complex defects—for example, d-TGA, ccTGA, pulmonary atresia, pulmonary stenosis, coarctation of the aorta, AV valve anomalies, PDA, ASD, tetralogy of Fallot, or truncus arteriosus communis.

Associated Syndromes

VSDs occur frequently in many genetic syndromes (e.g., trisomy 13, 18, 21, deletions, Goldenhaar syndrome). They also occur in connection with an alcohol embryopathy, but 95% of VSDs are not associated with chromosomal anomalies or syndromes.

15.2.2 Diagnostic Measures

Symptoms

The symptoms depend on the size of the defect and the pressures in systemic and pulmonary circulation. Small, not hemodynamically relevant VSDs are asymptomatic. They are generally noticed only due to the murmur on auscultation finding.

In large hemodynamically relevant VSDs, there are signs of congestive heart failure such as tachypnea or dyspnea, intercostal retractions, hepatomegaly, increased sweating, poor feeding, and failure to thrive. A systolic thrill can also be palpated at the left sternal border. The first symptoms usually occur when pulmonary vascular resistance decreases at around age 6 to 8 weeks.

Complications

If there is a large VSD, congestive heart failure can occur in early infancy. A large left-to-right shunt with excessive pulmonary blood flow leads to pulmonary hypertension. Due to the subsequent reduction of the shunt, there then appears to be an improvement in the clinical symptoms. The time at which pulmonary hypertension develops depends not only on the volume of the shunt, but also on the associated heart defects as well. Pulmonary hypertension becomes manifest especially early in children with an AV canal, d-TGA with VSD, or truncus arteriosus.

In VSD, a stenosis can also develop occasionally in the right ventricular outflow tract (double-chambered right ventricle). This obstruction sometimes does not develop until after corrective surgery. This stenosis of the right ventricular outflow tract is also described as the Gasul transformation.

Note

In infundibular or, more rarely, perimembranous VSDs there is a risk of developing aortic insufficiency, which in itself is an indication for surgery.

Bacterial endocarditis can occur, especially at the side of the right ventricle opposite the defect (jet lesion).

Auscultation

Note

If the pressure between the two ventricles is equalized—for example, in large nonrestrictive VSDs or already existing pulmonary hypertension—no typical systolic murmur can be auscultated.

There is a typical rough, band-shaped holosystolic murmur with PMI in the 3rd to 4th left parasternal ICS (frequently louder than 3/6) on auscultation. If there is a large left-to-right shunt, a low-amplitude, mesodiastolic murmur can be heard over the cardiac apex as a sign of a relative mitral stenosis. A pronounced second heart sound is a sign of pulmonary hypertension and must be interpreted as an alarm signal. In addition, a diastolic decrescendo murmur at the left sternal border, which can be a sign of aortic insufficiency, should be noted.

ECG

The ECG is unremarkable if the defect is small. In larger defects, there are signs of left ventricular volume overload. There is also frequently a P sinistroatriale. When the pressure increases in the right ventricle, signs of right ventricular hypertrophy also develop.

Chest X-ray

The X-ray is unremarkable if the defect is small. In larger VSDs, cardiomegaly develops in relation to the size of the shunt with dilatation of the left atrium and ventricle. There is lateral inferior displacement of the cardiac apex. The pulmonary artery segment is prominent due to volume overload; pulmonary vascular markings are increased and can be detected up to the periphery of the lungs. Additional right ventricular hypertrophy with prominent pulmonary arteries is an important indication of pulmonary hypertension.

Echocardiography

Echocardiography including color Doppler ultrasound is the diagnostic method of choice. It usually allows the number, size, and location of the defects to be reliably determined. Associated cardiac defects can also be ruled out.

Using CW Doppler and the Bernoulli equation, it is possible to estimate the pressure gradients across the defect. The VSD is said to be restrictive if the estimated restrictive ventricular pressure via the VSD flow is normal.

The pressure can also be calculated across the VSD (BP_{syst} -pressure gradient across the VSD) or estimated by the degree of valve insufficiency if the tricuspid valve is insufficient. The size of the left atrium and ventricle are indirect indications of the size of the shunt.

The typical sites of the VSD in echocardiography are listed in ▶ Fig. 15.9.

▶ **Perimembranous VSD.** This type can be best visualized in the parasternal long axis immediately below the aortic valve or in the parasternal short axis between the 9 and 12 o'clock positions. The apical five-chamber view also affords good visualization. These defects are sometimes concealed by a structure resembling an aneurysm. This is tissue from the septal tricuspid valve leaflet. This is sometimes called an "aneurysmal tissue tag (partially) obstructing a VSD" although the term "aneurysmal" is not correct from a pathological standpoint.

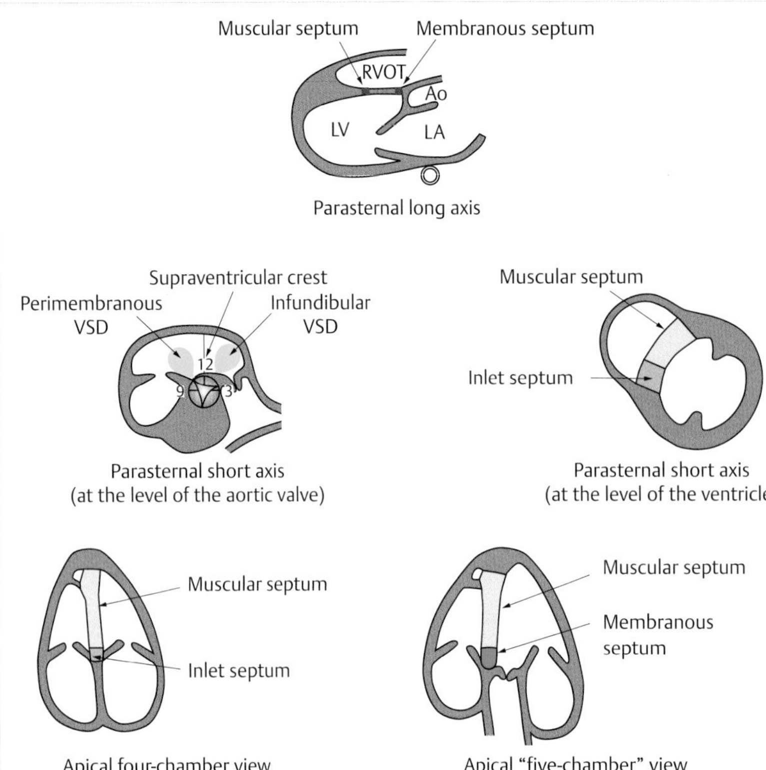

Fig. 15.9 Location of the ventricular septal defects (VSDs) in echocardiography. (Adapted from Eidem et al. 2009)[117]
The typical perimembranous VSD can be best visualized in the parasternal long axis below the aortic arch. Perimembranous and infundibular VSDs can be readily differentiated in the parasternal short axis—a perimembranous VSD is located between the 9 and 12 o'clock positions in the parasternal short axis, but an infundibular VSD between the 12 and 3 o'clock positions. Inlet VSDs can be readily visualized in the immediate vicinity of the AV valves in the four-chamber view by tilting in a posterior direction. Muscular VSDs can generally be detected in the four-chamber view or by following the ventricular septum in the parasternal short axes. Ao, aorta; LA, left atrium; LV, left ventricle; RVOT, right ventricular outflow tract.

▸ **Muscular VSD.** These VSDs can be readily visualized in the parasternal short axes and in the four-chamber view. With muscular defects, it is important to note whether there are one or more defects. Due to trabecularization of the right ventricle, larger muscular VSDs can appear as multiple defects in a color Doppler image.

▸ **Infundibular VSD.** Infundibular VSDs are located in the parasternal short axis between the 12 and 3 o'clock positions in the vicinity of the aortic valve. A leaflet of the aortic valve can prolapse into the defect and lead to aortic insufficiency.

▸ **Inlet VSD.** Inlet VSDs are located posteriorly in the area of the tricuspid valve annulus and can be readily visualized in the four-chamber view by tilting backward.

To assess the size of a VSD, its relation to the diameter of the aortic valve annulus can be used (see Hemodynamics above).

Cardiac Catheterization

Most VSDs can be reliably diagnosed using echocardiography. Cardiac catheterization is indicated only if the exact number or location of VSDs cannot be determined or there are presumed to be additional cardiac anomalies, or if the hemodynamic relevance (in particular increased pulmonary resistance) cannot be reliably assessed. Some VSDs can also be closed by interventional catheterization.

Pulse oximetry shows an increase in oxygen saturation in the right ventricle and pulmonary artery if there is a left-to-right shunt. Using the Fick principle, the shunt and the systemic-to-pulmonary blood flow ratio can be calculated. If there is a relevant VSD, there is an increase in left atrial pressure and left ventricular end-diastolic pressure. The pulmonary arterial pressure is also measured and the pulmonary vascular resistance calculated.

The VSD can be detected and precisely located in an angiography after injecting contrast medium into the left ventricle. It is important to note any potential aortic insufficiency.

In patients with elevated pulmonary vascular resistance, the examination may be supplemented by testing vasodilator responsiveness (Chapter 21).

MRI

An MRI is only rarely needed to clarify anatomical details in an isolated VSD.

15.2.3 Treatment

Conservative Treatment

In hemodynamically relevant defects, congestive heart failure is treated pharmacologically until surgery. The conservative treatment of an Eisenmenger reaction is discussed in Chapter 22.

Indications for Closure

- In a large left-to-right shunt with clinical symptoms (frequent pulmonary infections, failure to thrive, congestive heart failure that cannot be managed pharmacologically) the defect is closed in infancy.
- For older asymptomatic children with normal pulmonary pressures, surgery is indicated for a left-to-right shunt of over 40% of cardiac output if the Qp/Qs ratio is over 1.5, or if the left atrium and ventricle are dilated.
- In a VSD with secondary aortic insufficiency or aortic valve prolapse into the VSD, immediate surgery is always indicated; otherwise there is a risk that the valve may have to be replaced.
- Incipient pulmonary hypertension is also an indication for closure.

▸ **Contraindications.** VSD closure is contraindicated if there is fixed pulmonary hypertension (Eisenmenger reaction).

Surgery

The defect is usually closed with a patch; smaller defects may be closed by direct sutures. To avoid a ventriculotomy, a surgical access route across the right atrium and tricuspid valve (transtricuspid) is usually selected.

In isolated cases such as multiple defects ("Swiss cheese VSD") or complex accompanying cardiac anomalies, or if there are contraindications to cardiopulmonary bypass surgery, pulmonary artery banding may be performed as a palliative interim measure to reduce the excessive pulmonary blood flow.

The procedure if there is a VSD combined with coarctation of the aorta or a large PDA is controversial. In infancy, the aortic coarctation or the PDA may first be corrected without cardiopulmonary bypass. The VSD surgery is performed later, for example, at the age of 2 to 3 months. If there is a large, hemodynamically relevant VSD, a one-time procedure must also be considered. For Eisenmenger reaction, heart–lung transplant is the last treatment option.

Interventional Catheterization

Interventional catheterization closure using double umbrella occluder systems or special coils can be performed only for selected defects and is not yet a routine procedure in most centers (Chapter 24).

15.2.4 Prognosis and Outcome

▸ **Long-term outcome.** The rate of spontaneous closure is high, especially for smaller muscular defects and perimembranous defects. Within 2 years, 80 to 90% of small muscular defects and up to 50% of perimembranous defects close. Perimembranous VSDs are often (partially) covered by the growth of tricuspid valve tissue.

Note

VSDs do not become larger, but they occasionally become smaller or close spontaneously. Infundibular, inlet, and malalignment VSDs do not close spontaneously.

The perioperative mortality is less than 1% for uncomplicated cases, but can be considerably higher for critically ill neonates and infants.

There is a risk of a postoperative complete AV block, especially for perimembranous and inlet defects in which the bundle of His is in the vicinity of the defect border. This problem frequently occurs only temporarily in the first 1 to 2 weeks after surgery. A right bundle branch block occurs in 90% of cases after a ventriculotomy; in 20 to 50% of cases following transatrial/transtricuspid closure.

Tricuspid insufficiency can occur if the septal tricuspid leaflet had to be separated from the defect during surgery.

A residual defect occasionally remains, but is usually not hemodynamically relevant. There may also be a secondary residual defect due to suture rupture.

Tension on the septum can also cause postoperative obstruction of the outflow tract. This risk is present mainly in infundibular defects.

There may very rarely be a progressive increase in pulmonary vascular resistance and an Eisenmenger reaction despite closure of the VSD, mainly after a delayed operation.

▸ **Outpatient follow-up.** For small defects where no congestive heart failure develops during the first year of life and there are no signs of pulmonary hypertension, the examinations can be scheduled at greater intervals (e.g., every 1–2 years). At these checkups, the size of the VSD should be documented and special attention given to any indication of aortic insufficiency or prolapse of the aortic valve into the defect.

Hemodynamically relevant defects must be monitored more closely until surgery so that anticongestive medication can be adjusted if necessary to prevent the development of pulmonary hypertension.

Lifelong postoperative checkups are needed. Rhythm disorders (e.g., AV block), ventricular function, residual shunts, aortic insufficiency, and signs of pulmonary hypertension should be noted. Once a certain period has passed since surgery, checkups once or twice a year are enough. Endocarditis prophylaxis should be given postoperatively for the first 6 months if foreign material was used, and permanently if there are residual defects in the vicinity of the foreign material.

► **Physical capacity and lifestyle.** Physical capacity and development are not impaired after the timely successful closure of a small VSD. The patient may participate in sports without any restrictions 3 to 6 months after surgery if the defect was completely closed or only a small residual defect remains, ventricular function is good, and there is no evidence of pulmonary hypertension or relevant arrhythmias.

Pulmonary hypertension is a serious disease that impairs physical capacity significantly (Chapter 21).

► **Special aspects in adolescents and adults.** Fixed pulmonary hypertension (Eisenmenger reaction) usually develops in adolescence in patients with an isolated, uncorrected, and hemodynamically relevant VSD, but can occur much sooner in some heart defects associated with a VSD (e.g., d-TGA with VSD, complete AV canal). If corrective surgery is performed late, after moderate or severe pulmonary hypertension has already developed, the pulmonary hypertension is likely to progress. If the closure is performed late, there is also a greater risk of ventricular arrhythmias and sudden cardiac death.

15.3 Atrioventricular Septal Defect

15.3.1 Basics

Synonyms: AV canal, endocardial cushion defect

Definition

An atrioventricular septal defect (AVSD) is a development disorder of varying degrees affecting mainly the segments of the atrial and ventricular septum near the AV valve and the AV valves themselves. These structures arise from the endocardial cushion during embryonic development.

Typical features of an AVSD:

- Anomaly of the atrioventricular septum (segments of the atrial and ventricular septum near the AV valve)
- Common AV valve for both ventricles with a variable number of leaflets and openings
- Abnormal position and elongation of the ventricular outflow tract ("goose neck" deformity). In an AVSD, the aorta is located anterior to the single common AV valve, not wedged between the mitral and tricuspid valve.
- Displacement of the AV node and excitation conduction system

Epidemiology

AVSDs constitute 4 to 5% of all congenital heart defects. The incidence is 0.2 per 1,000 live births.

Note

An AVSD is frequently associated with Down syndrome (trisomy 21). Nearly half of patients with an AVSD suffer from Down syndrome and, conversely, around 40% of all patients with Down syndrome have a relevant heart defect, half of which involve an AVSD. Patients with Down syndrome usually have more favorable valve morphology for corrective surgery and fewer additional left heart defects.

Pathogenesis and Pathology

AVSD is caused by a developmental disorder of the embryonic endocardial cushion with anomaly of the segments of the atrial and ventricular septum near the AV valves (atrioventricular septum) and the AV valves including the leaflets, tendinous cords, and papillary muscles.

Only a single AV valve develops, which can, however, have one or two openings (see below: classification in partial and complete types). The AV valve usually consists of a total of five leaflets. The bridging leaflets are of particular significance. There is an anterior and a posterior bridging leaflet. These bridging leaflets bridge a defect in the segments of the atrial and ventricular septum and connect the left and right ventricular segments (► Fig. 15.10). The bridging leaflets play an important role in classifying the types of AVSD (► Fig. 15.11).

Classification

► **Partial AVSD.** In a partial AVSD there is only one hole in the atrial septum near the AV valve. The defect in the ventricular septum is closed by a tissue bridge that also connects the two bridging leaflets of the common AV valve. This results in a cleft in the mitral valve. Strictly speaking, the term "mitral valve" is incorrect, as even in a partial AVSD, there is only one AV valve with no separation into a mitral and a tricuspid valve. However, this common AV valve has two openings and this "cleft" leads to a hemodynamic "mitral valve insufficiency."

► **Intermediate AVSD.** In an intermediate AVSD there are two separate openings in a common AV valve. The two bridging leaflets are adjoined, similar to a partial AVSD. In addition, there is a defect in the atrial septum directly above the AV valve and a ventricular septal defect in the inlet septum directly below the AV valve level. The VSD is often restrictive in an intermediate AVSD.

► **Complete AVSD.** In a complete AVSD, there is an atrial septal defect directly above the AV valve level and a nonrestrictive VSD in the inlet septum directly below the AV valve level. The AV valve has a common opening. The left

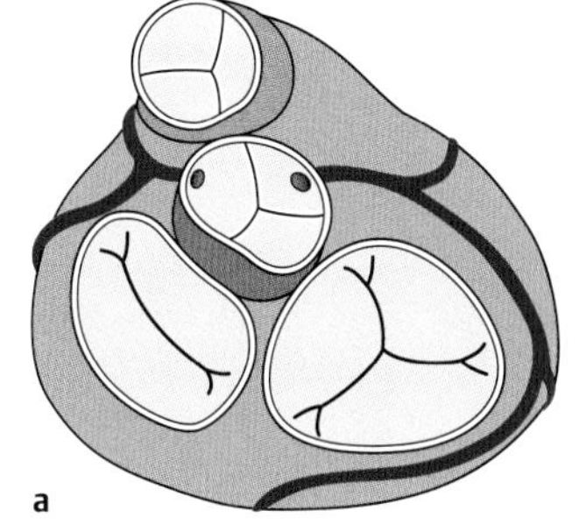

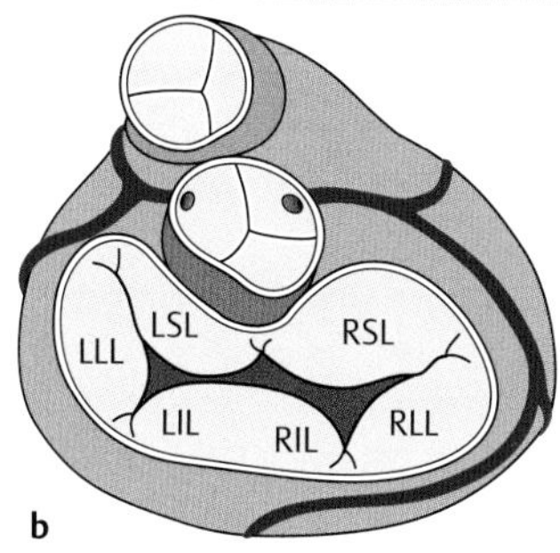

Fig. 15.10 AV and semilunar valves in a normal heart (**a**) and in a complete AVSD (**b**).[36]
In the view from above, two separate AV valves can be seen in a normal heart. The aortic valve is wedged between the mitral and tricuspid valves. In an AVSD, the aortic valve is located anterior to the single common AV valve. The anterior and posterior bridging leaflets bridge the septal defect and thus connect both ventricles. LSL, left superior leaflet (anterior bridging leaflet); LLL, left lateral leaflet; RSL, right superior leaflet (anterior leaflet); RLL, right lateral leaflet; LIL, left inferior leaflet; RIL, right inferior leaflet. (LIL and RIL together are also called the posterior bridging leaflet.)

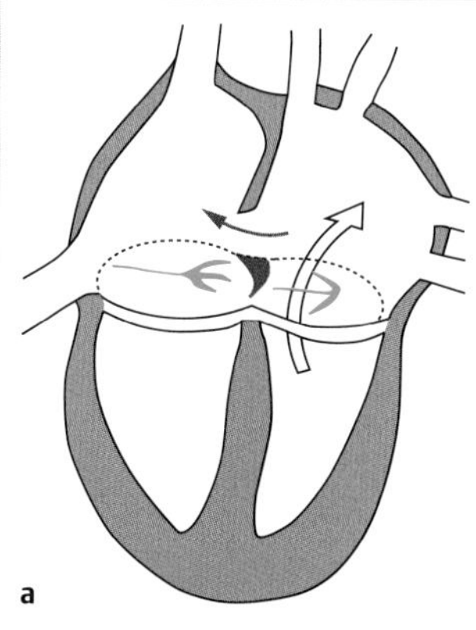

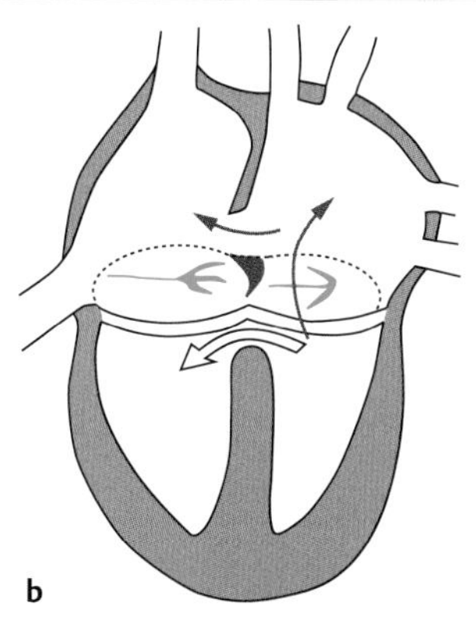

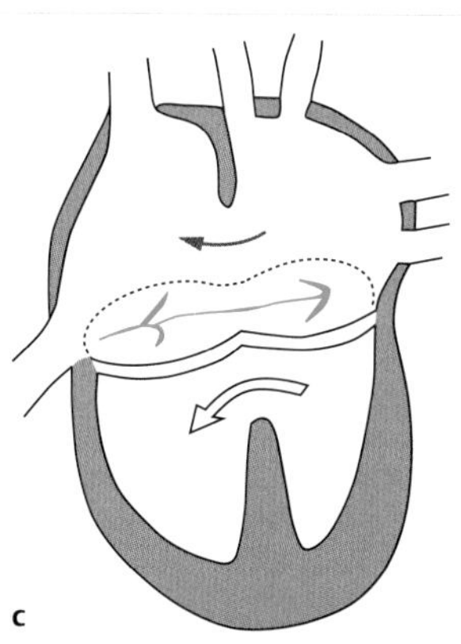

Fig. 15.11 Schematic drawing of partial, intermediate, and complete AVSDs. **a** In a partial AVSD there is a defect in the segment of the atrial septum near the AV valve. The AV valve has two openings. There is a cleft in the mitral valve. **b** An intermediate AVSD has defects in the atrial and ventricular septal segments near the AV valve. The defect in the ventricular septum is often restrictive. There are functionally two valve annuli. **c** In a complete AVSD there are defects in the segments of the atrial and ventricular septa near the AV valve. The defect in the ventricular septum is generally not restrictive. There is one AV valve with only one opening.

and right ventricular segments of the AV valve are connected by an anterior and a posterior bridging leaflet.

A complete AVSD is also subdivided into types A to C according to Rastelli (▶ Fig. 15.12 and ▶ Fig. 15.13). The location and attachment of the anterior bridging leaflet are important for this classification:

- Type A (most common type): The anterior bridging leaflet is separated immediately below the defect in the atrial and ventricular septum and is tethered to the septal crest by tendinous cords.
- Type B (least common type): The anterior bridging leaflet is tethered by tendinous cords that straddle the septal defect from the left to the right ventricle. The anterior bridging leaflet is oriented slightly toward the right ventricle. This type is frequently associated with a hypoplastic left ventricle (unbalanced AVSD, see below).
- Type C: A freely movable anterior bridging leaflet oriented far to the right that is attached to the anterior papillary muscle of the right ventricle.

There are also special forms of AVSD as described below.

▶ **Unbalanced AVSD.** In an unbalanced AVSD, one of the two ventricles is hypoplastic. By definition, the left ventricle is hypoplastic if it is not involved in forming the cardiac apex. Biventricular correction is usually not possible in this case.

Note

Due to the considerable consequences for surgical correction, it is absolutely necessary to check for an unbalanced AVSD preoperatively.

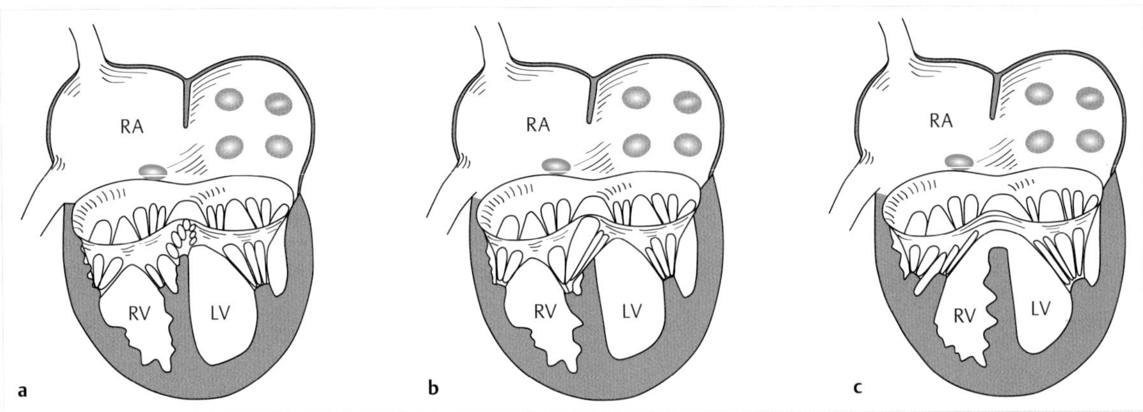

Fig. 15.12 Types of complete AVSD following Rastelli.[29] In the view from the front, the different attachments of the tendinous cords of the anterior bridging leaflet can be seen, which play an important role in the Rastelli classification and surgical correction. **a** Type A. **b** Type B. **c** Type C.
RA, right atrium, RV, right ventricle, LV, left ventricle.

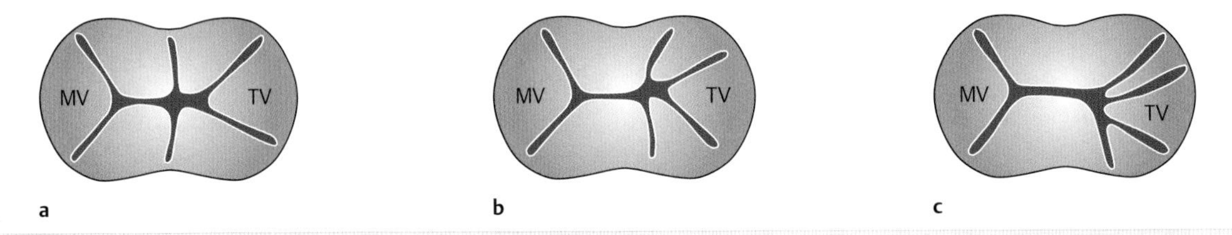

Fig. 15.13 AV valve leaflets in the Rastelli classification of complete AVSD. The view from above shows the arrangement of the bridging leaflets.[18] **a** Type A: The bridging leaflets are arranged nearly evenly across the two ventricles. **b** Type B: The bridging leaflets are oriented to the right. **c** Type C: The bridging leaflets are oriented far to the right.
TV, tricuspid valve; MV, mitral valve.

► **AV valve cleft.** This is a minimal variant of an endocardial cushion defect. There is only a cleft in an AV valve with no atrial or ventricular septal defect.

Hemodynamics

The hemodynamic situation depends on the extent of the left-to-right shunt at the atrial and ventricular levels, on the insufficiency of the AV valve, possible pulmonary hypertension, and accompanying anomalies.

► **Incomplete and intermediate AVSD.** Volume overload of the right atrium and ventricle and of pulmonary circulation (similar to an ASD).

► **Complete AVSD.** Depending on the size of the defects in the atrial and ventricular septum, there is usually a large left-to-right shunt at the atrial and ventricular level with excessive pulmonary blood flow and increasing congestive heart failure in early infancy. Insufficiency of the AV valve can complicate the situation. Obstructive pulmonary diseases and hypoventilation, which are often present in children with Down syndrome, aggravate the symptoms. Pulmonary hypertension with an increase in pulmonary resistance typically develops very soon in a complete AVSD. An Eisenmenger reaction usually looms within the first 6 months in the form of obstructive pulmonary vascular changes. Once an Eisenmenger reaction has occurred, a right-to-left shunt with cyanosis develops.

Associated Anomalies

The following cardiac defects occur frequently in conjunction with an AVSD:
- Patent ductus arteriosus (10%)
- Tetralogy of Fallot (10%)
- Double-outlet right ventricle
- Coarctation of the aorta (frequently associated with an unbalanced AVSD, almost never with Down syndrome)
- Heterotaxy syndromes
- Rarely: total anomalous pulmonary venous connection, persistent left superior vena cava

Associated Syndromes

An AVSD is the typical heart defect associated with trisomy 21 (Down syndrome). It is also frequently found with microdeletion of 22q11 or with the Ellis–van Creveld syndrome.

15.3.2 Diagnostic Measures

Symptoms

▶ **Partial and intermediate AVSD without mitral valve insufficiency.** The hemodynamic and clinical situation is similar to that of a large ASD with a large left-to-right shunt. The defect is usually asymptomatic in childhood, but later, congestive heart failure and in adulthood pulmonary hypertension can develop.

An exception is when there is a hypoplastic left ventricle and hypoplastic mitral valve annulus. In this case, there is a pronounced left-to-right shunt with excessive pulmonary blood flow and hypoperfusion in the systemic circulation early on so that congestive heart failure develops sooner.

▶ **Partial and intermediate AVSD with mitral valve insufficiency.** Congestive heart failure develops sooner in these patients because the regurgitation volume across the insufficient mitral valve leads to additional overload of the left ventricle.

▶ **Complete AVSD.** After the drop in pulmonary vascular resistance in the 2nd to 8th week of life, these patients rapidly develop congestive heart failure. There is frequently pronounced pulmonary blood flow. Problems are caused by pulmonary hypertension, failure to thrive, and recurrent pulmonary infections. Cyanosis during activity and later also at rest is a sign of pulmonary hypertension or an incipient Eisenmenger reaction.

Auscultation

▶ **Partial AVSD.** In a partial AVSD, the auscultation finding is largely consistent with that of an atrial septal defect: 2/6–3/6 systolic murmur with PMI in the 2nd left parasternal ICS as a sign of relative pulmonary stenosis. This is because a larger volume has to flow across the actually normal pulmonary valve as a result of the left-to-right shunt at the atrial level. There may also be a diastolic murmur due to the relative tricuspid valve stenosis. In addition, if there is mitral valve insufficiency, a clear bubbling (pouring) murmur can be heard over the cardiac apex. There is a fixed split second heart sound.

▶ **Intermediate and complete AVSD.** A loud holosystolic murmur can be heard with PMI in the 4th left parasternal ICS as a result of the left-to-right shunt across the septum and AV valve insufficiency. The second heart sound is loud as a sign of excessive pulmonary blood flow or hypertension. While the left-to-right shunt and therefore the intensity of the systolic murmur decreases as pulmonary hypertension increases, the second heart sound becomes steadily louder.

Complications

Irreversible pulmonary hypertension develops unusually early in patients with an AVSD, and in patients with trisomy 21, sometimes as soon as during the 6th to 12th month of life.

> **Note**
>
> In a complete AVSD, an irreversible increase in pulmonary resistance can develop within the 2nd year of life. Surgical correction should therefore be performed in the first year of life (generally at age 3 to 6 months).

ECG

There are indicative ECG findings associated with an AVSD that are enough to raise suspicion of the condition. Typical findings are:

- Left axis deviation: Left axis deviation arises due to displacement of the conduction system. Sometimes the axis "deviates" further up to right axis deviation. Moderate right axis deviation in an AVSD is found almost exclusively in connection with pulmonary hypertension or a pulmonary stenosis.
- I AV block: The PQ interval is frequently prolonged. Strictly speaking, this is not an AV block, since there is no delayed conduction in the AV node itself, but rather delayed intra-atrial conduction that leads to the extended PQ interval in the superficial ECG.
- Signs of right heart hypertrophy in the precordial leads (high R waves in $V_1 + V_2$ and a low S wave in $V_5 + V_6$): The signs of right heart hypertrophy can also be masked by left heart hypertrophy if there is simultaneous mitral valve insufficiency.
- Incomplete right bundle branch block (rsR′ or rR′ in $V_1 + V_2$): An incomplete right bundle branch block is found frequently, especially with a partial AVSD.

> **Note**
>
> A left axis deviation in the ECG should always make one think of an AVSD.

Chest X-ray

Typical X-ray findings are cardiomegaly with a prominent pulmonary segment and increased pulmonary vascular markings as a result of excessive pulmonary blood flow.

Echocardiography

The following findings are typical for an AVSD and should be investigated:

- Absence of the atrioventricular septum (defect in the lower segment of the atrial septum immediately above the AV valve and VSD in the inlet septum immediately below the level of the AV valve): In a partial AVSD, no shunt is found in the ventricular septum; in an intermediate AVSD the VSD is generally small and restrictive, and there is usually a large VSD in a complete AVSD.
- Assessment of the AV valve: Instead of two staggered valves, there is a common AV valve with all the leaflets at one level. In a partial or intermediate AVSD, there are two separate AV valve openings; in a complete AVSD only one valve opening is detected. In addition, the extent and location of AV valve insufficiencies must be investigated. The location and size of a cleft must also be determined.
- Assessment of ventricle sizes: It is also necessary to clarify whether the AVSD is balanced or unbalanced. If the left ventricle is not involved in forming the cardiac apex, there is a hypoplastic left ventricle by definition.
- Visualization of the bridging leaflets and attachments of the valve leaflets: Straddling tendinous cords and a single papillary muscle in the left ventricle should be noted.
- Assessment of the extent, site, and direction of the shunt at the atrial and ventricular level.
- Assessment of the left ventricular outflow tract: The "goose-neck" configuration due to the anterior and superior displacement of the aortic valve is typical. It should also be investigated whether there is a subaortic stenosis, which can be caused by a mitral valve leaflet.
- The pressure in pulmonary circulation should be estimated by Doppler ultrasonography to quantify the extent of pulmonary hypertension.
- Exclusion of additional anomalies, in particular PDA, tetralogy of Fallot, and coarctation of the aorta.

Cardiac Catheterization

Echocardiography is generally sufficient for diagnosing and assessing the individual anatomy. Cardiac catheterization is used primarily for the precise assessment of pulmonary vascular resistance, possibly including testing the responsiveness of the pulmonary vascular bed. Typical findings in an AVSD are:

- The left ventricle is easier to visualize than the right. The catheter reaches the left atrium and practically "falls" into the left ventricle after being advanced through the inferior vena cava and the right atrium.
- Large left-to-right shunt with elevated pressures in the pulmonary circulation.
- Angiography shows the "goose-neck" deformity due to the anterior displacement of the aortic valve in front of the common AV valve.

MRI

An MRI is not generally needed. In special cases, it can be used to clarify anatomical details and quantify shunts.

15.3.3 Treatment

Conservative Treatment

Digoxin, diuretics, beta blockers, and ACE inhibitors can be used as interim measures to treat congestive heart failure. A feeding tube may be inserted for a high-calorie diet to promote the child's growth until the operation. Oxygen should not be administered due to excessive pulmonary blood flow.

Indications for Surgery

There is practically always an indication for surgery. The timing of the operation is usually between the 3rd and 6th month of life for a complete AVSD. Early onset of obstructive pulmonary vascular changes and frequently pronounced congestive heart failure necessitate rapid corrective surgery.

For asymptomatic partial and intermediate AVSDs, the operation is generally performed between 2 and 4 years of age. If there are clinical symptoms of congestive heart failure, a pronounced shunt, or relevant AV valve insufficiency, the timing for operation may be earlier. In older patients, the operation is performed as an elective procedure after the diagnosis has been established.

► **Contraindications for an operative correction.** Operative correction is contraindicated after irreversible pulmonary hypertension (Eisenmenger reaction) has developed.

Surgery

The standard procedure is a patch closure of the atrial and ventricular septal defects using the one or two patch technique and reconstruction of the AV valve.

In an unbalanced AVSD, it is usually possible to perform only palliative operations for a univentricular heart in the sense of a Fontan procedure.

Pulmonary artery banding to protect against excessive pulmonary blood flow is performed only in exceptions as a palliative measure or as an interim measure until the definitive correction can be made, for example, if definitive surgery is not yet possible in very small premature infants with treatment-refractory congestive heart failure.

15.3.4 Prognosis and Outcome

► **Long-term outcome.** Spontaneous closure of an AVSD is not possible. Left untreated, 80% of children with a complete AVSD die within two years, the others develop an Eisenmenger reaction that makes surgical correction impossible. For reasons not yet understood, even patients who undergo successful timely surgery may still develop pulmonary hypertension and an Eisenmenger reaction in rare cases. Patients with an Eisenmenger reaction usually die in young adulthood.

The perioperative mortality rate for an early correction of a complete AVSD is less than 5%, but higher if there are additional complex anomalies. Postoperatively, a hemodynamically relevant AV valve insufficiency (rarely AV valve stenosis) can remain. Due to the elongation of the left ventricular outflow tract, there is also the risk of a postoperative subaortic stenosis.

The overall reoperation rate is approximately. 10%. Some of these patients require a mechanical valve. Pacemaker-dependent AV blocks and supraventricular and ventricular arrhythmias can sometimes occur, even years after corrective surgery.

► **Outpatient follow-up.** Frequent outpatient monitoring is necessary until surgery. In particular, development of congestive heart failure or pulmonary hypertension should be checked. Postoperatively, lifelong cardiac follow-up is needed. Residual defects in the vicinity of the septa, AV valve insufficiency, a subaortic stenosis, development of pulmonary hypertension, and arrhythmias (AV block, supraventricular and ventricular arrhythmias) should be noted.

Postoperative endocarditis prophylaxis should be given for at least 6 months and lifelong prophylaxis is needed if there are residual defects in the vicinity of prosthetic material.

► **Physical capacity and lifestyle.** The physical capacity of children with an isolated partial AVSD, similar to other atrial septal defects, is generally not impaired. However, if there is a complete AVSD, heart failure can develop in the first few months of life. Postoperatively, physical capacity depends primarily on residual defects such as AV valve insufficiency, a possible subaortic stenosis, and the regression of pulmonary hypertension. Physical capacity in everyday routine is usually good in most cases. The children can usually play sports if there are no or only small residual defects in the atrial and ventricular septa, no evidence of pulmonary hypertension, no relevant AV valve insufficiency, good ventricular function, and no relevant arrhythmias.

The quality of life and physical capacity is significantly impaired in patients with an Eisenmenger reaction (Chapter 22).

► **Special aspects in adolescents and adults.** An Eisenmenger reaction has almost always developed in untreated adolescents and adults with a complete AVSD. Since patients with trisomy 21 and an AVSD formerly did not generally undergo surgery, they today constitute a large percentage of the Eisenmenger patients. The special problems of an Eisenmenger reaction are summarized in Chapter 22.

15.4 Patent Ductus Arteriosus

15.4.1 Basics

Synonym: patent ductus Botalli

Definition

A patent ductus arteriosus (PDA) is a pathological persistence of the physiological prenatal shunt between the bifurcation of the pulmonary artery and the descending aorta (► Fig. 15.14).

Epidemiology

Approximately 10% of all congenital heart defects are PDAs. Girls are affected about twice as often as boys. Among mature neonates, the incidence of PDA is about 0.1 per 1,000 live births, but is considerably more frequent in premature neonates and following perinatal asphyxia. Almost half of all premature infants with a birth

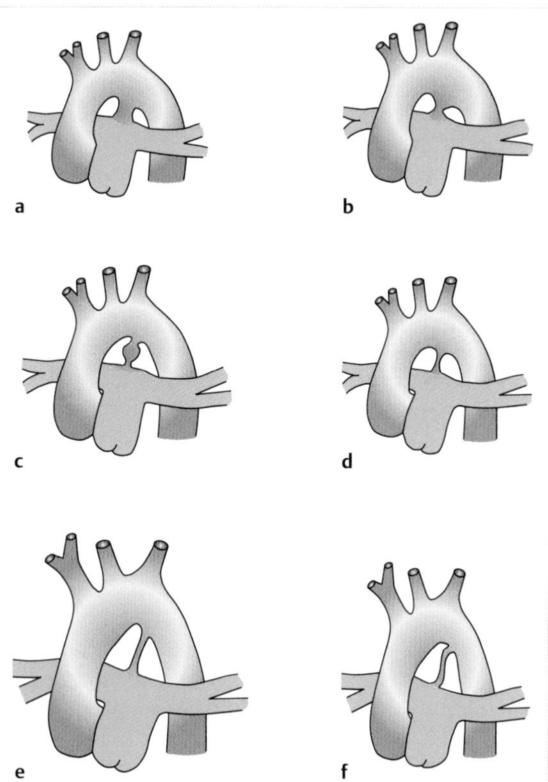

Fig. 15.14 a–f Patent ductus arteriosus (PDA) morphologies. The PDA is a communication between the descending aorta and the bifurcation of the pulmonary arteries. The morphology of the PDA can be varied. The length and width of a PDA determine the resistance in the systemic and pulmonary circulatory systems as well as the hemodynamic relevance of the ductus.

weight of less than 1750 g have a PDA. PDA is also more common among individuals living at high altitudes. This is probably due to the lower partial pressure of oxygen at high altitudes.

Pathogenesis

Prenatally, the ductus arteriosus exists as a shunt between the pulmonary artery and the descending aorta to bypass pulmonary circulation. The blood flows from the right ventricle through the pulmonary artery via the ductus arteriosus into the descending aorta, finally reaching the placenta via the umbilical artery. Intrauterine synthesis of endogenous prostaglandin E_2 maintains the patency of the ductus. If the mother takes prostaglandin synthesis inhibitors such as aspirin or ibuprofen during pregnancy, this can lead to premature intrauterine closure of the ductus, resulting in severe right ventricular pressure overload in the child.

Within the first hours of life, the increase in the partial pressure of oxygen and release of vasoactive substances normally results in the functional closure of the ductus. The actual anatomical closure from persistent contraction of the spiral arrangement of smooth muscle fibers and thickening of the intima usually takes several days to weeks. After the obliteration of the ductus, the remaining connective tissues are called ligamentum Botalli, which remains for the entire lifetime.

In neonates, all situations in which there is an inadequate postnatal increase in the partial pressure of oxygen are a risk factor for patent ductus arteriosus (PDA). Practically relevant are perinatal asphyxia and pulmonary diseases (e.g., meconium aspiration, pulmonary hypoplasia).

For some cardiac defects, there is no chance of survival after birth without a patent ductus arteriosus. This situation is termed ductal-dependent systemic circulation (e.g., associated with a critical aortic stenosis) or ductal-dependent pulmonary circulation (e.g., with critical pulmonary stenosis or pulmonary atresia). In patients with an obstruction of the right ventricular outflow tract (e.g., pulmonary atresia, tetralogy of Fallot) the ductus generally has an unusually tortuous course. This is probably due to the fact that there is retrograde blood supply to the pulmonary artery via the ductus arteriosus and not antegrade supply via the right ventricle as in a normal anatomical situation. The different flow direction in the ductus results in the unusual course of the ductus in cardiac defects with right heart obstruction.

Rarely occurring variants are a double ductus, an aneurysm of the ductus (particularly in Marfan patients), or a right-sided PDA.

Hemodynamics

When pulmonary vascular resistance drops after birth, there is a reversal of the shunt in the PDA. In an isolated PDA occurring without other cardiac anomalies, the fetal right-to-left shunt reverses to a left-to-right shunt through which blood from the descending aorta flows along the pressure gradient into the pulmonary artery. The blood flows though the pulmonary vessels and finally reaches the pulmonary circulation, the left atrium, and the left ventricle (volume overload from pulmonary circulation, left atrium and ventricle, and ascending aorta). The extent of the shunt depends on the width and length of the ductus and the resistance in the pulmonary and systemic circulation.

Classification

An isolated PDA is classified according to its hemodynamic relevance.

- Silent PDA: This is a very small, not hemodynamically relevant ductus that is detected as an incidental finding in a color Doppler examination and causes no heart murmur.
- Not hemodynamically relevant PDA: The PDA causes a typical continuous to-and-fro murmur, but does not lead to relevant volume overload of the left ventricle or pulmonary circulation. No pulmonary hypertension is present.
- Hemodynamically relevant PDA: In these cases, there is a moderate to large shunt across the ductus that causes symptoms of left ventricular and pulmonary volume overload.

Associated Anomalies

The PDA is a structure whose presence can be important for survival of patients having heart defects with:

- restrictive or absent pulmonary arterial flow (e.g., critical pulmonary stenosis, pulmonary atresia)
- restrictive or absent systemic arterial flow (e.g., critical aortic stenosis, critical aortic coarctation, interrupted aortic arch, hypoplastic left heart syndrome)

Associated Syndromes

A PDA frequently occurs in connection with the following syndromes:

- Congenital rubella syndrome
- Fetal alcohol syndrome

15.4.2 Diagnostic Measures

Symptoms

The symptoms of a PDA depend primarily on the shunt volume and age of the patient. A PDA in a premature infant is a special case with respect to the symptoms and therapy and is therefore discussed in a separate section (Chapter 15.5).

The effects of a large shunt across the PDA are perceptible in infancy. The symptoms of heart failure (tachypnea/dyspnea, feeding problems, failure to thrive, increased sweating) predominate. The peripheral pulses are noticeably strong (pulsus celer et altus, water hammer pulse) due to diastolic run-off of blood from the aorta into the pulmonary artery. The fontanelle pulse may be visible in infants. The pulse pressure is high. If the shunt is very large, a systolic or continuous thrill may be perceptible in the 1st to 3rd parasternal left ICS or in the suprasternal notch.

If elevated pulmonary resistance develops postnatally (e.g., associated with persistent fetal circulation due to asphyxia), there is a right-to-left shunt over the PDA with lower oxygen saturation in the lower half of the body distal to the junction of the ductus (differential cyanosis).

If the shunt is smaller, the children do not develop symptoms until later or not at all. Usually, the diagnosis in these cases is made only from an asymptomatic incidental finding. Increased susceptibility to infections can be the only symptom.

Complications

Depending on the size of the shunt, pulmonary hypertension may develop as a result of the excessive pulmonary blood flow, which is initially reversible but later becomes irreversible (Eisenmenger reaction). There is probably a slightly increased risk of endarteritis in the area around the PDA even if the shunt is not hemodynamically relevant. The development of a PDA aneurysm is extremely rare but involves the risk of a rupture.

Auscultation

In neonates, a purely systolic murmur with PMI in the 2nd to 3rd parasternal left ICS radiating into the back can usually be heard.

After pulmonary resistance drops (2nd to 8th week of life) the typical systolic–diastolic continuous machinery murmur is heard with PMI in the 1st to 2nd infraclavicular left ICS. The murmur can be heard both in systole and diastole because the pressure in the aorta is higher than in the pulmonary artery in systole and diastole. The maximum intensity of the murmur occurs simultaneously with the second heart sound and is softer again in the diastole (crescendo-decrescendo murmur).

If the ductus is very small, the murmur is clearer during inspiration and physical exertion. A silent ductus—as the name indicates—causes no conspicuous auscultation finding.

Differential diagnoses of a PDA based on the auscultation finding:

- "*Venous hum*" is a continuous murmur in the jugular veins with a maximum in early diastole. The murmur becomes softer during inspiration. It disappears when the jugular veins are compressed or the head is turned.
- An *aortopulmonary window* is sometimes difficult to distinguish from a PDA even using echocardiography. An aortopulmonary window always affects the ascending aorta and does not originate in the descending aorta like a PDA.
- In *pulmonary agenesis* a loud systolic–diastolic murmur is heard. The echocardiography finding with a typically massively dilated main pulmonary artery is indicative.
- *Coronary fistulas* originate in the coronary arteries and usually drain into the pulmonary artery or right ventricle.
- *Arteriovenous fistulas* are sometimes very difficult to distinguish using echocardiography. The exact visualization of the origin and drainage is important.
- *Peripheral pulmonary stenoses* often cause a murmur similar to PDA. The diagnosis is made using echocardiography.
- The *perforation of a sinus of Valsalva* into the right atrium or ventricle can sound similar to PDA on auscultation. The shunt in the region of the ruptured sinus to the right atrium or ventricle can be visualized using color Doppler.
- In *Bland–White–Garland syndrome* (anomalous origin of the left coronary artery from the pulmonary artery), a continuous murmur can only rarely be auscultated owing to a pronounced retrograde flow into the pulmonary artery. However, there are often changes in the ECG typical of ischemia. The anomalous origin of the coronary artery can sometimes be visualized in echocardiography.

ECG

A mid-sized left-to-right shunt will display signs of left heart hypertrophy. If there is a large shunt with pulmonary hypertension, the ECG will have signs of biventricular hypertrophy. When pulmonary hypertension becomes the prominent symptom later on (Eisenmenger reaction), signs of right heart hypertrophy will predominate.

Chest X-ray

If the shunt is large, there is cardiomegaly with left heart enlargement and dilatation of the ascending aorta. Pulmonary vascular markings are increased due to pulmonary recirculation. However, in pulmonary hypertension, only the central pulmonary vessels are dilated, while the peripheral vessels are narrow.

Echocardiography

Echocardiography including color Doppler is the method of choice to confirm the diagnosis and estimate the hemodynamic relevance of the PDA.

A PDA can generally be readily visualized in the parasternal short axis at the level of the 2nd left ICS; at the

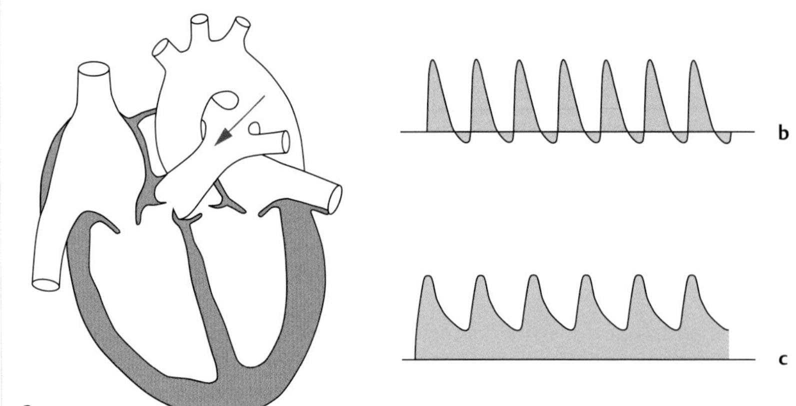

Fig. 15.15 Flow profile in the celiac trunk with otherwise normal anatomy (**a**) and a hemodynamically relevant PDA (**b**). The diastolic flow velocity in the celiac trunk is normally about one-third of the systolic velocity (**c**). In a hemodynamically relevant PDA, the diastolic flow velocity approaches zero or even negative flow (**b**).[28]

bifurcation of the pulmonary artery, the PDA can be visualized as a third vessel ("pulmonary trifurcation") in addition to the two pulmonary artery branches. By tilting the transducer in a posterior direction, the course of the ductus can be followed up to the descending aorta.

A color jet in the main pulmonary artery can be detected in the color Doppler scan. In a left-to-right shunt, a red color jet is directed toward the pulmonary valve.

Using CW Doppler, the pressure gradients across the ductus can be estimated—the ductus is restrictive if the pressure across the ductus is reduced by more than half of the systemic pressure (= systolic blood pressure).

Enlargement of the left atrium and left ventricle is an indication of hemodynamic relevance. A ratio left atrium/descending aorta of over 1.5 in the M mode is a sign of probable hemodynamic relevance.

In premature infants and neonates, the Doppler examination of the peripheral arteries (medial cerebral artery, celiac trunk) is the most sensitive method for evaluating the hemodynamic relevance of a PDA. An antegrade diastolic flow that is about one-third of the peak systolic flow (the diastolic flow is caused by the Windkessel function of the aorta) can normally be detected in these vessels. If there is a hemodynamically relevant PDA (i.e., requiring treatment), there is zero diastolic flow or negative diastolic flow in the peripheral vessels as a result of Windkessel leakage (▸ Fig. 15.15).

Note

Before deciding to close a PDA in a premature infant or neonate, surgically, ductal-dependent systemic or pulmonary circulation must be ruled out by echocardiography.

Cardiac Catheterization

Diagnostic cardiac catheterization is needed only if noninvasive findings are inconclusive, additional cardiac anomalies are present, or there are indications of an increase in pulmonary pressure. Typically, blood oximetry shows an increase in oxygen saturation in the pulmonary artery. It is usually possible to probe the ductus and the descending aorta directly. The catheter position is characteristic and is shaped like a treble clef. The pressure in the pulmonary artery is determined and pulmonary vascular response to vasoactive substances such as oxygen or NO may be tested.

However, cardiac catheterization is usually performed only for the interventional closure of a PDA.

MRI

An MRI is rarely indicated, but may be useful for providing anatomical details if there are associated anomalies or for quantifying a shunt.

15.4.3 Treatment

▸ **Conservative treatment.** In premature infants and neonates, an attempt can be made to close a hemodynamically relevant PDA in the first days of life by administering prostaglandin synthesis inhibitors (indomethacin, ibuprofen) (Chapter 15.5.3).

When the shunt is large, heart failure is treated symptomatically until the closure is definitive.

▸ **Indications.** Indications for closure of a PDA:
- Large PDA with signs of heart failure
- Signs of left atrial and left ventricular overload
- PDA with a typical heart murmur

For a silent asymptomatic PDA, the indication for closure is sometimes controversial. The theoretical risk of arteritis in the area of the PDA is an argument in favor of closure; the risk—albeit very small—of the procedure is an argument against closure.

▸ **Contraindications.** Contraindications for PDA closure:
- Large ductus with a right-to-left shunt and permanent pulmonary hypertension

- Ductal-dependent defects (unless correction or palliation of the heart defect is performed simultaneously)

Interventional Catheterization

Interventional catheterization for closure using an umbrella system or coils is the therapy of choice for a PDA. Children who weigh as little as 2 to 3 kg can now be successfully treated by interventional catheterization. At lower weights, the anatomical conditions are usually still too small for the relatively large catheter systems.

For patients without heart failure, preschool age is the preferred time for closure of the ductus (spontaneous closure is unlikely at this age). Older patients can be treated electively after the diagnosis is established.

Surgery

Surgical PDA closure is performed in small premature infants after the failure of pharmacological closure or if pharmacological closure is contraindicated. In older patients, the ductus is closed surgically if the PDA is so large that interventional catheter closure is unsuitable (e.g., a large window ductus).

Closure is made using a clip and ligation with or without transection via a lateral thoracotomy. It can sometimes be performed by thoracoscopy. It should be noted that prolonged treatment with prostaglandins makes the ductus tissue brittle and can complicate the operation.

15.4.4 Prognosis and Outcome

► **Long-term outcome.** After the third month of life, only 10% of PDAs close spontaneously. Formerly, patients with a relevant shunt usually died in young adulthood if untreated as a result of volume overload and Eisenmenger reaction.

An unclosed PDA entails a variable risk of endarteritis, which nowadays occurs very rarely in industrial nations.

The mortality rate is well under 1% for operative treatment and for interventional closure after age 2 years. Specific complications of a PDA closure are paresis of the left phrenic or recurrent laryngeal nerve or chylothorax if the thoracic duct is injured because of the close proximity of these structures to the ductus arteriosus. Very rarely, an adjacent vessel (e.g., the left pulmonary artery) can be accidentally ligated instead of the PDA. If the PDA was only ligated, there may be isolated cases of recanalization. In addition, a diverticulum of the ductus may form.

► **Outpatient follow-up.** Symptoms of heart failure in an untreated PDA must be noted in outpatient checkups. The size of the left atrium and left ventricle should be documented by echocardiography. In addition, the flow velocity across the ductus should be determined by Doppler ultrasonography (pressure gradient to pulmonary circulation?).

Outpatient monitoring after closure should focus especially on detecting the residual shunt and the specific complications listed above. If there is no residual shunt, the checkups can generally be discontinued after 2 years.

After PDA closure, endocarditis prophylaxis is required for 6 months, or for life if there is a residual shunt in the area around the foreign material.

► **Physical capacity and lifestyle.** After the timely, successful closure of a PDA, patients later almost always have normal physical capacity.

► **Special aspects in adolescents and adults.** In the rare cases in which a PDA is not diagnosed until adolescence or adulthood, irreversible pulmonary hypertension must be ruled out before it is closed. Calcification often develops in adults and can complicate the closure.

15.5 Patent Ductus Arteriosus in Premature Infants

15.5.1 Epidemiology

PDA (Chapter 15.4) is a frequent cause of morbidity and mortality in premature infants. The incidence of a PDA in premature infants weighing less than 1,750 g is about 45% and about 80% for those weighing less than 1,200 g.

► **Risk factors.** Aside from prematurity, the risk factors for a PDA are:

- Hypoxia, perinatal asphyxia
- Infusion of excessive fluid
- Hypocalcemia
- Furosemide (stimulates prostaglandin synthesis in the kidneys)
- Theophylline medication

15.5.2 Symptoms

Symptoms of excessive pulmonary blood flow develop when the pulmonary vascular resistance drops, with heart failure (frequently starting as soon as the 5th day of life) and deterioration of respiration.

Diastolic perfusion of the distal segments of the aorta (especially the abdominal organs and kidneys) deteriorates as a result of Windkessel leakage. There is a risk of developing necrotic enterocolitis and kidney failure. Cerebral perfusion is also impaired, increasing the risk of periventricular leukomalacia.

15.5.3 Treatment

Conservative Treatment

In premature infants and neonates, an attempt can be made to close a hemodynamically relevant PDA pharmacologically in the first days of life with prostaglandin synthesis inhibitors (indomethacin, ibuprofen, diclofenac).

► **Indications.** The indications for a pharmacological closure of the ductus are still controversial. In clinical practice, the following indications have been established:

- *Premature infants under 1,000 g:* In ventilated premature infants under 1,000 g, early treatment starting on the 2nd to 3rd day of life is recommended for a PDA with discrete symptoms.
- *Premature infants over 1,000 g*: Only hemodynamically significant or symptomatic PDAs should be treated. A PDA is considered hemodynamically significant or symptomatic if the following criteria are present:
  - Clinical signs of congestive heart failure
  - Substantial respiratory deterioration
  - Reduced, zero or retrograde diastolic flow in the cerebral arteries or the celiac trunk
  - Resistance Index (RI) in the anterior cerebral artery of over 0.9 (caution: RI alone is not a sufficient criterion).

► **Contraindications.** Contraindications for ductus closure are:

- Ductal-dependent defect (must be ruled out by echocardiography before the ductus is closed)
- Persistent pulmonary hypertension in the neonate
- Oliguria (< 1 mL urine/kg/h in the last 8 h), creatinine > 1.7 mg/dL
- Thrombocytopenia < 60,000/µL, pathological plasmatic coagulation
- Fresh cerebral, intestinal, or pulmonary hemorrhage
- Septic shock
- Necrotic enterocolitis
- Recent surgery

► **General measures associated with a PDA.** The following general measures must be noted for premature infants with a PDA:

- Exact fluid balance: A mild restriction of fluids is often propagated, but it should be noted that this impairs renal perfusion and increases the side effects of indomethacin treatment.
- Anemia (target Hct 0.45), hypoxemia, and hypocapnia must be avoided.
- Furosemide should be avoided, as it can have an unfavorable effect on the closure of the ductus by promoting renal synthesis of prostaglandin.

Pharmacological Closure

Ibuprofen and indomethacin, sometimes diclofenac as well, are used for pharmacological closure. The closure rate for ibuprofen and indomethacin is similar (65–80%). The frequency of side effects regarding bleeding, necrotic enterocolitis, and bronchopulmonary dysplasia is comparable for both substances. However, gastrointestinal, cerebral, and renal perfusion are affected less negatively by ibuprofen than by indomethacin. Based on the evidence from trials, the prophylactic treatment with indomethacin does not improve the respiratory situation or the neurological outcome but does lower the rate of cerebral hemorrhages. Ibuprofen is currently considerably more expensive than indomethacin.

► **Ibuprofen.** Ibuprofen is administered in three single doses:

- 1st single dose: 10 mg/kg as a bolus infusion over 30 min
- 2nd single dose (24 h after the 1st single dose): 5 mg/kg as a bolus infusion over 30 min
- 3rd single dose (24 h after the 2nd single dose): 5 mg/kg as a bolus infusion over 30 min

If the patient fails to respond to treatment, the ibuprofen cycle can be repeated or indomethacin therapy started.

► **Indomethacin.** Indomethacin is also administered in three single doses:

- 1st single dose: 0.2 mg/kg as a bolus infusion over 6 h
- 2nd single dose (12 h after the start of the 1st single dose): 0.2 mg/kg as a bolus infusion over 6 h
- 3rd single dose (12 h after the start of the 2nd single dose): 0.2 mg/kg as a bolus infusion over 6 h

Bolus infusions over 6 hours cause fewer renal side effects than 30-minute infusions.

The target indomethacin level 12 hours after the third single dose is 0.7 to 1 µg/mL.

After an initial treatment success with indomethacin, maintenance therapy for 3 to 5 days is currently recommended: 0.1 (to 0.2) mg/kg as a bolus infusion once a day for 6 hours. Maintenance therapy is started 24 hours after the start of the last single dose.

► **Side effects of indomethacin and ibuprofen.** The most important adverse effects of indomethacin and ibuprofen are:

- Kidney failure/oliguria (more frequent with indomethacin than with ibuprofen)
- Microhematuria
- Occult blood in stool, bowel perforation
- Increased risk of necrotic enterocolitis (especially in association with oliguria)
- Thrombocytopenia, platelet aggregation disorder

Operative Treatment

If pharmacological treatment is not successful, surgical closure of the ductus is indicated. In many hospitals, it is performed via a left lateral thoracotomy in the incubator on the intensive ward for premature infants.

15.6 Partial Anomalous Pulmonary Venous Connection

15.6.1 Basics

Synonym: "partial anomalous pulmonary venous return" (PAPVR)

Definition

In a partial anomalous pulmonary venous connection (PAPVC) one or more of the pulmonary veins drains into the right atrium or a systemic venous vessel connected to the right atrium instead of into the left atrium. The result is a hemodynamic situation comparable with an ASD.

Epidemiology

Partial anomalous pulmonary venous connections constitute less than 1% of all congenital heart defects. They seldom occur in isolation, but usually in combination with other cardiac anomalies.

Pathogenesis

During embryonic development, the blood supply and drainage of the lungs takes place via the splanchnic plexus. During the course of development, the common pulmonary vein bulges out of the left atrium and connects to the splanchnic plexus. The persistence of primitive connections that were previously responsible for venous drainage of the lung buds leads to partial anomalous pulmonary venous connections.

Classification

The partial anomalous pulmonary venous connections are classified according to the connections of the pulmonary veins. Many possible anomalies are conceivable. The clinically most important ones are described below.

► **Connection of the right pulmonary veins to the superior vena cava.** In this type, the right superior pulmonary veins typically drain into the superior vena cava below the azygos vein (► Fig. 15.17). The pulmonary vein of the middle lobe usually drains into the right atrium at the level of the junction of the superior vena cava. The right inferior pulmonary veins drain normally into the left atrium. An upper sinus venosus defect is almost always associated with this type of partial anomalous pulmonary venous connection. The superior vena cava is dilated below the azygos vein due to volume overload.

► **Connection of the right pulmonary veins to the right atrium.** In this case, all right pulmonary veins generally drain directly into the right atrium. There is almost always an ASD.

► **Connection of the right pulmonary veins to the inferior vena cava.** In this type, typically all of the right pulmonary veins (but sometimes only some of the right pulmonary veins) drain into the inferior vena cava. This anomaly is also called the *scimitar syndrome* (► Fig. 15.17) and is associated with other pulmonary anomalies such as hypoplasia of the right lung and lung sequestration. Aortopulmonary collaterals (connections between systemic arterial vessels and pulmonary veins) occur frequently with the scimitar syndrome. Often one or more segments of the right lobe of the lung are supplied via a collateral vessel from the descending aorta. The heart is displaced to the right by the right lung hypoplasia. The anomalous pulmonary vein proceeds downward parallel to the right atrium, passes through the diaphragm, and finally drains into the inferior vena cava. A direct connection with the right atrium is very rare. In more than one-third of cases, other heart defects are associated with a scimitar syndrome (e.g., ASD, PDA, VSD, tetralogy of Fallot, pulmonary stenosis, aortic coarctation).

The name scimitar syndrome stems from the curved opacity next to the cardiac silhouette in the chest X-ray, similar to a Turkish scimitar, made by the anomalous pulmonary vein (► Fig. 15.16).

► **Connection of the left pulmonary veins to the left innominate vein.** Left anomalous pulmonary venous connections usually drain through a vertical vein into the left innominate vein (► Fig. 15.17). There is usually an ASD. Left pulmonary veins rarely drain anomalously into the superior or inferior vena cava, the coronary sinus, the left subclavian vein, or directly into the right atrium vein.

Hemodynamics

The hemodynamics of the partial anomalous pulmonary venous connection corresponds with that of an ASD. The oxygenated blood from the anomalous pulmonary veins flows into the right atrium, reaches the left ventricle and finally the pulmonary circulation. This results in volume overload and dilatation of the right cardiac chambers and pulmonary recirculation. The size of the shunt depends on the number of anomalous pulmonary veins and on the resistance of the pulmonary vascular bed. An associated

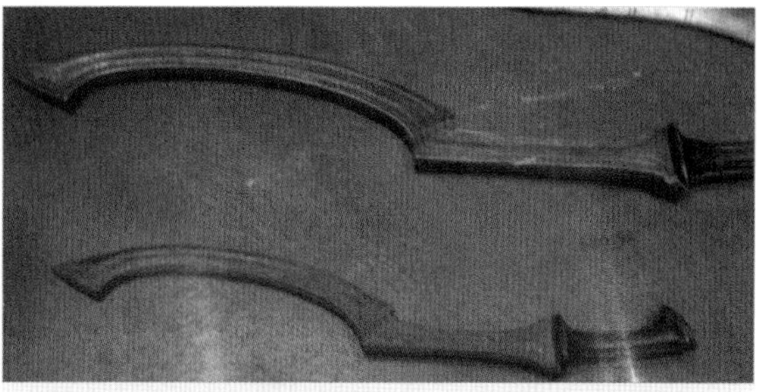

Fig. 15.16 Turkish scimitars.

ASD increases the volume overload and excessive pulmonary blood flow even further.

Associated Anomalies

Partial anomalous pulmonary venous connections are frequently associated with an ASD. Sinus venosus defects are practically always associated anatomically or functionally with a partial anomalous pulmonary venous connection. Anomalous pulmonary venous connections are also common in patients with a heterotaxy syndrome, especially left isomerism. They occur less frequently in combination with a tetralogy of Fallot.

> **Note**
>
> Sinus venosus defects are practically always associated anatomically or functionally with a partial anomalous pulmonary venous connection.

Associated Syndromes

Anomalous pulmonary venous connections have frequently been described in conjunction with Turner and Noonan syndromes.

> **Note**
>
> As a differential diagnosis, other cardiac anomalies that also lead to dilatation of the right ventricle and increased pulmonary blood flow must be distinguished from a partial anomalous pulmonary venous connection—primarily ASDs. But because an ASD can also be associated with anomalous pulmonary venous connections, they must be ruled out in every case of ASD.

15.6.2 Diagnostic Measures

Symptoms

The symptoms of a partial anomalous pulmonary venous connection are usually similar to those of an uncomplicated ASD. The majority of children with a partial anomalous pulmonary venous connection are asymptomatic. They may have breathing problems during exertion.

Patients with a scimitar syndrome frequently suffer from dyspnea, cyanosis, and pulmonary infections as a result of the associated bronchopulmonary anomalies.

Auscultation

If there is a simultaneous ASD, there is a fixed, split second heart sound independent of respiration. If the atrial septum is intact (very seldom) the second heart sound is unremarkable. A soft systolic murmur in the 2nd left parasternal ICS can be a sign of a relative pulmonary stenosis as a result of increased pulmonary circulation. A diastolic murmur in the right parasternal area generally corresponds with a relative stenosis of the tricuspid valve.

ECG

The ECG can be normal or similar to the finding of an uncomplicated ostium secundum ASD—incomplete right bundle branch block of the volume overload type (rSR′ in V_1). Signs of right atrial and right ventricular hypertrophy usually occur only in older patients.

Chest X-ray

Typical findings are an enlarged right ventricle and increased pulmonary vascular markings. Depending on the location of the anomalous pulmonary venous

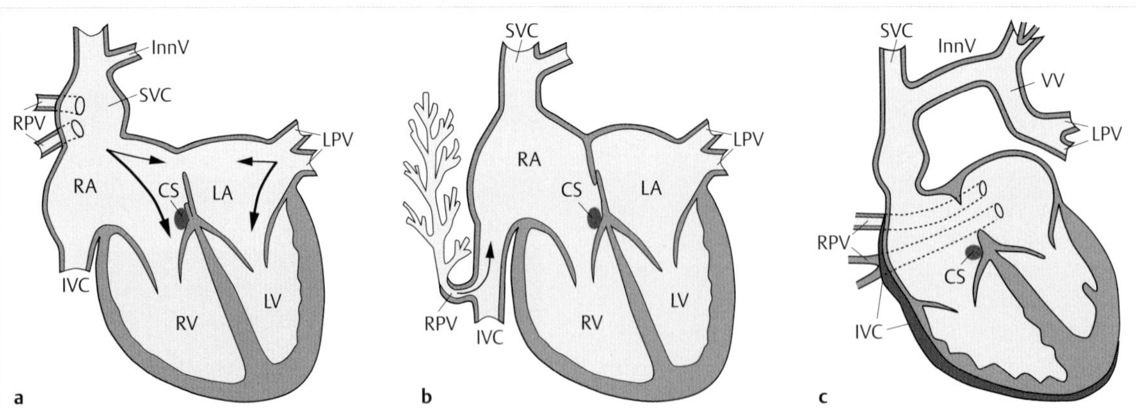

Fig. 15.17 The most frequent forms of a partial anomalous pulmonary venous connection. [1] **a** Connection of the right pulmonary veins to the superior vena cava. **b** Connection of the right pulmonary veins to the inferior vena cava (scimitar syndrome). **c** Connection of the left pulmonary veins to the left innominate veinc RA, right atrium; LA, left atrium; LV, left ventricle; RV, right ventricle; SVC, superior vena cava; IVC, inferior vena cava; CS, coronary sinus; LPV, left pulmonary veins; RPV, right pulmonary veins; InnV, innominate vein; VV, vertical vein.

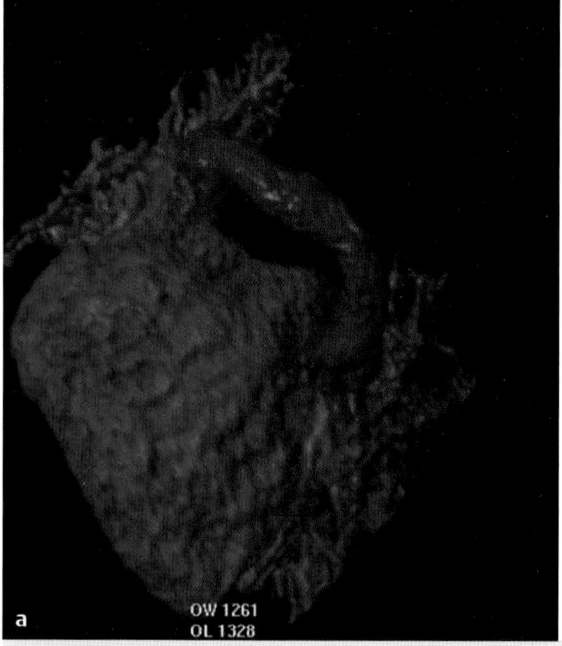

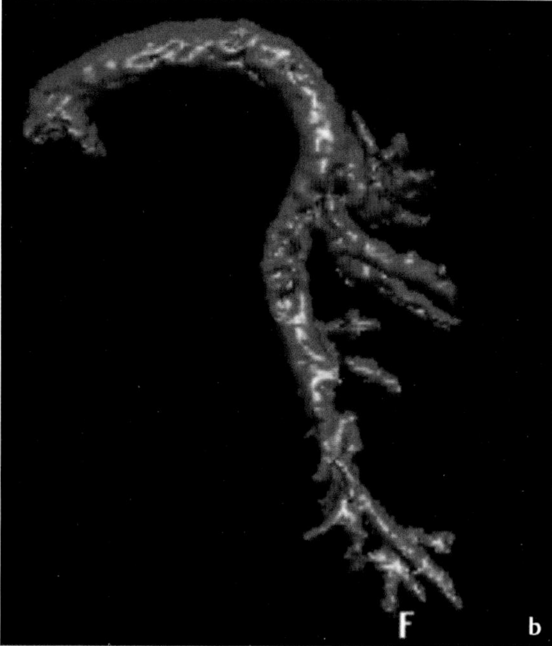

Fig. 15.18 3D reconstruction of a partial anomalous pulmonary venous connection (MRI). **a** The 3D reconstruction shows the anomalous connections of all left pulmonary veins into a vertical vein that drains the blood into the innominate vein. The blood from the pulmonary veins flows through the innominate vein into the superior vena cava. The pulmonary veins and the vertical and innominate veins are shown in red. The superior vena cava, the large right atrium, and the dilated right ventricle are blue. **b** 3D reconstruction of the left pulmonary veins, the vertical vein, and the innominate vein.

connection, the superior vena cava or the innominate vein may be dilated.

In the scimitar syndrome, there is typically a curved streaky opacity at the right of the heart. There is also hypoplasia of the right lung that displaces the cardiac silhouette to the right.

Echocardiography

It is difficult to visualize anomalous pulmonary vein connections. Every sign of right ventricular volume overload (dilated right atrium and ventricle) is suggestive of a partial anomalous pulmonary venous connection. Especially if an ASD is detected, a search must be made specifically for partial anomalous pulmonary venous connections. In a routine echocardiography, the connections of all pulmonary veins should always be visualized. If there is an anomalous pulmonary venous connection, the systemic veins distal to the anomalous connections are dilated; a color Doppler recording shows a conspicuously strong flow in this area.

When in doubt, a transesophageal echocardiography can be helpful, especially in larger patients.

MRI

MRI is now an ideal method for accurately diagnosing anomalous pulmonary venous connections. The 3D reconstruction of the pulmonary veins displays the anomalous connection(s) (▶ Fig. 15.18).

Cardiac Catheterization

Cardiac catheterization is not routinely needed to diagnose a partial anomalous pulmonary venous connection. It is indicated in individual cases if pulmonary hypertension is assumed to be the result of increased lung perfusion. Pulse oximetry shows a sudden increase in oxygen saturation in the vicinity of the connection.

Interventional catheterization to close aortopulmonary collaterals may be possible if there is a scimitar syndrome.

15.6.3 Treatment

▶ **Conservative treatment.** Pharmacological therapy is not indicated in asymptomatic patients. In patients with cardiac failure, anticongestive treatment (diuretics, afterload, possibly glycosides and beta blockers) is given to treat the symptoms until surgical correction can be performed.

▶ **Indications for surgical correction.** Surgical correction is indicated if there is evidence of excessive pulmonary blood flow or respiratory problems. Sometimes a Q_P/Q_S ratio of over 1.5 to 2 is given as the indication for

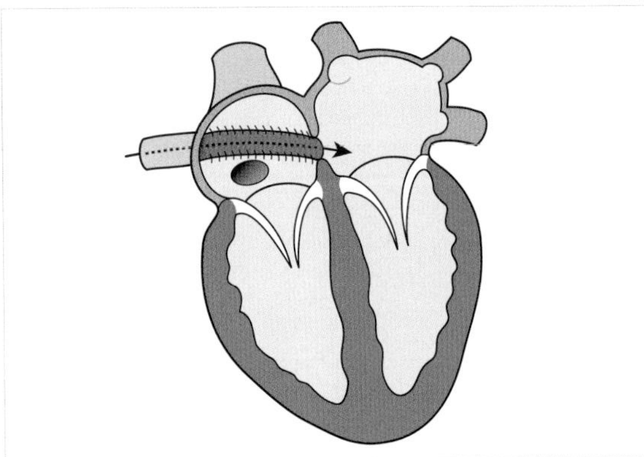

Fig. 15.19 Correction of a partial anomalous pulmonary venous connection with a patch tunnel. The anomalous pulmonary veins are redirected through a surgically formed tunnel at the back of the right atrium and through an ASD into the left atrium.

surgery. There is an indisputable indication for surgery if the right atrium or ventricle is dilated.

▸ **Contraindication for surgical correction.** Similarly to an ASD, surgical correction is contraindicated if pulmonary resistance is greatly elevated.

▸ **Operative treatment.** Surgical correction in which the anomalous pulmonary vein connections are redirected through a patch tunnel to drain into the left atrium is the definitive treatment. The ASD may have to be enlarged for this procedure (▸ Fig. 15.19). In a left pulmonary venous connection the pulmonary veins may be anastomized directly with the left atrial appendage. The surgery is performed as an elective procedure at preschool age if possible.

15.6.4 Prognosis and Outcome

▸ **Long-term outcome.** The anomalous connection of a single pulmonary vein associated with an intact atrial septum normally causes no problems. Otherwise, the natural outcome is similar to an uncomplicated ASD. Symptoms such as cardiac failure or pulmonary hypertension generally do not develop until adulthood. However, patients with a scimitar syndrome usually become symptomatic sooner (often in infancy), depending on the associated bronchopulmonary problems.

The perioperative mortality rate is extremely low (< 0.1%) in a majority of partial anomalous pulmonary vein connections, but higher for a scimitar syndrome. Patients who undergo surgical correction before pulmonary resistance develops have practically normal life expectancy. Rarely, postoperative atrial arrhythmias (sick sinus syndrome, sinus arrest, intra-atrial re-entrant tachycardias) occur due to the surgical manipulation near the sinus node and because of the patch material inserted.

In patients with a scimitar syndrome, the chronic bronchopulmonary problems usually persist even after surgery. The prognosis is least favorable in children who became symptomatic as neonates or in early infancy and have pulmonary hypertension.

▸ **Outpatient follow-up.** Regular postoperative monitoring is necessary, in particular to detect obstructions of the pulmonary veins and atrial arrhythmias (e.g., sick sinus syndrome).

Endocarditis prophylaxis is needed for the first 6 months postoperatively and lifelong prophylaxis is necessary if there are remaining defects in the vicinity of prosthetic material.

▸ **Physical capacity and lifestyle.** Patients who undergo correction in time generally have normal physical capacity. The course of the disease is similar to that in patients with a corrected ASD. In patients with a scimitar syndrome, physical capacity often remains clearly impaired even after correction of the anomalous pulmonary venous connection because of the associated bronchopulmonary problems.

▸ **Special aspects in adolescents and adults.** Cardiac failure usually does not develop in untreated patients until adulthood. Atrial arrhythmias can develop as a result of atrial overload. Cyanosis usually does not occur until the third or fourth decade of life. It is the result of the right-to-left shunt at the atrial level that develops when pulmonary vascular resistance increases due to excessive pulmonary blood flow. If an ASD is combined with a partial anomalous pulmonary vein connection, pulmonary hypertension develops sooner than in an isolated ASD.

15.7 Total Anomalous Pulmonary Venous Connection

15.7.1 Basics

Synonym: total anomalous pulmonary venous return (TAPVR)

Definition

A total anomalous pulmonary venous connection (TAPVC) is an anomalous connection of all pulmonary veins. The pulmonary veins drain into the right atrium or a vein connected to the right atrium instead of into the left atrium.

Epidemiology

Total anomalous pulmonary venous connections constitute approximately 1% of all congenital heart defects. Boys

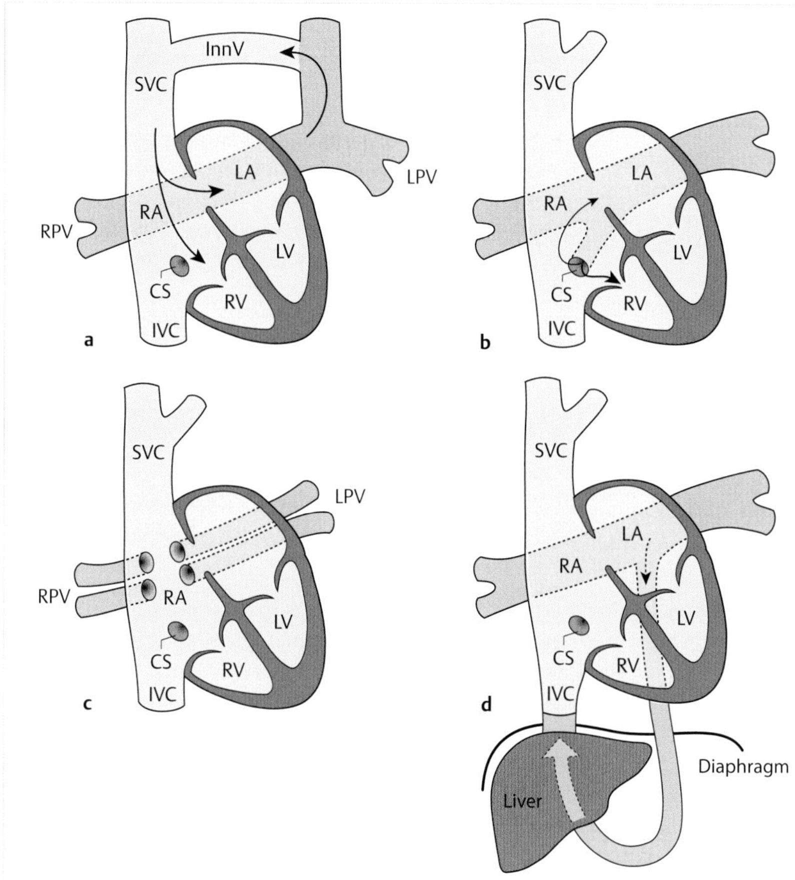

Fig. 15.20 The most common types of total anomalous pulmonary venous connection. **a** Supracardiac type with drainage of the pulmonary veins into a venous confluence behind the left atrium and drainage of the pulmonary venous blood through a vertical vein and the innominate vein into the superior vena cava. **b** Cardiac type with connection of the pulmonary veins in a venous confluence that drains the pulmonary venous blood into the coronary sinus. **c** Cardiac type with connection of the pulmonary veins directly to the right atrium. **d** Infracardiac type with connection of the pulmonary veins in a venous confluence that drains into a vein that runs in a caudal direction behind the heart, passes through the diaphragm, and connects to the portal vein. The pulmonary venous blood finally reaches the inferior vena cava through the portal vein and the hepatic veins.
RA, right atrium; LA, left atrium; LV, left ventricle; RV, right ventricle; SVC, superior vena cava; IVC, inferior vena cava; CS, coronary sinus; LPV, left pulmonary veins; RPV, right pulmonary veins; InnV, innominate vein.

are more often affected by an infracardiac-type total anomalous pulmonary venous connection; the other types affect both genders equally.

Pathogenesis

During embryonic development, a common pulmonary vessel develops into which all pulmonary veins drain. This pulmonary venous confluence normally fuses with the left atrium. In a total anomalous pulmonary venous connection, there is a faulty connection of the pulmonary venous confluence to a systemic vein instead of to the left atrium.

Classification

There are four types depending on the site of the anomalous connection (▶ Fig. 15.20), but there are also many anatomical variants:

- Supracardiac type (55%): The pulmonary venous blood collects in a common confluence of all pulmonary veins behind the left atrium. The confluence is connected with the innominate vein via a vertical vein running in cranial direction. The pulmonary venous blood flows through the innominate vein into the superior vena cava.
- Cardiac type (30%): The pulmonary veins drain via a short common trunk or with separate openings from posterior into the right atrium or the coronary sinus, which then drains the pulmonary venous blood into the right atrium.
- Infracardiac type (13%): The pulmonary venous blood flows through a common trunk behind the left atrium in a caudal direction through the diaphragm and then through the portal vein system or ductus venosus into the inferior vena cava. In the infracardiac type of total anomalous pulmonary venous connection, there is almost always a pulmonary venous obstruction that determines the hemodynamics.
- Mixed type: This type features various anomalous connections. This type is very rare and has a poor prognosis.

Note

Of particular significance in a total anomalous pulmonary venous connection is whether a pulmonary venous obstruction is also present. An obstruction is practically always present in the infracardiac type. Pulmonary venous obstructions can develop in up to 10% of cases even after corrective surgery due to intimal proliferation in the area of surgery and the veins themselves.

Hemodynamics

The pulmonary veins usually join in the retrocardiac area in a venous confluence located behind the left atrium from where the oxygenated pulmonary venous blood flows to the right atrium via various venous connections. There is a 100% left-to-right shunt that leads to volume overload in the right atrium and ventricle and in the pulmonary circulation system. Therefore, the right atrium and ventricle and the pulmonary artery are dilated; the left atrium is small. The only flow into the left ventricle comes through an ASD via a right-to-left shunt that is necessary for survival. The systemic circulation therefore receives mixed blood, but cyanosis may not be particularly pronounced due to the strong pulmonary recirculation.

The excessive pulmonary blood flow leads to pulmonary hypertension that can be additionally aggravated by a pulmonary venous obstruction and lead to pulmonary edema. Possible causes of such an obstruction are external compression (e.g., when passing through the diaphragm or from compression of the vertical vein between the left main bronchus and left pulmonary artery), intimal proliferation, or stenosis of the vein.

Associated Anomalies

A total anomalous pulmonary venous connection frequently occurs in isolation without any other cardiac anomalies. It can also occur in combination with what can be complex heart defects—for example, d-TGA, tetralogy of Fallot, truncus arteriosus communis, hypoplastic left heart syndrome, tricuspid atresia, coarctation of the aorta, AVSD, pulmonary atresia.

Associated Syndromes

A total anomalous pulmonary venous connection occurs frequently with heterotaxy syndromes. It has also been described in patients with a cat eye syndrome.

15.7.2 Diagnostic Measures

Symptoms

The presence or absence of a pulmonary venous obstruction is the most significant aspect of the clinical symptoms.

▸ **Total anomalous pulmonary venous connection without pulmonary venous obstruction.** In these types, the initial course is often relatively asymptomatic; at birth the children are usually unremarkable at first glance. Cyanosis is frequently not pronounced and not readily visible due to pulmonary recirculation; cyanosis should however be detected during routine neonatal pulse oximetry screening. Signs of heart failure (tachypnea, tachycardia, hepatosplenomegaly, delayed growth) develop in most children within the first weeks of life. Frequent respiratory infections are the result of excessive pulmonary blood flow.

▸ **Total anomalous pulmonary venous connection with pulmonary venous obstruction.** In these patients, pronounced cyanosis and dyspnea develop within the first hours of life. Pulmonary edema follows ("white" lung in an X-ray) with respiratory failure, rapidly developing cardiac failure, and metabolic acidosis.

Note

A total anomalous pulmonary venous connection with pulmonary venous obstruction is one of the few emergencies that requires immediate surgery.

Complications

The main feature of a pulmonary venous obstruction is rapidly developing pulmonary edema. However, if untreated, even patients without a pulmonary venous obstruction develop elevated pulmonary vascular resistance in the first months of life as a result of excessive pulmonary blood flow, which can make surgical correction impossible.

Auscultation

The auscultation finding is often nonspecific. The first heart sound is usually loud; there is a fixed split second heart sound that is also loud because of the volume overload of the right heart. There may be a functional pulmonary stenosis murmur or tricuspid regurgitation murmur.

ECG

The ECG shows signs of right atrial (P pulmonale) and right ventricular overload (e.g., of the volume overload type with rsR′ configuration in V_1, positive T wave in V_1 beyond the first days of life).

Chest X-ray

There is cardiomegaly due to the enlargement of the right atrium and ventricle with increased pulmonary vascular markings. If there is a pulmonary venous obstruction, there will already be signs of pulmonary congestion up to pulmonary edema (bilateral ground glass or fine reticular opacity extending to the periphery of the lungs) in the neonate.

In older children with a supracardiac anomalous pulmonary venous connection, the typical "snowman" or "figure 8" can often be seen, caused by the dilatation of veins (vertical vein, right superior vena cava).

Echocardiography

The diagnosis can usually be made easily by electrocardiography. Indicative findings are a conspicuously enlarged right atrium and ventricle and a right-to-left shunt at the atrial level. The left atrium is small. A venous confluence (3rd vessel in addition to the vena cava and aorta) can usually be visualized behind the left atrium. In a supracardiac anomalous pulmonary venous connection, massive flow can be seen in a dilated superior vena cava. In an anomalous pulmonary venous connection to the coronary sinus, the sinus is dilated. In the infracardiac type, dilated hepatic veins can be seen. Doppler ultrasonography is used to detect a pulmonary venous obstruction. Associated cardiac anomalies must be ruled out.

Cardiac Catheterization

A firm diagnosis can generally be made using echocardiography. Cardiac catheterization is needed only in isolated cases, for example, if there are associated complex cardiac anomalies. A typical finding in pulse oximetry is clearly elevated oxygen saturation in the right atrium with levels between 80% and 95%. Pressure is elevated in the right atrium, right ventricle, and pulmonary artery. If there is a pulmonary venous obstruction, high pulmonary capillary wedge pressure and generally suprasystemic right ventricular pressure are found. In a contrast medium angiography of the pulmonary artery, the flow path demonstrates the anomalous pulmonary venous connection.

MRI

An MRI can be used in individual cases to visualize unclear anatomical details. It is particularly valuable for assessing pulmonary vein stenoses that sometimes develop, even postoperatively.

15.7.3 Treatment

▸ **Conservative treatment.** Pharmacological treatment of heart failure is the most important measure for a total anomalous pulmonary venous connection without pulmonary venous obstruction until definitive surgical correction.

A total anomalous pulmonary venous connection with pulmonary venous obstruction is an emergency and requires immediate surgery. Until then, the children must be stabilized under intensive care. Because there is usually pulmonary edema, intubation and ventilation with a high PEEP (positive end expiratory pressure) is generally needed. To lower the elevated pulmonary resistance, the children are hyperventilated and in addition, inhaled NO or IV prostacyclin may be administered. Acidosis should be compensated. Diuretics are used to manage the pulmonary edema. Catecholamines are administered if there is low cardiac output, but can aggravate the pulmonary edema if there are severe pulmonary vein stenoses.

▸ **Interventional catheterization.** If there is a restrictive foramen ovale, interventional catheterization with a balloon atrial septostomy (Rashkind procedure) can be a palliative treatment option to maintain or enlarge the right-to-left shunt at the atrial level.

Another indication is a stenosis of the pulmonary venous connection to the superior vena cava. In such cases, a stent can first be placed in the superior vena cava as an interim measure. The corrective surgery is performed later.

▸ **Operative treatment.** Surgical correction is the only definitive treatment. It is performed electively within the first 3 months of life for nonobstructive pulmonary veins, but a total anomalous pulmonary venous connection with pulmonary venous obstruction is a cardiac surgery emergency and must be corrected immediately.

In this operation, depending on the type of the anomalous pulmonary venous connection, the widest possible anastomosis is created between the pulmonary vein confluence and the left atrium. A PDA is ligated and the atrial septum is closed.

15.7.4 Prognosis and Outcome

▸ **Long-term outcome.** If untreated, most of the patients die within the first year of life. If there is a pulmonary venous obstruction, the children generally survive only the first weeks of life. The surgical risk increases with the severity of the preoperative symptoms. An infracardiac-type anomalous pulmonary venous connection is a risk factor. The perioperative mortality rate is about 10 to 20%.

The postoperative course is particularly aggravated by new pulmonary venous obstructions, which can develop even long after the operation and can be surgically corrected only with difficulty or at a high risk. If this complication does not develop, the long-term prognosis is generally very good.

▸ **Outpatient follow-up.** Lifelong monitoring is necessary. In the postoperative period, particular attention must be given to pulmonary venous obstruction, anastomosis strictures, residual shunts in the atrial septum, and arrhythmias. Endocarditis prophylaxis is required in the first 6 postoperative months and lifelong prophylaxis is necessary if there are residual defects near the prosthetic material.

▸ **Physical capacity and lifestyle.** If there are no associated cardiac anomalies and no pulmonary venous obstructions, physical capacity is generally very good after correction.

▸ **Special aspects in adolescents and adults.** Patients who do not undergo corrective surgery hardly ever reach adolescence and adulthood. After correction, lifelong monitoring is required.

15.8 Aortopulmonary Window

15.8.1 Basics

Synonyms: aortopulmonary fenestration, aortopulmonary septal defect

Definition

An aortopulmonary window is a pathological nonrestrictive connection between the ascending aorta and the main pulmonary artery. Unlike a truncus arteriosus communis, there are always two distinct semilunar valves (aortic and pulmonary valves) (▸ Fig. 15.21).

Epidemiology

This is a rare condition that constitutes about 0.2% of all congenital heart defects.

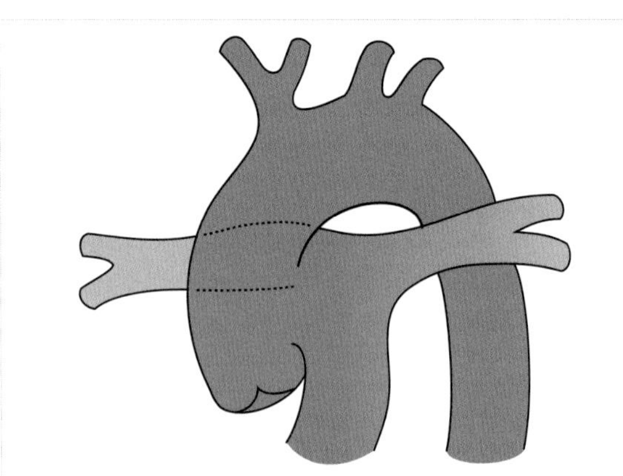

Fig. 15.21 Aortopulmonary window. The frontal view shows that in an aortopulmonary window, part of the ascending aorta and the main pulmonary artery are fused.

Pathogenesis

An aortopulmonary window is caused by an anomalous separation of the embryonic truncus arteriosus communis, from which the ascending aorta and the main pulmonary artery develop.

Classification

Depending on the site and the extent of the pathological connection between the ascending aorta and the main pulmonary artery, three types are distinguished (▸ Fig. 15.22):

- Type I (most common): This is a small defect midway between the semilunar valves and the bifurcation of the pulmonary arteries.
- Type II: The defect is further distal and includes the bifurcation of the pulmonary arteries. In this type the right pulmonary artery often originates directly from the aorta.
- Type III (very rare): This involves a large defect that affects almost the entire aortopulmonary septum, thus encompassing types I and II.

Hemodynamics

Like a PDA, the connection between the aorta and pulmonary artery leads to a left-to-right shunt with volume overload of the left heart and excessive pulmonary blood flow. If untreated, the defect leads to pulmonary hypertension, which can become irreversible within the first years of life.

Associated Cardiac Anomalies

There are associated cardiac anomalies in around half of the cases. The most common are VSDs, ASDs, PDA, anomalies of the aortic arch (interrupted aortic arch, coarctation of the aorta), tetralogy of Fallot, and a right aortic arch.

Coronary anomalies are also significant. An origin of the coronary arteries in the area of the aortopulmonary window has been described. Occasionally, individual coronary arteries can even originate from the pulmonary artery.

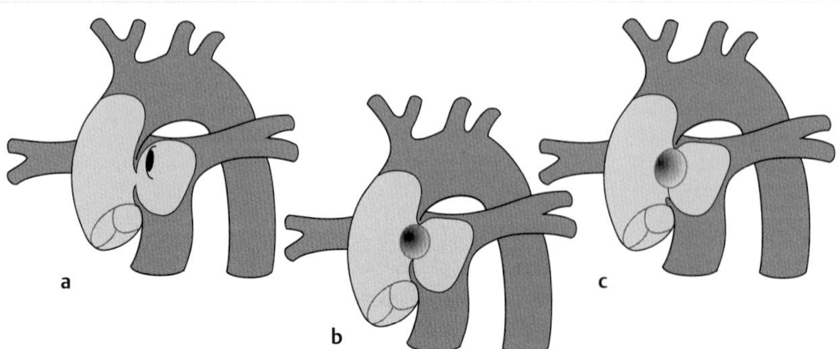

Fig. 15.22 Site and classification of aortopulmonary windows. **a** Type I: proximal defect. There is only a relatively small margin to the semilunar valves. **b** Type II: distal defect. There is a margin to the semilunar valves, but almost no upper margin. The right pulmonary artery sometimes arises from the aorta. **c** Type III: complete defect. Large, confluent defect that involves almost the entire aortopulmonary septum.

Associated Syndromes

Like all conotruncal anomalies, an aortopulmonary window is frequently associated with microdeletion of 22q11.

15.8.2 Diagnostic Measures

Symptoms

The symptoms of a large left-to-right shunt with excessive pulmonary blood flow develop when the pulmonary resistance drops, usually within the first weeks of life (tachypnea, dyspnea with intercostal retractions, failure to thrive). Similar to a PDA, there are strong pulses and a wide pulse pressure as a result of diastolic run-off into the pulmonary artery. Precordial activity is also increased depending on the volume of the shunt.

Complications

Large defects can quickly lead to pulmonary hypertension.

If there is a simultaneous interrupted aortic arch, closure of the PDA can lead to the development of cardiac shock with no pulses in the lower limbs and metabolic acidosis.

Auscultation

The auscultation finding depends on the size of the defect. A continuous systolic–diastolic machinery murmur, as in a PDA, is typical. In larger defects, a loud systolic ejection murmur is generally heard. A mid-systolic murmur at the cardiac apex is a sign of a relative stenosis of the mitral valve associated with increased pulmonary blood flow. A prominent second heart sound is indicative of pulmonary hypertension.

ECG

If the shunt is small, the ECG is unremarkable. Signs of biventricular overload can be seen if the shunt is large, in neonates, or if there is pulmonary hypertension.

Chest X-ray

Depending on the size of the shunt, there is cardiomegaly with enlarged left atrium and ventricle and increased pulmonary vascular markings. The pulmonary artery appears prominent, the aortic knob rather narrow.

Echocardiography

The defect can generally be diagnosed reliably using echocardiography. As a result of the left-to-right shunt, the left atrium and ventricle are enlarged and the pulmonary artery and its branches are dilated. The defect itself can be identified using color Doppler. Antegrade diastolic flow can be detected in the pulmonary artery. When rotating to visualize the intersecting great arteries, the 2D image shows an interruption of the contours of the vessels. Aside from the size of the defect, the relation to the branches of the pulmonary arteries should also be noted. Similar to a hemodynamically relevant PDA, there may be diastolic flow reversal in the abdominal aorta or celiac trunk.

Associated cardiac anomalies (in particular an interrupted aortic arch) must be ruled out.

PDA and truncus arteriosus communis should be considered as a differential diagnosis. However, a PDA does not originate from the ascending aorta. In truncus arteriosus communis, there is only one large semilunar (truncal) valve overriding a malalignment VSD.

Cardiac Catheterization

Cardiac catheterization is generally not required, but an isolated small aortopulmonary window can possibly be closed by interventional catheterization.

15.8.3 Treatment

▸ **Conservative treatment.** Cardiac failure is treated pharmacologically as an interim measure until definitive surgical correction can be performed.

▸ **Indications for surgical closure.** There is almost always an indication for surgery.

▸ **Contraindications for surgical closure.** Surgical closure is contraindicated if the diagnosis is not made before irreversible pulmonary hypertension has occurred.

▸ **Operative treatment.** The treatment of choice is closure of the defect with a patch via a transaortic access route. If there is a functional origin of the right pulmonary artery from the aorta, a tunnel-shaped patch can be sutured in place to allow the blood from the main pulmonary artery to flow into the right pulmonary artery ▸ Fig. 15.23.

Associated cardiac anomalies are usually corrected in the same operation, which is generally performed in the first weeks of life.

▸ **Interventional catheterization.** Interventional catheter closure is an alternative for some patients with isolated small defects that have an adequate margin to the semilunar valves and the bifurcation of the pulmonary arteries.

15.8.4 Prognosis and Outcome

▸ **Long-term outcome.** The prognosis is very good if the operation is performed in time, before irreversible pulmonary hypertension has developed.

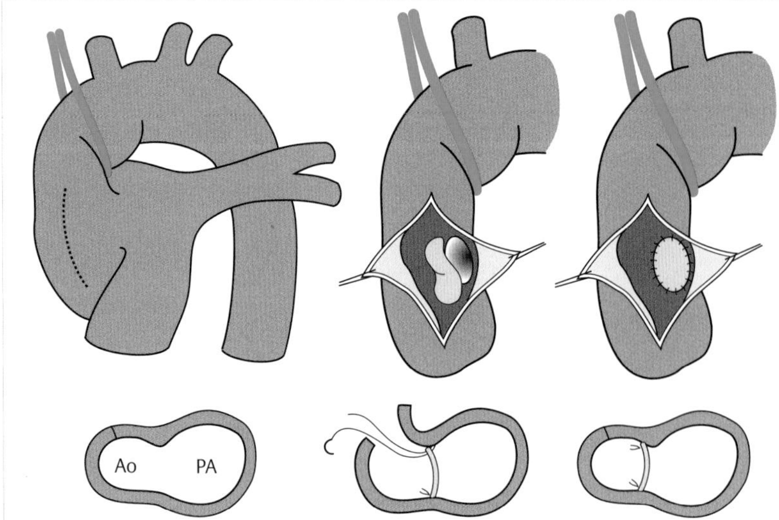

Fig. 15.23 Patch closure of an aortopulmonary window via an aortic access route. The defect in the aortopulmonary septum is closed with a patch via an incision in the ascending aorta.
Ao, aorta; PA, pulmonary artery.

► **Outpatient follow-up.** Postoperative monitoring to detect residual shunts in the vicinity of the patch or stenosis of the right pulmonary artery is important.

Endocarditis prophylaxis is required in the first 6 postoperative months and lifelong prophylaxis is necessary if there are residual shunts in the vicinity of the patch.

► **Physical capacity and lifestyle.** Physical capacity is not impaired if the defect is closed in time.

► **Special aspects in adolescents and adults.** Due to the standard of medical care in industrial nations, adolescent or adult patients with an undiagnosed aortopulmonary window are a rarity. If there is a significant shunt across the aortopulmonary window, these patients would have generally developed an Eisenmenger reaction. However, a few cases of adults have been described with a small aortopulmonary window without an increase in pulmonary vascular resistance. The hemodynamics and clinical symptoms of these patients are similar to those with a PDA.

15.9 Arteriovenous Fistulas

15.9.1 Basics

Definition

An arteriovenous fistula (AV fistula) is an abnormal connection between an artery and a vein that bypasses the capillary bed. There is either a direct connection between the two vessels or a network existing between them with a larger vascular lumen that offers lower resistance than the capillary bed. AV fistulas are generally congenital in children, but can be acquired (e.g., as a complication following a vein puncture).

The most common AV fistulas occurring in the brain, the liver, and the lungs are discussed here. Other typical sites are the thorax (usually proceeding from the mammary artery), neck (usually the external carotid artery or subclavian artery), limbs, and kidneys. AV fistulas can be isolated or occur in multiples. Multiple arteriovenous anomalies occur frequently in patients with Osler-Weber-Rendu syndrome.

Fistulas of the coronary arteries are described in Chapter 15.30.

Epidemiology

These anomalies occur rarely.

Pathology

Note

If no cardiac cause such as a congenital heart defect, arrhythmia, or myocarditis is found for cardiac failure, an AV fistula that leads to volume overload of the heart should be considered as a differential diagnosis. Clinical symptoms are strong pulses. The echocardiography shows enlargement of all cardiac chambers.

AV fistulas occur either as a direct connection between an artery and a vein or consist of a tangle of vessels of varying sizes (nidus) supplied by one or more arteries and drained by several veins. The reduced vascular resistance can lead to an increase in stroke volume with a large pulse pressure, increase in heart rate, cardiac volume overload, and if the shunt is large, to congestive heart failure. Blood flow can be reduced distal to the fistula. In neonates, cyanosis develops if the systemic vascular resistance is lower than the pulmonary vascular resistance and a right-to-left shunt develops across a still patent foramen ovale or PDA. In patients with cardiac failure, cyanosis can also be a sign of reduced peripheral blood flow that leads to cyanosis due to extraction.

15.9.2 Cerebral Fistulas

In cerebral fistulas, there are frequently multiple connections between arterial and venous vessels (AV angiomas). The vein of Galen malformation is a special form. This is an AV malformation with persistence of the precursor of the vein of Galen (the prosencephalic vein), with aneurysmal dilatation due to the high shunt volume. It can lead to compression phenomena (hydrocephalus, focal cerebral seizures, headaches, etc.). The left-to-right shunt causes a volume overload of all segments of the heart and can be so large that it can lead to intrauterine hydrops fetalis. The shunt often causes acute heart failure in the neonate.

► **Symptoms and physical examination.** Typical findings are signs of heart failure, a hyperactive heart, and a wide pulse pressure. A continuous systolic–diastolic pressure can be auscultated over the cranial vault. Cerebral hemorrhage, cerebral seizures, headaches, and focal neurological deficits can be the first signs of smaller cerebral AV malformations.

► **Echocardiography.** Enlargement of all cardiac chambers and excessive blood flow in the superior vena cava.

► **Chest X-ray.** Cardiomegaly with increased pulmonary vascular markings.

► **Cranial ultrasonography.** Visualization of a cystic malformation, detection of blood flow in the fistulas with Doppler ultrasound.

► **Cranial MRI.** Detailed visualization of the vascular architecture, the cerebral parenchyma, and cerebrospinal fluid spaces.

► **Cardiac catheterization and angiography.** A typical finding is increased oxygen content of venous blood in the superior vena cava. Selective angiographies aid in visualizing the inflow and outflow and extent of the AV malformation. Interventional catheter closure is an important treatment option.

► **Therapy.** An attempt is generally made to embolize the fistulas using interventional catheterization. However, this procedure is not unproblematic. Often previously minor fistula vessels gain significance after embolization of the main vessels. Another treatment option is the surgical elimination of the AV malformation. Sometimes both options need to be combined. The mortality rate is high, especially if there are multiple AV connections, and can be up 50%.

15.9.3 Hepatic Fistulas

AV fistulas occur in the liver generally as hemangioendotheliomas or in conjunction with Osler-Weber-Rendu syndrome. A hemangioendothelioma is a benign vascular tumor; multiple angiomatic telangiectasias in various organs occur in Osler-Weber-Rendu syndrome.

► **Symptoms and physical examination.** The clinical manifestations of hepatic fistulas are cardiac failure, gastrointestinal bleeding, and signs of portal hypertension. On auscultation, there may be a continuous systolic–diastolic murmur over the liver.

► **Chest X-ray.** In a hemodynamically relevant shunt, there is cardiomegaly with increased pulmonary vascular markings.

► **Echocardiography.** Enlargement of all segments of the heart, the inferior vena cava, and the hepatic vessels.

► **Sonography of the abdomen including Doppler ultrasound.** Visualization of the fistulas. Imaging may be supplemented by slice imaging.

► **Cardiac catheterization and angiography.** The typical finding is elevated oxygen content in the venous blood of the inferior vena cava. Selective angiographies can be made to visualize the inflows and outflows and the extent of the AV malformation.

► **Therapy.** Surgical excision is difficult unless it is a circumscribed lesion. Interventional catheter embolization generally is successful if only one arterial vessel is involved that connects directly with a vein. In complex AV malformations, the procedure is complicated considerably by the fact that after closure of the major supplying vessels, smaller vessels often supply the malformation with arterial blood.

15.9.4 Pulmonary Arteriovenous Fistulas

A pulmonary AV fistula is an abnormal connection that bypasses the pulmonary capillary bed. It involves a direct connection between a pulmonary artery and vein and may exist as single smaller areas in one lobe, or affect multiple locations usually located in both lungs. These diffuse AV malformations are frequently found in patients with Osler-Weber-Rendu syndrome, with hepatic diseases, or with an upper cavopulmonary anastomosis.

It is assumed that a hepatic factor produced in the liver that flows through the lungs counteracts pulmonary AV shunts such as this. This factor is possibly not produced in sufficient amounts in patients with liver disease. For patients with a cavopulmonary anastomosis, the mechanism is explained as follows: After an upper cavopulmonary anastomosis, the hepatic venous blood bypasses the lungs, as only venous blood from the upper half of the body flows into the lungs. For this reason, the hepatic factor does not take effect in the lungs and pulmonary AV shunts are opened.

► **Symptoms and physical examination.** The leading symptom is cyanosis, as deoxygenated blood bypasses the AV malformation at the lung alveoli and flows into the systemic bloodstream. If there is an isolated AV fistula, a continuous murmur can be auscultated over the fistula; the murmur is generally absent if there are multiple AV malformations. Furthermore, the AV fistulas can promote the development of paradoxical embolisms and cerebral abscesses.

► **Echocardiography.** A structurally unremarkable heart in cyanotic patients should always suggest a pulmonary AV fistula. The AV shunt may be detected using bubble echo. A few milliliters of a saline solution are shaken thoroughly and injected into a peripheral vein. (In patients with an upper cavopulmonary anastomosis, ensure that it is a vein for the upper half of the body.) Using echocardiography, bubbles can be detected in the right atrium and ventricle. During subsequent passage through the lungs, these bubbles are normally filtered out in the pulmonary capillary bed, but if there are pulmonary AV connections, bubbles can bypass the pulmonary capillary bed and reach the left atrium, where they can be visualized by echocardiography.

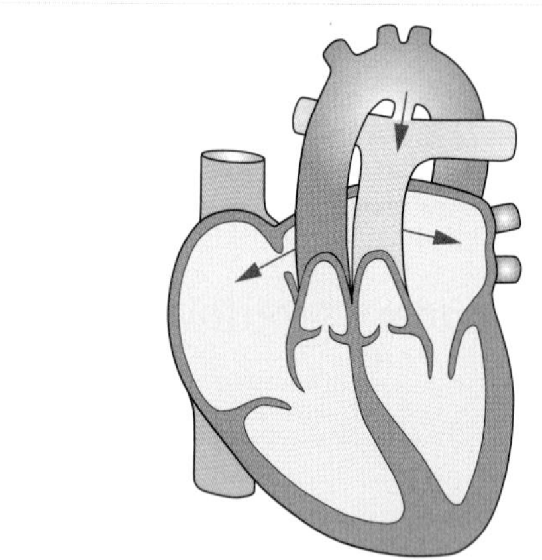

Fig. 15.24 Transposition of the great arteries (d-TGA). In d-TGA, the aorta originates from the right ventricle and the pulmonary artery from the left ventricle. The two large vessels run parallel to one another and do not intersect. The aorta is at the right of the pulmonary artery. The systemic and pulmonary circulations are arranged in parallel. Survival is possible only if there are shunt connections between the two circulations. A nonrestrictive communication at the atrial level is of particular significance.[15]

► **Cardiac catheterization.** Pulse oximetry shows arterial undersaturation. In an angiography, the intrapulmonary shunts can be visualized after injecting contrast medium into the right ventricle or pulmonary artery.

► **Treatment.** Interventional catheter closure of AV fistulas is the treatment of choice; a surgical procedure is only rarely needed. The procedure remains difficult if there are multiple intrapulmonary shunts. The situation is generally improved in patients who develop intrapulmonary shunts after an upper cavopulmonary anastomosis, when the hepatic venous blood flows through the lungs again, as is the case after completion of Fontan circulation.

15.10 Transposition of the Great Arteries

15.10.1 Basics

Definition

In dextro-transposition of the great arteries (d-TGA), the two great vessels (aorta, pulmonary artery) are "switched" (► Fig. 15.24 and ► Fig. 15.25). There is an anomalous origin of the aorta from the right ventricle and of the pulmonary artery from the left ventricle (ventriculoarterial discordance). The positions of the atria and ventricles relative to each other are normal (atrioventricular concordance). The result is a parallel and not connected circuit of systemic and pulmonary circulation. Deoxygenated blood is pumped from the right ventricle through the aorta back into the systemic circulation, while oxygenated blood from the left ventricle reaches the lungs. This leads to severe hypoxemia if no mixing of

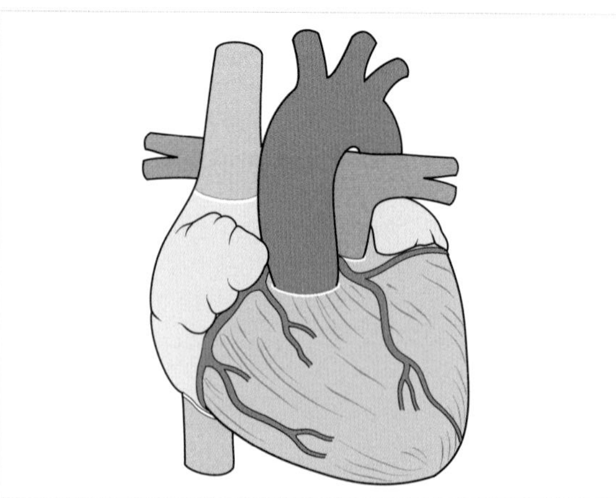

Fig. 15.25 External view of a heart with transposition of the great arteries (d-TGA). In d-TGA, the aorta is located in front of and somewhat to the right of the pulmonary artery. The aorta originates from the infundibulum of the right ventricle, the pulmonary artery from the left ventricle.

venous and arterialized blood can take place via additional connections (e.g., patent foramen ovale, PDA, VSD).

Epidemiology

A d-TGA constitutes about 5% of all congenital heart defects and is the second most common cyanotic defect after the tetralogy of Fallot. The incidence is approximately 20 to 30 per 100,000 live births. Boys are affected around twice as often as girls.

Pathogenesis

The details leading to a d-TGA are not fully understood. The cause may be a development disorder in the embryonic truncal septum that separates the originally common trunk into the aorta and pulmonary artery, or in the distal infundibulum (arterial cone).

Classification

A simple or complex TGA is distinguished depending on the presence of other cardiac anomalies:

- Simple d-TGA: The term "simple d-TGA" (d-TGA simplex) describes a d-TGA in which there are no other cardiac anomalies aside from a patent foramen ovale and PDA. Two-thirds of cases are d-TGA simplex.
- Complex d-TGA: In a complex d-TGA, additional cardiac anomalies such as a VSD or coronary anomalies are present.

Hemodynamics

The aorta arises from the right ventricle. It usually passes in front of the pulmonary artery, which arises behind the aorta from the left ventricle. Both vessels proceed upward parallel to each other and do not intersect. Generally, this means that the aorta is at the right (hence dextro-TGA, d-TGA) and in front of the pulmonary artery. Both circulations are arranged in parallel and are completely separate from each other. The right ventricle supplies the systemic circulation and the coronary arteries; the left ventricle supplies the pulmonary circulation. This can be survived only if there is a connection that results in oxygenated blood entering the aorta and thus systemic circulation. This connection is a defect at the atrial level that allows oxygenated blood from the left atrium to flow into the right atrium across a left-to-right shunt (▶ Fig. 15.26). The oxygenated blood then flows through the right ventricle into the aorta.

The pulmonary blood flow is increased by a PDA, leading to an increase in pressure in the left atrium, which encourages a left-to-right shunt at the atrial level. A VSD can have the same effect. It is important to understand that systemic circulation can generally be supplied with oxygenated blood only through a left-to-right shunt at the atrial level. A PDA or a VSD encourages a left-to-right atrial-level shunt by increasing pulmonary blood flow and thus increasing left atrial pressure.

An exception may be if there is a very large ASD with pressure equalization in both atria, where true

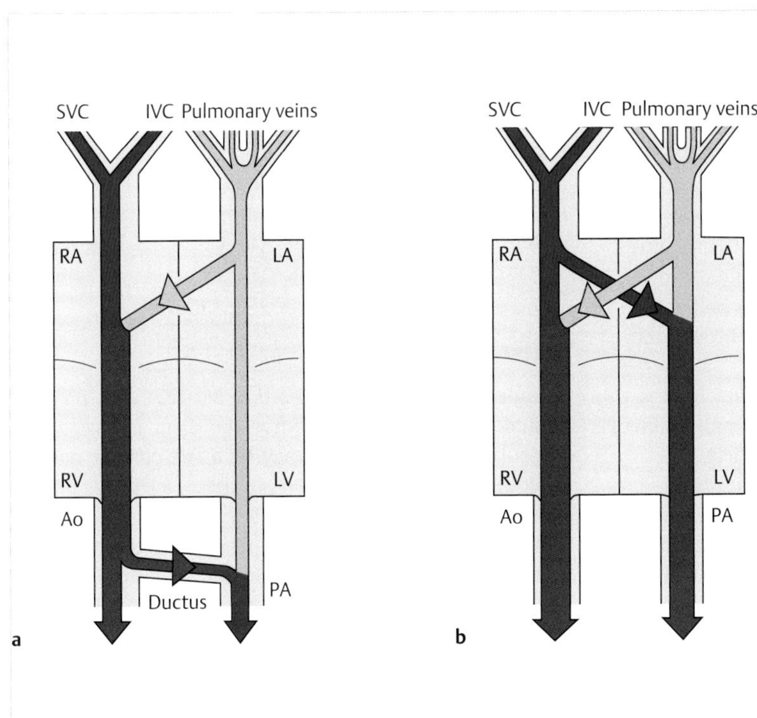

Fig. 15.26 Intracirculatory mixing of systemic and pulmonary blood in a d-TGA with a PDA and atrial communication (**a**) and in a d-TGA with a large, pressure-equalizing ASD (**b**). **a** Hemodynamics in a PDA and small atrial communication. Corresponding with the pressure gradient, the blood flows across the patent ductus into the pulmonary circulation. Due to the increased pulmonary blood flow, pressure increases in the left atrium and the left-to-right shunt at atrial level increases. Oxygenated blood from the pulmonary circulation mixes with deoxygenated blood from the systemic circulation through this left-to-right shunt at atrial level. **b** Hemodynamics of a large, pressure-equalizing atrial communication: If there is a large atrial communication that leads to pressure equalization between the two atria, there can be a true mixing of deoxygenated blood from the systemic circulation and oxygenated blood from the pulmonary circulatory system.
RA, right atrium, LA, left atrium, RV, right ventricle, LV, left ventricle, SVC, superior vena cava, IVC, inferior vena cava, Ao, aorta, PA, pulmonary artery. (Adapted from Wernowsky G et al. 1995)[111]

intracirculatory mixing of oxygenated and deoxygenated blood occurs at the atrial level. When the pulmonary vascular resistance is still elevated, a bidirectional shunt may form at the ductus level and also results in mixing oxygenated and venous blood. However, when the pulmonary vascular resistance drops, only a shunt from the systemic to pulmonary circulation occurs across the ductus.

In clinical practice, "poor mixers" are occasionally seen, in whom there is no satisfactory explanation for pronounced undersaturation despite a large atrial communication.

Associated Anomalies

Associated cardiac anomalies occur in around one-third of patients with a d-TGA (complex d-TGA) that sometimes have a considerable effect on the hemodynamics or consequences for the surgical procedure:

- A *ventral septal defect* (VSD) increases pulmonary blood flow and leads to an increase in left atrial pressure so the left-to-right shunt at atrial level is improved. In addition, if there is a very large VSD with equalization of the pressure in both ventricles, the left ventricle remains "fit," which can have a favorable effect on a later switch procedure.
- *Coronary anomalies* are frequent and are particularly significant for surgical correction. The most frequent coronary anomaly is an origin of the circumflex branch from the right coronary artery; less frequently, there is a single coronary ostium or an intramural course of the coronary arteries in the aortic wall. A coronary anomaly may make a switch procedure impossible, as the coronary arteries would have to be transplanted as part of the correction procedure.
- A *valvular* or *subvalvular pulmonary stenosis* becomes a functional aortic stenosis after a switch procedure. If there is a relevant pulmonary stenosis, a Rastelli procedure must be performed (see Chapter 15.10.3).
- The leading symptom of a d-TGA with *coarctation of the aorta* or *interrupted aortic arch* is dissociated cyanosis: the upper half of the body is cyanotic while the lower half is rosy. This occurs because the lower half of the body is supplied with oxygenated blood through the patent PDA.
- An *obstruction of the left ventricular outflow tract* is usually a dynamic stenosis caused by the protrusion of the ventricular septum into the left ventricle.
- *Mitral valve anomalies:* After a switch procedure, a previously existing mitral valve cleft can lead to severe mitral valve incompetence, so anomalies in the mitral valve must be diagnosed preoperatively and treated during the operation.

Associated Syndromes

A d-TGA is only rarely associated with genetic syndromes or extracardiac anomalies.

15.10.2 Diagnostic Measures

Symptoms

The clinical symptoms depend on the type and size of the shunt between the parallel circulatory systems and associated cardiac anomalies. Neonates are initially unimpaired in the immediate postnatal period and generally have a normal birth weight, as an intrauterine d-TGA has only a minimal hemodynamic effect.

The leading symptoms are severe central cyanosis that develops in the first hours or days of life that does not respond to oxygen and metabolic acidosis. This finding is in contrast to the relatively unremarkable auscultation finding of a d-TGA simplex.

Note

Increasing cyanosis, an unremarkable auscultation finding, and increased pulmonary blood flow in the chest X-ray in a neonate always suggest TGA.

In a d-TGA with large VSD, cyanosis may be less pronounced. Progressive heart failure is the main clinical symptom, which develops when pulmonary resistance drops and leads to increasing excessive pulmonary blood flow. In these cases, the symptoms of heart failure (poor feeding, tachypnea, tachycardia, hepatomegaly, and failure to thrive) are predominant.

Complications

The main problems are the developing severe systemic hypoxia and metabolic acidosis. Excessive pulmonary blood flow (d-TGA with large VSD) leads to increasing cardiac failure. In patients with a d-TGA and VSD, pulmonary vascular resistance develops sooner than in other defects associated with excessive pulmonary blood flow—often in infants as young as 3 to 4 months. The reasons are not yet fully understood.

Auscultation

A murmur is usually not heard in a d-TGA with no additional cardiac anomalies. After the drop in pulmonary vascular resistance, there may be a left parasternal systolic ejection murmur, which is a sign of a relative pulmonary stenosis associated with increased pulmonary blood flow. Because of the anterior position of the aorta, the second heart sound is prominent and seems to be unsplit because the closing sound of the pulmonary artery located to the posterior is not heard.

If there is a simultaneous VSD, a typical band-shaped holosystolic murmur with PMI in the 3rd or 4th left parasternal ICS can be heard after the drop in pulmonary vascular resistance.

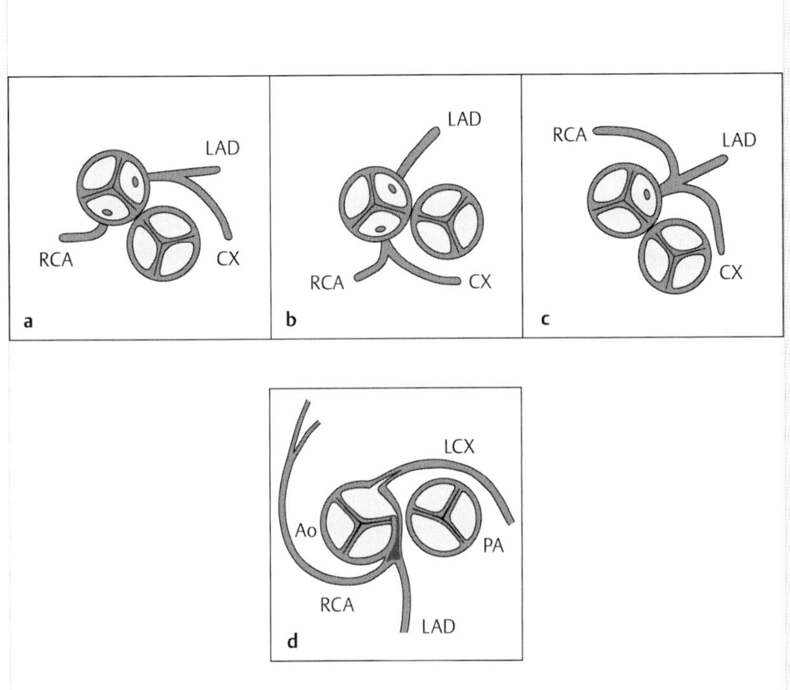

Fig. 15.27 The most common coronary anomalies associated with d-TGA. With d-TGA, the coronary arteries always arise from the "facing sinus," the sinus of Valsalva facing them immediately adjacent to the pulmonary valve. **a** The right coronary artery usually arises from the right-facing sinus at the right and the left coronary artery from the left-facing sinus. **b** In the most common coronary anomaly, the circumflex artery arises from the right coronary artery instead of from the left coronary artery. **c** A common coronary ostium of the two coronary arteries is another frequent anomaly. **d** An intramural course of the coronary arteries is particularly important for the surgeon. In this case, a coronary artery runs in the aortic wall between the aorta and pulmonary artery. This anomaly can make a coronary transfer in an arterial switch procedure impossible.
Ao, Aorta, PA, pulmonary artery, LAD, left anterior descending artery, RCA, right coronary artery, CX, circumflex branch, LCX, left circumflex artery (Adapted from Blume et al. 1999)[108].

ECG

The ECG has signs of (initially physiological, later pathological) right heart hypertrophy (moderate right axis deviation, high R waves in V_1/V_2, possibly a positive T wave in V_1 after the 1st day of life) and possibly signs of right atrial overload (P pulmonale).

If there is a large VSD or pulmonary stenosis, signs of biventricular hypertrophy develop.

Chest X-ray

The cardiac silhouette is generally slightly enlarged. The typical configuration of the cardiac silhouette is described as "egg on its side," an egg-shaped heart lying sideways in the thorax. The mediastinal vascular band is narrow; the pulmonary segment is absent. The pulmonary vascular markings are increased.

Echocardiography

A reliable diagnosis can be made using echocardiography. The following typical d-TGA findings should be assessed for every d-TGA:

- The parasternal long view shows the aorta arising from the right ventricle, which is in an *anterior* position. In the parasternal short axis view, the aorta lies anterior and to the right of the pulmonary artery. The two vessels run parallel to one another and do not intersect.
- The right ventricle is usually enlarged and compresses the banana-shaped left ventricle. The right ventricle normally curves around the left ventricle.
- Visualization of the coronary artery anatomy (▶ Fig. 15.27): The coronary arteries practically always originate from the "facing sinus," that is, from the two sinuses of Valsalva of the aorta located directly opposite the pulmonary artery. In a d-TGA, the right coronary artery usually originates in the right "facing sinus 1" and the left coronary artery with the circumflex branch arises from the left "facing sinus 2."
- Visualization of the atrial communication (patent foramen ovale, ASD II): A sufficiently large atrial shunt is necessary for survival. A protrusion of the atrial septum to the right and accelerated flow across the defect are signs of a restrictive atrial shunt.
- Visualization of the PDA: It is necessary to investigate whether the PDA is sufficiently wide or is occluded. The shunt direction must also be assessed. There is usually a bidirectional shunt until the drop in pulmonary vascular resistance, after which the flow is generally from the aorta to the pulmonary artery.
- Exclusion or detection of additional cardiac anomalies: especially VSD, valvular or subvalvular pulmonary stenosis, left ventricular outflow tract obstruction, coarctation of the aorta, and mitral valve cleft.

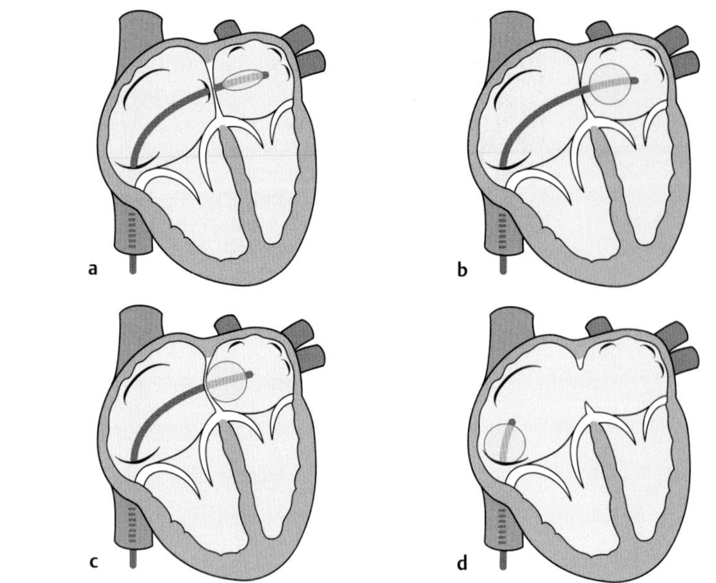

Fig. 15.28 Rashkind balloon atrial septostomy. **a** The balloon catheter is inserted through the foramen ovale into the left atrium. **b** The balloon is filled with fluid to expand it. **c** The filled balloon is then withdrawn forcefully. **d** The balloon tears the atrial septum when it is pulled out to greatly increase the size of the atrial connection.

Cardiac Catheterization

The diagnosis can usually be reliably made using echocardiography. Cardiac catheterization is indicated only to perform a Rashkind balloon atrial septostomy for a restrictive atrial connection (see Chapter 15.10.3) or in individual cases for the reliable visualization of the coronary arteries and associated cardiovascular anomalies.

MRI

A preoperative MRI is not usually needed, but can explain specific anatomical details. It is often performed postoperatively in older patients after an atrial baffle procedure (see Chapter 15.10.3).

15.10.3 Treatment

Conservative Treatment

Immediately after the diagnosis is made, *prostaglandin E infusion* should be started to keep the ductus arteriosus patent (initial dose: 50 [to 100] ng/kg/min). The dose can usually later be reduced considerably (5–10 ng/kg/min) or discontinued depending on the symptoms and the echocardiography findings.

Oxygen therapy should be given with caution. On the one hand, oxygen can provoke the closure of the ductus arteriosus and on the other hand, pulmonary resistance is also lowered when oxygen is given, which can result in an increase in the pulmonary blood flow and systemic saturation. After a successful balloon atrial septostomy, the pulse oximetry oxygen saturation should be over 70% without additional oxygen therapy or prostaglandin infusion to maintain the patency of the PDA.

The indication for volume treatment (e.g., fractionated 5 – 10 – 15 mL/kg IV) should be made generously, but volume overload must be avoided. If there are clear signs of excessive pulmonary blood flow (e.g., d-TGA with a large VSD), diuretics are indicated.

Interventional Catheterization

▸ **Rashkind balloon atrial septostomy.** If there is a restrictive atrial connection and systemic oxygen saturation below 70% despite a PDA, a Rashkind balloon atrial septostomy (▸ Fig. 15.28) is indicated. A special balloon catheter is inserted through the foramen ovale into the left atrium, filled with 2.5 to 3 mL of fluid, and retracted forcefully. This tears the atrial septum and enlarges the atrial connection. This procedure can generally also be performed in the intensive care unit under echocardiography guidance.

In older children with a rigid atrial septum, an alternative is blade atrial septostomy, which is performed using a special catheter with a blade at the tip.

Stent implantation in the ductus arteriosus is only rarely indicated to keep it patent for a long period.

Surgery

In principle, correction is possible at the atrial level (Mustard/Senning procedure), ventricular level (Rastelli procedure), or level of the great arteries (arterial switch operation). Today, the arterial switch procedure, which most closely approaches normal anatomy and gives the best long-term results, is generally preferred. Until the mid-1980s, before the more complicated switch procedure became routine, atrial baffle procedures were performed in most patients. The greatest surgical challenge

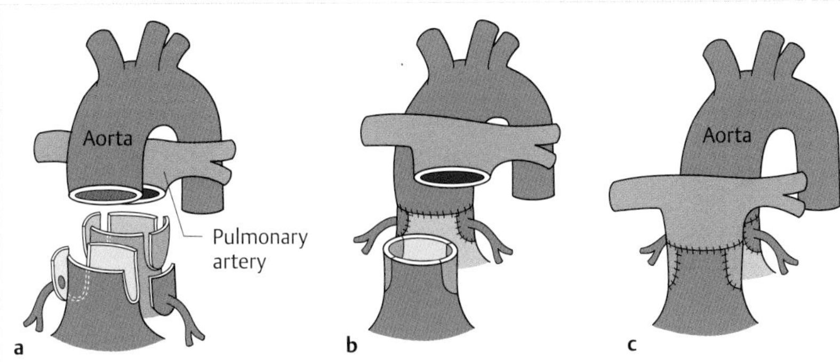

Fig. 15.29 Arterial switch operation (Jatene procedure). a First the aorta and pulmonary artery are transected and coronary arteries are separated from the aortic root. b Then the aorta is relocated posterior to the pulmonary artery (Lecompte maneuver) and the coronary arteries are implanted in the pulmonary artery root (neo-aorta). c Finally, the pulmonary artery is anastomosed with the aortic root (neo-pulmonary artery).

in the switch operation is transplanting the coronary arteries.

Arterial Switch Operation (Jatene procedure)

▸ **Indication.** Therapy of choice in the first 4 weeks of life, unless associated cardiac anomalies make this treatment option impossible.

▸ **Method.** After transecting the aorta and pulmonary artery, the great vessels must be transposed (▸ Fig. 15.29). In addition, the coronary arteries are excised with a "vascular cuff" and transplanted to the neo-aorta (coronary transfer). Usually the bifurcation of the pulmonary artery is relocated anterior to the aortic arch (Lecompte maneuver) to reduce the risk of tension in the pulmonary artery and its branches.

▸ **Timing of the operation.** After the patient has reached the age of 2 months the operation can no longer be easily performed without preparation of the left ventricle, which is no longer in adequate condition to function as a systemic ventricle after the drop in pulmonary resistance. If the operation has to be performed at a later time, pulmonary artery banding may be necessary as preparation, which leads to an increase in the muscular mass of the left ventricle.

Exception: If there is a large VSD, the left ventricle retains sufficient muscle strength due to the equalization of pressure between the right and left ventricles and may later be converted to a systemic ventricle, even without preparation.

Mustard or Senning Atrial Baffle Operation

▸ **Indication.** An atrial baffle operation may still be indicated today, especially when coronary anomalies make a coronary transfer impossible.

▸ **Method.** The blood from the superior and inferior vena cava is directed through a trousers-shaped baffle made of pericardial (Mustard) or atrial tissue (Senning) through the atria to the mitral and subpulmonary valve.

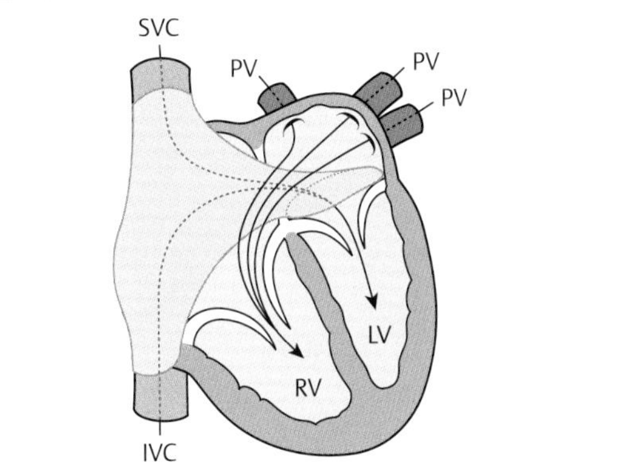

Fig. 15.30 Mustard or Senning atrial baffle procedure. See explanations in text.
RV, right ventricle; LV, left ventricle; SVC, superior vena cava; IVC, inferior vena cava; PV, pulmonary vein.

After the removal or modification of the atrial septum, the oxygenated blood from the pulmonary veins flows around the atrial baffle to the tricuspid and systemic valve (▸ Fig. 15.30).

Rastelli Procedure

▸ **Indication.** The Rastelli procedure is indicated for a d-TGA with VSD and severe pulmonary stenosis.

▸ **Method.** The pulmonary artery is transected at the trunk and the VSD is closed with a patch so that the left ventricle drains into the aorta (▸ Fig. 15.31). It may be necessary to enlarge the VSD prior to closure. The right ventricle is incised and connected with the pulmonary artery by a valved conduit.

Damus-Kaye-Stansel Procedure

▸ **Indication.** For a d-TGA with VSD and a relevant subaortic stenosis, a Damus–Kaye–Stansel procedure with implantation of an extracardiac conduit from the right ventricle to the pulmonary artery may be necessary. However, this operation is very rarely needed for d-TGA.

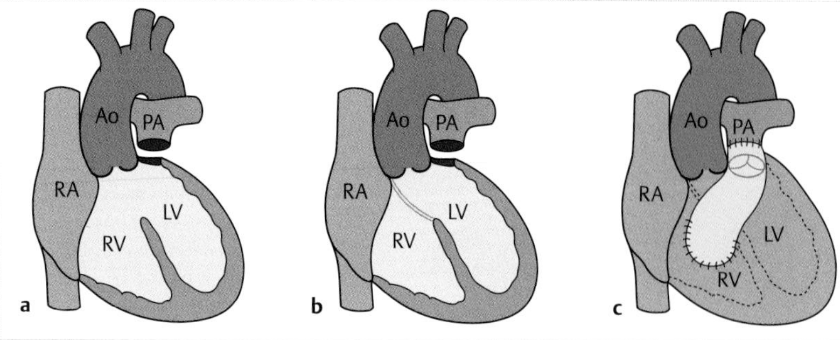

Fig. 15.31 Rastelli procedure for d-TGA with VSD and pulmonary stenosis. **a** The pulmonary artery is transected. **b** The VSD is closed with a patch. **c** The right ventricle and pulmonary artery are connected via a valved conduit.
RA, right atrium; RV, right ventricle; LV, left ventricle; Ao, aorta; PA, pulmonary artery.[29]

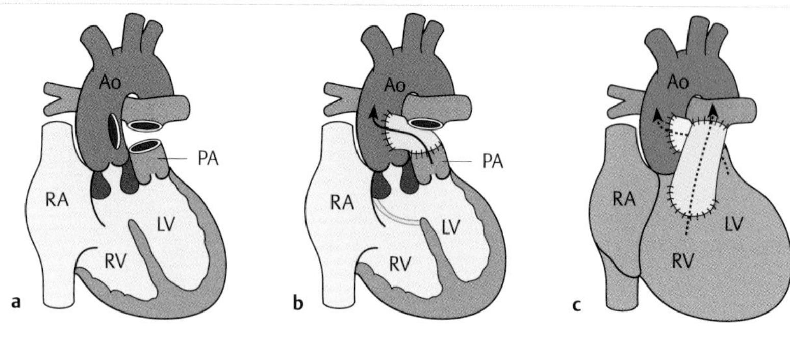

Fig. 15.32 Damus–Kaye–Stansel procedure for a d-TGA with VSD and relevant subaortic stenosis. **a** The pulmonary artery is transected. **b** End-to-side anastomosis between the ascending aorta and pulmonary artery and closure of the VSD. **c** An extracardiac conduit is implanted between the right ventricle and pulmonary artery.
RA, right atrium; RV, right ventricle; LV, left ventricle; Ao, aorta; PA, pulmonary artery.[29]

► **Method.** After transecting the main pulmonary artery, the pulmonary artery is anastomosed end-to-side with the ascending aorta (Damus–Kaye–Stansel anastomosis) and the VSD is also closed. The blood from the left ventricle then flows through the anastomosis via the main pulmonary artery into the aorta. The right ventricle is then connected with the pulmonary artery using an extracardiac conduit (► Fig. 15.32).

15.10.4 Prognosis and Outcome

► **Long-term prognosis.** Left untreated, 30% of the children die within one week, 50% within one month, and 90% within the first year of life.

After corrective surgery, the outcome depends primarily on the procedure used. The *arterial switch operation* yields the best results. The surgical risk is below 5% mortality for uncomplicated variants and about 10% for complicated situations. The late mortality rate is low. Tension in the vicinity of the transposed great arteries can lead to supravalvular stenosis, affecting mainly the pulmonary artery. Stenosis of the transplanted coronary arteries can cause myocardial ischemia with impaired ventricular function and/or ventricular arrhythmias. Complications in the coronary arteries contribute considerably to early mortality.

In a *Mustard or Senning atrial baffle procedure,* the surgical risk is less than 5%. There is, however, considerable late mortality and morbidity. Atrial arrhythmias occur frequently as a result of the extensive preparations in the atrial area. Typical arrhythmias are atrial tachycardias including atrial flutter and fibrillation or intra-atrial reentrant tachycardias, a sick sinus syndrome with a slow base rate, and AV conduction disorders. Pacemaker therapy and antiarrhythmic treatment are required relatively frequently. In addition, the right ventricle functions as a systemic ventricle after an atrial baffle procedure. Progressive dysfunction of the right systemic ventricle usually begins a few years after the operation. It is not rare for tricuspid insufficiency to develop, because the tricuspid valve functions as a systemic AV valve after atrial baffle surgery. Occasionally there are stenoses and leaks in the atrial baffle that require intervention. Depending on the site, baffle stenoses can lead to functional pulmonary or systemic venous stenoses.

After a *Rastelli procedure* a conduit stenosis or insufficiency frequently develops in the long term as a result of degeneration of the conduit, which can make it necessary to replace the conduit. A subaortic stenosis may also develop in the area of the conduit from the left ventricle to the aorta.

► **Outpatient follow-up.** Lifelong postoperative cardiac monitoring is necessary. After an arterial switch operation, particular attention must be paid to signs of coronary stenosis (myocardial ischemia) and supravalvular pulmonary or aortic stenoses and insufficiency of the semilunar valves.

Table 15.1 Typical and common long-term complications after surgical correction of a dextro-transposition of the great arteries

Method	Common complications
Arterial switch operation	• Coronary artery stenoses • Supravalvular pulmonary stenosis • Aortic insufficiency
Atrial baffle procedure	• Atrial arrhythmias (sick sinus syndrome, atrial tachycardias, atrial flutter/fibrillation, junctional rhythm, AV blocks) • Baffle stenosis, baffle leak • Tricuspid insufficiency (= systemic AV valve insufficiency) • Progressive dysfunction of the right ventricle (systemic ventricle)
Rastelli procedure	• Conduit degeneration (stenosis, insufficiency) • Subaortic stenosis (stenosis of the conduit between the left ventricle and aorta)
Damus–Kaye–Stansel procedure	• Stenosis of the anastomosis between the pulmonary artery and aorta • Conduit degeneration (stenosis, insufficiency) • Tendency to thrombosis in the area of the closed pulmonary valve

Following an *atrial baffle procedure*, monitoring should be directed in particular to atrial arrhythmias (Holter-ECG) and the function of the right systemic ventricle including the tricuspid valve.

Following a *Rastelli procedure,* the function of the conduit should be monitored closely and any stenosis in the conduit between the left ventricle and the aortic valve should be noted.

Endocarditis prophylaxis must be maintained for the first 6 postoperative months, and lifelong if there are residual defects near the foreign material or if valved conduits were used.

▶ **Physical capacity and lifestyle.** The results following an *arterial switch operation* have been so good that no serious impairment of physical capacity occurs in most cases. However, evidence of myocardial ischemia should be noted, which can be a sign of coronary stenosis. If supravalvular stenoses of the aorta or the pulmonary artery develop, the recommendations regarding physical capacity depend on the existing gradients (see Chapter 15.19 or Chapter 15.22).

Physical exercise capacity may sometimes be considerably impaired by progressive right ventricular dysfunction and tricuspid insufficiency in patients following an *atrial baffle procedure.* Pharmacological anticongestive treatment is often needed. The situation is sometimes further aggravated by an inadequate increase in the heart rate during exercise in a sick sinus syndrome. A pacemaker can often bring improvement of the symptoms. Most patients can engage in sports with low to moderate dynamic and low static stress levels. Participation in school sports can usually be allowed, but it may be helpful to excuse the patient from being graded.

▶ **Special aspects in adolescents and adults.** Since the atrial baffle operation was the standard procedure for correcting a d-TGA until the mid-1980s, most of the now adult patients were treated with this procedure. Accordingly, the main problems for these patients are rhythm disorders (atrial and also ventricle arrhythmias as a sign of a poor systemic ventricle), conduit obstructions, AV valve insufficiency, and in particular, progressively deteriorating function of the right systemic ventricles (▶ Table 15.1). A heart transplant is the last treatment option for some of these patients.

Since the first patients who were treated with a switch operation are just now reaching adulthood, there are no long-term results available for this procedure. However, the most likely potential long-term complications are expected to be coronary artery problems and dysfunction of the aortic valve (▶ Table 15.1).

15.11 Congenitally Corrected Transposition of the Great Arteries

15.11.1 Basics

Synonyms: levo-transposition of the great arteries (l-TGA), ventricular inversion

Definition

As in dextro-transposition of the great arteries (d-TGA), in congenitally corrected transposition of the great arteries (ccTGA), the aorta also arises from the right ventricle and the pulmonary artery from the left ventricle. However, there is a simultaneous "reversal" of the ventricles (ventricular inversion). The left ventricle is positioned in the position of the right ventricle (anterior and right) and vice versa. The right ventricle is thus connected to the left atrium and the left ventricle to the right atrium (▶ Fig. 15.33). The venous blood from the right atrium flows through the morphologic left ventricle into the pulmonary artery and arterialized blood flows from the left atrium through the morphologic right ventricle into the aorta. This is termed a discordant atrioventricular *and* ventriculoarterial connection. If no other cardiac anomalies are present, the hemodynamic features of a ccTGA are normal. Typically, in this heart defect the aorta runs to the left of the pulmonary artery. This characteristic has led to the designation l-TGA as a synonym for this heart defect (l is for levo = left).

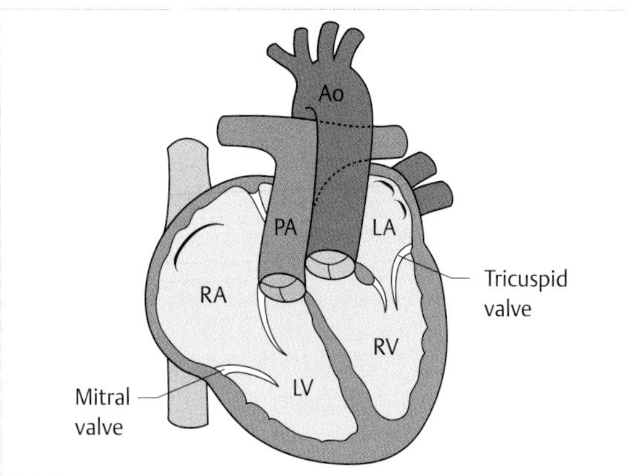

Fig. 15.33 Congenitally corrected transposition of the great arteries (ccTGA). In this abnormality the aorta arises from the right ventricle. Because there is a simultaneous inversion of the ventricles, the hemodynamic situation is normal as long as there are no other cardiac anomalies. However, associated heart defects such as tricuspid valve anomalies are very common. RA, right atrium; LA, left atrium; RV, right ventricle; LV, left ventricle; Ao, aorta; PA, pulmonary artery.

The term "l-TGA" has been established as a synonym for the heart defect described above. Strictly speaking, l-TGA means only that the aorta runs to the left of the pulmonary artery (l-transposition) and the term says nothing about the relationship of the atria to the ventricles or the ventricles to the major arteries. An l-transposition of the great vessels may also be found in association with other congenital heart defects—frequently with a double-inlet left ventricle, for example.

Pathogenesis

The cause is a faulty rotation of the left heart tube during embryonic development. This leads to a situation where the morphologic right ventricle is positioned to the left of the morphologic left ventricle.

Epidemiology

A ccTGA is a rare congenital anomaly and accounts for less than 1% of all congenital heart defects. Males are affected slightly more often than females.

Hemodynamics and Pathological Anatomy

The hemodynamic status in a ccTGA is normal if there are no other cardiac anomalies: the blood of the venous system flows through the right atrium into the left ventricle and from there through the pulmonary artery into the lungs. The blood flows through the pulmonary veins into the left atrium and from there through the right ventricle into the aorta.

The spatial relations are important. In a ccTGA, the morphologic left ventricle (subpulmonary) is usually located at the right and the morphologic right ventricle (subaortic) is located at the left of the chest. The ventricle with the characteristics of a right ventricle is called a morphologic right ventricle: The atrioventricular valve has three leaflets, the myocardium is clearly trabecular, and the inflow and outflow valves are separated by a muscle band (crista supraventricularis). The left ventricle has the following morphological features: The atrioventricular valve has two leaflets, the myocardium has a fine trabecular structure, and the inflow and outflow valves are merged (fibrous continuity).

In ccTGA, as in d-TGA, the aorta is located anterior to the pulmonary artery, but to the left of it. The ventricular septum is often located in the vertical/sagittal plane in a ccTGA. In 95% of cases there is a normal arrangement (situs solitus). Dextrocardia is found in around 20% of cases.

Clinically important is the fact that the AV node is located further anterior and superior than usual and that the bundle of His is a conspicuously long segment. These anatomical features may predispose to AV conduction disorders. In addition, accessory pathways are often found.

Note

In a ccTGA, the risk of AV blocks and accessory conduction pathways must always be considered.

Associated Anomalies

In around 90% of cases, there are accompanying cardiac anomalies that have a major effect on the clinical course. Most common are:

- Tricuspid valve anomalies (up to 90%): mostly tricuspid regurgitation, the Ebsteinlike anomaly of the tricuspid valve is also relatively common (in ccTGA, the tricuspid valve is found on the left side and functions as a systemic AV valve)
- VSD (75%)
- Subvalvular or valvular pulmonary stenosis (30–50%)
- Pulmonary atresia (10%)
- Preexcitation syndromes
- AV conduction problems

Less common are:

- Coarctation of the aorta, interrupted aortic arch
- Mitral valve anomalies
- Double-outlet right ventricle

Associated Syndromes

No frequent association with specific genetic syndromes has been described.

15.11.2 Diagnostic Measures

Symptoms

The clinical symptoms depend mainly on the accompanying cardiac anomalies. If there are no additional anomalies, patients may initially be completely free of symptoms. If there is a large VSD, the main symptom is excessive pulmonary blood flow and development of heart failure (tachypnea, hepatomegaly, poor feeding, failure to thrive). Patients with a relevant tricuspid regurgitation may also develop symptoms of heart failure, depending on its extent.

Patients with a ccTGA combined with a VSD and pulmonary stenosis may present with cyanosis as in tetralogy of Fallot.

Of particular importance is bradycardia. Due to the anatomical features of the AV node and the conduction system, one-third to almost one-half of the patients eventually develop a complete AV block.

Complications

Even with an isolated ccTGA, most patients develop clinical symptoms of heart failure—but often not until adulthood. These symptoms are due to the fact that the morphologic right ventricle is not suitable for the strains of a systemic ventricle. Increasing insufficiency of the tricuspid valve, which functions as a systemic AV valve, can have an unfavorable impact. Complete AV blocks make it necessary to implant a pacemaker. Supraventricular tachycardias can be the result of an accessory conduction pathway.

Auscultation

Due to the anterior location of the aorta, there is a single, loud second heart sound because the closing sound of the pulmonary artery can usually not be heard from its posterior location. A holosystolic left parasternal murmur can be caused by tricuspid regurgitation or a VSD. A systolic ejection murmur on the left upper sternal border suggests a pulmonary stenosis.

ECG

The inversion of Q waves that represent the left ventricle is a typical ECG finding. Normally, the Q waves are present in the left precordial leads (V_5, V_6)—however, in ccTGA, Q waves can be detected in the right precordial leads.

> **Note**
>
> Q waves in leads V_3R to V_1 suggest a ccTGA. In addition, AV blocks, pre-excitation, and supraventricular tachycardias should be noted.

Chest X-ray

A typical finding is an aorta that forms the upper left border. Cardiomegaly can be the result of tricuspid regurgitation or a VSD. The pulmonary blood flow is dependent on additional anomalies (VSD, pulmonary stenosis). Atrial dilatation or pulmonary edema is found if there is relevant tricuspid regurgitation. Dextrocardia is present in approximately 20% of cases.

Echocardiography

The diagnosis can be made reliably using echocardiography. In any event, accompanying cardiac anomalies must be noted. The following findings are typical:

- In the four-chamber view, the left AV valve (in this case, the tricuspid valve) is located further apical than the right one.
- The left ventricle has typical signs of a morphologic right ventricle (discontinuity between the AV valve and the semilunar valve from a muscle band, strong trabeculation, moderator band, attachment of the tendinous cords of the AV valve in the ventricular septum).
- The position of the great vessels in relation to each other can be visualized in the parasternal short axis. The aorta is located anterior and to the left of the pulmonary artery. The two vessels are parallel and do not intersect.
- The course of the ventricular septum is unusual in ccTGA with a rather vertical orientation.
- For the further procedure, it is important to assess the coronary arteries, which usually arise from the "facing sinus" as in a d-TGA (▸ Fig. 15.27).
- Associated cardiac anomalies must be ruled out or identified, especially VSD, tricuspid anomalies, and obstructions of the outflow tracts.

> **Note**
>
> Every Ebstein anomaly of a left AV valve suggests a ccTGA.

Cardiac Catheterization

Cardiac catheterization is generally indicated only if there are additional anomalies. In these cases, cardiac catheterization can answer questions, for example, as to the size of the shunt and whether pulmonary hypertension is present in a VSD. In the angiography, the connection between the right atrium and the morphologic left ventricle as well as the connection of the left atrium to the morphologic right ventricle can be visualized. The aorta is located anterior and to the left.

MRI

In an MRI, detailed and often complex anatomical spatial relations and additional cardiac anomalies can be visualized. In addition, the shunt in a VSD can be quantified and function and size of the systemic ventricle can be evaluated.

15.11.3 Treatment

Conservative Treatment

If necessary, heart failure can be treated pharmacologically. If there is tricuspid regurgitation, ACE inhibitors are used to reduce the afterload.

Surgical Treatment

The surgical procedure for a ccTGA is made difficult by the specific anatomy including abnormal location of the AV node and the unusual orientation of the ventricular septum.

Two different surgical options are available. In a conventional surgical intervention, the individual associated cardiac anomalies are corrected or are treated palliatively. In an anatomical correction, associated heart anomalies are corrected in addition to a correction of the left ventricle so that it later functions as a systemic ventricle. This requires the complex double switch procedure, which is expected to give a better long-term prognosis.

► **Conventional surgical procedures.** The following conventional surgical procedures may be indicated:

- VSD closure: Postoperatively there is a high risk of a complete AV block. Due to the specific anatomy, closure via a transatrial access can be difficult. To minimize the risk of a complete AV block, the sutures of the VSD patch should be placed from the morphologic right ventricle. However, in a ccTGA, the morphologic right ventricle is located on the left side so that it can be more readily reached via an access through the aortic valve.
- Banding the pulmonary artery: If there is a large VSD, banding the pulmonary artery may be useful as an interim measure to reduce excessive pulmonary blood flow.
- Tricuspid valve reconstruction or replacement: depending on the severity of tricuspid regurgitation, a tricuspid valve reconstruction or replacement may be necessary.
- Tricuspid valve annuloplasty.
- Aortopulmonary anastomosis (modified Blalock–Taussig shunt): In a VSD with severe pulmonary stenosis, an aortopulmonary anastomosis can be indicated as an interim measure to ensure pulmonary perfusion. At a later stage, a VSD patch closure and implantation of a valved conduit can be performed.
- Univentricular palliation (modified Fontan procedure): If there is significant hypoplasia of the right systemic ventricle, a univentricular palliative Fontan procedure may be needed in individual cases.

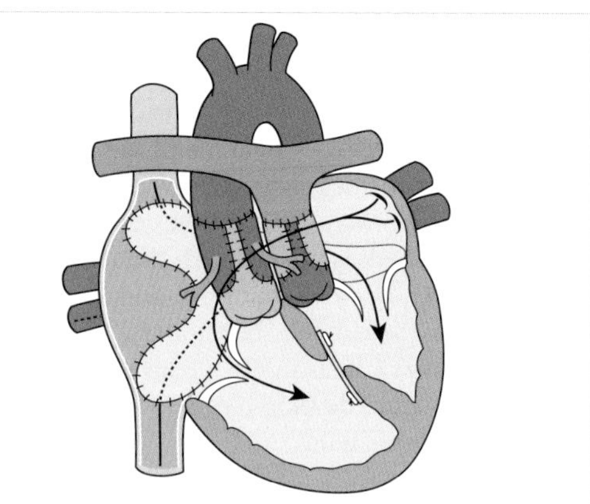

Fig. 15.34 Double switch procedure (atrial baffle and arterial switch). The venous blood from the venae cavae is conducted to the tricuspid valve through a conduit. The arterialized blood from the pulmonary veins flows outside the conduit to the mitral valve. The atrial septum must first be removed (atrial septectomy). Because both great arteries including the coronary arteries are transplanted in an arterial switch procedure, the morphologic left ventricle ultimately functions as a systemic ventricle.

► **Double switch procedure.** The aim of the double switch operation is to transform the left ventricle into a systemic ventricle. This is possible using a combination of an atrial baffle procedure with an arterial switch operation (► Fig. 15.34). In the atrial baffle procedure, the blood of the systemic veins is conducted to the morphologic right ventricle and the blood of the pulmonary veins is conducted to the morphologic left ventricle. In order to allow the blood of the systemic veins to reach the aorta from the morphologic left ventricle, an additional arterial switch procedure to transplant the great vessels must be performed.

In a ccTGA with VSD and severe pulmonary stenosis, it is also possible to perform a double switch procedure in which, instead of the arterial switch, a Rastelli procedure is performed with implantation of a conduit between the morphologic right ventricle and the pulmonary artery (► Fig. 15.35). Details of the individual surgical procedures are found in Chapter 15.10.

► **Pacemaker.** Implantation of a pacemaker is indicated if there is a complete AV block or symptomatic bradycardia.

► **Cardiac transplant.** A cardiac transplant is the last treatment option for progressive failure of the systemic ventricle.

15.11.4 Prognosis and Clinical Course

► **Long-term outcome.** The spontaneous course of a ccTGA can vary considerably. There have been reports of

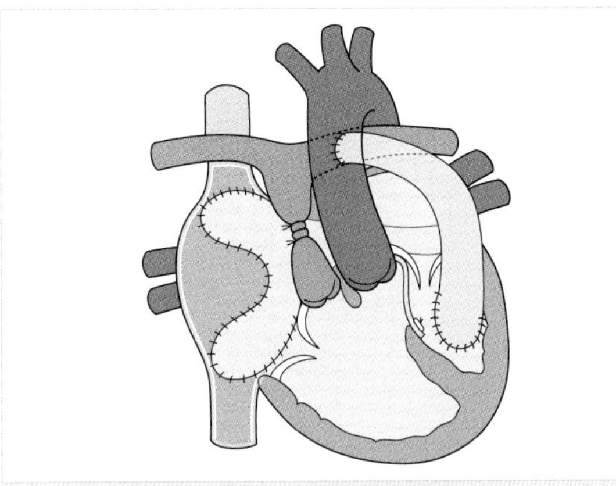

Fig. 15.35 Double switch procedure (atrial reverse and Rastelli procedure) for a ccTGA with VSD and relevant pulmonary stenosis. If there is a relevant obstruction of the right ventricular outflow tract, the patient is not suitable for an arterial switch procedure, as this would lead to obstruction of left ventricular outflow. In these cases, the morphologic right ventricle is therefore connected by a conduit with the pulmonary artery, thus bridging the right ventricular outflow tract obstruction. The VSD is closed with a patch so that the morphologic left ventricle drains into the aorta. The double switch procedure is completed by the atrial baffle procedure.

patients who remained asymptomatic until adulthood. Usually, however, in the long term there is failure of the morphologic right ventricle, which functions as a systemic ventricle and is not designed to withstand the overload. Accompanying anomalies have a considerable effect on the long-term outcome. There is also the risk of developing a spontaneous or postoperative AV block.

A double switch procedure should counteract the development of morphologic right systemic ventricular failure over time, but long-term results are still pending.

▸ **Outpatient checkups.** Even asymptomatic patients without additional anomalies should have a checkup at least once a year in order not to overlook developing systemic ventricular failure, tricuspid regurgitation, and an AV block. Moreover, postoperatively, it is important to check for the specific complications of the various conventional methods. After a double switch procedure, because of the atrial baffle procedure, special attention should be given to atrial arrhythmias, drainage disorders of the systemic venous and pulmonary venous blood caused by stenosis of the conduit, and leakage of the conduit. In the combination with the arterial switch procedure, coronary and supravalvular pulmonary stenosis may develop. After the Rastelli procedure, the conduit must be checked for possible degeneration.

▸ **Physical capacity and lifestyle.** In an untreated ccTGA, physical capacity is usually increasingly impaired by the long-term development of ventricular failure and the tricuspid regurgitation often associated with it. In certain circumstances, however, symptom-free survival is possible with the morphologic right ventricle as a systemic ventricle.

▸ **Special aspects in adolescents and adults.** Many of the typical long-term problems of an untreated ccTGA do not develop until adulthood. Heart failure as a result of systemic ventricular dysfunction often develops between the ages of 30 to 40 years. Progressive tricuspid regurgitation may also have an adverse effect. Almost 50% of adult patients with a ccTGA require a pacemaker due to a complete AV block. Atrial arrhythmias including atrial flutter/fibrillation and supraventricular tachycardias affect nearly 40% of patients. There is not yet sufficient data to assess the long-term results of a double switch procedure.

15.12 Double-Outlet Right Ventricle

15.12.1 Basics

Synonym: origin of both great arteries from the right ventricle

Definition

In a double-outlet right ventricle (DORV), the pulmonary artery as well as the aorta arises completely, or at least mainly, from the right ventricle. A VSD is practically always present. When both great arteries originate entirely in the right ventricle, a VSD is the only outlet from the left ventricle.

The hemodynamic status depends primarily on the location of the VSD in relation to the great vessels and the presence or absence of a pulmonary stenosis.

The definition of DORV is not always consistent. For some authors, a sufficient criterion is that one artery originates entirely and the other originates at least predominantly from the right ventricle (50% rule), but this definition is not correct from an embryological standpoint.

Another definition requires the presence of a bilateral conus. A conus (synonym for infundibulum) is a muscular ring or a tunnel located below the semilunar valve. Normally only the right ventricle has a conus or a muscular infundibulum. Therefore, in normal anatomy, a muscular infundibulum is found only below the pulmonary artery. By contrast, it is typical for a DORV that such a muscular conus is found below the pulmonary valve as well as below the aortic valve. This results in muscle tissue being present between the two semilunar valves (conus septum). There is also a typical discontinuity between the mitral valve and the adjacent semilunar valve. By contrast, in normal anatomy there is fibrous continuity

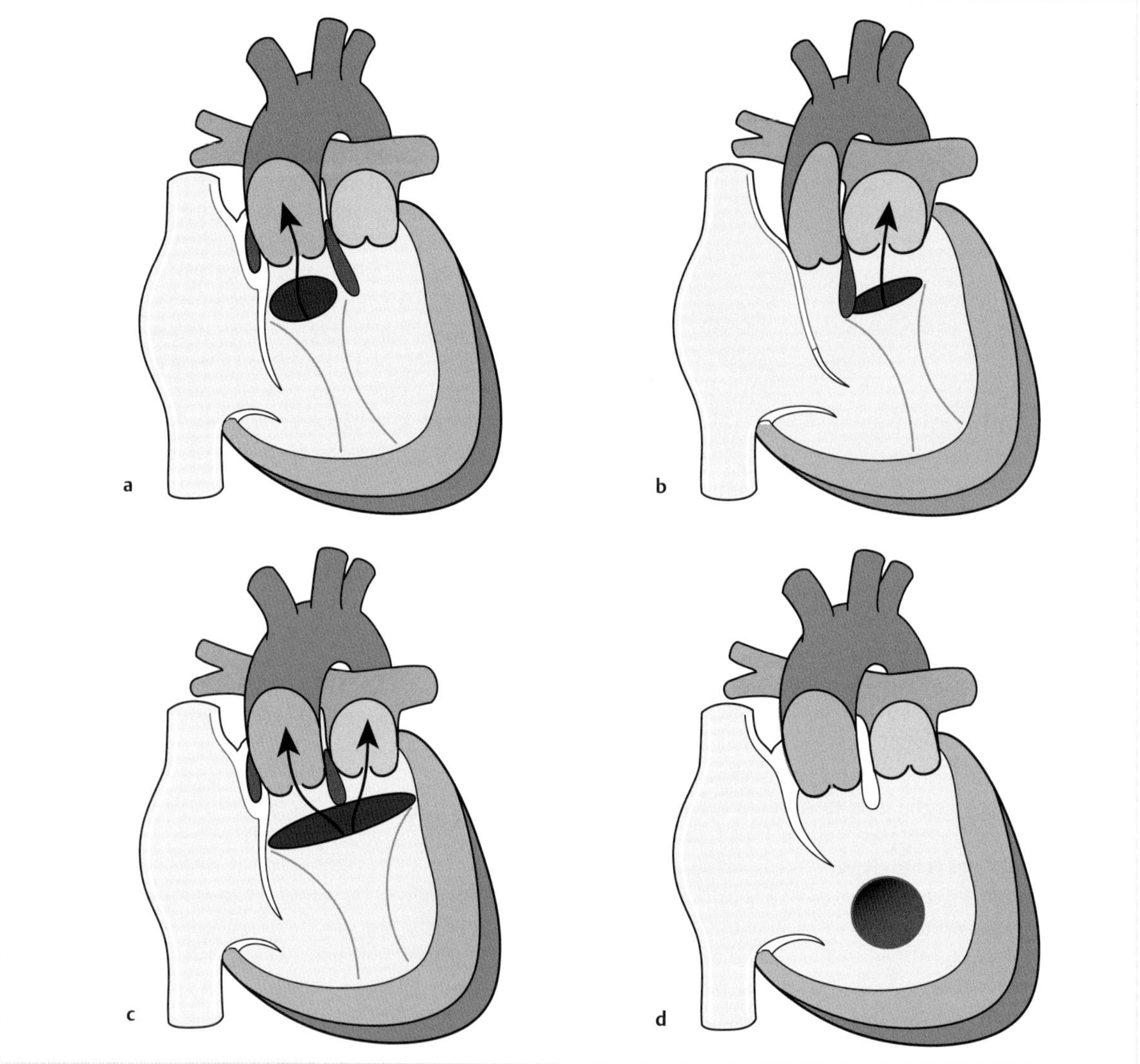

Fig. 15.36 Types of double-outlet right ventricle (DORV) depending on the opening of the right ventricle. The respective displacement of the conus septum that leads to subpulmonary or subaortic stenosis is shown in (**a**) and (**b**). **a** DORV with a subaortic VSD. **b** DORV with a subpulmonary VSD (Taussig–Bing anomaly). **c** DORV with a doubly committed VSD. **d** DORV with an uncommitted VSD.

between the mitral valve and the aortic valve, which means that the aortic valve and the mitral valve merge into each other and are not separated by a muscle band.

Epidemiology

DORVs constitute 1 to 1.5% of all congenital heart defects. The incidence is 0.1 per 1,000 live births.

Pathogenesis

The cause is probably a development disorder of the embryonic conotruncal septation.

Classification

DORVs are classified depending on the location of the VSD in relation to the great vessels, which is crucial for the hemodynamics (▸ Fig. 15.36):

- DORV with subaortic VSD (50%): The VSD is located just below the aortic valve. It is often associated with a pulmonary stenosis (Fallot-type DORV). The pulmonary stenosis is usually a subvalvular stenosis caused by the conus septum.
- DORV with a subpulmonary VSD (25%): This is also called Taussig–Bing anomaly. The VSD is located just below the pulmonary artery. This form is often associated with a subaortic stenosis caused by the conus

septum. The subaortic stenosis leads to impaired development of the aortic arch so that an interrupted aortic arch or coarctation of the aorta often occurs.
- DORV with a doubly committed VSD (5%): The VSD is connected to both great vessels.
- DORV with an uncommitted (remote) VSD (20%): The VSD has no direct connection to the great vessels.

Hemodynamics and Pathology

DORV does not present a uniform clinical picture. The major differences in the hemodynamic situation depend on the location of the VSD in relation to the great vessels and the presence or absence of a pulmonary stenosis.

In principle, the aorta and the pulmonary artery may have any spatial relation to each other. Most common is the side-to-side position, where both vessels originate next to each other from the heart and have a parallel course, with the aorta usually at the right of the pulmonary artery. Other possibilities are a normal position (rare), a d-malposition (the aorta originates from the pulmonary artery and runs parallel to the pulmonary artery at its right), and an l-malposition (the aorta originates from the pulmonary artery and runs parallel to the pulmonary artery at its left).

The correct term used for a DORV is malposition, not transposition of the great vessels, because the pulmonary artery always originates from the "correct" right ventricle.

Aortic and pulmonary valves are located at the same level and are typically separated by the conus septum. There is typically also a bilateral conus.

Hemodynamically, the different types of DORV are similar to three defects:
- Tetralogy of Fallot (leading symptom: cyanosis)
- Large VSD (leading symptom: excessive pulmonary blood flow / heart failure)
- d-TGA with VSD (leading symptoms: cyanosis, excessive pulmonary blood flow / heart failure)

A pulmonary stenosis is commonly associated with a subaortic stenosis and, very rarely, associated with a subpulmonary VSD (Taussig–Bing anomaly). In a subpulmonary VSD, there is often a subaortic stenosis caused by the conus septum, which may lead to incomplete development of the aortic arch resulting in aortic coarctation or an interrupted aortic arch.

► **Subaortic VSD with a pulmonary stenosis (Fallot type).** The hemodynamic situation is similar to tetralogy of Fallot: The oxygenated blood flows from the left ventricle through the VSD primarily into the aorta, while the deoxygenated blood passes from the right ventricle to the pulmonary artery. Because of pulmonary stenosis, the pulmonary blood flow is reduced, causing cyanosis, depending on the extent of pulmonary stenosis.

► **Subaortic VSD without pulmonary stenosis (rare).** The hemodynamic situation is similar to a large VSD: Due to the large VSD, the pressure between the two ventricles is usually equalized. There is excessive pulmonary blood flow, leading to heart failure, and a risk of pulmonary hypertension developing.

► **Subpulmonary VSD (Taussig–Bing anomaly) without pulmonary stenosis.** The hemodynamic situation is similar to d-TGA with VSD: The oxygenated blood from the left ventricle crosses the VSD to reach the pulmonary artery, while the deoxygenated blood from the right ventricle flows primarily into the aorta and from there into the systemic circulation. There is excessive pulmonary blood flow due to the VSD. Initially, cyanosis is not pronounced, but heart failure and pulmonary hypertension can develop rapidly.

► **Subpulmonary VSD (Taussig–Bing anomaly) with pulmonary stenosis (very rare).** The hemodynamic situation and clinical features are similar to tetralogy of Fallot. There is often severe cyanosis and ductal-dependent pulmonary blood flow.

► **Doubly committed VSD without pulmonary stenosis.** The hemodynamic situation is similar to large VSD.

► **Doubly committed VSD with pulmonary stenosis.** The hemodynamic situation is similar to tetralogy of Fallot.

► **Uncommitted VSD without pulmonary stenosis.** The hemodynamic situation is similar to large VSD.

► **Uncommitted VSD with pulmonary stenosis.** The hemodynamic situation is similar to tetralogy of Fallot.

Associated Anomalies

Associated cardiac anomalies are common with DORV. A VSD is almost always present. Subvalvular obstruction of the outflow tract occurs mostly through displacement of the conus septum. The most important associated anomalies, which often also have an effect the surgical procedure, are listed below:
- VSD (almost always present)
- Malposition of the great vessels (typically side-to-side position of the great vessels, rarely also l- or d-malposition)
- Anomalies of the AV valves (AV canal, often with unbalanced ventricles as well)
- Pulmonary stenosis (usually subpulmonary and caused by conus tissue, hemodynamically relevant)
- Pulmonary atresia (ductal-dependent pulmonary blood flow)
- Mitral stenosis/atresia with hypoplasia of the left ventricle

- "Straddling" mitral valve (mitral valve chordae pass through the VSD into the right ventricle)
- Subaortic stenosis, coarctation of the aorta, interrupted aortic arch (especially with a Taussig–Bing anomaly in which the subaortic region may be obstructed by the conus septum)
- Coronary anomalies: single origin of both coronary arteries, origin of the anterior interventricular branch from the right coronary artery
- Anomalies of the conduction system (AV nodes, bundle of His)

Associated Syndromes

DORV occurs more frequently in children born to diabetic mothers and a more frequent occurrence in association with certain chromosomal diseases (CHARGE association, trisomy 13, trisomy 18, tetrasomy 8p, microdeletion of 22q11) has also been described. DORV also occurs often in heterotaxy syndromes.

15.12.2 Diagnostics

Symptoms

There are various clinical manifestations corresponding with the different hemodynamic features described above:

- Fallot type: leading symptom is cyanosis depending on the severity of the pulmonary stenosis
- VSD type: mainly signs of heart failure due to excessive pulmonary blood flow (primarily poor feeding, failure to thrive, increased sweating, tachypnea/dyspnea, hepatomegaly)
- TGA with VSD type: leading clinical findings are signs of heart failure due to excessive pulmonary blood flow; due to pulmonary recirculation, cyanosis is initially usually relatively mild

If there is also aortic coarctation or an interrupted aortic arch, the pulses are absent in the lower limbs after the closure of the ductus arteriosus, and heart failure develops.

Auscultation

The second heart sound is loud if there is excessive pulmonary blood flow or an anterior position of the aorta. If there is pulmonary stenosis, there is a rough holosystolic murmur with PMI in the 2nd left intercostal space. A band-shaped holosystolic murmur with PMI in the 4th left intercostal space is a sign of a VSD. A low-frequency diastolic murmur over the cardiac apex indicates a relative tricuspid stenosis associated with excessive pulmonary blood flow.

ECG

There is almost always a right axis deviation, sometimes a marked right axis deviation. Often there is a first degree AV block. If pulmonary stenosis is present, there are signs of a right ventricular hypertrophy, often a complete right bundle branch block, and a P dextrocardiale. Signs of biventricular hypertrophy are predominant if no pulmonary stenosis is present. Isolated signs of left ventricular hypertrophy are rare in these cases. Typically left axis deviation occurs if there is an associated AV canal.

Chest X-ray

The radiological appearance of the different types of DORV varies depending on the hemodynamics:

- DORV with pulmonary stenosis: usually normal-sized cardiac silhouette and decreased pulmonary vascular markings depending on the extent of the pulmonary stenosis
- DORV without pulmonary stenosis: usually significantly enlarged cardiac silhouette, prominent pulmonary artery segment, and increased pulmonary vascular markings
- Taussig–Bing anomaly: similar to TGA ("egg lying on its side"), but with a wider waist

Echocardiography

The diagnosis can usually be reliably made using echocardiography. The examination shows the following typical findings or can clarify the following questions:

- In the parasternal long axis, the posterior great artery overrides the VSD by more than 50%; the anterior artery arises entirely from the right ventricle
- No fibrous continuity between the anterior mitral leaflet and the adjacent semilunar valve (substantiating evidence)
- Assessment of the position of the great vessels to each other (side-to-side position), l- or d-malposition (i.e., the aorta is located anterior to and at the left or the right of the pulmonary artery)
- Location and size of the VSD (subaortic, subpulmonary, doubly committed, uncommitted)
- Subpulmonary or subaortic obstruction of the outflow tract
- Visualization of the conus septum (muscle tissue between the two great arteries shaped like a teardrop or the head of a match)
- Size of the left ventricle
- Presence of a PDA (especially important if there is a pulmonary stenosis: ductal-dependent pulmonary blood flow?)
- Assessment of the aortic arch: detection or exclusion of hypoplasia of the aortic arch, an interrupted aortic arch, or coarctation of the aorta (especially important if there is a Taussig–Bing anomaly)
- Visualization of the coronary arteries (origin, course)

Table 15.2 Summary of the most important surgical options for the various types of double-outlet right ventricle (DORV)

DORV type	Associated anomaly	Surgical procedure
Subaortic VSD	–	VSD patch tunnel
	Severe pulmonary stenosis	Rastelli procedure or "réparation à l'étage ventriculaire" (REV)
Subpulmonary VSD (Taussig–Bing anomaly)	–	Arterial switch procedure
	Coronary anomalies	Atrial baffle procedure
	Large distance between aorta and pulmonary artery (coronary transfer not possible)	Atrial baffle procedure
	Severe subaortic stenosis	Damus–Kaye–Stansel anastomosis, conduit implantation between right ventricle and pulmonary artery, VSD patch tunnel
Doubly committed VSD	–	VSD patch tunnel
Uncommitted VSD	–	VSD patch tunnel, if a patch tunnel is not possible, Fontan completion

Cardiac Catheterization

Cardiac catheterization is indicated when important questions remain unanswered despite echocardiography, for example:

- Measurement of pressure, flow and resistance in the pulmonary circulation
- Assessment of the pressure gradient across an outflow tract stenosis
- Exclusion of associated anomalies
- Visualization of the origin and course of the coronary arteries

MRI

An MRI can provide a detailed visualization of the anatomy. It is used in individual cases, for example, to clarify the relationship between the VSD and great arteries. Shunt and flow volumes can be quantified.

15.12.3 Treatment

Conservative Treatment

If the patient has progressive cardiac failure, anticongestive treatment may bridge the time until surgery. If there is a critical pulmonary stenosis, pulmonary atresia, severe aortic coarctation, or an interrupted aortic arch, prostaglandin E (initially 50 ng/kg/min, later possibly reduced) may be necessary to ensure pulmonary and systemic perfusion.

Interventional Catheterization

If there are hemodynamic features of a TGA and a restrictive atrial shunt, a Rashkind maneuver (balloon atrial septostomy) may be required. In individual cases, balloon dilation of a pulmonary stenosis can also be indicated.

Surgical Treatment

Due to the many variations and different hemodynamic features, the surgical procedure must always be decided on a case-by-case basis depending on:

- Location of the VSD with respect to the great arteries
- Position of the great arteries with respect to each other
- Presence or absence of a pulmonary stenosis
- Associated anomalies (coronary anomalies, coarctation of the aorta, interrupted aortic arch)

Palliative Measures

Today, primary correction is generally attempted. Palliative surgery is considered on a case-by-case basis, for example, to achieve more favorable conditions for corrective surgery. The palliative procedures include banding the pulmonary artery if there is excessive pulmonary blood flow and creating an aortopulmonary shunt if there is insufficient pulmonary blood flow.

Corrective Surgery

The surgical procedure depends mainly on the location of the VSD in relation to the great arteries (▶ Table 15.2). Sometimes a subaortic VSD can be corrected, similar to tetralogy of Fallot. Extensive surgeries are necessary for a subpulmonary VSD (Taussig–Bing anomaly). The aim in these cases is to perform an arterial switch operation including a VSD closure. In cases with a great distance between the VSD and the great vessels (uncommitted VSD), a biventricular correction is often not possible. The situation frequently becomes more favorable after the children are more than 2 years old.

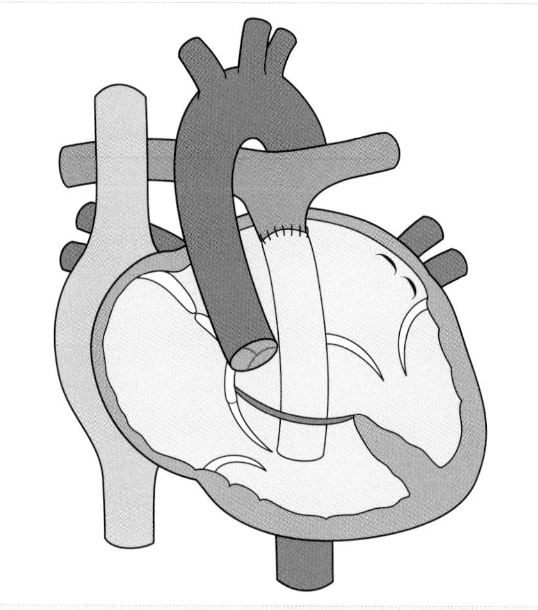

Fig. 15.37 Correction of a DORV with pulmonary stenosis by a Rastelli procedure. See explanation in text.

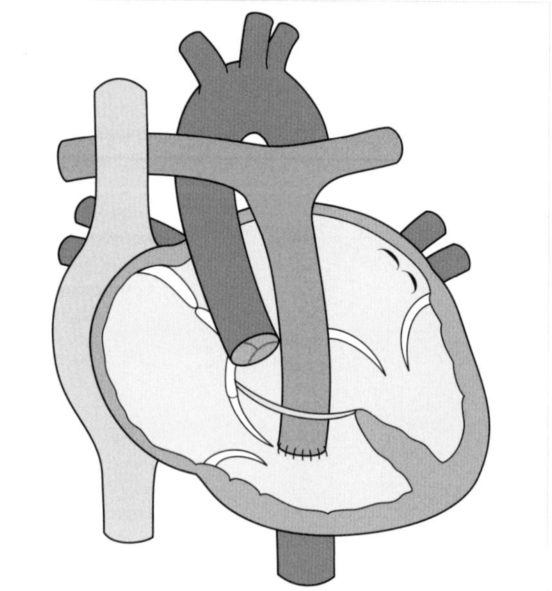

Fig. 15.38 Correction of a DORV with pulmonary stenosis using a "réparation à l'étage ventriculaire" (REV procedure). See explanation in text.

Subaortic VSD

► **Intraventricular tunnel.** The correction is similar to that for tetralogy of Fallot. The VSD is closed with a tunnel patch so that the left ventricle drains through the aorta. Under certain circumstances, the VSD must be enlarged (complication: AV block). If there is pulmonary stenosis, the right ventricular outflow tract must be widened.

Without pulmonary stenosis, this procedure must be performed as early as in the first year of life—sometimes even in the neonatal period—due to the risk of increased pulmonary resistance. In children with pulmonary stenosis, the timing of the surgical procedure is based on the degree of cyanosis.

► **Rastelli procedure.** This operation is necessary if the patient has a severe subvalvular or valvular pulmonary stenosis. The right ventricle is connected to the pulmonary artery by a conduit. Blood from the left ventricle flows into the aorta through an intracardiac patch tunnel. The patch also closes the VSD (► Fig. 15.37).

► **"Réparation à l'étage ventriculaire" (REV).** This surgical procedure is an alternative procedure for DORV with a severe valvular or subvalvular pulmonary stenosis. In an REV, the pulmonary artery is directly anastomosed to the right ventricle through a ventricular incision (► Fig. 15.38). The pulmonary artery bifurcation is brought forward anterior to the aorta (Lecompte maneuver).

Subpulmonary VSD

The arterial switch procedure including closure of the VSD is the treatment of choice. This procedure is usually performed in the neonatal period. Additional anomalies such as coronary anomalies or obstructions of the left outflow tract make other surgical procedures necessary. An associated hypoplasia of the aortic arch, aortic coarctation, or an interrupted aortic arch is usually corrected in the same session.

► **Switch procedure and VSD closure.** If the coronary anatomy is more favorable and no outflow obstruction is present, an arterial switch procedure can be performed as for a d-TGA. In addition, the VSD is closed with a tunnel patch so that the left ventricle drains into the aorta (► Fig. 15.39).

► **Mustard or Senning atrial baffle.** If a switch procedure is not possible owing to a coronary anomaly or the relationship of the great arteries to each other, a Mustard or Senning atrial baffle procedure operation must be considered (► Fig. 15.40). In this procedure, foreign material (Mustard) or atrial tissue (Senning) is excised to allow systemic venous blood to flow through the trousers-shaped atrial tunnel into the left ventricle and from there into the pulmonary artery. The pulmonary venous blood flows past the tunnel into the right ventricle (see Chapter 15.10). In addition, the VSD is closed with a tunnel patch that conducts the blood from the left ventricle to the pulmonary artery.

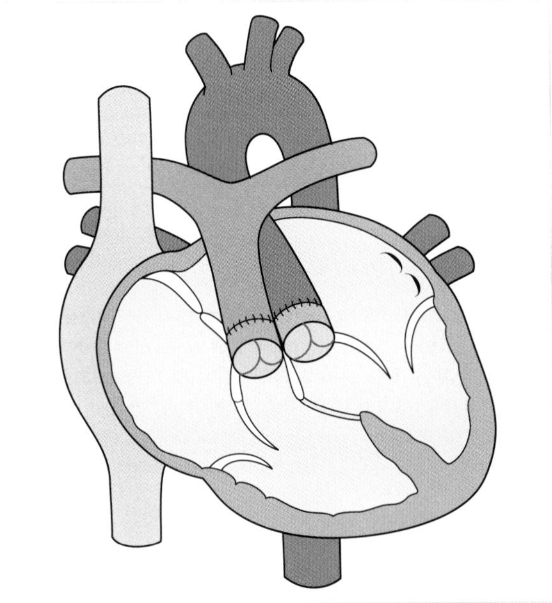

Fig. 15.39 Correction of a Taussig–Bing anomaly with an arterial switch procedure. See explanation in text.

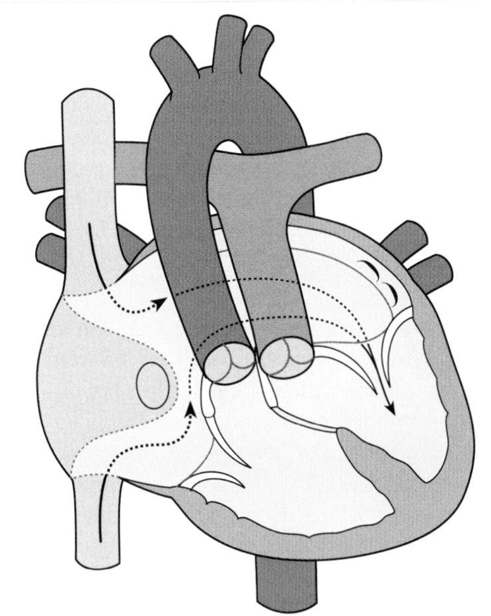

Fig. 15.40 Correction of a Taussig–Bing anomaly with an atrial baffle procedure. See explanation in text.

► **Damus–Kaye–Stansel (DKS) procedure with VSD patch closure and implantation of a conduit between the right ventricle and the main pulmonary artery.** A severe subaortic stenosis may require this elaborate procedure. In this operation, the main pulmonary artery trunk is anastomized with the aortic root (DKS anastomosis). The former pulmonary valve becomes the neo-aortic valve. In addition, the VSD is closed with a patch so that the left ventricle drains in the neo-aortic valve (former pulmonary valve). Pulmonary blood flow is ensured by the implantation of a conduit between the right ventricle and the distal end of the main pulmonary artery (► Fig. 15.41).

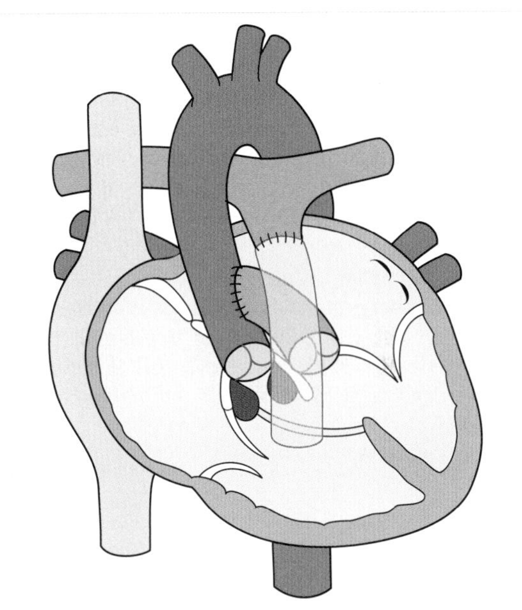

Fig. 15.41 Correction of a Taussig–Bing anomaly with a subaortic stenosis by a Damus–Kaye–Stansel (DKS) anastomosis, implantation of a conduit between the right ventricle and the main pulmonary artery and closure of the VSD. See explanation in text.

Doubly Committed VSD

An attempt is made to divert the blood through the patch tunnel from the left ventricle into the aorta.

Uncommitted VSD

Due to the large distance between the VSD and the great vessels, it is often not possible to redirect the left ventricular blood to the aorta via a patch tunnel, so that in many cases, Fontan completion is the only treatment option.

15.12.4 Prognosis and Clinical Course

► **Long-term course.** Left untreated, children with DORV without pulmonary stenosis develop severe heart failure and pulmonary hypertension as a result of excessive pulmonary blood flow.

If a severe pulmonary stenosis is not treated, in the long term the typical complications of cyanotic heart failure (e.g., polycythemia, tendency to bleed, risk of brain abscess) develop.

After surgical correction, the 15-year survival rate for unproblematic cases is above 90%. Reoperations are required in up to one-third of the patients, mainly due to obstruction of the right or left ventricular outflow tract and conduit problems. Obstructions of the left ventricular outflow tract are caused by a developing subaortic stenosis or a too narrow patch tunnel in a small VSD. In addition, the course can be complicated by ventricular arrhythmias.

▶ **Outpatient checkups.** Postoperatively, lifelong monitoring is necessary. In particular, it is important to note obstructions in the region of the outflow tracts, a residual VSD, and (ventricular) arrhythmias. If the right ventricular outflow tract had to be widened, pulmonary regurgitation can be expected. After a switch procedure, it is important to look specifically for supravalvular pulmonary stenosis and for signs of coronary stenosis. After an atrial baffle procedure, patients can develop systemic and pulmonary venous outflow stenosis (baffle stenosis). Supravalvular arrhythmias are also common in these patients. After a conduit implantation, stenoses, calcification, and insufficiency of the conduit should be noted. The typical long-term problems of Fontan circulation are predominant after univentricular palliation (Chapter 15.18).

▶ **Physical capacity and lifestyle.** Patients who have had an intracardiac completion usually have normal physical capacity for everyday activities. The problems that arise after a Fontan procedure are described in Chapter 15.18.

▶ **Special aspects in adolescents and adults.** If there is no pulmonary stenosis, patients who have not undergone surgery usually develop irreversible pulmonary hypertension with severe cyanosis (Eisenmenger reaction) and a poor prognosis by adolescence or adulthood.

15.13 Truncus Arteriosus Communis

15.13.1 Basics

Synonym: persistent truncus arteriosus

Definition

In a truncus arteriosus communis, only one large arterial vessel with a semilunar valve (truncus valve) arises from the heart. This vessel supplies the systemic, pulmonary, and coronary circulation. The truncus overrides a high VSD (malalignment VSD) that is almost always present. The truncus valve generally has three or four dysmorphic, thickened leaflets and is frequently insufficient.

Epidemiology

This is a relatively rare defect, constituting 1% to 2% of all congenital heart defects.

Pathogenesis

The intrauterine separation of the embryonic truncus into the aorta and pulmonary artery by the aortopulmonary septum in the 4th to 5th week of gestation fails to occur or is only partial. The infundibular septum of the right ventricular outflow tract and pulmonary valve tissue are also absent.

Classification

The anatomy of the pulmonary vessels depends on the stage when the separation of the embryonic truncus came to a halt. There are two commonly used classifications:

▶ **Classification by Collet and Edwards.** This classification comprises three types (▶ Fig. 15.42):

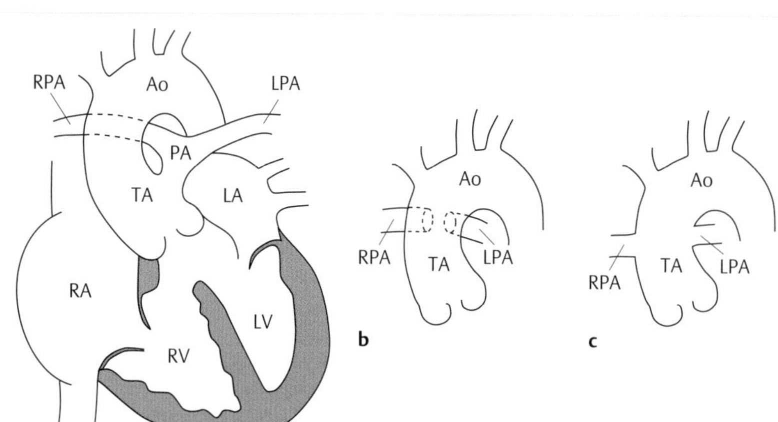

Fig. 15.42 Classification of truncus arteriosus communis by Collet and Edwards. **a** Type I: Aorta and pulmonary artery arise from a common trunk. **b** Type II: Both pulmonary arteries arise jointly or separately from the posterior wall of the trunk. **c** Type III: Both pulmonary arteries arise from the lateral aspect of the trunk. RA, right atrium; LA, left atrium; RV, right ventricle; LV, left ventricle; Ao, aorta; LPA, left pulmonary artery; RPA, right pulmonary artery; PA, pulmonary artery; TA, truncus arteriosus.[29]

- Type I (approx. 60%): Aorta and pulmonary artery arise from a common trunk. The pulmonary artery branches into a left and a right branch shortly after its origin.
- Type II (approx. 20%): The right and left pulmonary arteries arise jointly or separately from the posterior wall of the trunk.
- Type III (approx. 10%): Both pulmonary arteries originate independently of one another from the lateral aspect of the trunk.

Earlier, a type IV was also defined. In this type, both pulmonary arteries are absent. The lungs are perfused exclusively via aortopulmonary collaterals. In terms of pathogenesis, this cardiac defect ("truncus IV" in medical jargon) is not a truncus arteriosus, but a pulmonary atresia with VSD (Chapter 15.26).

► **Classification by van Praagh.** Van Praagh divides the different truncus types into the main classes A and B (► Fig. 15.43). Class A has a VSD; class B has an intact ventricular septum. Since an intact ventricular septum has been described only in a few isolated cases of truncus arteriosus, class B has little practical relevance. The van Praagh and the Collet and Edwards classifications overlap in some areas:

- A1: Corresponds with type I by Collet and Edwards (see Classification by Collet and Edwards).
- A2: Corresponds with type II by Collet and Edwards (see Classification by Collet and Edwards).
- A3: Only one pulmonary artery arises from the truncus, the other pulmonary artery is supplied via a ductus arteriosus or from collaterals from the aorta ("hemitruncus").
- A4: There are additional anomalies of the aortic arch (coarctation of the aorta, atresia of the aortic arch, interrupted aortic arch). The lower half of the body is supplied with blood via a PDA.

Note

The most common form of a truncus arteriosus communis is a mixture of types I and II or of A1 and A2. In most cases, there is a short pulmonary artery, which makes it difficult to distinguish between types I and II or types A1 and A2 (known as "type 1.5").

Hemodynamics

The blood from the two ventricles flows into the truncus. Due to the large VSD, the pressure is equalized in the two ventricles. The truncus thus contains mixed arterialized and venous blood. The mixed blood then flows into the pulmonary and systemic circulation as well as to the

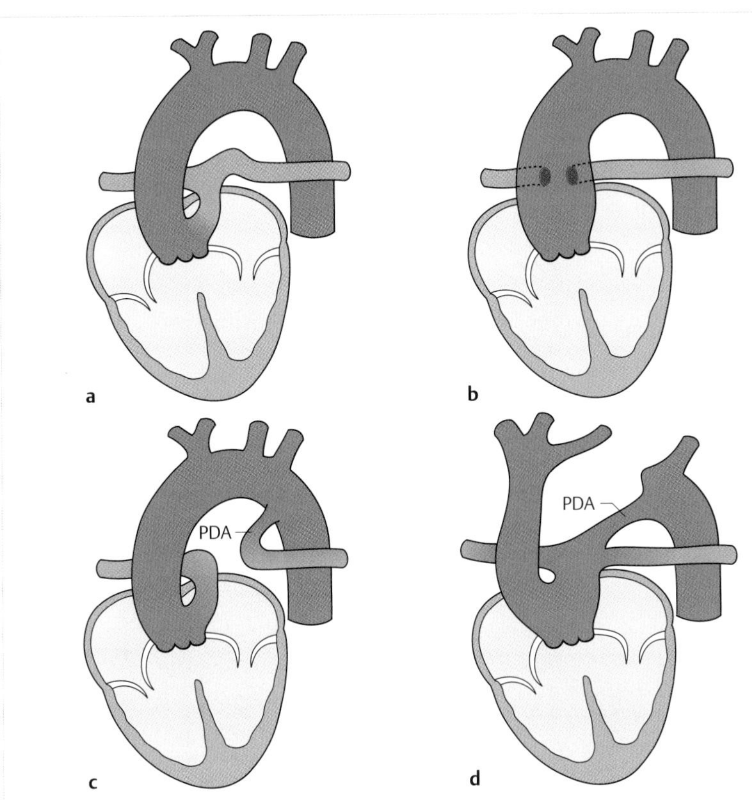

Fig. 15.43 Classification of the truncus arteriosus communis by van Praagh. **a** A1: Aorta and pulmonary artery arise from a common trunk. **b** A2: Both pulmonary arteries arise jointly or separately from the posterior wall of the trunk. **c** A3: Only one pulmonary artery arises from the trunk. The other pulmonary artery is supplied via a PDA or collaterals from the aorta ("hemitruncus"). **d** A4: There are additional anomalies of the aortic arch (coarctation of the aorta, atresia of the aortic arch, interrupted aortic arch). The lower half of the body is supplied with blood via a PDA. PDA, patent ductus arteriosus.

coronaries. Oxygen saturation is generally identical in the aorta and pulmonary artery. There may, however, be "directed flow" that causes the arterialized blood from the left ventricle to flow into the aorta, resulting in very low mixing of the blood.

When pulmonary vascular resistance drops in the first few days after birth, pulmonary perfusion increases greatly. The blood takes the path of least resistance and flows mainly into the pulmonary circulation. As in other cyanotic defects, arterial oxygen saturation is dependent on the pulmonary blood flow. If pulmonary perfusion is reduced (e.g., due to a stenosis at the origin of the pulmonary arteries), there is considerable cyanosis. If pulmonary perfusion is increased, both ventricles are subject to considerable volume overload that may be further aggravated by insufficiency of the truncus valve.

Associated Anomalies

- VSD: a malalignment VSD that the truncus valve overrides – similar to the aorta in a tetralogy of Fallot – is practically always present. Sometimes almost the entire ventricular septum can be missing.
- Truncus valve anomalies: There is frequently truncus valve insufficiency, less often truncus valve stenosis. The truncus valve can have a varying number of leaflets (between two and six truncus valve leaflets have been described in the literature, but in most cases there are three or four).
- A right aortic arch is relatively common (25–60%).
- ASDs are present in 20% of cases.
- Stenoses at the origin or hypoplasia of the pulmonary arteries: Stenoses at the origin of the pulmonary artery can have a favorable hemodynamic effect, as they protect the pulmonary circulation from excessive blood flow and pulmonary hypertension.
- Coronary anomalies (15–30%): The left coronary artery may arise unusually far distally. In addition, the left anterior descending artery may arise from the coronary artery.
- Coarctation of the aorta, hypoplasia of the aortic arch, or an interrupted aortic arch (type A4 by van Praagh): In these cases, systemic perfusion depends on a PDA (extremely rare).
- Left persistent superior vena cava.

A ductus arteriosus is usually not present in most cases of a truncus arteriosus. Intrauterinely, it is also not hemodynamically relevant except for types A3 and A4.

Associated Syndromes

Like all conotruncal anomalies, a truncus arteriosus communis is frequently associated with microdeletion of 22q11. Frequent cases have also been observed in connection with maternal diabetes mellitus.

15.13.2 Diagnostic Measures

Symptoms

Symptoms usually appear shortly after birth and depend mainly on pulmonary perfusion, which is increased in most patients. Leading symptoms are *mild cyanosis* and *increasing congestive heart failure* (tachypnea/dyspnea, hepatomegaly, failure to thrive, pulmonary edema) as a result of excessive pulmonary blood flow. Due to increased pulmonary perfusion, cyanosis is often not pronounced.

If pulmonary perfusion is reduced (e.g., due to stenosis at the origin of the pulmonary artery) cyanosis is a major symptom, but the lungs are at least partially protected from excessive blood flow.

The peripheral pulses are strong (pulsus celer et altus) and pulse pressure is wide.

Complications

As a result of increased pulmonary perfusion, pulmonary hypertension develops early with a truncus arteriosus communis, often between the 3rd and 6th month of life. A fixed increase in pulmonary resistance makes any correction impossible.

Auscultation

There is a single prominent second heart sound. A systolic click can often be auscultated over the cardiac apex and at the upper left and sternal area. Usually, a rough, loud systolic murmur is heard in the left parasternal area. A systolic murmur can also be heard if a pulmonary stenosis is present. If there is truncus valve insufficiency, an early diastolic murmur occurs; a relative mitral stenosis (sign of increased blood flow across the mitral valve) causes a mid-diastolic murmur.

ECG

The ECG is usually uncharacteristic. There are frequently signs of biventricular hypertrophy.

Chest X-ray

In most cases (increased pulmonary blood flow), there is cardiomegaly with increased pulmonary vascular marking. The heart is wide at the diaphragm and the cardiac apex is upturned. If there is a right aortic arch (30%), it forms a border to the upper right mediastinum.

Note

Mild cyanosis, increased pulmonary vascular markings in combination with a right aortic arch suggest a truncus arteriosus communis.

Echocardiography

The diagnosis can generally be reliably made by echocardiography. A dilated vessel (truncus vessel) that overrides a malalignment VSD can be identified in the parasternal long axis. The coronary and pulmonary arteries arise from this vessel. In the parasternal short axis, the usually thickened semilunar valve can be visualized. It typically has three or four leaflets. The valve can be assessed with respect to insufficiency or stenosis by Doppler sonography.

The assessment of the origins of pulmonary arteries is important for classification: Is there evidence of one pulmonary artery? Do the branches of the pulmonary artery arise jointly or separately from the trunk? Are there any stenoses at the origins of the pulmonary artery branches?

The left atrium and ventricle are typically dilated; there is hyperdynamic contractility of the left ventricle as a sign of volume overload.

A right aortic arch can best be visualized from a suprasternal direction. It is important to rule out or identify an interrupted aortic arch or other aortic anomalies. It is indispensable to visualize the origins and course of the coronary arteries in order to plan surgery.

Note

In echocardiography, the first impression is of a dilated vessel that overrides a malalignment VSD. The right ventricular outflow tract is absent.

Cardiac Catheterization

Routine cardiac catheterization is not necessary. In unclear cases, it is useful for assessing anomalies of the coronary arteries, origin and course of the pulmonary arteries, stenoses of the pulmonary arteries, pressure and peripheral resistance in the pulmonary vessels, and additional anomalies.

MRI

An MRI can be helpful for visualizing anatomical details.

15.13.3 Treatment

▶ **Conservative treatment.** The early onset of congestive heart failure usually necessitates anticongestive treatment until the operation. If there is simultaneously an interrupted aortic arch, prostaglandin E must be administered to keep the ductus arteriosus patent.

▶ **Indication for surgical correction.** There is nearly always an indication for surgical correction.

▶ **Contraindication for surgical correction.** Corrective surgery is contraindicated if there is a fixed increase in pulmonary resistance.

Note

Despite cyanosis, the application of oxygen is generally contraindicated in a truncus arteriosus communis as it lowers pulmonary resistance and thus increases pulmonary blood flow and heart failure.

Surgical Treatment

Today, early surgical correction is preferred. Palliative measures such as banding the pulmonary artery to reduce the pulmonary blood flow or creating an aortopulmonary shunt if pulmonary blood flow is reduced are performed only in isolated cases when corrective surgery cannot (yet) be performed for other reasons (e.g., extremely low weight, severe infection).

The definitive correction is usually performed within the first two months of life due to heart failure and the early onset of an Eisenmenger reaction. Only in the rare cases of balanced hemodynamics, in which the pulmonary circulation is protected from excessive blood flow by pulmonary stenoses, can surgery be delayed.

The correction is performed using the Rastelli procedure (▶ Fig. 15.44). The VSD is closed so that the left ventricle drains into the truncus vessel. The truncus vessel becomes the neo-aorta in this case. The right ventricle is connected with the pulmonary artery or arteries via a valved conduit, which was previously separated from the pulmonary artery or truncus.

If there are simultaneous anomalies of the aortic arch (coarctation of the aorta, interrupted aortic arch), the aortic arch is reconstructed in the same session. Severe truncus valve insufficiency may necessitate valve replacement.

15.13.4 Prognosis and Course

▶ **Long-term prognosis.** Without surgery, almost all children die within the first year of life. The early postoperative mortality is about 10%; the 10-year survival rate is about 80%. Since relatively small conduits are used in infancy, they must be replaced later. A conduit replacement becomes necessary within 5 years in more than half of the patients. Postoperatively, as a result of the right ventriculotomy and the VSD patch, there is almost always a right bundle branch block and sometimes ventricular arrhythmias. A postoperative complete AV block occurs rarely. Pulmonary hypertension can persist or even progress, especially in patients who were operated on after infancy.

▶ **Outpatient checkups.** Cardiac monitoring is necessary for the entire lifetime. Particular attention must be paid

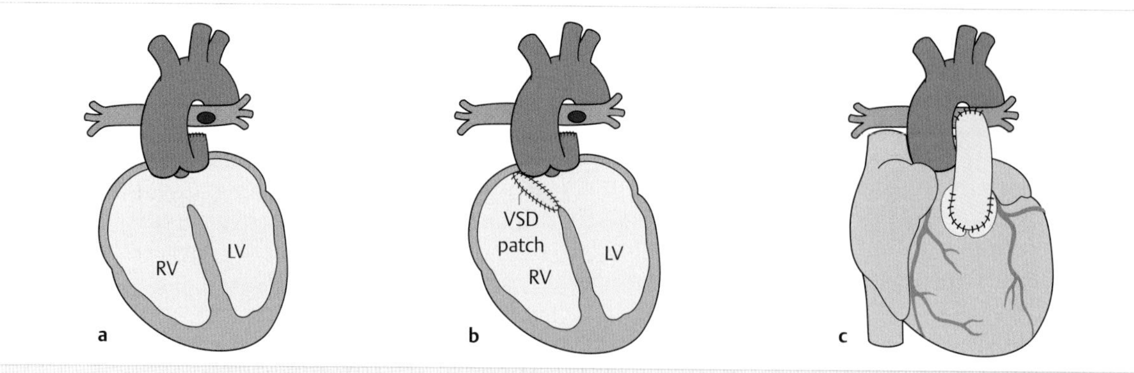

Fig. 15.44 Rastelli procedure for correcting a truncus arteriosus communis. First the pulmonary arteries are separated from the truncus arteriosus communis and the truncus is closed at the separation site (a). The VSD is then closed so that the left ventricle drains into the truncus vessel (b), which becomes the neo-aorta. After the pulmonary arteries have been separated, a valved conduit is implanted between the right ventricle and the bifurcation of the pulmonary artery (c). If separate pulmonary arteries arise from the truncus, a bifurcation of the pulmonary arteries must first be surgically made.[37]
LV, left ventricle; RV, right ventricle.

to the function of the conduit (stenoses, calcification, insufficiency), ventricular arrhythmias, and pulmonary hypertension. In addition, truncus valve insufficiency can increase over time. Lifelong endocarditis prophylaxis is needed.

▶ **Physical capacity and lifestyle.** The quality of life of most patients who have had corrective surgery is good. Recommendations regarding physical capacity must take the function of the conduit, the truncus valve, and the ventricle, arrhythmias, and the extent of possible pulmonary hypertension into consideration.

▶ **Special aspects in adolescents and adults.** There is almost always an Eisenmenger reaction in adolescent or adult patients who have not had corrective surgery. Other than this, the already described postoperative complications (conduit problems, arrhythmias, pulmonary hypertension) and progression of truncus valve insufficiency should be noted. Most late deaths probably occur as a result of arrhythmias.

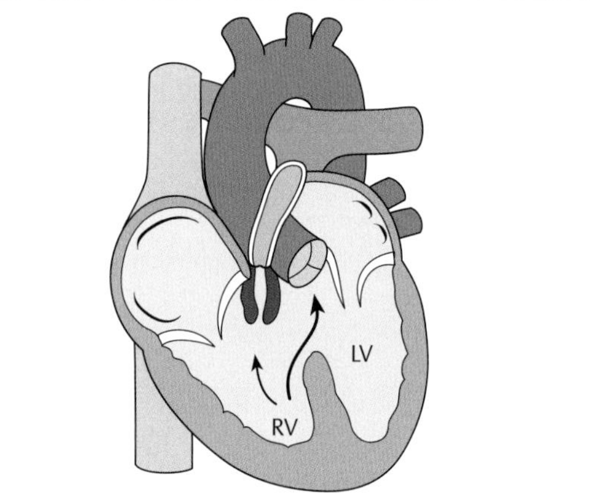

Fig. 15.45 Tetralogy of Fallot: combination of a large VSD with an overriding aorta and an obstruction of the right ventricular outflow tract in the form of an infundibular and/or valvular pulmonary stenosis. As a result of the right ventricular obstruction, there is right ventricular hypertrophy.[15]
LV, left ventricle; RV, right ventricle.

15.14 Tetralogy of Fallot

15.14.1 Basics

Definition

Tetralogy of Fallot (TOF) (▶ Fig. 15.45) is a complex heart defect with the following combination of anomalies:

- Large ventricular septal defect (malalignment VSD)
- Aorta overriding the VSD (dextro and anterior position of the aorta)
- Obstruction of the right ventricular outflow tract (infundibular and/or valvular pulmonary stenosis, often a narrow pulmonary valve annulus)
- Right ventricular hypertrophy (result of obstruction of the right ventricular outflow tract)

Epidemiology

Tetralogy of Fallot is the most common cyanotic heart defect. It constitutes approximately 10% of all congenital heart defects. Boys are affected somewhat more often than girls.

Pathogenesis

The underlying cause is an anomaly of the infundibular septum. This septum is displaced in a right anterior direction. The muscular and infundibular septa are thus no longer at the same level and cannot fuse together during embryonic development. This results in a VSD (malalignment VSD). The dislocation of the infundibular septum also leads to an obstruction of the right ventricular outflow tract and displacement of the aortic roof. A pronounced obstruction of the right ventricular outflow tract can lead to intrauterine hypoperfusion and hypoplasia of the pulmonary arteries.

Classification

Depending on the degree of the right ventricular outflow tract obstruction, two types are differentiated:
- Pink Fallot: Relatively small obstruction of the right ventricular outflow tract; patients are not cyanotic.
- Blue Fallot: Pronounced obstruction of the right ventricular outflow tract with relevant pulmonary hypoperfusion; therefore, cyanosis is present.

Hemodynamics

The degree of obstruction of the right ventricular outflow tract is decisive for the hemodynamics. The right ventricular obstruction is caused by an infundibular and/or valvular pulmonary stenosis. The pulmonary valve annulus and main pulmonary artery are usually hypoplastic. Various degrees of pulmonary vascular hypoplasia and peripheral pulmonary stenoses can develop secondarily.

Due to the large VSD, the pressure is equalized between the two ventricles, so there is functionally only one pumping chamber. If there is pronounced stenosis of the right ventricular outflow tract, the blood flows primarily into the aorta due to the high resistance to pulmonary circulation. Very little blood reaches the pulmonary circulation, resulting in cyanosis.

In patients with less pronounced stenosis of the right ventricular outflow tract, there is sufficient blood flow into the pulmonary circulation. Such children are not cyanotic. However, the obstruction of the right ventricular outflow tract generally increases within the first few months of life. Cyanosis initially develops only under exertion, but later at rest as well.

Associated Anomalies

Associated anomalies often occur with a tetralogy of Fallot. The most common is a right aortic arch. Coronary anomalies are very significant for surgical correction. For example, it is not uncommon for the left anterior descending artery (LAD) to arise from the right coronary artery and cross the right ventricular outflow tract. These anomalies can make the incision of the right ventricle in the corrective operation considerably more complicated. The most common associated anomalies are listed below:
- Right aortic arch (30%)
- ASD II ("pentalogy of Fallot," 25%)
- Left persistent superior vena cava
- Coronary anomalies (e.g., LAD from the right coronary artery crossing the right ventricular outflow tract)
- AV canal
- Additional muscular VSD
- Subaortic stenosis, supravalvular mitral stenosis
- PDA
- Aortopulmonary collaterals (MAPCA)

If there is pulmonary atresia, the clinical picture can be considered to be an extreme variant of a tetralogy of Fallot according to hemodynamic criteria. However, since it is a different clinical picture from the pathogenesis aspect, this entity is discussed separately (Chapter 15.15).

The special form of a tetralogy of Fallot with agenesis of the pulmonary valve (Miller–Lev–Paul syndrome) has a few special features and is described in more detail at the end of this chapter.

Associated Syndromes

A tetralogy of Fallot, like all conotruncal deformities, is frequently associated with a microdeletion of 22q11, which can be confirmed in around 10% of cases of tetralogy of Fallot.

15.14.2 Diagnostic Measures

Symptoms

The clinical symptoms can vary considerably depending on the degree of stenosis of the right ventricular outflow tract. In most cases, there is only mild to moderate cyanosis in neonates. Cyanosis increases later with the development of hypertrophy of the infundibulum muscles.

Due to the large VSD, there is only rarely excessive pulmonary blood flow with signs of congestive heart failure. Pulmonary circulation is generally sufficiently protected due to the stenosis of the right ventricular outflow tract. If there are symptoms of excessive pulmonary blood flow, the diagnosis of a tetralogy of Fallot should be reconsidered.

Complications

The course of the disease can be complicated by cyanotic spells. These are paroxysmal episodes in which the children become deeply cyanotic, lose muscle tone, and can lose consciousness or develop seizures. This is thought to be caused by a spasm of the hypertrophic infundibulum muscles due to sympathicotonia or a sudden drop in systemic resistance. These cyanotic spells occur in particular after awakening and after physical or psychological stress (e.g., feeding, crying, playing roughly) or due to a drop in systemic resistance (e.g., hot bath, after feeding). Earlier, when no surgical treatment was yet available, cyanotic spells were a major cause of death in Fallot patients.

Older children who have not had corrective surgery assume a typical squatting position, especially after physical exertion. The children squat down and remain in this position. Squatting causes the systemic resistance to increase so that the flow of blood out of the ventricles into the systemic circulation is counteracted by greater resistance, more blood reaches the pulmonary circulation, and cyanosis decreases.

Clubbing (drumstick fingers and toes and watch-glass nails), gingival hyperplasia, and polyglobulia are signs of chronic hypoxemia in young children who have not undergone corrective surgery and are only rarely observed today because of early correction.

Endocarditis occurs in a tetralogy of Fallot more frequently than in other cyanotic heart defects. Cyanotic patients also tend to develop brain abscesses.

Auscultation

A 2/6 to 4/6 loud, rough, spindle-shaped systolic murmur with PMI in the 2nd to 3rd left parasternal ICS is indicative. It corresponds to the murmur of the right ventricular outflow tract obstruction. The VSD generally does not cause a murmur because the pressure is equalized. The second heart sound is soft and single, as the closing of the pulmonary valve cannot be heard.

ECG

If there is a relevant obstruction of the right ventricular outflow tract, the ECG presents signs of right heart stress: right axis deviation, tall R waves in the right precordial leads V_1 and V_2, and deep S waves in the left precordial leads V_5 and V_6. A P dextrocardiale is rather unusual in children.

> **Note**
>
> Left axis deviation in Tetralogy of Fallot always suggests an associated AV canal.

Chest X-ray

The heart is usually of normal size in the X-ray but has a conspicuous shape ("boot-shaped heart," "coeur en sabot"): rounded, upturned cardiac apex, decreased pulmonary vascular marking, prominent waist (empty pulmonary artery segment). If there is a right aortic arch, the mediastinum has a convex right border.

Echocardiography

An indicative finding is an aorta overriding a large malalignment VSD. This finding can be best visualized in the parasternal long axis. The location and extent of the obstruction of the right ventricular outflow tract must be determined. Is there an infundibular, valvular, or supravalvular stenosis or a combination of these? It may be difficult to visualize the frequently hypoplastic pulmonary arteries. The diameter of the pulmonary valve, the infundibulum, and the pulmonary arteries should be carefully documented.

The pressure gradient across the right ventricular outflow tract can be estimated by Doppler sonography. In a neonate it is usually 50 to 70 mmHg, in an infant 70 to 90 mmHg. If the pressure gradient is lower, the diagnosis of tetralogy of Fallot should be questioned. In addition, the VSD including the shunt is visualized and the extent of right ventricular hypertrophy is determined. It is important to assess anomalies of the coronary arteries. In particular, branches that cross the right ventricular outflow tract must be ruled out or identified. In tetralogy of Fallot, a possible right aortic arch must always be investigated. Other associated anomalies are documented or ruled out.

A possible differential diagnosis is double-outlet right ventricle (DORV) with a pulmonary stenosis. In this case, there is typically a discontinuity between the aorta and the pulmonary artery due to a muscle collar (conus tissue).

If there is a truncus arteriosus communis, only a single large vessel arises from the ventricles, which overrides the malalignment VSD. The branches of the pulmonary arteries or the main pulmonary artery arise from this truncus vessel.

Cardiac Catheterization

Diagnostic cardiac catheterization is required preoperatively only if there is any uncertainty with respect to the pulmonary vessels, the coronary arteries, or associated anomalies such as MAPCAs or for interventional measures.

The pressure is typically equalized between the two ventricles. The extent and exact location of the pressure gradient across the right ventricular outflow tract is measured when the catheter is withdrawn.

Contrast medium is injected into the right ventricle to visualize the right ventricular outflow tract, the pulmonary valve annulus, and the VSD with the overriding aorta. To visualize the coronary arteries, the contrast medium is injected into the aortic root, or a direct coronary angiography is performed.

MRI

Anatomical details can often be clarified in an MRI. Postoperatively, it is performed primarily in older patients for precise quantification of postoperative pulmonary insufficiency and to assess the size of the right ventricle.

15.14.3 Treatment

Conservative Treatment

In neonates with a severe obstruction of the right ventricular outflow tract and a systemic oxygen saturation of less than 70%, prostaglandin E is administered to keep the ductus arteriosus patent and improve pulmonary perfusion. Endocarditis prophylaxis is always indicated for tetralogy of Fallot.

Note

Digoxin, diuretics, and vasodilators are generally contraindicated in tetralogy of Fallot. Digoxin increases the infundibular stenosis. Vasodilators lower the resistance in the systemic circulation and thus increase the right-to-left shunt and cyanosis. Diuretics can induce volume depletion that can lead to cyanotic spells.

Acute treatment of a cyanotic spell:

- Immediate sedation (e.g., Ketamin 2 mg/kg IV or 5 mg/kg IM; or morphine 0,1-0,2 mg/kg IV, SC or IM; alternatively, diazepam rectal gel for example)
- Oxygen administration
- Increase the resistance in the systemic circulation: Press the child's flexed knee against the chest, squatting position, possibly infusion of vasoconstrictors (noradrenaline)
- Volume bolus (20 – 40 – 60 mL/kg)
- Compensate metabolic acidosis by buffering
- Beta blocker (e.g., propranolol 0.01–0.1 mg/kg very slowly IV under monitor guidance)

To prevent a recurrence after the first cyanotic spell, a beta blocker (e.g., propranolol 1–2 mg/kg/d in three or four individual doses) can be administered to bridge the period before surgery. The beta blocker reduces the risk of an infundibulum spasm. Basic sedation may be useful.

Interventional Catheterization

Balloon dilation is useful only for predominantly valvular pulmonary stenosis. It can lead to intermittent improvement of oxygen saturation and to "catch-up" growth if there is a hypoplastic pulmonary vascular bed.

Balloon dilation of an infundibular stenosis is not effective. In individual cases, pulmonary perfusion can be improved by stent implantation in the right ventricular outflow tract, but this is not yet a routine procedure in many centers.

In pronounced cases in which pulmonary blood flow is dependent on a PDA, a stent can be implanted as an interim measure to keep the ductus patent.

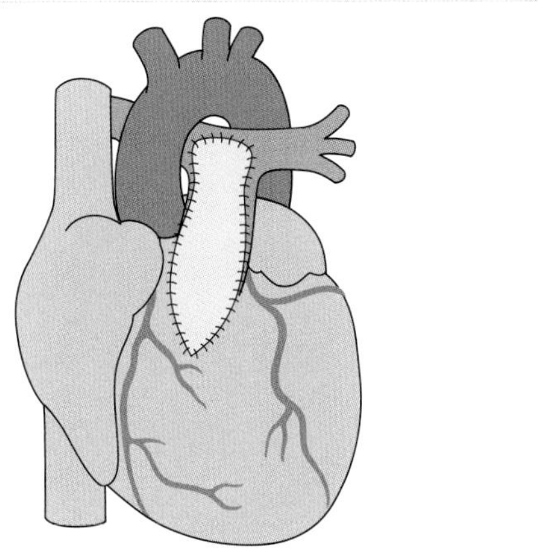

Fig. 15.46 Correction of a tetralogy of Fallot including a transannular patch. The obstruction of the right ventricular outflow tract is expanded with a transannular patch of autologous pericardium. The patch expands the right ventricular outflow tract, the pulmonary valve annulus, and the pulmonary artery. The disadvantage of this method is that pulmonary insufficiency generally develops.

Surgical Treatment

The treatment goal today is primary surgical correction. There is almost always an indication for surgery in children with a tetralogy of Fallot. Palliative surgery is only rarely needed. The corrective surgery is generally performed between the 3rd and 6th month of life. After a cyanotic spell has occurred, surgery is indicated promptly, and even sooner if severe cyanosis occurs.

In this surgery, the VSD is closed with a patch so the overriding aorta is assigned to the left ventricle. This maneuver is usually performed via a tricuspid access route after opening the right atrium, rarely via a right ventricular incision. To relieve the obstruction of the right ventricular outflow tract, the infundibular stenosis is resected. A valvular pulmonary stenosis is treated by commissurotomy or valvulotomy. The pulmonary valve annulus is left intact if possible so valve function is not impaired. However, sometimes the pulmonary valve annulus must be incised and expanded with a patch (transannular patch, ▶ Fig. 15.46). This patch, (usually made from autologous pericardium) extends from the right ventricular outflow tract across the pulmonary valve annulus into the pulmonary artery. Sometimes this patch must be sutured even beyond the bifurcation of the pulmonary artery.

Initial palliative surgery is generally indicated only if there is an extremely hypoplastic pulmonary vascular bed or if there are coronary anomalies, which pose a high risk in small children if an incision is made in the right ventricular outflow tract. In these cases, first an aortopulmonary shunt (▶ Fig. 15.47) is made to improve pulmonary blood flow before the actual correction is made later.

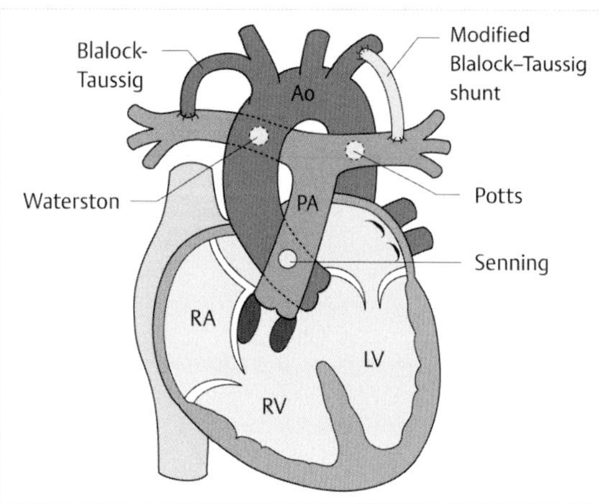

Fig. 15.47 Various aortopulmonary shunts. Aortopulmonary shunts are today used only rarely as interim measures to ensure pulmonary blood flow in a tetralogy of Fallot.
The *Waterston shunt* is an anastomosis between the ascending aorta and the right pulmonary artery; the *Potts shunt* is a direct connection between the descending aorta and the left pulmonary artery. A *Senning anastomosis* is a connection between the pulmonary artery and the proximal ascending aorta. In the original *Blalock–Taussig shunt*, the subclavian artery was anastomosed with the ipsilateral pulmonary artery. These days a *modified Blalock–Taussig shunt* is made more frequently. In this shunt, a Gore-Tex tube connects the subclavian artery with the ipsilateral pulmonary artery.
LV, left ventricle; RV, right ventricle; RA, right atrium; PA, pulmonary artery; Ao, aorta.

15.14.4 Prognosis and Outcome

► **Long-term prognosis.** Left untreated, most patients die in childhood. The survival rate without treatment is 75% after one year, 40% after 4 years, and 5% after 40 years.

The early mortality rate of the corrective surgery is less than 5%. The great majority of corrected patients can lead a nearly normal life afterward. The survival rate at 35 years after the operation is around 85%.

Important late complications are:

- Arrhythmias: Ventricular arrhythmias are particularly feared. Risk factors for ventricular arrhythmias are pulmonary insufficiency, patients who were operated on late, widened QRS complex in the ECG (> 180 ms), and impaired ventricular function. Ventricular arrhythmias are associated with an increased risk of sudden cardiac death. In adult patients, supraventricular arrhythmias such as atrial flutter and fibrillation also occur frequently.
- Pulmonary insufficiency, right ventricular dilatation and dysfunction: There is almost always significant pulmonary insufficiency if a transannular patch was needed for the correction. Mild or moderate pulmonary insufficiency is generally well tolerated, but severe chronic pulmonary insufficiency leads to dilation of the right ventricle and impaired right ventricular function in the long term. Tricuspid insufficiency can develop as a result of right ventricular dilatation.
- Residual obstruction of the right ventricular outflow tract
- Aneurysm of the right ventricular outflow tract after patch expansion
- Residual VSD
- Dilatation of the aortic root, aortic insufficiency
- Left ventricular dysfunction

Repeat surgery is needed primarily as a result of pulmonary insufficiency.

► **Outpatient checkups.** Lifelong cardiac follow-up is needed at annual intervals or more frequently even years after the corrective surgery. The major focus of the examinations should be on the long-term complications described above, especially assessment of the pulmonary valve (pulmonary insufficiency, stenosis), the size and function of the right ventricle, and any arrhythmias. There is almost always a right bundle branch block after the corrective operation.

Endocarditis prophylaxis is always necessary for the first 6 postoperative months, and lifelong if defects later develop in the vicinity of the prosthetic material.

► **Physical exercise capacity and lifestyle.** The quality of life and physical exercise capacity in everyday activities is good for most patients. Around 80 to 90% of patients are classified as NYHA (New York Heart Association) class I according to clinical symptoms. Competitive sports are not recommended for most patients. Unlimited physical activity can be recommended only if the following conditions are fulfilled: no relevant residual VSD, normal size of the right ventricle, only mild pulmonary insufficiency, good ventricular function, normal pressure in the right ventricle, no relevant arrhythmias, and good capacity in an exercise test. In most cases, sports with low to moderate dynamic and static stress are possible.

► **Special aspects in adolescents and adults.** Most adolescent and adult patients have undergone surgical correction. Frequently, the main problem of these patients is residual pulmonary insufficiency with subsequent enlargement of the right ventricle and a right ventricular systolic dysfunction. These changes lead to widening of the QRS complex in the ECG and a predisposition for ventricular arrhythmias. There is an increased risk of sudden cardiac death. It is often difficult to determine the proper time for pulmonary valve replacement. The improvement of right ventricular function must be weighed against the necessity of a later reoperation if valve replacement is performed too soon. An MRI is the ideal method for

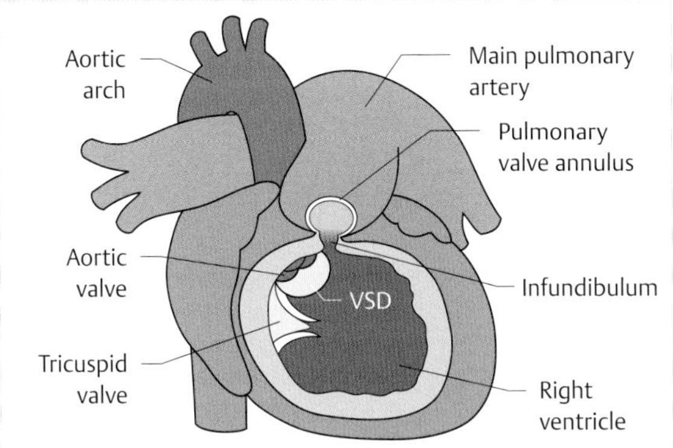

Fig. 15.48 Tetralogy of Fallot with agenesis of the pulmonary valve (Miller–Lev–Paul syndrome). The typical Fallot findings are present: large VSD with an overriding aorta, stenosis of the right ventricular outflow tract, and consecutive hypertrophy of the right ventricle. There is only a rudimentary fibrous ring or membrane for the pulmonary valve. As a result of the oscillating flow, there is massive dilatation of the pulmonary artery and its main branches.

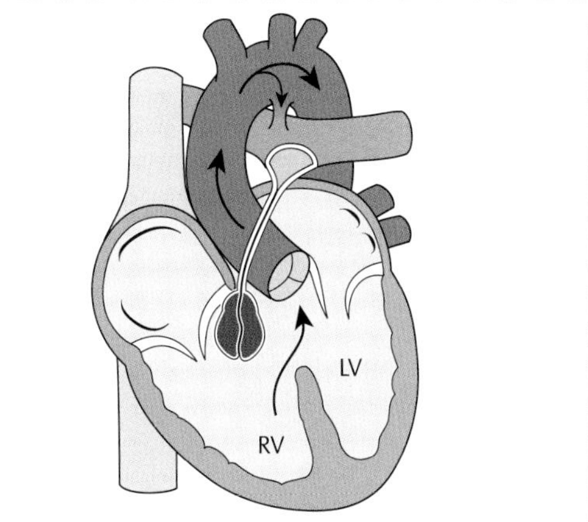

Fig. 15.49 Pulmonary atresia with ventricular septal defect (VSD). The pulmonary valve is atretic and the right ventricular outflow tract is clearly hypoplastic. In addition, similar to tetralogy of Fallot, there is a large malalignment VSD with an overriding aorta. The configuration of the pulmonary artery and the central pulmonary vessels is quite variable.[15]

assessing the size and function of the right ventricle, the extent of pulmonary insufficiency, and stenosis of the pulmonary artery.

15.14.5 Tetralogy of Fallot with Agenesis of the Pulmonary Valve (Miller–Lev–Paul Syndrome)

Around 2% of all patients with tetralogy of Fallot have agenesis of the pulmonary valve (▶ Fig. 15.48). These children have only a fibrous ring or membrane that serves as a rudimentary pulmonary valve. This generally leads to a relevant stenosis and severe insufficiency of the rudimentary pulmonary valve. Because of the considerable insufficiency and the oscillating flow in the pulmonary artery, the pulmonary artery is sometimes massively enlarged and can lead to compression of the bronchia and trachea. The main branches of the pulmonary artery can also be dilated, but the peripheral pulmonary arteries are often typically very thin. NB: There is no PDA in most cases.

Cyanosis and respiratory problems such as stridor and dyspnea are the most prominent *clinical symptoms* in neonates. On *auscultation,* a systolic–diastolic murmur ("to-and-fro murmur") can be heard with PMI in the left parasternal area, which sounds like sawing wood.

The dilatation of the pulmonary artery and possibly its branches is conspicuous in *radiology.* As a result of the compression of the trachea and bronchia, atelectasis, and hyperinflation of areas of the lungs can occur.

In *echocardiography,* the typical findings of tetralogy of Fallot with malalignment VSD and an aorta overriding the defect can be detected. In addition, there is sometimes a massively dilated pulmonary artery. Using Doppler ultrasound, accelerated flow across the rudimentary pulmonary valve and pronounced insufficiency can be seen. The rudimentary pulmonary valve itself is a fibrous band with no opening or closure movement.

In the operation, first the pulmonary valve is replaced and the dilated pulmonary artery is plicated if necessary. In addition, the VSD is closed. A Lecompte maneuver is generally also performed to reposition the right pulmonary artery anterior to the aorta and decompress the bronchi.

15.15 Pulmonary Atresia with Ventricular Septal Defect

15.15.1 Basics

Synonym: Pulmonary atresia with ventricular septal defect was formerly also known as "pseudotruncus" or "truncus arteriosus Type IV." Some authors also speak of a tetralogy of Fallot with pulmonary atresia. However, from the pathogenetic standpoint, a pulmonary atresia with ventricular septal defect is neither a variant of truncus arteriosus communis nor an extreme variant of tetralogy of Fallot.

Definition

Pulmonary atresia with ventricular septal defect (PA-VSD) is a complex heart defect with the following features (▶ Fig. 15.49):

- Atresia of the pulmonary valve (sometimes there is also atresia of the main pulmonary artery and/or the central pulmonary arteries)

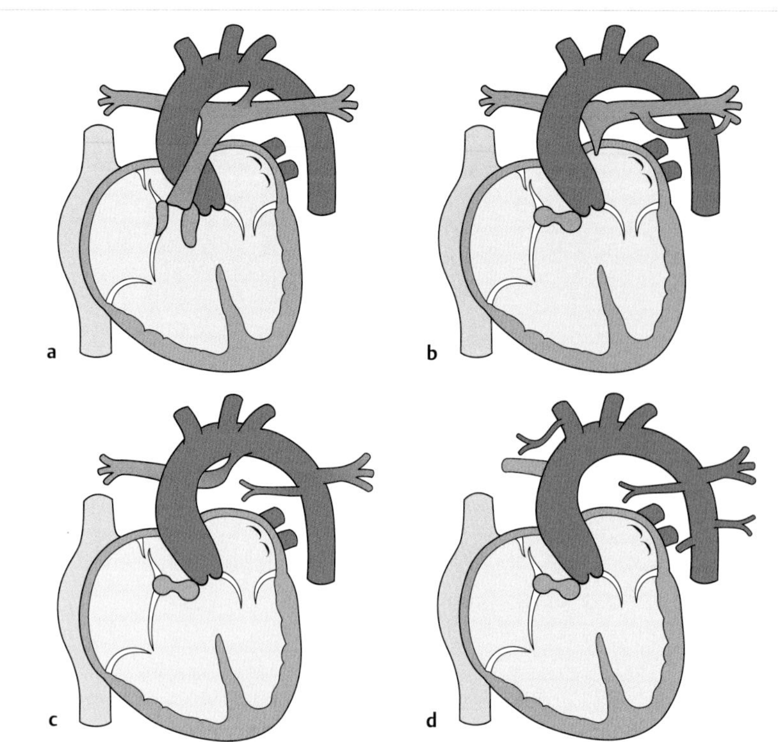

Fig. 15.50 Classification of pulmonary atresia with ventricular septal defect. **a** Group I: normally developed central and peripheral pulmonary arteries, ductal-dependent pulmonary blood flow. **b** Group II: normally developed central and peripheral pulmonary arteries, but no main pulmonary artery ductal-dependent pulmonary blood flow. **c** Group III: narrow or hypoplastic central pulmonary vessels, pulmonary blood flow mainly via aortopulmonary collaterals, ductus is absent or narrow. **d** Group IV: no central pulmonary vessels, pulmonary blood flow only via usually multifocal aortopulmonary collaterals.[37]

- Underdevelopment of the right ventricular outflow tract
- Large malalignment VSD
- VSD with overriding aorta

Another common feature is MAPCAs (major aortopulmonary collateral arteries, aortopulmonary collaterals, see section on Pathogenesis below).

The extent of development of the pulmonary artery is decisive for the surgical correction and outcome. In most patients, the atresia is limited to the pulmonary valve and the pulmonary artery, but other branching anomalies and stenoses of the pulmonary vessels and pronounced hypoplasia of the pulmonary vascular bed may also occur.

Epidemiology

PA-VSDs constitute about 3% of all congenital heart defects.

Pathogenesis

The genesis of a PA-VSD is not fully understood. A few cases of intrauterine transition of a pulmonary stenosis to a pulmonary atresia have been documented. In a pulmonary atresia, the lungs are supplied by the ductus arteriosus or the aortopulmonary collaterals (MAPCAs, persistent embryonic vascular connections between the lung buds and the aorta).

Classification

The classification is based mainly on the degree of development of the pulmonary arteries and the type of pulmonary blood flow (▶ Fig. 15.50). The main pulmonary artery and central pulmonary arteries are present in most cases. However, there is a wide range of different morphologies. In an extreme case, the central pulmonary arteries are absent and the lungs are perfused only via aortopulmonary collaterals.

Hemodynamics and Pathology

From the hemodynamic standpoint, this heart defect can be considered an extreme variant of tetralogy of Fallot. However, the underlying disease is different; the decisive difference is the configuration of pulmonary artery systems (see also Classification below).

Pulmonary atresia can be variable in extent. If it is a membranous atresia, the pulmonary artery and its branches are normally developed, but there is an impermeable membrane instead of the pulmonary valve. In a muscular atresia, there is no valve system at all: the right ventricular outflow tract is usually rudimentary in such cases. In the most severe forms, the central pulmonary arteries are completely absent.

The only outlet from the right ventricle is a VSD, through which the right ventricular blood reaches the aorta. The systemic circulation thus contains missed blood.

If pulmonary arteries are present, the lungs are perfused via a PDA. If central pulmonary vessels are absent, the lungs are perfused via collaterals. In these cases, the ductus arteriosus is frequently not developed at all.

Pulmonary blood flow is possible via the following connections:

- PDA
- Major aortopulmonary collateral arteries (MAPCAs): These are aortopulmonary collaterals that usually arise from the thoracic aorta, but also from the subclavian artery, mammary artery, or intercostal arteries, and drain into the pulmonary arteries
- Coronary fistulas (extremely rare)
- Dilated bronchial arteries

MAPCAs tend to develop stenoses. If there are no stenoses, excessive pulmonary blood flow may develop with pulmonary hypertension and difficult-to-control pulmonary bleeding from the collateral vessels.

The ductus arteriosus has a few special features in a pulmonary atresia. Since intrauterine blood flow does not occur normally via the pulmonary artery, but retrograde via the aorta, the ductus arises at an unusual angle from the aorta; it is narrow, and often has a tortuous course.

Associated Anomalies

- ASD II or patent foramen ovale (approx. 80%)
- Right aortic arch (40%)
- Left persistent superior vena cava
- AV canal
- Tricuspid atresia
- Coronary anomalies (rare)
- d- or l-TGA

Associated Syndromes

As with all conotruncal anomalies, a PA-VSD is frequently associated with microdeletion of 22q11, occurring in about one-quarter of cases. PA-VSD also occurs frequently with heterotaxy syndromes.

15.15.2 Diagnostic Measures

Symptoms

The leading symptom is cyanosis that depends on the extent of pulmonary blood flow and is usually already present at birth. Cyanosis is especially pronounced when the ductus threatens to close in ductal-dependent forms.

If excessive pulmonary blood flow is the main symptom—for example, in patients whose lungs are supplied by non-stenotic aortopulmonary collaterals—there are signs of congestive heart failure (tachypnea/dyspnea, hepatomegaly, failure to thrive).

Complications

When pulmonary perfusion occurs via aortopulmonary collaterals, there is generally increasing cyanosis due to the increasing stenosis of the collaterals.

If the collateral vessels are large without stenosis, pulmonary hypertension develops in the affected areas of the lungs with the risk of more severe pulmonary hemorrhage from the collateral vessels. The clinical correlate is hemoptysis.

Auscultation

There is a single, loud second heart sound. Depending on the location, a continuous systolic–diastolic murmur is a sign of PDA or aortopulmonary collaterals. The latter can often also be auscultated over the back.

ECG

There are typically signs of right ventricular and right atrial hypertrophy: right cardiac axis deviation, P dextrocardiale, tall R waves in the right precordial leads, and deep S waves in the left precordial leads. Positive T waves, later ST segment depression, and T wave inversion can be found in the right precordial leads even in infancy.

If there is pronounced collateral circulation with volume overload of the left ventricle, signs of biventricular hypertrophy develop.

Chest X-ray

The X-ray usually shows a normal sized heart with a conspicuous shape ("boot-shaped heart," "coeur en sabot") as in tetralogy of Fallot: rounded, upturned cardiac apex, narrow waist in the pulmonary segment (empty pulmonary segment). If there is a right aortic arch, the mediastinum has a right convex border. The pulmonary vascular markings are often asymmetrical and decreased due to difference in blood flow through the collaterals.

If there is excessive pulmonary blood flow, the pulmonary vascular markings are increased and the heart has a spherical shape.

Echocardiography

An indicative finding is a large malalignment VSD with an overriding aorta and a blind right ventricular outflow tract. The VSD with overriding aorta can be seen in the parasternal long axis. The blind right ventricular outflow tract can often be best viewed in the parasternal short axis. The extent of the pulmonary vascular system must be determined: Is the main artery present? Is there a pulmonary artery bifurcation? Pulmonary stenosis? If there is a main pulmonary artery, the retrograde perfusion of the pulmonary artery can be visualized using color Doppler imaging. The ductus frequently has a tortuous course.

It is often difficult to visualize aortopulmonary collateral vessels, and usually it is easiest from a suprasternal view. Associated cardiac anomalies (right aortic arch, ASD II, patent foramen ovale, coronary anomalies) must be ruled out by echocardiography.

Cardiac Catheterization

There is almost always an indication for diagnostic cardiac catheterization. The examination is useful, especially for:

- visualizing the pulmonary vascular situation
- assessing pulmonary blood flow (evidence of PDA and/or collateral vessels, selective visualization of the collateral vessels and their supply territories, differentiation between unifocal and multifocal pulmonary blood flow)
- determining pulmonary vascular resistance
- coronary angiography to exclude coronary anomalies or fistulas

MRI

MRI is very useful for obtaining an exact 3D visualization of the pulmonary vessels and aortopulmonary collaterals.

15.15.3 Treatment

Conservative Treatment

If there is ductal-dependent pulmonary blood flow, prostaglandin E (initially 50 ng/kg/min, later reduced) is administered in addition to ample fluids to keep the ductus arteriosus patent until definitive treatment.

In case of heart failure (excessive pulmonary blood flow associated with a wide PDA or unobstructed pulmonary perfusion from collaterals), anticongestive therapy and fluid restriction are required until definitive treatment.

Interventional Catheterization

If there is only membranous valve atresia (imperforate valve), an attempt can be made to open the atretic valve using high-frequency current. For muscular atresias, a stent may also be implanted in the right ventricular outflow tract to prevent restenosis.

If there is ductal-dependent pulmonary blood flow, pulmonary perfusion can be ensured by implanting a stent in the ductus, but this is only a palliative measure so that the pulmonary vessels increase in size before the definitive surgical correction.

Should there be excessive pulmonary blood flow through the aortopulmonary collaterals, coil embolization of those collaterals providing a double supply to areas of the lung. If pulmonary hemorrhage from the collaterals occurs, an attempt can also be made to occlude the affected collateral vessels by interventional catheterization.

▸ **Surgical Treatment.** The goal of surgical treatment is to create the absent continuity between the right ventricle and the pulmonary arteries. In addition, the VSD is closed to separate the circulation systems. It is primarily the extent of pulmonary vascular hypoplasia that determines the surgical options. Sometimes surgical correction is not possible until previous measures have led to catch-up growth of the pulmonary vessels.

If there is ductal-dependent pulmonary blood flow, first an aortopulmonary anastomosis is created in infancy (e.g., modified Blalock–Taussig shunt) or the right ventricular outflow tract is enlarged with a patch, without closing the VSD. These measures improve pulmonary perfusion and lead to "catch-up" growth of the hypoplastic pulmonary vascular bed. When the pulmonary vessels have reached an adequate size, the definitive correction is made using a Rastelli procedure (▸ Fig. 15.51). A conduit is implanted between the right ventricle and the pulmonary arteries, and the VDS and aortopulmonary shunt are closed.

If there is multifocal pulmonary blood flow from several aortopulmonary collaterals, anomalous branches of the pulmonary arteries or peripheral pulmonary stenoses, *unifocalization* is required: The aortopulmonary collaterals are connected to each other and bundled in one common vessel that is functionally equivalent to a pulmonary artery. Simultaneously, a valved conduit or homograft is implanted as a connection between the right ventricle and the unifocalized vessel (pulmonary artery). Due to the increased resistance in the unifocalized pulmonary arteries, the VSD must often be left as an "overflow" valve and possibly may not be closed until a later time.

To estimate the size of the pulmonary vessels, the Nakata index and the McGoon ratio are used:

$$\text{Nakata index} = \frac{A_{left}(mm^2) + A_{right}(mm^2)}{\text{Body surface area}(m^2)}$$

with

A_{left} = Cross section of the left pulmonary artery, and

A_{right} = Cross section of the right pulmonary artery

Normal: $300 \pm 30\ mm^2/m^2$

$$\text{McGoon ratio} = \frac{A_{left}(mm) + A_{right}(mm)}{B(mm)}$$

with

A_{left} = Diameter of the left pulmonary artery,

A_{right} = Diameter of the right pulmonary artery, and

B = Diameter of the descending aorta

Normal: > 2

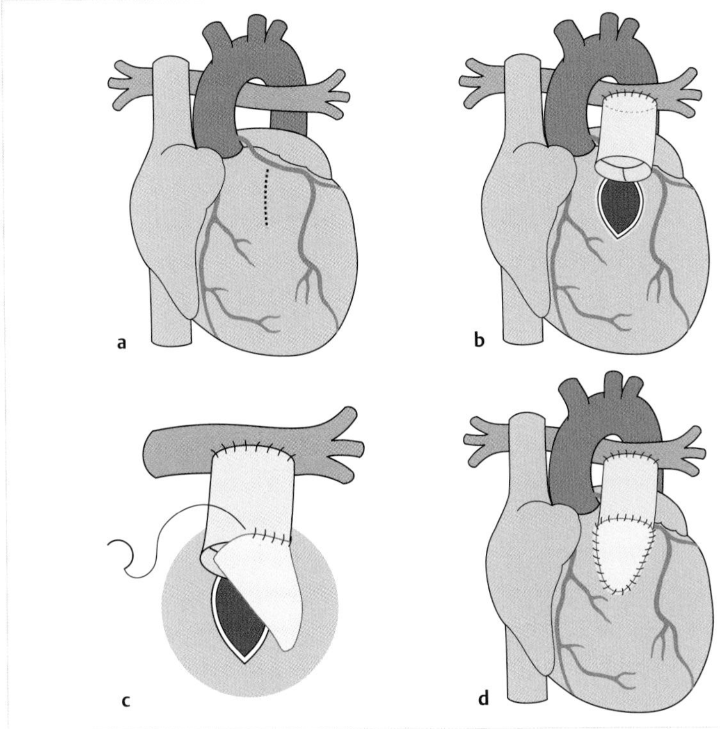

Fig. 15.51 Correction of a pulmonary atresia with ventricular septal defect in a Rastelli procedure. In addition to closing the VSD, a valved conduit is implanted as a connection between the right ventricle and the central pulmonary arteries. First an incision of the infundibulum and possibly resection of infundibular muscle tissue is required for this.
a Incision of the pulmonary artery and infundibulum. **b** The distal end of the valved conduit is attached at the incision of the pulmonary arteries. **c** After wedge-shaped expansion of the infundibular incision, the proximal end of the conduit is implanted here. **d** Postoperative situation.

15.15.4 Prognosis and Outcome

▶ **Long-term prognosis.** Left untreated, many children with a PA-VSD die within the first two years of life. If there is ductal-dependent pulmonary blood flow, the children die when the duct closes. Patients who have pronounced aortopulmonary anastomoses may survive until young adulthood in rare cases.

Depending on the study, 60 to 90% of patients with a PA-VSD can have their defects corrected by surgery. As a rule of thumb, the greater the hypoplasia of the central pulmonary arteries, the less favorable the long-term prognosis is.

The major long-term problems are arrhythmias, stenosis of the pulmonary arteries, persistent pulmonary hypertension in the inadequately developed vascular bed, and complications with the conduit (stenosis, insufficiency), which frequently require repeat surgery or interventional catheterization.

▶ **Outpatient checkups.** Lifelong postoperative outpatient monitoring is needed. After the palliative implantation of an aortopulmonary shunt, the shunt function must be checked regularly. The growth of the central pulmonary artery must be documented in order to make a decision on the definitive corrective surgery.

After implantation of the conduit between the right ventricle and the pulmonary artery, regular tests of conduit function are required so the conduit can be replaced when necessary. Special attention should also be paid to arrhythmias and pulmonary hypertension that may develop. Lifelong endocarditis prophylaxis is needed.

▶ **Physical exercise capacity and lifestyle.** After palliative procedures, physical exercise capacity is usually clearly limited. After corrective surgery, the patients are generally able to handle normal everyday activities. No competitive sports should be played.

▶ **Special aspects in adolescents and adults.** Severe cyanosis is the major problem for patients of this age group who are inoperable or treated palliatively. Complications include hypoxic heart failure, disposition for thromboembolic events, cerebral abscesses, and increased tendency to bleed.

Some of these patients benefit from interventional catheterization to implant stents in the aortopulmonary collaterals. This palliative measure leads to a decrease in cyanosis and an increase in oxygen saturation. If there are large aortopulmonary collaterals, the rupture of collateral vessels can cause pronounced hemoptysis. In this case, it is sometimes useful to occlude the respective vessels by coil embolization in interventional catheterization.

Regular cardiac monitoring is necessary for adolescents and adults who have undergone corrective surgery.

15.16 Pulmonary Atresia with Intact Ventricular Septum

15.16.1 Basics

Definition

In pulmonary atresia with intact ventricular septum (PA/IVS), the right ventricular outflow tract is completely obstructed (▶ Fig. 15.52). The ventricular septum is intact. The right ventricle therefore has no "normal" outflow. It is drained across an insufficient tricuspid valve, occasionally also through fistulas between the right ventricle and the coronary arteries (myocardial sinusoids). An interatrial communication with a right-to-left shunt across an atrial septal defect (ASD) or a patent foramen ovale (PFO) is necessary for survival. The pulmonary blood flow is usually across a patent ductus arteriosus (PDA), rarely also through aortopulmonary collaterals (major aortopulmonary collateral arteries, MAPCAs).

The degree of hypoplasia of the right ventricle and the presence or absence of connections between the right ventricle and the coronary arteries are decisive for the prognosis and therapy.

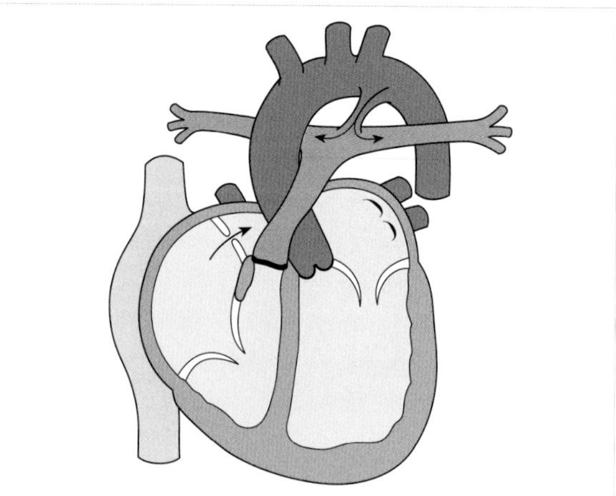

Fig. 15.52 Pulmonary atresia with intact ventricular septum. In a pulmonary atresia with intact ventricular septum, the right ventricular outflow tract is completely obstructed. In most cases, there is a membrane instead of the pulmonary valve. The right ventricle cannot drain normally. The size of the right ventricle varies widely. There is always a right-to-left shunt at the atrial level. Pulmonary perfusion is ensured by a patent ductus arteriosus.

Epidemiology

Less than 1% of all congenital heart defects are PA/IVS. Boys and girls are affected equally.

Pathogenesis

The genesis is not fully understood. An intrauterine disease or possibly an inflammatory disease may lead to the obstruction of the pulmonary artery or the right ventricular outflow tract. There are varying severities of impaired development of the right ventricle, likely depending on the time when the atresia occurred.

Classification

Classification is based on the size of the right ventricle. There are fluid transitions:

- Type I (85%): hypoplastic right ventricle ("peach pit right ventricle")
- Type II (15%): normal-sized right ventricle with accompanying tricuspid insufficiency

Hemodynamics and Pathology

The right ventricle normally has three parts (tripartite right ventricle) and consists of an inlet portion, trabecular portion, and outlet portion (= infundibulum). Variants of PA/IVS range from an almost normal-sized or only slightly hypoplastic right ventricle with a well-developed infundibulum and pulmonary valve closed only by a membrane, up to a unipartite ventricle with no inlet portion and an atretic infundibulum having only a rudimentary pulmonary valve. In the latter variant, myocardial sinusoids are almost always present.

The tricuspid valve is frequently dysplastic or hypoplastic and often manifests tricuspid insufficiency. The right atrium is usually clearly dilated due to the inflow congestion into the right ventricle and the presence of the frequently insufficient tricuspid valve.

Due to the lack of normal outflow from the right ventricle, blood collects in the right ventricle. Therefore, most of the blood from the right atrium flows into the left atrium across a right-to-left shunt at the atrial level (ASD or PFO). There, the venous blood is mixed with the oxygenated blood from the pulmonary veins. This leads to volume overload of the left atrium and ventricle. The systemic circulation receives mixed blood.

Pulmonary blood flows almost exclusively across a PDA (ductal-dependent pulmonary blood flow). Sometimes aortopulmonary collaterals ensure pulmonary blood flow.

The right ventricle can be drained only via two abnormal pathways:

- *Tricuspid insufficiency:* In systole, blood returns to the right atrium via an insufficient tricuspid valve, then flows to the left atrium across an ASD or a PFO, finally reaching the systemic circulation through the left ventricle. The size of the right ventricle correlates with the extent of tricuspid insufficiency: the more pronounced the tricuspid insufficiency is, the better the right ventricle can develop.
- *Myocardial sinusoids*: These are fistulas between the right ventricle and the coronary arteries (▶ Fig. 15.53).

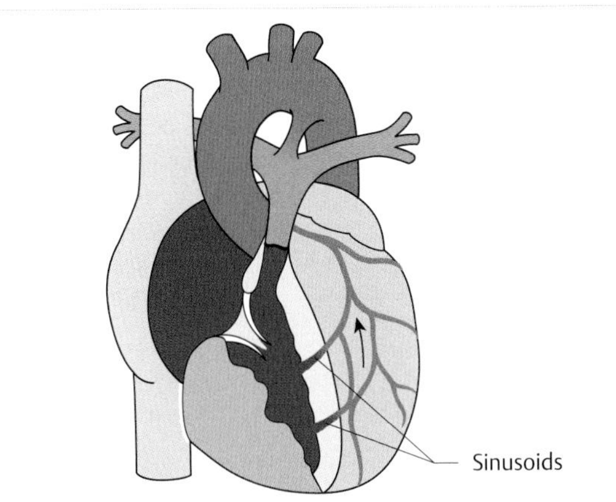

Fig. 15.53 Myocardial sinusoids associated with pulmonary atresia with intact ventricular septum. Myocardial sinusoids are persistent connections between the right ventricle and the coronary arteries (arrow). In an extreme case, blood flow of the coronary arteries depends on these myocardial sinusoids or fistulas in pulmonary atresia with intact ventricular septum.

Since the right ventricle has no outlet if there is no tricuspid insufficiency, suprasystemic pressures arise in the right ventricle. As a result, embryonic connections between the right ventricle and the coronary arteries (myocardial sinusoids) persist. They are frequently associated with stenoses of the coronary arteries or atresia of the coronary sinus ostia. If there is severe stenosis or atresia of the coronary sinus ostia, the coronaries are perfused exclusively from the right ventricle ("right ventricular dependent coronary circulation").

Associated Anomalies

- ASD, PFO (necessary for survival).
- Tricuspid regurgitation: In pulmonary atresia with intact ventricular septum, tricuspid regurgitation provides the outlet from the right ventricle. Generally, the greater intrauterine tricuspid regurgitation is, the better the right ventricle can develop.
- Myocardial sinusoids: Myocardial sinusoids occur in particular with a very hypoplastic right ventricle and can then also provide an outlet from the right ventricle.
- Stenosis and atresia of the coronary arteries: Stenoses and atresias of the coronary arteries are particularly significant. In these cases, coronary perfusion may be completely dependent on myocardial sinusoids.
- Right aortic arch (rare).
- Uhl anomaly (extremely rare).

Associated Syndromes

No increased frequency of genetic syndromes has been reported.

15.16.2 Diagnostic Measures

Symptoms

The leading symptom is cyanosis from birth. Closure of the ductus arteriosus causes a hypoxic crisis. If there is a restrictive atrial septal shunt or pronounced tricuspid regurgitation, this results in manifest right heart failure with hepatomegaly and reduced cardiac output.

Auscultation

There is a single, pronounced second heart sound. If there is tricuspid regurgitation, a dull systolic decrescendo murmur with PMI in the 4th left parasternal ICS can be heard. A PDA, and possibly myocardial sinusoids as well, cause a continuous systolic–diastolic murmur with PMI in the 2nd left parasternal ICS.

ECG

Typically, there are signs of right atrial overload (P dextrocardiale). If there is a hypoplastic right ventricle, there will be deep R waves in the right precordial leads and tall R waves in the left precordial leads (signs of left heart hypertrophy). Abnormal repolarization in the right precordial leads can occur as a sign of pressure overload of the right ventricle.

Very rarely, signs of myocardial ischemia are found in association with myocardial sinusoids and atresia of the coronary sinus ostia.

Chest X-ray

The heart can be of normal size or it may be enlarged with a dilated right atrium. A typical finding is a missing pulmonary segment. The pulmonary vascular markings depend on the width of the PDA and are usually decreased.

Echocardiography

The diagnosis can be reliably made using echocardiography. The examination should cover the following points:

- Evaluation of the pulmonary valve: There is typically a membranous pulmonary valve that does not open. A pulmonary atresia can be differentiated from a pronounced critical pulmonary stenosis using color Doppler. If there is a pulmonary atresia, color Doppler detects no blood flow across the valve. Retrograde perfusion of the pulmonary artery occurs across a PDA.
- Evaluation of the right ventricular outflow tract: Is there an infundibulum or is it absent? How wide is the right ventricular outflow tract?
- Evaluation of the size and function of the tricuspid valve: The valve diameter is often smaller than normal for age. Tricuspid regurgitation must be urgently investigated. If necessary, the right ventricular pressure

across the tricuspid regurgitation can be estimated using the Bernoulli equation. The tricuspid valve can also exhibit Ebstein-type anomalies; sometimes a tricuspid stenosis can be detected.

- Evaluation of the right ventricle: The external diameter is usually normal, but the cavity is clearly hypoplastic.
- Detection of a right-to-left shunt at the atrial level with an atrial septum that protrudes to the left.
- Visualization of the PDA: Origin from the descending aorta, often tortuous course in the direction of the confluence of the pulmonary arteries, left-to-right shunt across the ductus.
- Search for myocardial sinusoids and coronary fistulas: Dilated coronary arteries can be a sign of coronary fistulas. Color Doppler can be used in an attempt to visualize retrograde systolic perfusion of the coronaries.
- Determine the diameter of the branches of the pulmonary arteries (important for making a decision on treatment).

Cardiac Catheterization

Diagnostic cardiac catheterization is indicated in almost all patients. In particular, it can identify or rule out coronary anomalies. Retrograde systolic filling of coronary arteries after injection of contrast medium is a sign of myocardial sinusoids and atretic coronary sinus ostia. In these cases, there is also no diastolic washout of the coronaries by the normally antegrade coronary perfusion. These findings suggest that coronary perfusion stems mainly from the right ventricle.

In addition, visualization and evaluation of the size and development of the right ventricle and the tricuspid valve are an important part of the examination. The pressure in the right ventricle is usually suprasystemic.

15.16.3 Treatment

Conservative Treatment

Prostaglandin (initially 50 ng/kg/min IV, gradual reduction is usually possible later) is given to neonates to maintain patency of the ductus arteriosus.

Interventional Catheterization

High frequency perforation of the atretic valve followed by balloon dilation can be performed in patients with a right ventricle large enough to permit biventricular correction. Stents may be implanted in the right ventricular outflow tract. Since the right ventricle is usually not immediately strong enough to handle pulmonary blood flow alone, additional pulmonary perfusion via the ductus arteriosus must be ensured. Either a stent is implanted in the ductus or the prostaglandin treatment to maintain patency of the ductus is temporarily continued.

If there is a restrictive foramen ovale, the atrial shunt can be enlarged with a Rashkind balloon atrial septostomy. However, this method should be used only if hypoplasia of the right ventricle allows only univentricular palliation over the long term. In biventricular correction, the right ventricle is initially dependent on increased preload. A large atrial shunt would function as an overflow valve in this case and could possibly mean that sufficient volume may not be available for the right ventricle.

Surgical Treatment

The surgical procedure is determined largely by the size of the right ventricle and the presence or absence of myocardial sinusoids or coronary anomalies (▶ Fig. 15.54).

The size of the right ventricle correlates with the size of the tricuspid valve. The Z value has been established as a measure for the size of the tricuspid valve. Biventricular correction appears to be possible if the size of the tricuspid valve is not less than a Z value of –3. In neonates, a valve annulus diameter of 7 mm is frequently given as the threshold. Otherwise, the goal is univentricular palliation in the sense of Fontan circulation or a 1.5-ventricle solution (see insufficient size of the right ventricle (p. 158), below).

$$\text{Z score} = \frac{A_{left} - A_{right}}{B}$$

with

A_{left} = Measured diameter of the tricuspid valve,

A_{right} = Mean normal diameter, and

B = Standard deviation of the mean normal diameter

▶ **Sufficient size of the right ventricle.** This group includes around one-third of patients. They are treated by a commissurotomy of the pulmonary valve and possibly enlargement of the infundibulum with an infundibulectomy or patch enlargement (if the infundibulum cannot be reconstructed, possibly implantation of a valved conduit or homograft as well). In addition, it is usually necessary first to create an aortopulmonary shunt. Pulmonary blood flow is initially ensured by this shunt, as the right ventricle is often not strong enough to handle the pulmonary blood flow alone. The shunt and the atrial septum can later be closed in some patients, creating a biventricular situation.

▶ **Insufficient size of the right ventricle.** First, an aortopulmonary anastomosis is created to ensure pulmonary blood flow. Usually, the pulmonary valve is also opened by a commissurotomy and the outflow tract is widened. Later, when the pulmonary arteries are large enough, univentricular palliation (Fontan completion, two-stage procedure: upper cavopulmonary anastomosis, then total cavopulmonary anastomosis [TCPC]) is performed. If

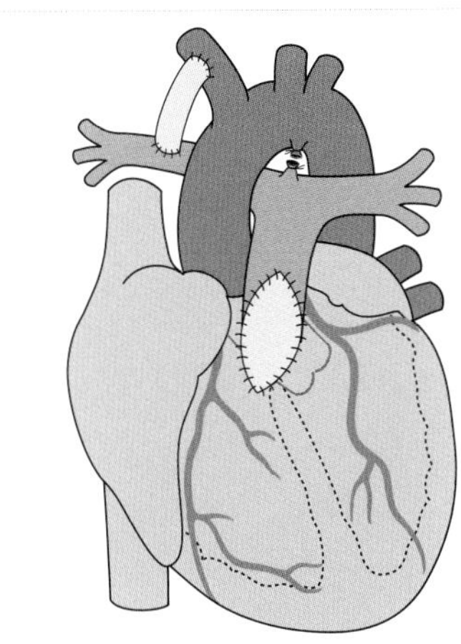

Fig. 15.54 Typical surgical palliation in a neonate with pulmonary atresia and intact ventricular septum. In the first step, the pulmonary valve is often opened surgically and the right ventricular outflow tract may be enlarged (patch and/or infundibulectomy). Since the hypoplastic, stiff right ventricle is usually not yet capable of ensuring sufficient pulmonary perfusion, an aortopulmonary shunt is made. Later, there may be catch-up growth of the pulmonary circulatory system and growth of the right ventricle. Depending on the size and function of the right ventricle, a biventricular correction, "1.5-ventricle palliation," or univentricular palliative Fontan completion can be performed.

conditions are more favorable, a 1.5-ventricle solution ("one-and-a-half Fontan") may be attempted. For this, an upper cavopulmonary anastomosis is made without obstructing the pulmonary artery, so that the pulmonary circulation is supplied via the upper cavopulmonary anastomosis as well as antegrade via the right ventricle. However, there is less volume to the right ventricle due to the upper cavopulmonary anastomosis, as the blood from the upper half of the body flows through the anastomosis directly to the lungs.

In some cases, growth of the right ventricle can be achieved by creating an aortopulmonary shunt and opening the right ventricular outflow tract, so that after closure of the shunt, it may be possible to achieve biventricular correction. Prior to this, a trial occlusion is made during cardiac catheterization to test whether occlusion of the shunt is tolerated.

▸ **Right ventricular dependent coronary perfusion.** In this case, the coronaries are supplied with blood exclusively, or at least mostly, via myocardial sinusoids or fistulas from the right ventricle. Relieving pressure in the right ventricle (by opening the valve or widening the infundibulum) would lead to flow reversal in the coronaries with outflow into the right ventricle and subsequent myocardial ischemia. In these cases, only univentricular palliation (Fontan completion) is possible.

15.16.4 Prognosis and Clinical Course

▸ **Long-term prognosis.** Without treatment, half of the patients die within the first month of life and 85% within the first year. The long-term prognosis depends on the size and configuration of the right ventricle and tricuspid valve and on anomalies of the coronary arteries such as stenoses, fistulas, or myocardial sinusoids. Currently, biventricular correction can be performed for only 30 to 40% of patients. Reoperations are frequently required, often within the first year of life. The 10-year survival rate of all patients who have had corrective surgery is only 40%.

Later complications after widening the right ventricular outflow tract or commissurotomy of the pulmonary valve are pulmonary insufficiency and supraventricular arrhythmias as a result of tricuspid insufficiency.

▸ **Outpatient checkups.** After implantation of an aortopulmonary shunt, the shunt function must be monitored on a regular basis. In addition, the size and function of the right ventricle, function of the tricuspid valve, and morphology of the right ventricular outflow tract must be checked. After the widening of the right ventricular outflow tract or commissurotomy of the pulmonary valve, pulmonary insufficiency and right ventricular function must be monitored in order to assess the proper time for valve replacement, should it become necessary. Especially if there is tricuspid insufficiency, supraventricular arrhythmias can develop as a result of right atrial overload, so regular ECG monitoring is recommended.

Atrial arrhythmias, thromboembolic events, protein-losing enteropathy, and increasing cyanosis should be noted in patients who have undergone Fontan palliation.

Endocarditis prophylaxis is indicated in patients with an aortopulmonary shunt or in cyanotic patients—for 6 months after corrective surgery, and lifelong if there are residual defects in the vicinity of foreign material or after valve replacement.

▸ **Physical exercise capacity and lifestyle.** If biventricular correction was successful, the patient's physical exercise capacity is usually good. Patients with Fontan palliation are usually able to handle everyday activities, but should not participate in competitive sports. Fontan patients who must maintain oral anticoagulation should avoid contact sports.

▸ **Special aspects in adolescents and adults.** The now-adult patients who were formerly treated only with an aortopulmonary shunt as a palliative measure show the following overriding symptoms of chronic hypoxemia: polyglobulia, disposition for thromboses, risk of cerebral abscesses, high risk of endocarditis, and complications due to hemorrhage.

15.17 Ebstein Anomaly

15.17.1 Basics

Synonyms: Ebstein disease, Ebstein malformation

Definition

The Ebstein anomaly is an anomaly of the tricuspid valve, in which the tricuspid valve is displaced toward the apex of the right ventricle (▶ Fig. 15.55). The resulting situation is that part of the right ventricle has the function of an atrium ("atrialized right ventricle"). The functional right ventricle is thus smaller. There are widely varying forms.

Etiology

The etiology is unclear. However, a higher risk for Ebstein anomaly has been reported if the mother took lithium during pregnancy.

Epidemiology

Ebstein anomaly is a rare deformity. It occurs in around 1 of 20,000 live births and constitutes approximately. 0.05% of all congenital heart defects.

Pathology

The morphology of the tricuspid valve varies greatly in the Ebstein anomaly. The leaflets are frequently dysplastic. The displacement of the tricuspid valve is usually caused by fusion of the septal and the posterior leaflets with the endocardium of the right ventricle. However, these two leaflets may be only rudimentary or they may be absent entirely.

The anterior leaflet is often oversized ("redundant") and is usually attached normally to the tricuspid valve annulus.

The displacement of the tricuspid valve leaflets leads to functional atrialization of part of the right ventricle. This part is functionally part of the right atrium, but contracts with the right ventricle. The size of the remaining right ventricle varies. In extreme cases, practically only the right ventricular outflow tract is present. The myocardium of the inlet segment is often markedly thin. Due to the leaflet malformations, there may also be an obstruction of the right ventricular outflow tract.

The deformity of the leaflets leads to varying degrees of tricuspid regurgitation, but in rare cases, fusion of the individual leaflets can also lead to a functional stenosis or even atresia of the tricuspid valve.

Hemodynamics

As a result of the tricuspid regurgitation, pressure is increased in the right atrium. An atrial septal defect (ASD) or patent foramen ovale (PFO), which is almost always present, leads to a right-to-left shunt at the atrial level and to cyanosis. The right atrium is dilated.

In addition to tricuspid regurgitation and the small functional right ventricle, other mechanisms can lead to a decrease in the antegrade blood flow to the lungs. Examples of this are a pulmonary stenosis or atresia or displacement of the right ventricular outflow tract by tissue from the tricuspid valve. In neonates, the increased pulmonary vascular resistance further hinders ejection from the right ventricle.

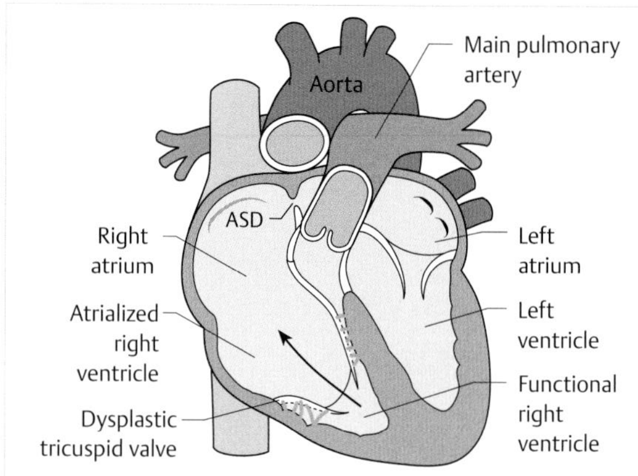

Fig. 15.55 Ebstein anomaly. The tricuspid valve is displaced far toward the apex of the right ventricle. In most cases, this is due to the fact that the septal and posterior leaflets of the tricuspid valve are fused to the wall of the right ventricle, resulting in "atrialization" of the right ventricle.

Associated Anomalies

There is usually a shunt at the atrial level. Of particular importance are stenoses and obstructions of the right ventricular outflow tract, which further obstruct blood flow to the lungs. There are also frequently accessory conduction pathways in Ebstein anomaly. The most important associated anomalies are listed below:

- ASD or PFO (nearly always present)
- Pulmonary stenosis or atresia
- Obstruction of the right ventricular outflow tract by tricuspid valve tissue
- VSD
- l-TGA
- Accessory conduction pathways: Accessory conduction pathways are a predisposing factor for the WPW syndrome or paroxysmal supraventricular tachycardias. In the Ebstein anomaly, several accessory conduction pathways are sometimes present simultaneously.

Associated Syndromes

No association with specific genetic syndromes has been described.

15.17.2 Diagnostic Measures

Symptoms

The clinical symptoms vary widely depending on the different pathological anatomy, and extend from intrauterine symptoms to adults with no major problems. Typical manifestations in the various age groups are:

- *Prenatal:* hydrops fetalis, miscarriage, supraventricular tachycardias, lung hypoplasia. Usually, however, the pregnancy is unremarkable.
- *Neonate:* rapidly developing signs of congestive heart failure (hepatomegaly, edema, metabolic acidosis, respiratory failure), cyanosis as a result of the right-to-left shunt at the atrial level.
- *Older children, adolescents, and adults*: Impaired physical capacity, increasing heart failure, paroxysmal supraventricular tachycardias associated with accessory conduction pathways, atrial flutter associated with atrial overload.

Auscultation

The systolic regurgitation murmur of tricuspid insufficiency can be heard at the lower left sternal border. There may be a loud-split first heart sound as a result of delayed closure of the tricuspid valve. The second heart sound is typically widely split as well. There is also frequently a gallop rhythm. A mid-diastolic murmur is a sign of a functional or actual tricuspid stenosis.

ECG

Typical findings are a P dextrocardiale, a right ventricular conduction delay up to a complete right bundle branch block, pre-excitation (shortened PQ interval, delta wave), supraventricular tachycardia, and with increasing age other atrial arrhythmias as well (atrial flutter or fibrillation) and ventricular extrasystoles.

Chest X-ray

In pronounced cases, there may be massive cardiomegaly with marked dilatation of the right atrium and decreased pulmonary vascular markings (▶ Fig. 15.56).

Echocardiography

The diagnosis of Ebstein anomaly can be reliably made using echocardiography (▶ Fig. 15.57). The following findings can be typically visualized and should be documented:

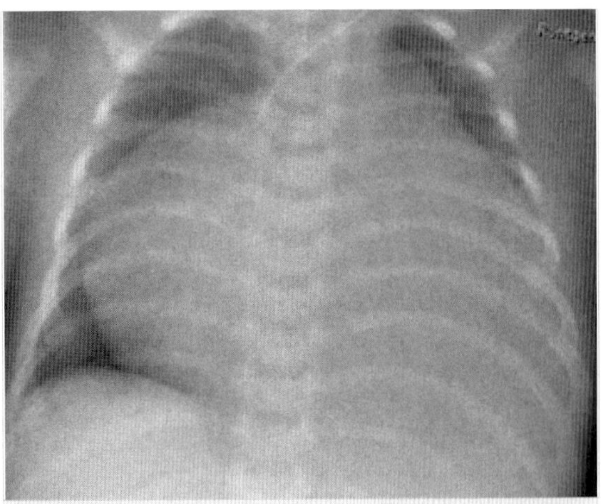

Fig. 15.56 Chest radiograph in Ebstein anomaly. There is massive cardiomegaly with pronounced dilatation of the right atrium.

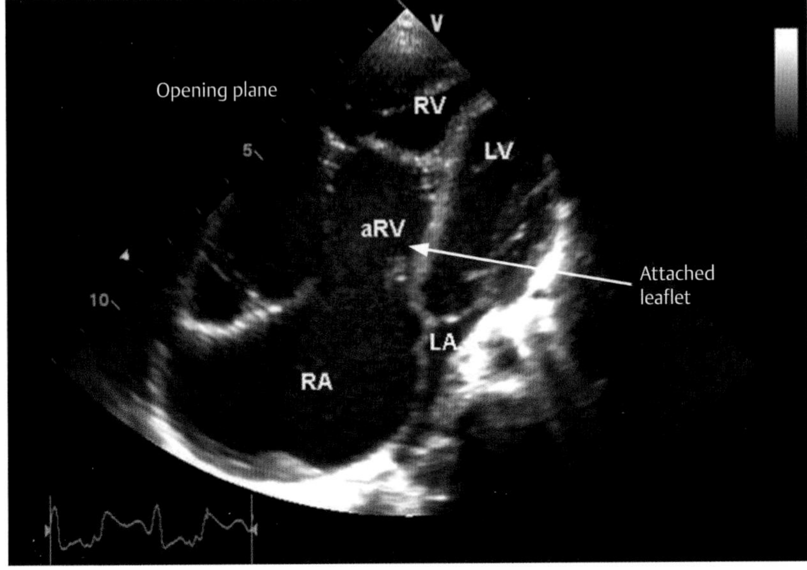

Fig. 15.57 Echocardiography finding in an Ebstein anomaly. The four-chamber view shows the apical displacement of the tricuspid valve. The right atrium is clearly dilated; the functional right ventricle is considerably reduced in size.
RV, right ventricle; LV, left ventricle; RA, right atrium; LA, left atrium; aRV, atrialized right ventricle.

- Displacement of the tricuspid valve leaflets toward the apex in the right ventricle
- Apical displacements of the tricuspid valve by more than 8 mm/m^2 body surface area compared with the mitral valve
- Visualization of the various tricuspid valve leaflet attachments on the wall of the right ventricle or at the tricuspid valve annulus
- Marked dilatation of the right atrium, small right ventricle
- Determination of the size of the right ventricle (atrialized segment of the right ventricle, functional right ventricle) and of the diameter of the tricuspid valve annulus
- Doppler ultrasound verification of tricuspid insufficiency
- Visualization of the right-to-left shunt at the atrial level
- Estimate of a possible obstruction of the right ventricular outflow tract (obstruction from tricuspid valve tissue)
- Assessment of the size and function of the left ventricle
- Usually, paradoxical motion of the ventricular septum
- Exclusion or assessment of associated anomalies, especially a pulmonary stenosis or atresia, a PDA, or a VSD

Cardiac Catheterization

Cardiac catheterization is not routinely required. It may be indicated if there are additional anomalies—for example, interventional catheterization of a pulmonary stenosis or atresia, or to rule out an ASD.

Electrophysiological Examination

If there are recurrent supraventricular tachycardias, tachycardia with a wide QRS complex, or syncopes, an electrophysiological examination with the option of ablating accessory conduction pathways may be necessary.

15.17.3 Treatment

Conservative Treatment

Individuals with severe forms of Ebstein anomaly require treatment as neonates. The situation frequently improves when the increased pulmonary resistance in the immediate postnatal period falls. If there is pronounced cyanosis, prostaglandin E_1 is given to maintain patency of the ductus arteriosus to improve pulmonary perfusion. Pulmonary resistance can be additionally lowered by hyperventilation and compensating metabolic acidosis. To increase systemic resistance, noradrenaline, for example, can be given. Among the available options for treating congestive heart failure are catecholamines, digoxin, and diuretics. Some supraventricular tachycardias require appropriate antiarrhythmic treatment (Chapter 18).

Surgical Treatment

Surgical treatment is indicated in symptomatic neonates who respond inadequately to conservative measures. Sometimes palliative measures such as creating an aortopulmonary shunt are first initiated to ensure pulmonary perfusion. If biventricular therapy does not appear to be possible in the long term, other measures can supplement the aortopulmonary shunt, for example, reducing the size of the right atrium, atrial septectomy, and closure of the tricuspid valve with a patch. This means that a tricuspid atresia is created artificially. This procedure is made in preparation for a univentricular palliative Fontan procedure.

Indications for surgery in older patients are manifest heart failure (NYHA III and IV), an increase in cyanosis, and signs of right heart obstruction. Surgery may also be appropriate in asymptomatic patients with increasing cardiomegaly and severe tricuspid insufficiency.

The goal is to reconstruct the tricuspid valve. The numerous surgical techniques and their modifications reflect the great variability of this disease. The most frequently used are the Danielson and the Carpentier techniques. In the Danielson annuloplasty, the atrialized portion of the right ventricle and the septal and posterior tricuspid valve leaflets are pulled up toward the atrium (▶ Fig. 15.58). This moves the displaced valve leaflets into their normal position. Then the ostium of the tricuspid valve is plicated. The large anterior tricuspid leaflet closes the ostium of the tricuspid valve in

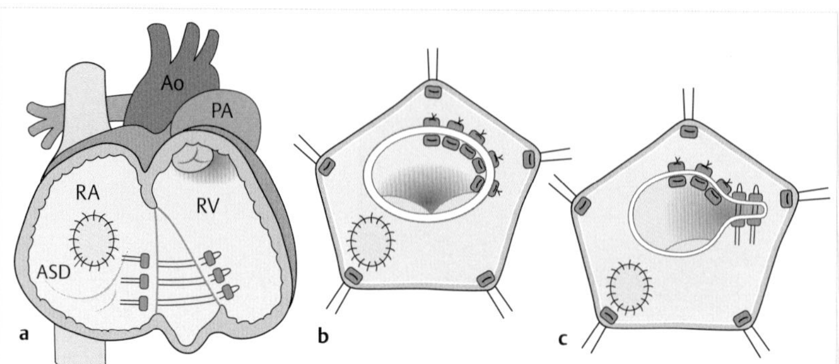

Fig. 15.58 Tricuspid valve reconstruction using the Danielson method. By means of single mattress sutures, the posterior and septal tricuspid valve leaflets are pulled up to the original valve annulus and attached (**a, b**). The valve annulus is also plicated (**c**). The result is a functionally monocuspid valve.[29]

systole, like a monocuspid valve. More recently, the so called "cone procedure" has been reported as producing promising results.

Tricuspid valve replacement with an artificial or bioprosthetic valve is necessary if valve reconstruction is not possible.

If the right ventricle is perceptibly hypoplastic, univentricular palliation is indicated. First an upper cavopulmonary anastomosis is made, followed later by complete separation of the systemic and pulmonary circulatory systems using the Fontan procedure.

In the event that catheter ablation of an accessory conduction pathway is not possible, the pathway may be transected during the operation. In extreme cases, a cardiac transplant may be the last treatment option.

15.17.4 Prognosis and Outcome

► **Long-term course.** The long-term course of patients with the Ebstein anomaly varies greatly and ranges from pronounced symptoms that lead to intrauterine death to mild forms with an almost normal life expectancy. Important risk factors are early onset of manifestations, a functional small right ventricle, cardiomegaly (cardiothoracic ratio > 0.6), and obstruction of the right ventricular outflow tract. The perioperative mortality rate in neonates is high.

► **Outpatient checkups.** Lifelong outpatient follow-up is necessary for all patients with the Ebstein anomaly. Particular attention should be paid to signs of congestive heart failure and cyanosis and to the arrhythmias described above. The size of the heart and severity of tricuspid insufficiency and the function of both ventricles must be checked regularly. Reoperations are quite often needed at some point after surgical tricuspid valve reconstruction.

► **Physical capacity and lifestyle.** Physical capacity depends on the severity of the anomaly and can vary widely. Increasing impairment of capacity is an indication for surgery.

The ability to engage in sports depends on the severity of the Ebstein anomaly. Patients with mild forms (no cyanosis, normal size of the right ventricle, no arrhythmias) have no restrictions with respect to sports. Patients with moderate tricuspid insufficiency may engage in less intensive sports if they have no arrhythmias. Patients with severe forms (severe tricuspid insufficiency, enlarged right ventricle, arrhythmias) may not play sports.

► **Special aspects in adolescents and adults.** Adolescents and adults with uncorrected Ebstein anomaly must be monitored for the development or increase of congestive heart failure. An increasing impairment of capacity, progressive tricuspid insufficiency, and cyanosis are an indication for surgery. In addition, supraventricular tachycardias may arise as a result of accessory conduction pathways and require pharmacological therapy or catheter ablation. However, the success rate of catheter ablation in patients with Ebstein anomaly is lower than in other patients. Atrial arrhythmias such as atrial flutter or fibrillation can also occur as a result of right atrial overload. Over time, patients occasionally develop ventricular arrhythmias, usually stemming from the right ventricle. Later, left ventricular dysfunction may develop.

Pregnancy infrequently leads to complications in noncyanotic Ebstein patients, but the pregnancy can be complicated by arrhythmias; heart failure occurs rarely. As a result of the increasing intravasal volume during pregnancy, the right atrial pressure increases and a right-to-left shunt at the atrial level may arise or increase. Maternal cyanosis is associated with a higher risk for the child. In women with an artificial valve replacement that necessitates anticoagulation, the teratogenic effect of coumarin derivatives (Coumadine, warfarin) should be noted.

15.18 Tricuspid Atresia

15.18.1 Basics

Definition

Tricuspid atresia refers to agenesis or only rudimentary development of the tricuspid valve and the right ventricular inflow tract, so there is no direct connection between the right atrium and the right ventricle (► Fig. 15.59). Instead of the tricuspid valve there is usually a fibromuscular diaphragm with a central recess (dimple), less often a fibrous membrane.

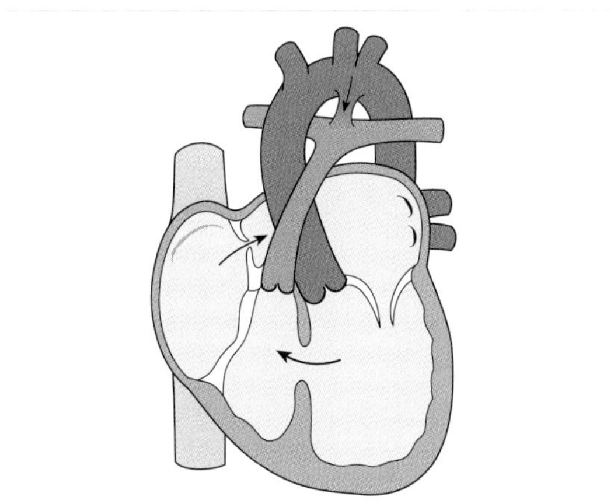

Fig. 15.59 Tricuspid atresia. There is no connection between the right atrium and the right ventricle in tricuspid atresia. The tricuspid valve is atretic or only rudimentary. There must be a right-to-left shunt at the atrial level. The right ventricle can be filled with blood only via a ventricular septal defect.

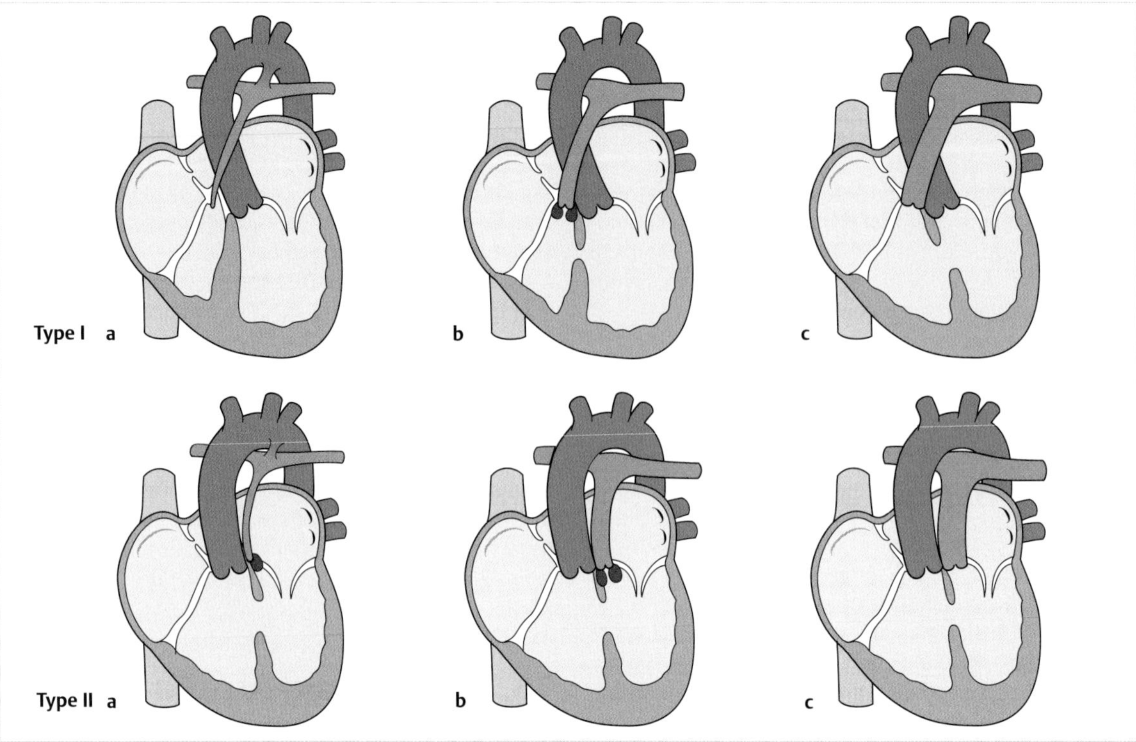

Fig. 15.60 Forms of tricuspid atresia. Type I describes a normal position of the vessels, type II, d-transposition, and type III an abnormal position of the arteries (except d-transposition). Most frequent are types Ib (with normal position of the great arteries, pulmonary stenosis, and a small VSD) and IIc (with d-TGA, without pulmonary stenosis). Together, these two types (II b and II c) constitute around 70% of all tricuspid atresias. Type III (abnormal position of the great arteries except d-TGA) is not illustrated.

Epidemiology

Tricuspid atresia constitutes approximately 1% to 3% of all congenital heart defects. The incidence is around 1 per 10,000 live births. Boys are affected somewhat more often than girls. It is the third most common cyanotic heart defect after tetralogy of Fallot and d-TGA.

Pathogenesis

The presumed cause is a complete fusion of the developing segments of the tricuspid valve during the embryonic period. Whether a muscular or a fibrous atresia results depends on when the fusion occurs. A muscular atresia develops at an earlier time than a fibrous atresia.

Classification

The classification is based mainly on the position of the great arteries (▶ Fig. 15.60). Classification into subgroups is determined by the extent of pulmonary blood flow:

- Type I: Normal position of the great arteries
  a) Intact ventricular septum with pulmonary atresia
  b) Small VSD with pulmonary stenosis
  c) Large VSD without pulmonary stenosis
- Type II: d-Transposition of the great arteries
  a) VSD with pulmonary atresia
  b) VSD with pulmonary stenosis
  c) VSD without pulmonary stenosis
- Type III: Abnormal position of the great arteries except d-TGA

The subgroups a to c reflect the extent of pulmonary perfusion:

- Subgroup a: Pulmonary atresia (ductal-dependent pulmonary blood flow)
- Subgroup b: Pulmonary valve or subpulmonary stenosis (decreased pulmonary blood flow)
- Subgroup c: Unremarkable pulmonary arteries (increased pulmonary perfusion)

The most frequent type, constituting around half of all cases, is type Ib (tricuspid atresia with normal position of the great vessels and pulmonary stenosis/hypoplasia); the second most common (20%) is type IIc (tricuspid atresia with d-TGA and unremarkable pulmonary arteries).

Hemodynamics

In tricuspid atresia, venous blood flows from the right to the left atrium through an atrial shunt, which is necessary for survival. The right atrium is dilated and hypertrophic. From the left atrium, the blood reaches the left ventricle through the mitral valve. Since all the systemic venous blood and all the oxygenated blood of the pulmonary venous return drains into the left atrium, the left atrium and ventricle are large and contain mixed blood. Flow to the right ventricle is possible only across a VSD. The size of the right ventricle is related to the extent of the VSD, which already determines the blood flow to the right ventricle in the intrauterine period. The pulmonary and systemic perfusions depend on the position of the great arteries:

- Normal position of the great arteries (type I): The lungs are perfused from a VSD. The mixed blood reaches pulmonary circulation via the right ventricle and the pulmonary arteries. If the ventricular septum is intact (type Ia, rare) pulmonary perfusion takes place across a left-to-right shunt via a PDA.
- d-Transposition of the great arteries (type II): The pulmonary artery arises from the left ventricle, which is thus responsible for pulmonary perfusion. The aorta comes out of the right ventricle, which is supplied with blood from the left ventricle across a VSD.

In patients with a normal position of the great arteries, the VSD is generally small. If there is a d-transposition, the VSD must be large to supply the systemic circulation with enough blood from the right ventricle.

Note

If the great vessels are in the normal position, pulmonary perfusion is usually reduced by a pulmonary stenosis and/or a restrictive VSD. In a d-TGA position, pulmonary blood flow is usually increased. There is also frequently a hypoplastic aortic arch and/or coarctation of the aorta. As a result of the excessive pulmonary blood flow, congestive heart failure and pulmonary hypertension frequently develop.

Associated Anomalies

Tricuspid atresia is practically always associated with other cardiac anomalies. An atrial shunt is necessary for survival. A VSD is the only inlet to the right ventricle and is almost always present. The major associated cardiac anomalies are:

- Atrial septal defect / patent foramen ovale: An atrial shunt is necessary for survival. It ensures that blood can flow out of the right atrium.
- VSD: Almost always present (except in type Ia). The VSD ensures the perfusion of the right ventricle and correlates with its size.
- Pulmonary stenosis, hypoplasia, atresia: The extent of the obstruction of the pulmonary valve is decisive for the extent of pulmonary blood flow.
- d-Transposition of the great arteries: A d-TGA is present in 30% of patients with tricuspid atresia (type IIa–c).
- l-Transposition of the great arteries: An l-TGA is present in approximately 3% of all tricuspid atresias (type III).
- Coarctation of the aorta or interrupted aortic arch: Anomalies of the aortic arch are present, especially in tricuspid atresias with d-TGA of the great vessels.
- Left persistent superior vena cava.
- Juxtaposition of the atrial appendages.

Associated Syndromes

Tricuspid atresias have been frequently observed in connection with the following syndromes: cat eye syndrome, trisomy 21, and heterotaxy syndromes.

15.18.2 Diagnostic Measures

Symptoms

Around two-thirds of patients become symptomatic within the first week. The leading symptom is cyanosis caused by the obligatory right-to-left shunt at the atrial level. The extent of cyanosis depends on pulmonary perfusion.

Cyanosis is less pronounced in children with increased pulmonary blood flow (type Ic or IIc). In these cases, due to excessive pulmonary flow, the main symptoms are signs of congestive heart failure (tachypnea/dyspnea, increased sweating, poor feeding, failure to thrive).

Cyanotic spells may occur if the size of the VSD decreases or subpulmonary stenosis increases. If there is pulmonary atresia, closure of the ductus arteriosus leads to critical deterioration.

Hepatomegaly can be a sign of a restrictive atrial shunt. The absence of pulses in the groin is a sign of an associated coarctation of the aorta or an interrupted aortic arch.

Auscultation

A heart murmur can be auscultated in almost all patients with a tricuspid atresia. The first heart sound is typically single and usually prominent. The second heart sound is soft or missing entirely if there is a pulmonary stenosis or pulmonary atresia. If there is excessive pulmonary blood flow, the second heart sound can also be widely split.

A rough systolic murmur in the 3rd/4th left parasternal ICS is a sign of a VSD. If there is a pulmonary stenosis or an obstruction of the right ventricular outflow tract, a systolic ejection murmur can also be auscultated with PMI in the 2nd left parasternal ICS.

If there is clearly excessive pulmonary blood flow, the murmur of a relative mitral stenosis ("rumbling" diastolic murmur over the cardiac apex) can be auscultated.

ECG

The characteristic ECG feature of a tricuspid atresia is a mild or moderate left axis deviation. A P dextrocardiale (tall, narrow P wave) is a sign of right atrial overload. If there is excessive pulmonary blood flow, a P mitrale (wide, notched P wave) may occur.

Signs of left ventricular hypertrophy are apparent in the precordial leads: tall R waves and prominent Q waves in the left precordial leads with deep S waves in the right precordial leads. There are no signs of physiological right heart hypertrophy in neonates.

Note

Differential diagnosis of a left axis deviation in neonates: tricuspid atresia or AV canal.

Chest X-ray

The size and shape of the heart depend on the pulmonary blood flow:

- *Reduced pulmonary blood flow*: normal or slightly enlarged heart with decreased pulmonary vascular markings
- *Excessive pulmonary blood flow*: enlarged cardiac silhouette and increased pulmonary vascular markings

The right cardiac border is typically enlarged as a sign of enlargement of the right atrium. This finding is especially pronounced if there is a restrictive atrial shunt. If there is transposition of the great vessels, an egg-shaped cardiac silhouette ("egg lying on its side") with a narrow mediastinal vascular band is typical in the anteroposterior image. A concave pulmonary artery segment associated with pulmonary atresia results in a narrow cardiac waist.

Echocardiography

The diagnosis can be reliably made using echocardiography. The leading symptoms are absence of the tricuspid valve and a perceptibly small right ventricle. A right-to-left shunt at the atrial level is obligatory. The typical echocardiography findings and clinical questions that must be investigated by echocardiography are:

- No connection between the right atrium and the right ventricle: Instead of the tricuspid valve, Doppler ultrasonography shows a dense connective tissue structure or a thin membrane without valve opening movements.
- Large right atrium with a right-to-left shunt across an atrial communication (patent foramen ovale or ASD). If the shunt is restrictive, the atrial septum protrudes clearly to the left.
- Small, rudimentary right ventricle: The size of the right ventricle correlates with the extent of the VSD.
- Visualization of the ventriculo-arterial connections: Normal position or transposition or the great vessels?
- Visualization and evaluation of the VSD: This is usually a muscular VSD. The gradient across the VSD can be estimated by Doppler ultrasonography. The VSD is particularly important if there is transposition of the great arteries, as the hemodynamic function of a restrictive VSD is similar to that of a (sub)aortic stenosis. If the diameter of the VSD is smaller than the diameter of the aortic valve, a decrease in size of the VSD can be expected. Hemodynamically, it corresponds to increasing subaortic stenosis.
- Evaluation of the pulmonary valve and the right ventricular outflow tract: Exclusion or visualization of an atresia; Doppler ultrasound evaluation of the pulmonary valve and the right ventricular outflow tract with respect to stenosis.
- Doppler ultrasonographic estimate of the pressure in the pulmonary circulation across the VSD using the Bernoulli equation.
- The left ventricle may be dilated, especially if there is excessive pulmonary blood flow.
- Exclusion of accompanying anomalies, especially hypoplasia of the aortic arch or coarctation of the aorta.

Cardiac Catheterization

Diagnostic cardiac catheterization is now no longer needed on a routine basis. It can be useful in unclear cases, especially for excluding associated cardiac anomalies and evaluating a restrictive atrial or ventricular septum and to assess the pulmonary vessels. The following findings and clinical questions may need to be visualized or clarified:

- Discontinuity between the right atrium and right ventricle: The right ventricle cannot be probed directly via the right atrium; the catheter passes into the left atrium through the shunt in the atrial septum instead.
- Visualization and evaluation of the atrial shunt (ASD, patent foramen ovale): If there is a difference in pressure of more than 5 mmHg between the left and right atria, a restriction must be assumed. The A wave is pronounced if this is the case. A Rashkind procedure is indicated if there is a restrictive atrial shunt.
- Origin and course of the great arteries: Normal or TGA position?
- Visualization of the VSD: Especially if there is a TGA, a restriction across the VSD must be excluded.
- Evaluation of the pulmonary vessels: Quantification using the McGoon ratio and Nakata index.
- Detection or exclusion of a pulmonary stenosis or atresia (valvular, subvalvular stenosis?).
- Exclusion of associated cardiac anomalies, in particular of anomalies of the aortic arch (especially with TGA) and a left persistent superior vena cava.
- Quantification of the pulmonary and systemic blood flow and the shunt.
- Determination of pulmonary vascular resistance.
- Pulse oximetry reveals similar oxygen saturation levels in the left atrium, left and right ventricle, and in the pulmonary arteries and aorta (complete mixing of the systemic venous, pulmonary venous, and coronary venous blood in the left atrium).

MRI

MRI hardly plays any role in primary diagnostics thus far, but can provide information about specific questions such as associated cardiac anomalies. The major significance of MRI is in the postoperative follow-up examinations.

15.18.3 Treatment

Conservative Treatment

If there is ductal-dependent pulmonary or systemic blood flow, it is necessary to administer prostaglandin E.

- Pulmonary atresia (types Ia and IIa) with ductal-dependent pulmonary blood flow:
  - Prostaglandin IV to maintain patency of the ductus arteriosus (initially 50 ng/kg/min, gradual reduction is usually possible later)
  - Compensation of metabolic acidosis by buffering with sodium bicarbonate and volume substitution (target base excess [BE] + 2 to + 4 to reduce pulmonary resistance)
  - Ample fluids
  - Possibly intubation and ventilation with hyperventilation and increased FiO_2 to reduce pulmonary resistance
  - Possibly increasing peripheral resistance (e.g., with adrenaline or noradrenaline)
  - Possibly inotropic treatment with catecholamines
- Severe coarctation of the aorta with ductal-dependent systemic blood flow:
  - Prostaglandin IV to maintain the patency of the ductus arteriosus (initially 50 ng/kg/min, gradual reduction is usually possible later)
  - Possibly lowering systemic resistance (e.g., with sodium nitroprusside)
- Signs of congestive heart failure as a result of excessive pulmonary blood flow (e.g., type Ic, IIc):
  - Anticongestive treatment with diuretics and reduction of afterload (ACE inhibitor, sodium nitroprusside)

Note

Caution: Digoxin is contraindicated in a restrictive VSD and for stenosis of the right ventricular outflow tract (subpulmonary stenosis, subaortic stenosis), because the restriction or outflow tract stenosis can increase under digoxin.

► **Cyanotic spell.** A restrictive VSD and normal position of the great arteries can result in stenosis of the right ventricular outflow tract that is expressed clinically as a cyanotic spell similar to tetralogy of Fallot.

The therapy corresponds to that for a cyanotic spell in tetralogy of Fallot: Press the knee against the chest (increases systemic resistance), administer oxygen, volume substitution, sedation, possibly beta blockers (propranolol, esmolol).

Interventional Catheterization

If there is a restrictive atrial shunt, a Rashkind balloon atrial septostomy or a blade septostomy is indicated in order to improve the right-to-left shunt at the atrial level.

If there is a valvular pulmonary stenosis, a balloon valvuloplasty can improve pulmonary perfusion and thus oxygenation.

In individual cases, a stent implantation in the ductus arteriosus can improve or ensure pulmonary or systemic perfusion, but this is not yet a routine procedure.

Surgical Treatment

Palliative Treatment

Most patients require a palliative procedure before definitive surgery in the form of univentricular Fontan completion is possible. Palliation depends mainly on the extent of pulmonary perfusion (reduced or increased pulmonary blood flow) and on a possible intracardiac restriction (restrictive VSD). The procedure is summarized in ► Table 15.3).

► **Reduced pulmonary perfusion.** If there is reduced pulmonary blood flow, an aortopulmonary shunt is created in the neonatal period. This is usually a modified Blalock–Taussig shunt (Gore-Tex tube between the subclavian artery and the ipsilateral pulmonary artery).

► **Increased pulmonary perfusion.** In patients with d-TGA and increased pulmonary perfusion (type IIc), banding of the pulmonary artery was formerly performed to reduce pulmonary perfusion. However, the disadvantage of this procedure is that the size of the VSD may be reduced due to ventricular pressure overload and ensuing hypertrophy, and it then becomes restrictive. In such cases, the hemodynamic result is a subaortic stenosis.

Therefore, today a Damus–Kaye–Stansel (DKS) anastomosis is created in these patients and systemic perfusion may possibly be ensured by a graft to widen the frequently hypoplastic aortic arch. In a DKS anastomosis, the ascending aorta and the pulmonary artery are anastomosed. The pulmonary artery is transected at the base. To ensure pulmonary perfusion, an aortopulmonary shunt is created (usually a modified Blalock–Taussig shunt). Pulmonary perfusion is controlled by the selection of the shunt (diameter, length, position).

► **Restrictive VSD and d-TGA.** Systemic perfusion is jeopardized by the restriction of the ventricular septum. A DKS anastomosis is therefore created to ensure systemic perfusion. Pulmonary perfusion is ensured by the simultaneous creation of an aortopulmonary shunt.

Table 15.3 Summary of the surgical procedures for various forms of tricuspid atresia

Hemodynamic situation	Palliative measures in the neonatal period	Definitive treatment	
Tricuspid atresia and reduced pulmonary perfusion (e.g., type Ib)	Aortopulmonary shunt	Upper cavopulmonary anastomosis (usually between the 2nd and 6th month of life)	Total cavopulmonary anastomosis (usually between age 2 and 4 years)
Tricuspid atresia and TGA and restrictive VSD	Damus–Kaye–Stansel anastomosis and aortopulmonary shunt		
Tricuspid atresia and increased pulmonary perfusion	Damus–Kaye–Stansel anastomosis and aortopulmonary shunt		

Fontan Completion Procedure to Separate the Circulatory Systems

Tricuspid atresia is the classic indication for separation of the pulmonary and systemic circulatory systems using the Fontan procedure. After this procedure, the lungs are passively perfused without the support of a pumping ventricle. The separation of the circulatory systems is generally performed in two stages.

▸ **Bidirectional upper cavopulmonary anastomosis.** The superior vena cava is anastomosed with the right pulmonary artery so that the venous blood of the upper half of the body flows passively into the lungs. The pulmonary artery is transected. In addition, an atrial septectomy is performed to improve the shunt at the atrial level (▸ Fig. 15.61).

The operation is usually performed after pulmonary resistance drops, that is, at the age of 2 to 6 months.

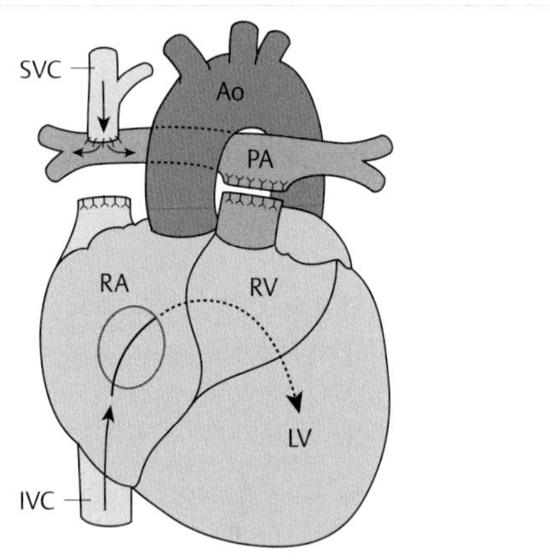

Fig. 15.61 Bidirectional upper cavopulmonary anastomosis. The superior vena cava is anastomosed directly with the pulmonary artery. The venous blood from the upper half of the body can then flow passively into the lungs. In addition, an atrial septectomy is performed so that the venous blood from the lower half of the body can flow unobstructed into the left atrium and reach the systemic circulation via the left ventricle. The pulmonary artery is transected. After this operation, arterial oxygen saturation ranges from 75% to 85%.
LV, left ventricle; RV, right ventricle; RA, right atrium; PA, pulmonary artery; Ao, Aorta; SVC, superior vena cava; IVC, inferior vena cava. [29]

▸ **Total cavopulmonary anastomosis (modified Fontan procedure).** In this procedure, the inferior vena cava and the hepatic veins are connected to the right pulmonary artery via an intracardiac or extracardiac tunnel, so that the venous blood from the lower half of the body can also flow passively into the lungs (▸ Fig. 15.62). The result is a complete separation of the circulatory systems. Often, first a window is left between the tunnel and the atrium ("fenestrated Fontan"), which functions as an overflow valve when venous pressure is elevated (disadvantage: residual cyanosis due to right-to-left shunt). This window can usually be closed later on using interventional catheterization.

This operation is generally performed after age 2 years. An extracardiac tunnel probably has the most favorable long-term outcome. This procedure can be performed in children with a weight of 12 to 15 kg using a tunnel prosthesis measuring 18 to 20 mm, which is equivalent to 70 to 80% of the diameter of the vena cava in an adult, so the disadvantage due to the lack of growth potential of the prosthesis is probably no longer crucial.

▸ **Preconditions for a Fontan procedure.** In 1978, Choussat formulated a total of 10 criteria that should be fulfilled to perform a Fontan procedure. Now some of these criteria have been proven to be irrelevant (e.g., age between 4 and 15 years, normal systemic venous connections). With respect to pulmonary vascular resistance, however, the criteria have become even stricter. Originally, pulmonary vascular resistance of up to 4 Wood units per m^2 body surface area was accepted; today

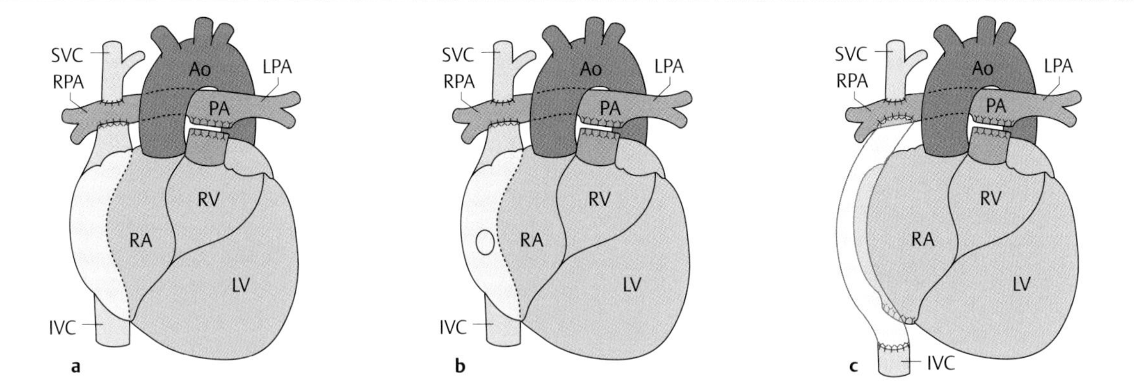

Fig. 15.62 Forms of a total cavopulmonary anastomosis (TCPC). In a TCPC, the inferior vena cava is also connected to the pulmonary artery. There are different methods available (intracardiac or extracardiac tunnel). Subsequently, the venous blood from the lower and upper halves of the body reaches the lungs passively. The systemic and pulmonary circulations are thus completely separated and the patients are no longer cyanotic. If a tunnel fenestration were made, arterial oxygen saturation would be around 85 to 90%, that is, lower than normal, due to the right-to-left shunt. **a** TCPC with intra-atrial tunnel without fenestration. **b** TCPC with intra-atrial tunnel and fenestration. **c** TCPC with extra-cardiac tunnel.
LV, left ventricle; RV, right ventricle; RA, right atrium; PA, pulmonary artery; LPA, left pulmonary artery; RPA, right pulmonary artery; Ao, aorta; SVC, superior vena cava; IVC, inferior vena cava.[29]

pulmonary vascular resistance of below 2 Wood units per m² body surface area is required.

Note

The current recommendations are:

- Adequate size of the pulmonary arteries (McGoon ratio > 1.8 or Nakata index > 250 mm²/m²)
- Normal pressure and resistance conditions in the pulmonary circulation (mean pressure in the pulmonary artery < 15 mmHg, pulmonary vascular resistance < 2 Wood units per m²)
- Normal function of the left ventricle (ejection fraction > 60% with normal end-diastolic pressure) and of the mitral valve (mitral valve reconstruction may be necessary)
- Central pulmonary stenosis and distorsions of the pulmonary vessels (untreated or iatrogenic as a result of banding the pulmonary artery or creating an aortopulmonary shunt) must be ruled out or eliminated (preoperatively by interventional catheterization or intraoperatively)

15.18.4 Prognosis and Clinical Course

► **Long-term prognosis.** Without treatment, approximately 70% of patients die within the first year of life. Patients with sufficient or increased pulmonary blood flow have the most favorable prognosis in a natural course. There are isolated cases of patients with balanced pulmonary perfusion who reach adolescence without treatment. The perioperative mortality rate for a Fontan procedure is about 5%; the 10-year survival rate is about 90%.

The Fontan procedure and its modifications have typical long-term complications:

- *Arrhythmias:* The underlying rhythm is markedly bradycardic. A sinus node dysfunction occurs relatively frequently. In addition, an AV block can occur postoperatively. Therefore, a permanent pacemaker electrode is sometimes implanted in the right atrium during the TCPC to spare a later re-sternotomy, as the pacemaker electrodes cannot be simply inserted transvenously in Fontan patients. In addition, there are frequently atrial arrhythmias such as atrial flutter/fibrillation and supraventricular tachycardias. The rate of occurrence arrhythmias has been improved, however, through new surgical procedures in which an intra-atrial lateral or extracardiac tunnel is made.
- *Thrombosis risk:* The cause of the increased risk of thrombosis is the slow blood flow in the right atrium. The risk is increased considerably by atrial flutter or fibrillation. In addition, impaired liver function or the loss of coagulation-inhibiting proteins via the intestine (protein-losing syndrome) can increase the risk of developing a thrombosis. Anticoagulation is therefore recommended for Fontan patients in many centers. However, anticoagulation should be started at doses lower than usual owing to a possible impairment of liver function and potential tendency to hemorrhage.
- *Protein-losing enteropathy (PLE):* Clinical signs are watery diarrhea with the loss of proteins and

electrolytes, edema, pleural and pericardial effusions, and ascites. The risk of thrombosis increases due to the loss of anticoagulants. PLE is a major cause of late mortality in Fontan patients. The cause of the syndrome is not fully understood. It often occurs in patients with high venous pressure, but can also occur in patients with low venous pressure. To treat it, an attempt can be made to reduce venous pressure by fenestration of the Fontan tunnel or to improve the hemodynamics by switching an "old" Fontan tunnel to a lateral or extracardieac tunnl.
- Plastic bronchitis: Plastic bronchitis is a rare but severe complication after a Fontan operation. The known risk factors are mainly the same as for protein-losing enteropathy. It is characterized by the formation of casts of rubber-like consistency in the tracheobronchial tree which mainly consist of fibrin. The endobronchial casts can lead to airway obstruction and pulmonary failure. The patients often appear to have recurrent episodes of bronchitis or pneumonia which is difficult to distinguish. Smaller casts are not recognized for a while because the patients tend to swallow them like sputum. Treatment is often difficult and includes, for example, optimizing cardiac function, using bronchodilators, corticosteroids, aerosolized tissue plasminogen activator, or urokinase and bronchoscopic extraction of the bronchial casts. In addition repeat catheter investigation is indicated to rule out and/or treat additional blood supply via aortopulmonary collaterals, measure pressures and create a Fontan fenestration if indicated.

Note

Recurrent wheezing, pneumonia or bronchitis in Fontan patients is highly suspicious for plastic bronchitis

- *Excessive venous pressure:* If there is excessive venous pressure, fenestration of an unfenestrated Fontan tunnel may be useful. In an extreme case, return to an upper cavopulmonary anastomosis may be necessary.
- *Stenosis of the anastomosis between the superior vena cava and the pulmonary artery:* Stenoses of the anastomosis may develop over time and can lead to an increase in venous pressure and signs of congestive heart failure. Sometimes interventional dilation or reoperation is necessary.
- *Dysfunction of the systemic ventricle:* The cause may be insufficiency of the AV valve. In addition, if the operation was performed at a late stage, the myocardium is likely to be already so damaged that it can no longer recover sufficiently.
- *Cyanosis:* Cyanosis can arise due to the development of intrapulmonary arteriovenous collaterals or due to connections between the two circulations (e.g., fenestration of the tunnel or venovenous collaterals). Treatment is usually by interventional catheterization. In addition, cyanosis can be a sign of a dysfunction of the systemic ventricle or of stenosis of the anastomosis between the venae cavae and the pulmonary artery.

► **Outpatient checkups.** Lifelong outpatient follow-up is necessary for all patients with tricuspid atresia. After the creation of an aortopulmonary anastomosis in the neonatal period, the function of the anastomosis must be checked at frequent intervals. The desired oxygen saturation level is 75 to 85%.

For patients with an upper cavopulmonary anastomosis, there is the same target saturation level. Because of the postoperatively increased blood pressure in the superior vena cava, venovenous collaterals between the upper and lower halves of the body can develop in these patients, which lead to an increase in cyanosis. Intrapulmonary arteriovenous shunts can also increase cyanosis.

After a Fontan procedure, reduced physical capacity, recurrent cyanosis and edema, hepatomegaly, ascites, and pleural or pericardial effusions are signs of a deteriorating hemodynamical situation.

The ventricular and AV valvular function must be assessed by echocardiography. The Fontan tunnel should also be visualized (obstruction, tunnel leakage?). Intracardiac or venous thromboses must be ruled out. Blood flow in the vena cavae and pulmonary arteries should be breath-dependent (a continuous flow pattern is a sign of a stenosis of the anastomosis). Dilated vena cavae and hepatic veins are also indications of a stenosis of the anastomosis or pulmonary hypertension. A search should always be made for pericardial or pleural effusions and ascites. In case of doubt, there should be a generous indication made for diagnostic cardiac catheterization or MRI.

The necessity of anticoagulation in patients with an aortopulmonary anastomosis and upper or total cavopulmonary anastomosis has not been conclusively clarified. Many centers treat patients with aortopulmonary anastomoses with ASA (aspirin) as a platelet aggregation inhibitor. Patients with upper and total cavopulmonary anastomoses are often given ASA or Phenprocoumon/warfarin depending on their individual risk profile.

Endocarditis prophylaxis is required for all patients with an untreated tricuspid atresia and after palliative measures (aortopulmonary shunt, DKS anastomosis, banding of the pulmonary artery, upper cavopulmonary anastomosis). After a TCPC, endocarditis prophylaxis should be maintained for at least 6 more months, and lifelong if there are any residual defects in the area around foreign material.

► **Physical exercise capacity and lifestyle.** After a Fontan operation, most patients can handle activities of daily living well. Most of the patients are classified as NYHA I or II for many years. Physical exercise capacity is improved in over 75% of the patients after the Fontan procedure, but normal levels are not achieved in objective tests of capacity (an approximate maximum of 50-70%. in comparison with healthy individuals). Competitive sports should be avoided. Participation in school sports is generally possible, but the child must be allowed to take breaks as needed.

Physical exercise with low to moderate dynamic and low static stress is possible if the following criteria are fulfilled:

- Good ventricular function
- No relevant AV valve insufficiency
- No pronounced arrhythmias
- Oxygen saturation > 80%
- Adequate increase in blood pressure during exercise

Years later, many patients develop reduced physical exercise capacity. This is partly due to (atrial) arrhythmias and partly due to decreasing ventricular function.

► **Special aspects in adolescents and adults.** The Fontan procedure and its modifications have been performed for more than three decades and many Fontan patients have now reached adulthood. The late complications after a Fontan procedure have already been described above. In adolescent or adult patients who were treated only palliatively with an aortopulmonary shunt or pulmonary banding, the most important complications involve chronic cyanosis (chronic hypoxemia, polyglobulia, risk of thrombosis, risk of hemorrhage, disposition for cerebral abscesses).

Women who have Fontan hemodynamics and desire to conceive should be aware of the following: pregnancy leads to an increase in intravasal volume, which leads to volume overload of the single ventricle and to an increase in systemic venous pressure. As a result of deteriorating ventricular function, AV valve insufficiency, and arrhythmias, congestive heart failure can develop. In addition, there is an increased tendency for coagulation during pregnancy, so there is a greater risk of thrombosis. It should also be noted that certain drugs have a teratogenic potential (e.g., coumarin derivatives, ACE inhibitors). There is an increased risk of miscarriage for women with Fontan hemodynamics. Nevertheless, the risk appears to be acceptable for patients with a stable hemodynamic situation and no tachycardias or previous embolic events. Thorough obstetric and cardiac monitoring during pregnancy must be ensured.

15.19 Single Ventricle

15.19.1 Basics

Synonyms: univentricular heart, univentricular atrioventricular connection; depending on the morphology of the main ventricle, also "double-inlet left ventricle" (DILV), "double-inlet right ventricle" (DIRV), "common-inlet ventricle"

Definition

In single ventricle physiology, the blood flows from both atra across one common or two AV valves into a single ventricular chamber. If this ventricle is a morphological left ventricle, this is termed a "doublE-Inlet left ventricle" (DILV). If there is a morphological right ventricle, it is called a "doublE-Inlet right ventricle" (DIRV). Only rarely is it not possible to clearly determine the morphology of the ventricle.

In most cases, there is an additional outlet ventricle that is a rudimentary remainder of the other ventricle connected with the main ventricle via a foramen bulboventriculare (ventricular septal defect). In this case, one great vessel arises from the main ventricle and the other from the rudimentary outlet ventricle. Only rarely do both great vessels arise directly from the main ventricle.

The term "single ventricle" is frequently used more broadly in literature and includes all cardiac defects that are not suitable for biventricular correction (e.g., also tricuspid atresia or a hypoplastic left heart syndrome).

> **Note**
>
> In single ventricle physiology, the VSD between the main ventricle and the rudimentary outlet ventricle is called a foramen bulboventriculare.

Epidemiology

This is a rare defect that constitutes less than 1% of all congenital heart defects.

Pathogenesis

The anomaly arises because of impaired development of the embryonic ventricular separation and/or AV valve formation.

Classification

The nomenclature depends on the anatomy and morphology of the main ventricle (▶ Table 15.4). The main ventricle can usually be classified as a left (DILV) or right (DIRV) ventricle based on morphological criteria. In around 80% of cases, there is a left main ventricle. In rare cases, the main ventricle cannot be classified morphologically as either a left or a right ventricle.

The van Praagh or Anderson classifications use the corresponding criteria:

► **Double-inlet left ventricle (80%).** The main ventricle has the morphological criteria of a left ventricle. The right ventricle is only rudimentary and functions merely as an outlet ventricle, which drains either into the aorta or the

Table 15.4 The most important features for differentiating between a morphologic left and right ventricle

Right ventricle	Left ventricle
Tricuspid valve (3 leaflets), 3 papillary muscles	Mitral valve (2 leaflets), 2 papillary muscles
Discontinuity between the AV and semilunar valve	Continuity between the AV and semilunar valve
Muscular outflow tract (infundibulum)	No infundibulum
Gross trabeculation	Fine trabeculation
Septal and parietal muscle bands, moderator band	No septal and parietal muscle bands

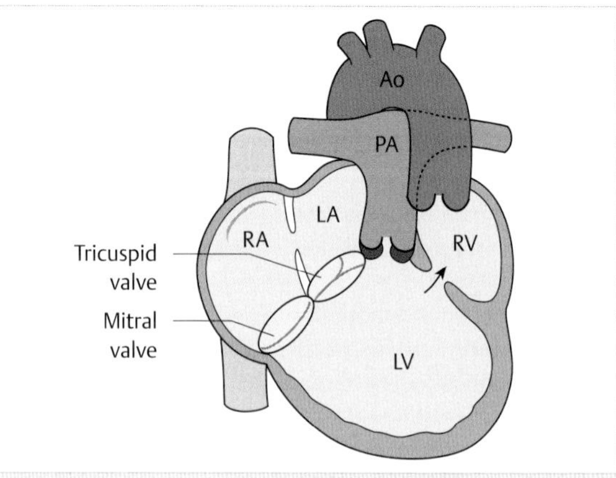

Fig. 15.63 Most common form of a single ventricle: double-inlet left ventricle (DILV) with l-TGA. In this case, the rudimentary right ventricle is located in front and to the left of the left ventricle. The aorta, which is located to the left and in front of the pulmonary artery, arises from the rudimentary ventricle.[29]
LV, left ventricle; RV, right ventricle; LA, left atrium; RA, right atrium; PA, pulmonary artery; Ao, aorta.

pulmonary artery. The two ventricles are connected with each other via a VSD, which in this case is termed “foramen bulboventriculare.” The foramen bulboventriculare is often obstructive and thus hinders outflow from the main ventricle into the rudimentary ventricle and the vessel that arises from it. In most cases the rudimentary morphological right ventricle is located *anterior* to and *at the left* of the main ventricle.

The most common type of a single ventricle is the left ventricular type with l-transposition of the great arteries (DILV with l-TGA position, ▶ Fig. 15.63). The aorta arises from the rudimentary morphological right ventricle and passes to the left of the pulmonary artery. The rudimentary right ventricle is located at the *left* and *anterior* to the main ventricle. The mitral valve is located at the right and the tricuspid valve at the left. However, the AV valves frequently have changes and cannot be clearly identified as tricuspid or mitral valve. Therefore, they are often referred to as the left or right AV valve. A subpulmonary stenosis is present in about half of cases. If the foramen bulboventriculare is restrictive, a hemodynamic subaortic stenosis arises. This type of single ventricle constitutes about 75% of all cases.

▶ **Double-inlet right ventricle** (5%). Both atria drain into a morphological right ventricle. No left ventricle has developed or it is so extremely hypoplastic that it can often be identified only by the pathologist. This means that both great arteries generally arise from the morphological right ventricle. This form is frequently associated with an AV canal. There is also frequently a pulmonary stenosis or atresia.

▶ **Double-inlet ventricle of indeterminate type.** The myocardium of the single ventricle cannot be clearly identified as a typical right or a typical left ventricle. There is no outlet ventricle. There are frequently malpositions of the great vessels, anomalies of the AV valves, and pulmonary stenosis or atresia.

▶ **Common-inlet ventricle.** In a common-inlet ventricle, the atria drain via a common AV valve with a single ventricle. This form is typically associated with an ASD I. The atrial septum is frequently entirely absent. The most common type is associated with heterotaxy (situs ambiguus, asplenia) and consists of a common atrium, a common AV valve, and a common ventricle. In some ways, this anomaly is an extreme form of an unbalanced AV canal. An extremely hypoplastic second ventricle can sometime be identified. There is frequently a pulmonary stenosis or atresia.

▶ **Single-inlet ventricle.** In a single-inlet ventricle, there is only one AV valve, which is connected with the dominant ventricle. Examples of this are tricuspid atresia or mitral atresia, which are discussed in more detail in the respective chapters.

Hemodynamics

The right and left atrial blood is mixed in the common main ventricle. Both great vessels arise functionally from this ventricle so that aorta and pulmonary artery contain mixed blood, and oxygen saturation is identical in the two vessels. Therefore, transposition or a normal position of the great vessels is of lesser importance for the hemodynamics in this defect.

However, the common main ventricle must supply both the systemic and the pulmonary circulation, which leads to a pronounced overload of this ventricle and eventually to congestive heart failure.

The extent of the pulmonary blood flow is decisive for the hemodynamics and the clinical situation:

- If the pulmonary blood flow is reduced (e.g., as a result of a pronounced pulmonary stenosis, extreme form: pulmonary atresia with ductal-dependent pulmonary blood flow) cyanosis results; if the pulmonary blood flow is increased, the symptoms of congestive heart disease predominate.
- Frequently, a single ventricle is combined with a pulmonary stenosis, which can lead to balanced pulmonary perfusion and can maintain a stable hemodynamic situation (ratio of pulmonary to systemic perfusion) for a long time. If there is no pulmonary stenosis, systemic pressure prevails in the pulmonary circulation (pulmonary hypertension).
- A restrictive foramen bulboventriculare leads hemodynamically to a subaortic stenosis in the most common type of single ventricle (DILV with l-TGA). Occasionally there are obstructions of the aortic arch that can lead to a ductal-dependent systemic blood flow.

Associated Anomalies

Associated anomalies occur in the great majority of single ventricles. They are often very significant for the hemodynamics:

- Transposition of the great arteries: In 85% of cases, there is a d-TGA or l-TGA of the great vessels
- Subvalvular or valvular pulmonary stenosis (extreme form: pulmonary atresia): A pulmonary stenosis has a decisive effect on the extent of the pulmonary blood flow
- Subaortic stenosis or stenosis of the aortic arch (rare)
- Atrioventricular septal defect / AV canal
- Atrial septal defect
- Anomalous heart positions (dextrocardia, mesocardia)
- Anomalous pulmonary venous connection
- Anomalies of the systemic veins (e.g., left persistent superior vena cava, atretic right superior vena cava)

Associated Syndromes

Single ventricle physiology often occurs in combination with heterotaxy syndromes.

15.19.2 Diagnostic Measures

Symptoms

Corresponding with the different hemodynamic situations described above, there are various clinical pictures depending on the pulmonary resistance:

- *With a relevant pulmonary stenosis:* The most prominent symptom is central cyanosis. The extent of the cyanosis depends on pulmonary perfusion.
- *Without a relevant pulmonary stenosis:* The typical signs of congestive heart failure develop (poor feeding, failure to thrive, increased sweating, tachypnea/dyspnea, hepatomegaly).

Complications

In patients without pulmonary stenosis, obstructive pulmonary vascular disease and pulmonary hypertension develop due to excessive pulmonary blood flow.

If the patient has the most common form of single ventricle physiology (DILV with l-TGA), in which the aorta arises from the rudimentary ventricle, increasing restriction of the foramen bulboventriculare can develop. This causes a reduction of systemic perfusion and an increase of pulmonary perfusion.

Increasing AV valve insufficiency often creates a difficult hemodynamic situation. In addition, some of the patients develop a complete AV block.

Auscultation

Typical auscultation findings are as follows:

- Pronounced single second heart sound. If there is transposition of the great vessels, the closing sound of the aortic valve, which is in an anterior position, is loud. If there is pulmonary hypertension, the closing sound of the pulmonary valve is pronounced. If there is congestive heart failure, a third heart sound can sometimes be auscultated (gallop rhythm).
- If there is a pulmonary stenosis, a rough, spindle-shaped systolic murmur with PMI in the 2nd to 3rd left parasternal ICS can be auscultated.
- If there is excessive pulmonary blood flow, the diastolic murmur of a relative mitral stenosis may be auscultated over the cardiac apex.

ECG

In the ECG, there is an unusual ventricular hypertrophy pattern: There are frequently similar QRS complexes in most precordial leads. The Q waves are often deformed as a result of the abnormal septum excitation. There may be a first to second degree AV block. In addition, arrhythmias such as supraventricular tachycardias or a wandering pacemaker can sometimes be found.

Chest X-ray

If there is no pulmonary stenosis, a large cardiac silhouette with a large left atrium and excessive pulmonary blood flow can be seen in the radiograph.

If there is a pulmonary stenosis, the cardiac silhouette is of normal size; the pulmonary vascular markings tend to be decreased.

If there is TGA, a narrow mediastinum will be seen.

Echocardiography

The indicative finding is a main ventricle into which both AV valves drain. This can be best visualized in the parasternal long axis or in the four-chamber view. The following should also be visualized or investigated:

- Visualization of the rudimentary ventricle: If there is a DILV, the rudimentary ventricle is in anterior position, with a DIRV it is posterior. Sometimes it cannot be visualized at all by echocardiography. If there is a common inlet ventricle and in a single ventricle of indeterminate type, typically no rudimentary ventricle can be visualized.
- Assessment of ventricular function.
- Determination of the ventriculoarterial connection: In 85% of cases, there is either an l-TGA or d-TGA.
- Visualization and measurement of the foramen bulboventriculare: If the pressure gradient determined by Doppler ultrasonography is greater than 10 mmHg, the foramen bulboventriculare is classified as restrictive.
- Estimate of a possible pulmonary stenosis by Doppler ultrasonography.
- Color Doppler ultrasound visualization of possible AV valve insufficiencies.
- Doppler sonographic estimate of the pressure in the pulmonary circulation (especially in association with excessive pulmonary blood flow).
- Exclusion or visualization of anomalous pulmonary or systemic venous connections
- Visualization of the aortic arch and aortic isthmus (exclusion of hypoplasia of the aortic arch or coarctation of the aorta).
- Visualization of the situs abdominalis (situs ambiguus associated with heterotaxy syndromes).

Cardiac Catheterization

Cardiac catheterization is not urgently required if the anatomy can be sufficiently clarified using echocardiography. In unclear cases, it can be used to visualize and evaluate the following:

- Location and connection of the atriums with ventricles.
- Main and rudimentary ventricles (angiographic evaluation of the main ventricles and classification as right or left ventricle). If there is a DILV, the rudimentary ventricle may be visualized superior/anterior to the main ventricle; if there is a DIRV, the rudimentary ventricle is usually inferior/posterior or cannot be distinguished from the main ventricle at all.
- Foramen bulboventriculare (pressure gradient between the main and rudimentary ventricle associated with a restrictive foramen bulboventriculare).
- Course of the great vessels (normal or transposition).
- AV valves.
- Evaluation of a possible obstruction of the outflow tract: Measurement of pressures over the aorta and pulmonary artery. If there is no subpulmonary obstruction, there is systemic pressure in the pulmonary circulation (pulmonary hypertension).
- Measurement of pressure and resistance in pulmonary circulation.
- Exclusion of anomalous systemic and pulmonary venous connections.
- Exclusion of a hypoplastic aortic arch or coarctation of the aorta.

MRI

In unclear cases, the anatomy can be clearly visualized using MRI. Some indications for MRI are findings with respect to anomalous pulmonary and systemic venous connections that cannot be clarified by echocardiography.

15.19.3 Treatment

Conservative Treatment

If there is critical pulmonary stenosis or pulmonary atresia or an interrupted aortic arch, severe coarctation of the aorta, or hypoplastic aortic arch, prostaglandin is administered until surgery can be carried out to ensure pulmonary and systemic perfusion. Pharmacological treatment is also given for incipient congestive heart failure. Long-term penicillin prophylaxis is required for heterotaxy syndromes with asplenia.

► **Surgical Treatment.** The aim of surgical treatment is to separate the circulatory systems using the Fontan procedure. Before an upper cavopulmonary anastomosis (upper bidirectional Glenn anastomosis) can be made as the first step of Fontan palliation, palliative measures are usually needed if pulmonary and systemic perfusion are not balanced (► Table 15.5):

- If there is *reduced pulmonary blood flow* (pulmonary stenosis, pulmonary atresia) an aortopulmonary shunt is made first.
- If there is *unmanageable excessive pulmonary blood flow, banding of the pulmonary artery* was formerly performed relatively frequently to reduce pulmonary perfusion. However, there is a risk that the size of the foramen bulboventriculare may be reduced as a result of the developing ventricular hypertrophy. The foramen bulboventriculare would then be restrictive and obstruct blood flow to the rudimentary ventricle and the great artery that arises from it. Because of this risk, banding the pulmonary artery is usually avoided and a DKS anastomosis is made, if possible. In this procedure, the pulmonary artery is transected and the proximal segment is anastomosed with the aorta. The lungs are perfused via an aortopulmonary shunt. Pulmonary blood flow can be controlled by selecting a suitably sized shunt (► Fig. 15.64).
- If there is a *restrictive foramen bulboventriculare with no pulmonary or subpulmonary stenosis*, a DKS procedure is performed first. This ensures perfusion of the systemic circulation via the pulmonary artery and the aorta despite the restrictive foramen bulboventriculare. Pulmonary perfusion is ensured by the creation of an aortopulmonary shunt (► Fig. 15.64).

Table 15.5 Summary of the surgical procedures for the most common constellations of a single ventricle

Hemodynamic situation	Palliative step in the neonatal period	Definitive palliation	
Single ventricle and reduced pulmonary perfusion	Aortopulmonary shunt	Upper cavopulmonary anastomosis (usually between the 4th and 6th month of life)	Total cavopulmonary anastomosis (usually between age 2 and 4 years)
Single ventricle and uncontrolled excessive pulmonary blood flow	Damus–Kaye–Stansel procedure and aortopulmonary shunt		
Single ventricle and restrictive foramen bulboventriculare	Damus–Kaye–Stansel procedure and aortopulmonary shunt		
Single ventricle and restrictive foramen bulboventriculare and pulmonary stenosis	Widening the foramen bulboventriculare		

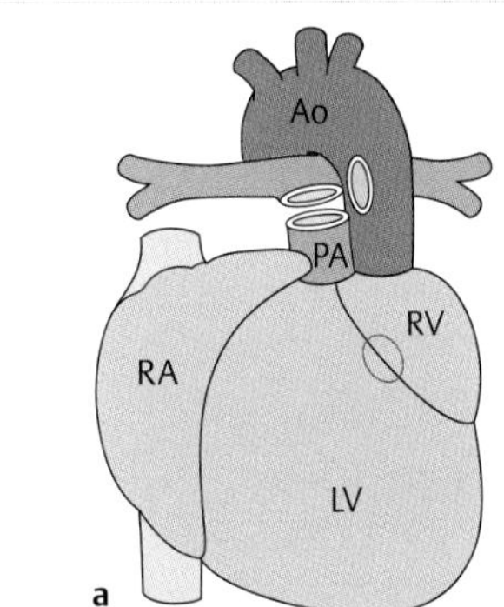

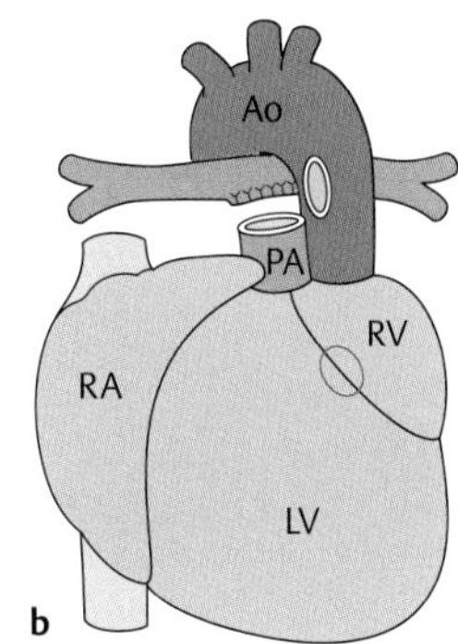

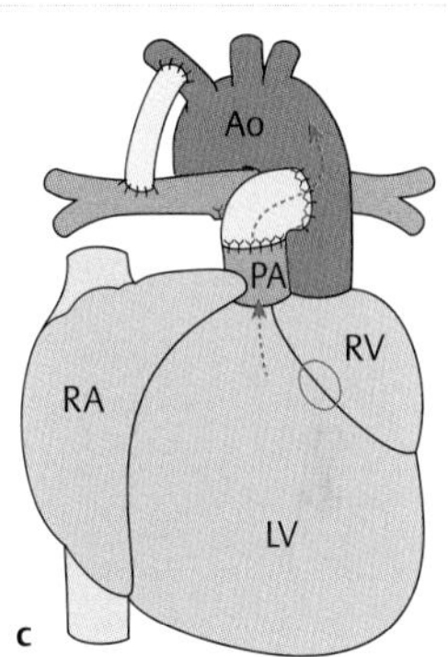

Fig. 15.64 Damus–Kaye–Stansel anastomosis in a DILV with l-TGA and restrictive foramen bulboventriculare. In this procedure, the pulmonary artery is transected and the proximal segment of the pulmonary artery is anastomosed with the ascending aorta. This ensures perfusion of the systemic circulation via the proximal pulmonary artery despite the restrictive foramen bulboventriculare, which functions as a subaortic stenosis. An aortopulmonary shunt is also necessary for perfusion of the lungs. **a** The pulmonary artery is transected. **b** The distal pulmonary artery is occluded at the transection site. **c** The stump of the proximal pulmonary artery is anastomosed with the ascending aorta. A shunt is made from an aortic arch vessel to the right pulmonary artery to allow perfusion of the lungs.[29]
LV, left ventricle; RV, right ventricle; RA, right atrium; PA, pulmonary artery; Ao, aorta.

- If there is a *foramen bulboventriculare with pulmonary or subpulmonary stenosis,* it may be necessary to surgically enlarge the foramen bulboventriculare. However, this involves a not insignificant risk including the danger of a complete AV block.

The actual separation of circulatory systems by Fontan completion involves two operative stages (▶ Table 15.5):

- *Bidirectional upper cavopulmonary anastomosis:* The superior vena cava is anastomosed with the right pulmonary artery. After this, the venous blood from the upper half of the body reaches the lungs passively without passing through a ventricle. If an aortopulmonary shunt was previously made, it is eliminated in this same session. This is an initial step to separate pulmonary and systemic circulation. The arterial oxygen saturation is then around 75 to 85%. This procedure is made at the age of 2 to 6 months after the drop in pulmonary resistance.
- *Total cavopulmonary anastomosis (modified Fontan procedure):* The inferior vena cava and hepatic veins are connected to the right pulmonary artery via an intracardiac or extracardiac conduit. This means that the pulmonary and systemic circulatory systems are completely separated. The lungs are perfused passively with systemic venous blood without involving any ventricle. Sometimes a window is initially left between the Fontan conduit and the atrium, which functions as an overflow valve when venous pressure is increased (disadvantage: residual cyanosis due to the right-to-left shunt). This procedure is generally scheduled after age 2 years. Details of the Fontan procedure are described in Chapter 15.18.

There have been isolated reports of septation of the main ventricle in the literature. In these cases, an artificial interventricular septum is made from a synthetic patch that divides the main ventricle into two compartments.

However, the akinetic synthetic patch can never fulfill the function of a "real" muscular septum. In some cases, only a cardiac transplant remains as a last treatment option.

15.19.4 Prognosis and Clinical Course

▸ **Long-term prognosis.** The spontaneous course depends primarily on the pulmonary blood flow: If there is a pulmonary stenosis with balanced hemodynamics between the pulmonary and systemic circulation, there may be a relatively few symptoms until late adulthood in some cases. However, the majority of patients with a single ventricle die in infancy from the consequences of congestive heart failure or hypoxia.

The later complications after separation of the circulatory systems by Fontan completion are described in Chapter 15.18. They include arrhythmias, dysfunction of the systemic ventricle, protein loss syndrome, and the risk of thrombosis. The 10-year survival rate after a Fontan procedure is 60 to 80%.

▸ **Outpatient follow-up.** Lifelong outpatient follow-up is necessary for patients with a single ventricle. In the rare cases of balanced hemodynamics, surgical methods can be postponed initially. However, frequent monitoring is indicated to check for increasing cyanosis and signs of congestive heart failure and for the development of pulmonary hypertension.

The typical problems after an upper cavopulmonary anastomosis is made and after Fontan circulation is completed are discussed in Chapter 15.18.

▸ **Physical exercise capacity and lifestyle.** After completion of Fontan circulation, most patients are able to handle normal everyday activities. However, objective exercise tests generally show reduced capacity. Competitive sports should be avoided. Contact sports are not suitable for patients who are given oral anticoagulation.

▸ **Special aspects in adolescents and adults.** The typical complications after a Fontan procedure are described in Chapter 15.18. The few patients who have reached adolescence or adulthood without a surgical procedure generally have chronic hypoxia as a result of an Eisenmenger reaction or pulmonary stenosis.

15.20 Hypoplastic Left Heart Syndrome

15.20.1 Basics

Definition

The hypoplastic left heart syndrome (HLHS) is a congenital cardiovascular defect involving hypoplasia of the left ventricle. It is associated with critical stenosis or atresia of the mitral and/or aortic valve and hypoplasia of the ascending aorta and the aortic arch.

In a deviation from this definition, the term HLHS is sometimes also used to include all heart defects with anatomic or functional hypoplasia of the left ventricle, that is, when it is not involved in forming the cardiac apex (e.g., also for an unbalanced AV canal with a hypoplastic left ventricle or the inability to create a biventricular repair (e.g. DORV with a small left ventricle, etc.).

Epidemiology

HLHS constitutes 1 to 2% of all congenital heart defects. It is one of the most frequent causes of heart failure in neonates and is the most common cause of cardiac death in the first week of life. Two-thirds of cases involve boys.

Pathogenesis

The primary anomalies are likely stenosis or atresia of the left ventricular outflow tract. Due to the resulting reduced perfusion of the left ventricle, the ascending aorta, and the aortic arch up to the site where the ductus enters it, their development is inadequate and they remain hypoplastic.

Note

Not every atresia of the aorta is associated with HLHS. For example, if there is also a large VSD, the left ventricle can develop better and there may be other treatment options.

Pathology and Hemodynamics

The main feature is hypoplasia of the left ventricle, which in an extreme case is only as large as a grain of rice. In addition, there is an atretic or severely stenotic aortic valve with a hypoplastic annulus, a hypoplastic ascending aorta, a hypoplastic mitral valve including the tendinous cords and papillary muscles, or mitral valve atresia. There may be endocardial fibroelastosis of the left ventricle and possibly of the left atrium. The extent of the hypoplasia of the left ventricular and aortic structures can vary considerably (▸ Fig. 15.65).

In an HLHS, the left heart is not able to produce sufficient cardiac output. There is no or only minimal antegrade blood flow from the left ventricle to the ascending aorta. Intrauterinely, the ascending aorta, the head and neck vessels, and the coronary arteries are perfused by retrograde flow across the PDA. An adequate intrauterine blood supply is thus ensured, so that an HLHS is relatively well tolerated by the fetus. Postnatally, two factors in particular lead to rapid decompensation—one is the drop in

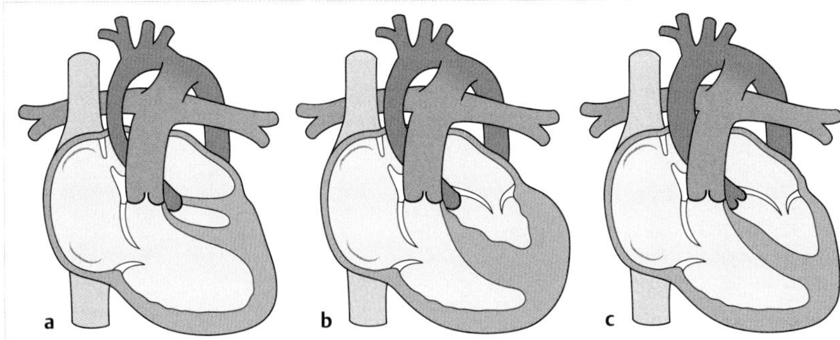

Fig. 15.65 Forms and severity of a hypoplastic left heart syndrome (HLHS). The size of the left ventricle can vary considerably. **a** Aortic and mitral valve atresia. **b** Aortic atresia and normal mitral valve. **c** Aortic stenosis and normal mitral valve.[1]

pulmonary resistance that leads to a reduction of the right-to-left shunt across the ductus arteriosus for retrograde perfusion of the ascending aorta including the head and neck vessels and the coronary arteries, and the other is the closure of the ductus arteriosus that is necessary for survival. This results in a drastic reduction of perfusion of the systemic circulation and coronary arteries, leading to cardiac shock and the development of severe metabolic acidosis.

The ductus arteriosus must remain patent and there must be an adequate left-to-right shunt at the atrial level for the individual to survive. The oxygenated blood from the pulmonary veins cannot drain through the left ventricle into the systemic circulation in an HLHS, but can flow only across a patent foramen ovale or across an ASD from the left to the right atrium. In the right atrium, the arterialized blood mixes with the venous blood from the venae cavae. The mixed blood flows through the right ventricle to the pulmonary artery. Some of this blood supplies the pulmonary circulation; the remainder flows across the ductus arteriosus to the systemic circulation with retrograde flow to the ascending aorta. The right ventricle thus supplies the pulmonary, coronary, and systemic circulation. Excessive pulmonary blood flow develops. Restricted outflow of the blood from the left atrium (restrictive atrial shunt) leads to pulmonary edema.

Associated Anomalies

Around 25% of patients have additional cardiovascular anomalies:

- Coarctation of the aorta: can have an unfavorable effect on retrograde blood flow to the ascending aorta and thus lead to deterioration of coronary and cerebral perfusion
- Coronary anomalies, anomalies of the coronary sinus
- Anomalies of the venae cavae
- VSD (10%)
- Anomalies of the pulmonary veins
- Anomalies of the tricuspid valve

Extracardiac anomalies that have been described include, in particular, anomalies of the central nervous system (e.g., agenesis of the corpus callosum, holoprosencephaly). In addition, there may be gastrointestinal anomalies such as diaphragmatic hernias, duodenal atresia, or intestinal malrotation.

Associated Syndromes

Extracardiac anomalies and genetic syndromes occur in 15 to 30% of patients in association with an HLHS. Some of the genetic syndromes and genetic anomalies that have been described are Turner syndrome, Noonan syndrome, Smith–Lemli–Opitz syndrome, Holt–Oram syndrome, Ellis–van Creveld syndrome, CHARGE syndrome, and trisomy 13, 18, and 21.

15.20.2 Diagnostic Measures

Symptoms

Immediately postnatally, neonates are usually unremarkable. Marked cyanosis directly after birth indicates a restrictive foramen ovale that obstructs the outflow from the left atrium and can lead to congestive pulmonary edema.

Complications

Within the first hours to days of life, when the ductus arteriosus closes and the pulmonary resistance is reduced, acute deterioration occurs with tachycardia, pale gray skin tone, and weak pulses (clinical picture similar to sepsis). Global heart failure with peripheral edema, pulmonary edema, increasing cyanosis, low blood pressure, and hepatomegaly quickly develops. Finally, cardiogenic shock develops with oligouria or anuria and metabolic acidosis.

Auscultation

Auscultation is usually not very indicative. As heart failure increases, neonates have tachycardia, possibly with a gallop rhythm. The second heart sound is loud and single (pulmonary artery component). There is often no heart murmur. It may be possible to auscultate a 2/6–3/6 systolic murmur with PMI in the left parasternal area as a sign of a relative pulmonary or tricuspid valve stenosis.

ECG

The ECG has low or absent left ventricular potentials (low R wave, deep S wave in V_5/V_6). Typically, there are signs of right ventricular hypertrophy (pathologic right axis deviation, tall R wave in V_1/V_2), and signs of right atrial overload (P dextrocardiale). ST segment changes and T inversions can be a sign of more severe myocardial ischemia.

Chest X-ray

There is usually cardiomegaly. The heart has a rounded shape; the right ventricle forms the left border of the heart and the cardiac apex is upturned. There is increased pulmonary vascular marking in the perihilar region. There may be the typical signs of pulmonary edema.

Echocardiography

Indicative findings are a small, hypoplastic left ventricle that is not involved in forming the cardiac apex and large right atrium and ventricle with a large pulmonary artery. In an extreme case, the left ventricle can be identified as a tiny structure behind the right ventricle only after detailed analysis. The echogenicity of the left ventricle is often increased as a result of endocardial fibroelastosis. A significant finding is also a hypoplastic ascending aorta with retrograde perfusion across the PDA. The ascending aorta typically has a narrow thread or ribbon shape. The aortic and mitral valves are hypoplastic and severely stenotic or atretic. There is a left-to-right shunt at the atrial level. A restrictive atrial shunt must be ruled out. The left atrium is small. There is a right-to-left shunt across the PDA that supplies the systemic circulation, with retrograde perfusion of the ascending aorta and the coronary arteries. It is important to assess the function of the right ventricle and the tricuspid valve, which function as a systemic ventricle and systemic AV valve.

Associated anomalies (especially coarctation of the aorta and coronary anomalies) must be ruled out by echocardiography.

Cardiac Catheterization

Cardiac catheterization may be risky in an HLHS. It is therefore indicated only for particular clinical questions that cannot be answered by echocardiography (e.g., coronary anomalies) or by a planned intervention.

MRI

MRI is of only secondary importance as a primary diagnostic tool. It is used especially for postoperative follow-up after a Norwood procedure and for an upper, lower, or total cavopulmonary anastomosis.

15.20.3 Treatment

HLHS is the heart defect with the most unfavorable prognosis. If the defect is left untreated, 80% of the children die within the first week of life. The perioperative risk is high: The survival rate for the three-stage operative procedure is around 50 to 70%. There is a similar prognosis for a cardiac transplant.

The parents must therefore be informed comprehensively of all possible options (stopping treatment and compassionate care, Norwood procedure, hybrid procedure, cardiac transplant, if available).

Conservative Treatment

Immediately after the diagnosis is made, a prostaglandin E infusion must be started (initially 50 ng/kg/min, later reduced to the lowest possible dose) to maintain patency of the ductus arteriosus (ductal-dependent systemic and coronary blood flow!). To improve perfusion of the systemic circulation, an attempt is made to increase pulmonary resistance and reduce systemic resistance. The targets are oxygen saturation of 70 to 80%, a PaO_2 of around 40 mmHg, normal arterial blood pressure, and a $PaCO_2$ of 40 (up to 50) mmHg.

Additional administration of oxygen is contraindicated, as it leads to excessive pulmonary blood flow and deterioration of systemic and coronary perfusion by reducing the pulmonary resistance. Buffering should not be initiated until the BE is below –5.

Catecholamines, phosphodiesterase inhibitors, and diuretics are used to treat congestive heart failure. Intubation and mechanical ventilation are often required (see above for target levels under ventilation). Ventilation should be avoided, however, if at all possible, because it almost always leads to an increase in pulmonary perfusion. To improve systemic perfusion, afterload reducers such as sodium nitroprusside are administered.

Initial treatment of HLHS:

- Prostaglandin E infusion (initially 50 ng/kg/min, later reduced to a maintenance dose)
- Avoid intubation and mechanical ventilation if possible; but this is indicated if there is a restrictive atrial shunt and pulmonary edema
- FiO_2 0.2 L, avoid additional oxygen
- Target oxygen saturation of 70 to 80%
- Target $PaCO_2$ is 40 mmHg, target PaO_2 is 40 mmHg (if saturation is higher—that is, if there is excessive pulmonary blood flow—target $PaCO_2$ is 50 mmHg)
- Achieve normal arterial blood pressure (if necessary, volume therapy, catecholamines, milrinone)
- Buffering only if the BE is below –5

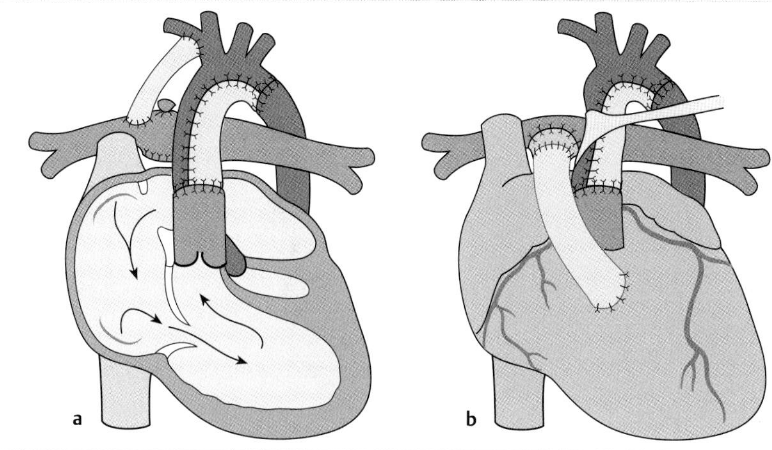

Fig. 15.66 Norwood I procedure with modified Blalock–Taussig shunt (a) or Sano shunt (b). A "neo-aorta" is created by anastomosing the pulmonary artery with the hypoplastic ascending aorta and patch repair of the aortic arch. The pulmonary perfusion is ensured either via an aortopulmonary shunt (e.g., with a modified Blalock–Taussig shunt [**a**]), or implanting a conduit between the right ventricle and the pulmonary artery (with Sano shunt [**b**]). [1]

Note

The "normal reaction" to hypoxia and circulatory depression in the form of hyperoxygenation, hyperventilation, and blind buffering can be fatal in HLHS!

Interventional Catheterization

If there is a restrictive atrial shunt (barely patent foramen ovale or small ASD), a Rashkind balloon atrial septostomy or blade atrial septostomy is indicated. In a restrictive atrial shunt, the blood cannot drain sufficiently out of the left atrium and there is a risk of pulmonary congestion and pulmonary edema.

Surgical Treatment

The standard surgical treatment for HLHS is Norwood palliation. This procedure includes a total of three operations that result in a complete separation of the circulatory systems by a Fontan procedure. The alternative is a cardiac transplant, which is possible only to a limited extent because very few donor organs are available.

▸ **Norwood I procedure.** Timing: usually from the 5th to 7th day of life. A major stage in this procedure is the formation of a "neo-aorta" to enable unrestricted systemic perfusion (▸ Fig. 15.66). This goal is achieved by anastomosing the hypoplastic aorta with the pulmonary artery. In addition, the aortic arch is widened. The systemic circulation is then supplied via the neo-aorta. To ensure pulmonary perfusion, an aortopulmonary shunt (e.g., a modified Blalock–Taussig shunt) is also made. In some centers, a Sano shunt between the right ventricle and pulmonary artery is made instead of the aortopulmonary shunt. The advantage of the Sano shunt is higher diastolic pressure (less diastolic run-off), but the disadvantage is that a ventriculotomy is needed to create the Sano shunt and the pulmonary arteries require more extensive reconstruction later on.. The ductus arteriosus is closed during the Norwood I procedure. The atrial septum is resected (atrial septectomy) to ensure mixing at the atrial level.

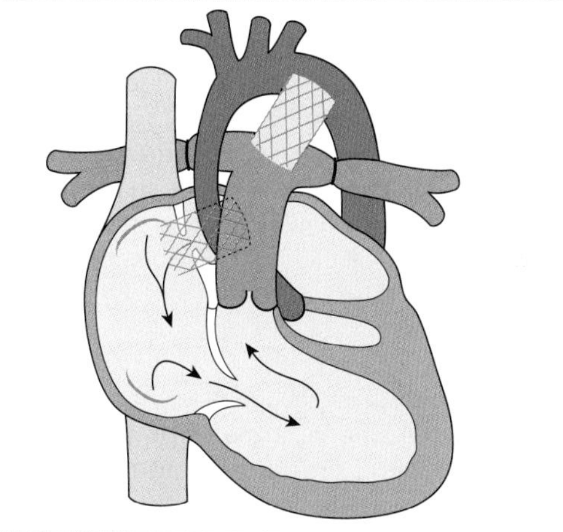

Fig. 15.67 Hybrid procedure as an alternative to the Norwood I procedure. In this procedure, the ductus arteriosus is kept patent with a stent to ensure the systemic and coronary perfusion. The atrial shunt may also be stented. Banding of the pulmonary arteries is performed in the same session to protect against excessive pulmonary blood flow.[1]

One alternative to the Norwood I procedure is to initially implant only a stent to keep the ductus arteriosus patent (▸ Fig. 15.67). This measure must be supplemented by banding the pulmonary artery due to the risk of excessive pulmonary blood flow. This hybrid procedure (combination of interventional catheterization and surgery) can be a preparatory step for further treatment by Fontan completion or to bridge the period until a cardiac transplant.

▸ **Norwood II procedure.** Timing: usually in the 4th to 6th month of life. The Norwood II procedure corresponds with an upper bidirectional cavopulmonary anastomosis (bidirectional Glenn procedure or alternatively hemi-Fontan procedure). The superior vena cava is anastomosed with the right pulmonary artery (▶ Fig. 15.68). The venous blood from the upper half of the body then flows passively into the lungs. The aortopulmonary shunt is no longer necessary to ensure pulmonary perfusion and is removed.

▶ **Norwood III procedure.** Timing: usually in the 2nd or 3rd year of life. The Norwood III procedure corresponds with a total cavopulmonary anastomosis (TCPC, modified Fontan procedure). In this procedure, the inferior vena cava is connected to the right pulmonary artery through a surgically formed tunnel through the right atrium. Today, a Gore-Tex conduit is frequently used to create an extracardiac tunnel that passes next to the right atrium. The advantage of such a tunnel is that it is likely that fewer atrial arrhythmias will occur later. Sometimes the Fontan tunnel is fenestrated so it serves as an "overflow valve" in the event of outflow tract obstruction in the pulmonary circulation (e.g., if there is high pulmonary pressure). It may be a disadvantage that this can lead to mixing with venous blood in the systemic circulation, resulting in mild cyanosis. Sometimes the fenestration can be closed at a later time by interventional catheterization.

▶ **Cardiac transplant.** In an HLHS, in addition to the heart, the ascending aorta and aortic arch up to beyond the isthmus must also be replaced.(▶ Fig. 15.69) This must be noted when removing the donor organ. The mortality rate after transplant is comparable with that after a Norwood procedure. However, this treatment option is considerably limited in Europe due to the lack of donor organs.

15.20.4 Prognosis and Clinical Course

▶ **Long-term outcome.** HLHS has the poorest prognosis of all congenital heart defects. If the defect is left untreated, 80% of the patients die within the first week of life. Only 5% of children survive the first month of life. HLHS is the most frequent cause of cardiac death in the first weeks of life.

Despite the introduction of Norwood palliation, the mortality rate is still high, although the postoperative results have clearly improved in recent years. The overall 5-year survival rate is currently just under 70%.

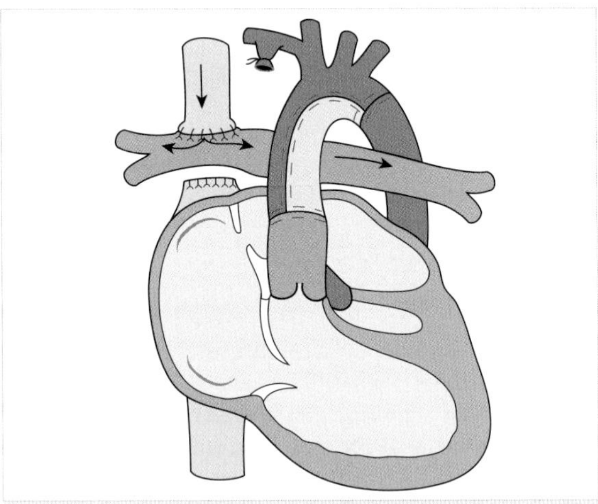

Fig. 15.68 Bidirectional upper cavopulmonary anastomosis in an HLHS. In this procedure, the superior vena cava is anastomosed to the pulmonary artery, after which the blood from the upper half of the body flows passively into the lungs.[1]

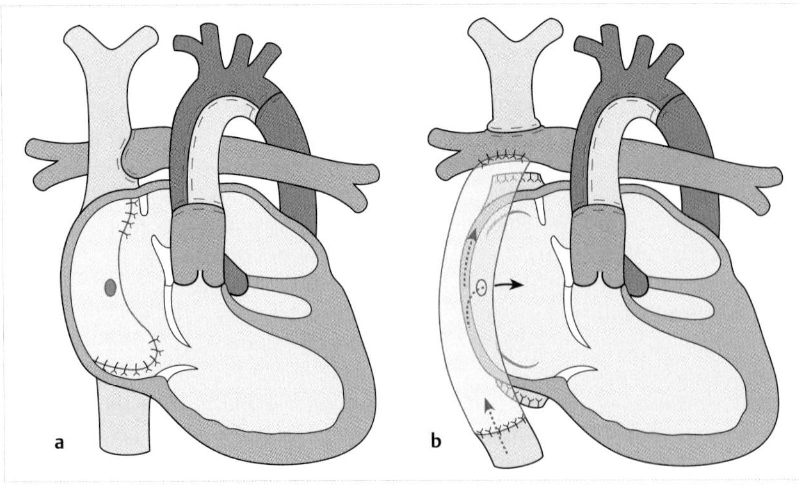

Fig. 15.69 Total cavopulmonary anastomosis with a lateral atrial tunnel or an extracardiac tunnel in an HLHS. In the last stage to complete separation of the circulatory systems, the inferior vena cava is anastomosed to the pulmonary artery, for example, via a tunnel in the lateral segment of the right atrium (**a**) or via an extracardiac tunnel (**b**) using a tube graft. **a** Total cavopulmonary anastomosis with lateral atrial tunnel. **b** Total cavopulmonary anastomosis with extracardiac tunnel.[1]

More than half of the children later have neurological problems or mental retardation of varying degrees. At age 3 years, fewer than 25% of patients have age-appropriate development.

The later problems after a Fontan procedure include arrhythmias (often bradycardia, supraventricular arrhythmias), dysfunction of the right systemic ventricle, a protein loss syndrome, tendency to thromboembolisms, and development of cyanosis (right-to-left shunt across a tunnel fenestration, pulmonary AV shunts; see Chapter 15.29).

► **Outpatient checkups.** Frequent outpatient checkups (e.g., weekly or fortnightly) are needed between the Norwood I and Norwood II procedures. After a Norwood I procedure, there is volume overload of the systemic ventricle (it receives the blood from the systemic and pulmonary circulation) and has to pump the blood into both circulatory systems. The target arterial oxygen saturation level is 75 to 85%. A higher saturation is a sign of excessive pulmonary blood flow, a lower level of reduced pulmonary perfusion (e.g., shunt stenosis, "outgrowing" the shunt). If there are signs of reduced systemic perfusion and increased pulmonary perfusion, afterload reduction, with ACE inhibitors for example, is useful. If there is excessive pulmonary blood flow, diuretics may be used with caution to treat heart failure. However, hypovolemia must be avoided.

For thromboembolism prophylaxis, ASA is generally administered as a platelet aggregation inhibitor (3–5 mg/kg/d).

Gastrointestinal or respiratory infections can be life-threatening to Norwood patients due to the fluid loss or hypoxemia.

Outpatient checkups after upper or total cavopulmonary anastomosis are described in Chapter 15.18.

Endocarditis prophylaxis is required for all patients with HLHS until at least 6 months after Fontan completion, lifelong if there is a prosthetic valve or residual defects in the vicinity of foreign material.

► **Physical exercise capacity and lifestyle.** After a Fontan procedure, most patients can cope with activities of daily living. However, they are objectively considerably impaired in comparison with their age group (about 50-60% compared with healthy individuals). Competitive sports should be avoided. Participation in physical education is generally possible, but patients must be allowed to take breaks at their own discretion. Some patients develop a loss of physical capacity after years. This is partially due to (atrial) arrhythmias and reduced function of the right systemic ventricle.

► **Special aspects in adolescents and adults.** Until the 1980s, HLHS was considered untreatable. Only a few patients have thus far reached adulthood, so there is little experience with adult patients.

15.21 Pulmonary Stenosis

15.21.1 Basics

Definition

A pulmonary stenosis is an incomplete obstruction of the right ventricular outflow tract. The obstruction can involve the pulmonary valve itself or the pulmonary artery or its branches. It can also be located below the pulmonary valve in the area of the infundibulum.

Epidemiology

A pulmonary stenosis is a relatively common anomaly, constituting around 10% of all congenital heart defects. It can occur in isolation or more often as an accompanying anomaly with other congenital defects. Boys and girls are affected approximately equally. Family clusters have been described.

Pathogenesis

Faulty development of the distal bulbus cordis or intrauterine endocarditis have been postulated as causes. The association of supravalvular pulmonary stenosis with numerous syndromal conditions makes a genetic factor likely.

Classification

Classification depends on the location of the stenosis (► Fig. 15.70):

► **Valvular pulmonary stenosis (90%).** A valvular pulmonary stenosis is by far the most common type of pulmonary stenosis, at 90%. The valve is typically thick; the leaflets are frequently fused together and obstruct the valve opening (► Fig. 15.70 **a**). The fused semilunar valves open incompletely and like a funnel into the pulmonary artery. This leads to the typical doming of the pulmonary valve in systole. The valve can be bicuspid or unicommissural, less often tricuspid. The pulmonary valve annulus is sometimes hypoplastic. The severity of stenosis ranges from insignificant to severe "buttonhole stenosis."

A *dysplastic pulmonary valve* is a special form of valvular pulmonary stenosis. The leaflets are extremely thick due to myxomatous tissue. The annulus of a dysplastic valve is generally hypoplastic. A dysplastic pulmonary valve is frequently associated with Noonan syndrome.

► **Subvalvular pulmonary stenosis (infundibular pulmonary stenosis).** In a subvalvular or infundibular

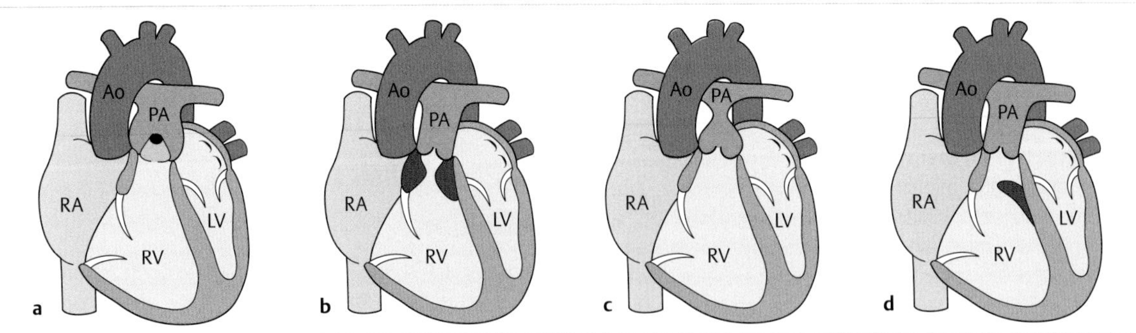

Fig. 15.70 Forms of pulmonary stenosis. **a** Valvular pulmonary stenosis: The valve opens incompletely and like a funnel into the pulmonary artery (doming). **b** Subvalvular pulmonary stenosis: The obstruction occurs below the valve in the area of the muscular right ventricular outflow tract, the infundibulum. **c** Supravalvular pulmonary stenosis: The stenosis is located above the valve in the area of the pulmonary artery (central supravalvular pulmonary stenosis). Peripheral supravalvular pulmonary stenoses can also occur in the branches of the pulmonary artery. **d** Double-chambered right ventricle: The right ventricle is divided into two segments by a muscle bundle.
LV, left ventricle; RV, right ventricle; RA, right atrium; PA, pulmonary artery; Ao, aorta.

pulmonary stenosis, thick and often hypercontractile muscles of the right ventricular outflow tract (infundibulum) lead to obstruction (▶ Fig. 15.70 **b**). An infundibular pulmonary stenosis occurs only rarely in isolation. It is frequently associated with a VSD (e.g., in tetralogy of Fallot). It is usually a secondary result of a (possibly reversible) myocardial hypertrophy of various causes (e.g., due to a valvular pulmonary stenosis). It is sometimes a dynamic obstruction that can increase acutely (typical example: Fallot crisis with cyanotic spells).

The *double-chambered right ventricle* is a special form of a subvalvular stenosis (▶ Fig. 15.70 **d**). The right ventricle is divided into two segments—the proximal high-pressure and the distal low-pressure ventricle—by an abnormally large muscle bundle located below the infundibulum. It is usually associated with a VSD. The obstruction generally increases over time.

▶ **Supravalvular pulmonary stenosis (central and peripheral).** Supravalvular pulmonary stenosis can be central, affecting the main pulmonary artery, or peripheral, affecting the branches of the pulmonary artery (▶ Fig. 15.70 **c**). Supravalvular pulmonary stenoses can occur in isolation or in multiples. It is frequently associated with valvular pulmonary stenosis, a VSD, or tetralogy of Fallot.

Peripheral pulmonary stenoses often occur in syndromal diseases. Typical examples are Williams–Beuren syndrome, Noonan syndrome, Alagille syndrome, and rubella embryopathy.

Supravalvular pulmonary stenoses can occur postoperatively after a TGA switch procedure or after surgical correction of a tetralogy of Fallot or a truncus arteriosus communis.

Table 15.6 Severity of pulmonary stenosis

Severity	Systolic pressure gradient	Valve opening size
I (insignificant)	< 25 mmHg	1.0–2.0 cm^2/m^2 BSA
II (mild)	25–49 mmHg	< 1 cm^2/m^2 BSA
III (moderate)	50–79 mmHg	< 0.5 cm^2/m^2 BSA
IV (severe)	> 80 mmHg	< 0.25 cm^2/m^2 BSA

BSA = body surface area.

▶ **Severity.** The severity of a pulmonary stenosis is determined based on pressure gradients (▶ Table 15.6).

Pathology and Hemodynamics

As a result of the increased pressure in the right ventricle, right ventricular hypertrophy including muscular hypertrophy of the infundibulum develops. A valvular stenosis causes poststenotic dilatation of the pulmonary artery due to the turbulent blood flow.

Even severe stenoses with a right ventricular pressure over 200 mmHg are often tolerated for a long time without leading to right heart failure. At rest, the cardiac output can be maintained for a long time. Only during exertion or in the presence of right ventricular insufficiency is the heart no longer able to produce sufficient cardiac output. A long-term increase in right ventricular pressure leads to endocardial fibrosis and impaired right ventricular compliance.

In a critical pulmonary stenosis, pulmonary blood flow is ductal dependent. (Ductal-dependent pulmonary blood flow is part of the definition of critical pulmonary stenosis.) If there is severe pulmonary stenosis with a patent foramen ovale, an ASD, or a VSD, cyanosis over a right-to-left shunt can occur.

Associated Anomalies

Pulmonary stenoses are often associated with other cardiac anomalies, for example:

- Patent foramen ovale or ASD
- VSD
- PDA
- Tetralogy of Fallot
- Single ventricle

Infundibular or supravalvular pulmonary stenoses sometimes occur in combination with valvular pulmonary stenoses.

Associated Syndromes

Supravalvular pulmonary stenoses in particular occur in combination with syndromal diseases.

- Williams–Beuren syndrome (supravalvular pulmonary stenoses, often in combination with a supravalvular aortic stenosis)
- Noonan syndrome (valvular or supravalvular pulmonary stenoses, dysplastic pulmonary valve)
- Alagille syndrome (supravalvular pulmonary stenoses)
- Rubella embryopathy (supravalvular pulmonary stenoses)

15.21.2 Diagnostic Measures

Symptoms

Most patients are asymptomatic or have few symptoms. Even if there is severe stenosis, the patients are often relatively free of symptoms for a long time.

Complications

Patients with more severe stenoses may develop reduced physical capacity, rapid fatigability, or dyspnea on exertion. If there are severe stenoses, syncopes or chest pain may occur after physical exertion. Cyanosis occurs only rarely if the pulmonary stenosis is severe and a right-to-left shunt develops across a still patent foramen ovale, an ASD, or a VSD.

Tachypnea/dyspnea and general cyanosis will occur in the neonatal period if there is a critical pulmonary stenosis with ductal-dependent pulmonary blood flow. Hepatomegaly is a sign of right heart failure.

Auscultation

Indicative auscultation findings are:

- Ejection click: In a mild to moderate valvular stenosis, an extra sound can be heard shortly after the first heart sound in the 2nd left parasternal ICS.
- The second heart sound is split; splitting increases as the severity of the stenosis increases. The pulmonary component of the second heart sound is soft.
- Loud, rough, spindle-shaped systolic ejection murmur of medium frequency with PMI in the 2nd/3rd left parasternal ICS radiating over the entire precordial area, to the back, the axilla, and the jugular notch (but not to the carotids).
- It may be possible to auscultate the systolic regurgitation murmur of tricuspid insufficiency.

Note

The severity of a pulmonary stenosis can be estimated on the basis of the auscultation finding. The more pronounced the pulmonary stenosis is, the louder the murmur is, and the later it reaches its maximum. As the severity of the pulmonary stenosis increases, the split of the second heart sound increases, but if there is severe valvular pulmonary stenosis, the very thick valve may not produce a closing sound.

ECG

The ECG is normal in a mild pulmonary stenosis. In more severe stenoses, there are signs of right ventricular and right atrial hypertrophy: tall R waves in the right precordial leads, deep S waves in the left precordial leads, tall, narrow P wave. The height of the R wave in V_1 correlates with the severity of the stenosis.

If there is a severe stenosis, abnormal repolarization in the form of ST segment depression and T wave inversion also occurs.

Chest X-ray

The heart usually has a normal size in a radiograph. The cardiac apex is typically upturned as a result of the right ventricular concentric hypertrophy. In the lateral image, the right ventricle occupies much of the retrosternal space. The pulmonary segment is sometimes prominent (poststenotic dilatation). The pulmonary vascular marking is usually normal, but reduced if pulmonary stenosis is severe.

If the pulmonary stenosis is critical, cardiomegaly with decreased pulmonary vascular marking may already be apparent in a neonate.

Echocardiography

Echocardiography is used to make the diagnosis and assess the severity. The following points should be investigated in the echocardiography:

- Location of the stenosis: subvalvular (best visualized in the parasternal tilted long axis), valvular (best

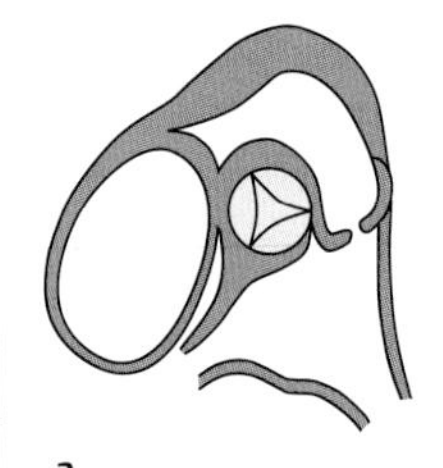

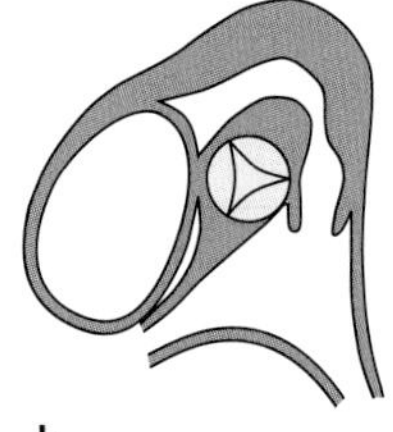

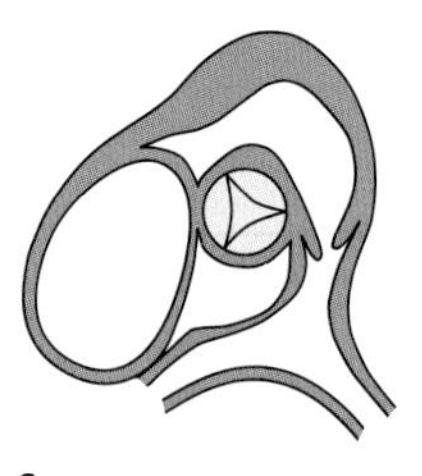

Fig. 15.71 Valvular (**a**), subvalvular (**b**), and supravalvular stenosis (**c**) in echocardiography (parasternal short axis.)[31]

visualized in the parasternal short axis, ▶ Fig. 15.71) or supravalvular (possibly best visualized from a suprasternal direction). It is important to examine the entire right ventricular outflow tract, the valve, the pulmonary artery, and its branches thoroughly for stenoses, as the different forms of pulmonary stenosis occur not only in isolation, but in combination as well.

- Visualization of valve morphology (best visualized in the parasternal or subcostal short axis): Is there valve dysplasia and/or myxomatous thickening? Are the commissures fused together? In doming of the valve, the leaflets protrude into the pulmonary artery during systole instead of opening completely.
- Pulmonary valve annulus: If there is an isolated valvular stenosis, the annulus is usually of normal width; if the stenosis is critical or the valve dysplastic, the annulus is often hypoplastic.
- Pulmonary artery and branches: If the valvular stenosis is severe, there is usually poststenotic dilatation.
- Assessment of the right ventricle: Is there right ventricular hypertrophy? It is often associated with an increasing obstruction of the right ventricular outflow tract. If there is pronounced right ventricular hypertrophy, the septum may protrude into the left ventricle and impair left ventricular function.
- Assessment of the size of the right atrium.
- Measurement of the pressure gradient using Doppler ultrasound: The gradient across the stenosis can be estimated by the flow velocity using the simplified Bernoulli equation. If right ventricular function is impaired, however, the gradient does not correlate with the degree of stenosis.
- Color Doppler: Visualization of the turbulent flow at the stenosis, exclusion or detection of pulmonary or tricuspid insufficiency.

Cardiac Catheterization

Purely diagnostic cardiac catheterizations are usually needed only for supravalvular stenoses owing to the reliability of echocardiography. In most cases, cardiac catheterization is performed only for therapeutic purposes.

The pull-back pressure curve from the pulmonary artery to the right ventricle exhibits a distinct jump depending on the location of the stenosis. A two-stage jump in pressure occurs in a valvular stenosis combined with an additional infundibular stenosis. If there is a valvular stenosis, the angiography shows the typical doming of the rigid margins of the valve, which barely move. In infundibular stenoses, constriction of the infundibulum can be seen during systole.

For better visualization of the pulmonary artery and the bifurcation, the sagittal plane is tilted 30° in a cranial direction (view of the pulmonary artery and bifurcation from above). In addition, for a specific assessment of the left pulmonary artery, an RAO (right anterior oblique) visualization and, to assess the right pulmonary artery, a LAO (left anterior oblique) visualization may be used.

MRI

MRI is used in particular for adult patients or for supravalvular pulmonary stenoses when the limits of echocardiography are reached. Potential associated cardiac anomalies can be ruled out.

15.21.3 Treatment

Conservative Treatment

▶ **Neonates with critical pulmonary stenosis.** In neonates with a critical pulmonary stenosis, the ductus arteriosus must be kept patent with a prostaglandin E infusion (initially 50 ng/kg/min, dose later adjusted) to ensure pulmonary perfusion. To improve the left-to-right shunt across the ductus, the peripheral systemic resistance can be increased (e.g., with noradrenaline) and the pulmonary vascular resistance can be lowered (oxygen, hyperventilation, alkalization with sodium bicarbonate [target BE + 2 to + 4]).

▶ **Indications for interventional catheterization or surgical treatment**

- Pressure gradient over 50 mmHg at rest or over 70 mmHg under exertion (for a balloon valvuloplasty, a resting gradient of over 40 mmHg applies)
- Symptoms: exertional dyspnea, syncopes, failure to thrive due to the pulmonary stenosis, reduced capacity
- Cardiomegaly
- Abnormal repolarization in the ECG

▶ **Timing of treatment.** Treatment of critical pulmonary stenoses is begun immediately after the diagnosis is made in the neonatal period. The best results for a balloon valvuloplasty or surgical treatment are achieved at preschool age. A double-chambered right ventricle should be corrected early, as the symptoms can be expected to deteriorate.

Interventional Catheterization

▶ **Balloon valvuloplasty/angioplasty.** Balloon valvuloplasty is considered the treatment of choice for isolated valvular pulmonary stenoses. Due to the high rate of restenosis, in supravalvular stenoses it is often supplemented by a stent implantation in the stenotic area (peripheral pulmonary stenoses that are surrounded by lung parenchyma cannot be operated on). Balloon angioplasty or valvuloplasty is less promising for subvalvular stenoses and dysplastic valves.

▶ **Procedure.** For a valvular pulmonary stenosis, a dilation balloon is selected with a diameter 1.2 to 1.5 times larger than that of the pulmonary valve. For dysplastic valves and supravalvular stenoses, an even larger balloon diameter is often needed.

Especially in neonates with a critical pulmonary stenosis, a reactive stenosis of the hypercontractile infundibulum occasionally occurs postinterventionally, which does not resolve for days or weeks. In such cases, temporary treatment with a beta blocker can be considered.

▶ **Complications.** A typical complication of a balloon valvuloplasty of a stenotic valve is the occurrence of pulmonary insufficiency, but this is rarely clinically relevant. Other possible complications are an incomplete or complete right bundle branch block (sometimes temporary), increasing (temporary) obstruction of the infundibulum, rupture of the papillary muscle, and balloon rupture.

Surgical Treatment

Elective surgery is indicated for patients with a dysplastic pulmonary valve that cannot be improved by interventional catheterization (▶ Table 15.7). It is rarely needed for an isolated valvular pulmonary stenosis, which can usually be treated by interventional catheterization.

Table 15.7 Summary of the most important surgical procedures for the various forms of pulmonary stenosis

Form of pulmonary stenosis	Surgical treatment	Remarks
Isolated valvular pulmonary stenosis	Commissurotomy (incision of the fused valves in the area of the commissures)	Results are comparable with those of balloon valvuloplasty, so balloon valvuloplasty is generally the preferred option
Dysplastic valve	Commissurotomy or valvulotomy is often not sufficient. If the valve is severely dysplastic, it may be necessary to resect the entire valve. The resulting "free" pulmonary insufficiency may necessitate an early reoperation or the immediate implantation of a valved conduit or homograft. If the valve annulus is narrow, it must also be widened (e.g., with a transannular patch—Disadvantage: pulmonary insufficiency can often not be avoided)	
Infundibular pulmonary stenosis	Infundibulectomy (resection of infundibular muscle tissue), possibly patch expansion of the infundibulum	
Double-chambered right ventricle	Resection of the anomalous muscle bundle and closure of an associated VSD	Caution: cardiac conduction system
Supravalvular pulmonary stenosis	Patch expansion of the pulmonary artery or bifurcation	Peripheral pulmonary stenoses of the branches of the pulmonary artery can generally not be treated surgically, but are a typical indication for interventional catheterization and stenting
Critical pulmonary stenosis with a hypoplastic right ventricle	Biventricular correction is sometimes not possible. In these cases, an aortopulmonary shunt is created in the neonate period, followed later by univentricular palliation in a Fontan procedure or a "one-and-a-half Fontan" (Chapter 15.27)	

Typical indications for surgery are also an infundibular pulmonary stenosis and a double-chambered right ventricle with a relevant pressure gradient.

In some neonates with a critical pulmonary stenosis, the antegrade flow across the pulmonary valve dilated by interventional catheterization is not sufficient because of a hypoplastic right ventricle or low compliance of the right ventricle, so an aortopulmonary shunt must be implanted in these children to ensure pulmonary perfusion.

15.21.4 Prognosis and Clinical Course

▸ **Long-term outcome.** The long-term outcome depends mainly on the severity and form of the stenosis. Severe heart failure develops as early as the neonatal period if there is a *critical pulmonary stenosis*. These children die if left untreated. If there is a *mild valvular pulmonary stenosis* with a gradient below 50 mmHg, the stenosis does not generally increase over the long-term course. However, if there is already a moderate or even severe stenosis with gradients over 50 mmHg (indication for treatment) in the first two years of life, progression can be expected.

Supravalvular stenoses are not usually progressive; they even tend to spontaneous resolution. In a double-chambered right ventricle, the obstruction often increases rapidly.

The prognosis is very good after the successful balloon valvuloplasty or commissurotomy of a *valvular pulmonary stenosis*. A possible secondary infundibular stenosis usually resolves over time. Possible restenosis can be treated by interventional catheterization.

▸ **Outpatient checkups.** After the diagnosis is made, regular cardiac checkups are needed. An increase in the gradient and, for more severe stenoses, right ventricular function and size should be noted in particular. If the gradient is over 50 mmHg, progression can be expected which may eventually lead to an indication for interventional catheterization or surgery.

Postinterventionally or postoperatively, the patient should be monitored for the development of restenosis and possible pulmonary insufficiency. The right ventricular size and function should also be assessed. Lifelong endocarditis prophylaxis is needed after the implantation of valve replacements. After valve reconstruction using foreign material or a balloon dilatation, endocarditis prophylaxis is recommended for 6 months after the procedure, but it should be given for a longer period if there are residual defects at or near prosthetic material.

▸ **Lifestyle and physical exercise capacity.** In most cases, children have age-appropriate physical exercise capacity. Restrictions on physical activity and sports are not necessary unless the gradients are over 50 to 70 mmHg.

After a balloon valvuloplasty or surgery, the patient can participate in physical education or organized sports 1 to 3 months after the procedure if the following conditions are met:

- Peak gradient under 50 mmHg
- No relevant pulmonary insufficiency
- Reduction of the right ventricular overload

If the remaining gradient is more than 50 mmHg or there is more severe pulmonary insufficiency, the patient can engage in sports with a low to medium dynamic and static stress level.

▸ **Special aspects in adolescents and adults.** Balloon valvuloplasty is the treatment option of choice, just as for children with isolated valvular pulmonary stenoses. There is definitely an indication for symptomatic patients and those with gradients over 50 mmHg. Active patients are often treated even if the pressure gradients are lower.

15.22 Aortic Stenosis

15.22.1 Basics

Definition

An aortic stenosis is an incomplete obstruction of the left ventricular outflow tract. The stenosis can be at the valvular level or be located below or above the valve, and is termed valvular, subvalvular, or supravalvular aortic stenosis accordingly.

Epidemiology

Aortic stenoses constitute around 3 to 5% of all congenital heart defects. Boys are affected considerably more often than girls (4:1). A bicuspid aortic valve, which is often associated with an aortic stenosis ("minimal variant of an aortic stenosis"), is the most common cardiac anomaly of all (approx. 1% of all individuals).

Pathogenesis

The cause is probably a development disorder during the formation of the primitive left ventricle and the outflow tracts in early pregnancy. Fetal endocarditis has also been discussed as the cause of an aortic stenosis.

Classification

Classification of aortic stenoses is based on their location (▸ Fig. 15.72).

▸ **Valvular aortic stenosis.** A valvular aortic stenosis is by far the most common form of aortic stenosis (approx. 75%). In most cases, it is associated with a *bicuspid aortic valve* (▸ Fig. 15.73). A bicuspid aortic valve is present in

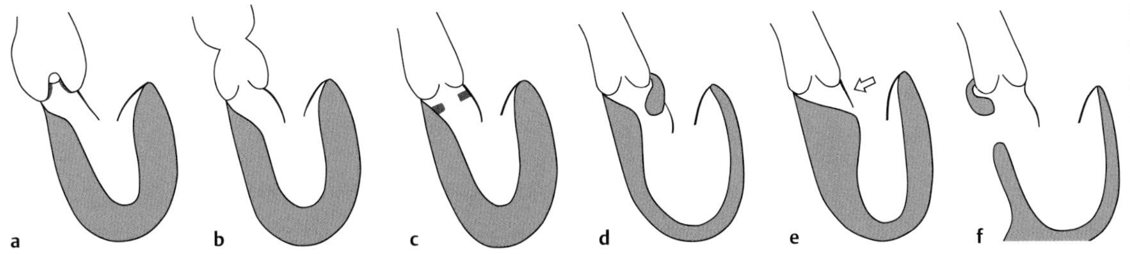

Fig. 15.72 Valvular, supravalvular, and subvalvular aortic stenosis.
a Valvular aortic stenosis with the typical doming of the aortic valve and poststenotic dilatation of the ascending aorta. **b** Supravalvular aortic stenosis. **c** Subvalvular aortic stenosis due to a fibrous membrane. **d** Subvalvular aortic stenosis due to a tunnel-like fibromuscular collar. **e** Subvalvular aortic stenosis associated with hypotrophic obstructive cardiomyopathy. **f** Subvalvular aortic stenosis associated with a malalignment VSD.

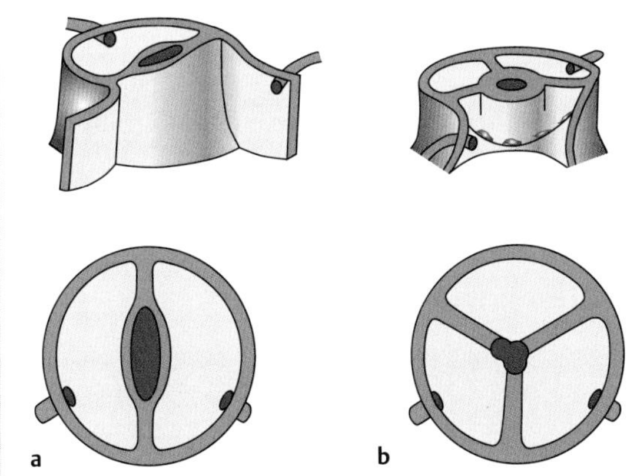

Fig. 15.73 Bicuspid aortic valve in the lateral view and from above (**a**) and stenotic tricuspid aortic valve with typical doming (**b**). [Adapted from Goor, Lillehei, 1975][109]

1% of all individuals. Without adhesions or thickening of the leaflets, a bicuspid aortic valve is a normal variant, but the risk of endocarditis is slightly increased. The morphology of the bicuspid valve can vary considerably; the valve opening is often eccentric. A bicuspid aortic valve usually does not cause any problems in childhood, but in adulthood, a relevant aortic stenosis may develop due to calcification or endocarditis. A bicuspid aortic valve is frequently associated with coarctation of the aorta; the valve is less often monocuspid in valvular aortic stenosis.

In *critical aortic stenosis* of the neonate, the valve often has thickened myxomatous leaflets, the lumen of the valve is severely obstructed ("buttonhole stenosis"), and the annulus is hypoplastic. In a critical aortic stenosis, there is a fluid transition to a hypoplastic left heart syndrome, as the intrauterine development of the left ventricle and the ascending aorta is generally not normal. Systemic blood flow is ductal dependent because insufficient cardiac output is pumped across the severely stenotic aortic valve.

► **Subvalvular aortic stenosis.** Subvalvular aortic stenosis is the second most common form of aortic stenosis (approx. 20%). The subvalvular outflow tract can be obstructed by:

- Fibrous membrane
- Tunnel-like fibromuscular collar
- Segments of the ventricular septum of a malalignment VSD

Subvalvular aortic stenoses are often not yet present at birth and do not develop until later. Circumscribed membranous subvalvular stenoses are more common and are possibly a result of turbulent blood flow in an unusually shaped left ventricular outflow tract. They are often associated with other cardiac anomalies such as VSD, PDA, or coarctation of the aorta. Such a membranous subvalvular stenosis can also develop secondarily after correction of certain defects (e.g., after closure of a VSD).

A tunnel-like fibromuscular obstruction is often associated with hypoplasia of the aortic valve annulus and the ascending aorta and with other left ventricular anomalies. For example, it is one component of the Shone complex (mitral stenosis due to a supravalvular annulus, parachute mitral valve, subaortic stenosis, and coarctation of the aorta).

Causes of subvalvular left ventricular outflow tract obstructions that should be differentiated from this are hypertrophic obstructive cardiomyopathy or a malalignment VSD, in which the ventricular septum can protrude into the left ventricular outflow tract.

Note

The otherwise normal aortic valve can be damaged and aortic insufficiency can develop as a result of the "stenosis jet" of a subvalvular aortic stenosis that hits the aortic valve.

► **Supravalvular aortic stenosis.** Supravalvular aortic stenosis is the least common form of aortic stenosis (under 5%). The obstruction is located above the

Table 15.8 Severity of aortic stenosis

Severity	Systolic pressure gradient	Valve opening size
I (insignificant)	<25 mmHg	<2.0 cm^2/m^2 BSA
II (mild)	25–49 mmHg	0.8–2.0 cm^2/m^2 BSA
III (moderate)	50–69 mmHg	0.5–0.8 cm^2/m^2 BSA
IV (severe)	>70 mmHg	<0.5 cm^2/m^2 BSA

BSA = body surface area.

unremarkable aortic valve. Up to 50% of cases of supravalvular aortic stenosis are associated with Williams–Beuren syndrome.

Isolated supravalvular aortic stenoses with an autosomal dominant inheritance pattern or sporadic occurrences are also possible.

▸ **Severity.** The severity of an aortic stenosis is determined based on the pressure gradients (▸ Table 15.8).

Hemodynamics

Left ventricular hypertrophy develops as a result of the increased pressure in the left ventricle. Poststenotic dilatation often develops in a valvular stenosis because of the turbulent blood flow. Aortic insufficiency can develop in a subvalvular stenosis as a result of the stenosis jet that hits the aortic valve.

Mild and moderate stenoses are usually well tolerated (slight hypertrophy, normal cardiac pump function). However, aortic stenosis is a progressive disease, in which stenosis often increases with growth. This leads to an increase in left ventricular hypertrophy, reduced ejection fraction, and diminished coronary blood flow with increased myocardial oxygen demand. This ultimately results in myocardial ischemia, which in turn causes an impaired cardiac output response to exercise. The patients are at risk of a stress-related syncope or sudden cardiac death.

Associated Cardiac Anomalies

Subvalvular stenoses in particular are associated with other cardiac anomalies (VSD, PDA, coarctation of the aorta).

Note

A bicuspid aortic valve is often associated with coarctation of the aorta.

The *Shone complex* is a combination of various left heart anomalies. The complete syndrome includes supravalvular mitral stenosis, mitral valve anomalies, subvalvular aortic stenosis, valvular aortic stenosis, aortic arch hypoplasia, and coarctation of the aorta.

In a critical aortic stenosis, intrauterine development of the left heart is abnormal, so the transition to a hypoplastic left heart syndrome is fluid.

Associated Syndromes

Supravalvular aortic stenoses occur in more than half of patients with Williams–Beuren syndrome. Other symptoms of this syndrome are peripheral pulmonary stenosis, stenoses of the aortic arch vessels and renal arteries, facial dysmorphism ("elfin" facial appearance, small or unusually shaped teeth), mental retardation, and a conspicuously deep, husky voice and cheerful demeanor.

15.22.2 Diagnostic Measures

Symptoms

Neonates with a *critical aortic stenosis* are already symptomatic and severely ill shortly after birth. They present the main symptoms of heart failure: tachypnea, tachycardia, poor feeding, cyanosis (right-to-left shunt across the ductus arteriosus), edema, hepatosplenomegaly, and arterial hypotension.

Note

The clinical picture of a critical aortic stenosis can be mistaken for sepsis. The diagnosis is made more difficult by the fact that no indicative cardiac murmur can be auscultated in the stage of cardiogenic shock because of reduced left ventricular ejection.

Children with *mild* or *moderate aortic stenoses* are usually asymptomatic in the first years of life and feel they have normal physical capacity (caution: danger of stress-related excessive increase of left ventricular pressure during sports resulting in infarction, arrhythmias / ventricular fibrillation, syncopes, or sudden cardiac death).

Aortic stenosis is usually diagnosed during investigation of a heart murmur.

Possible clinical symptoms of an aortic stenosis are easy fatigability, exercise-related dyspnea, angina pectoris, ventricular arrhythmias, and syncopes.

Patients with a supravalvular aortic stenosis can develop the *Coanda effect*: Since the stenosis jet is aimed directly into the brachiocephalic trunk and thus into the right subclavian artery, the blood pressure is higher in the right arm than in the left.

Auscultation

The indicative auscultation finding is a rough, spindle-shaped systolic ejection murmur with PMI in the 2nd/3rd right parasternal ICS, radiating into the carotid arteries.

The maximum sound is in the early systole in mild stenoses, and in the late systole as the obstruction increases. The murmur is usually relatively loud (3/6–5/6).

An ejection click is also typical for valvular stenoses. This is an extra early systolic extra sound (opening sound of the stenotic valve) that follows the first heart sound. The second heart sound is finely split, sometimes also paradoxically split in more severe stenosis.

Note

In neonates with critical aortic stenosis, the heart murmur is very soft and sometimes cannot be heard at all due to the reduced left ventricular ejection fraction.

ECG

In mild aortic stenoses, the ECG is unremarkable. More severe stenoses present with signs of left ventricular hypertrophy: tall R waves in the left precordial leads and deep S waves in the right precordial leads. There may be T wave inversion and ST segment depression (strain pattern) in the left precordial leads as a sign of subendocardial ischemia.

Overall, however, there is only a moderate correlation between the extent of the changes in the ECG and the severity of the stenosis.

Chest X-ray

The radiograph usually shows a normal-sized heart. A valvular stenosis typically presents with dilatation of the ascending aorta and/or a prominent aortic knob. The cardiac apex may be rounded and displaced in a caudal direction.

Neonates with a critical aortic stenosis present with cardiomegaly and signs of pulmonary edema.

Echocardiography

The diagnosis is made by echocardiography. Echocardiography can also be used to assess the severity. The following points must be investigated for every form of aortic stenosis:

- Number of leaflets (tricuspid, bicuspid, monocuspid)
- Assessment of possible aortic insufficiency
- Measurement of the aortic valve annulus (indispensable prior to planned balloon dilation or valve replacement)
- Determination of the pressure gradient by CW Doppler. The mean pressure gradient correlates much better with the actual gradient than the maximum gradient (V_{max}), because the maximum gradient overestimates the gradient
- Assessment of ventricular function and hypertrophy (septum thickness, left ventricular posterior wall)

Note

In a critical aortic stenosis, the gradient across the aortic valve is not informative.

The other typical findings for the various types of aortic stenosis are listed below.

► **Valvular stenosis.** Thickened leaflets with impaired movement, parachutelike doming of the fused leaflets with a turbulent central jet of color in the color Doppler sonogram during systole. In a bicuspid aortic valve, only two leaflets can be identified in the parasternal short axis. In the M mode across the bicuspid aortic valve, the coaptation line that represents valve closure is eccentric (► Fig. 15.74).

► **Subvalvular stenosis.** The subvalvular narrowing of the outflow tract may have a circumscribed ring shape (fibrous membrane) or a longer tunnel-like shape (fibromuscular collar). In the Doppler scan, flow acceleration begins below the aortic valve in the left ventricular outflow tract. The anterior leaflet of the mitral valve may be pulled into the outflow tract during systole by suction caused by the rapid flow in the outflow tract. This phenomenon is called "systolic anterior movement" (SAM).

► **Supravalvular stenosis.** A circumscribed or diffuse narrowing of the ascending aorta and flow acceleration can be detected in the CW Doppler scan.

Cardiac Catheterization

Cardiac catheterization may be indicated for a reliable assessment of the pressure gradient and before deciding on a corrective procedure. There is also the option of balloon valvuloplasty or angioplasty. Additional cardiac or coronary anomalies can also be ruled out.

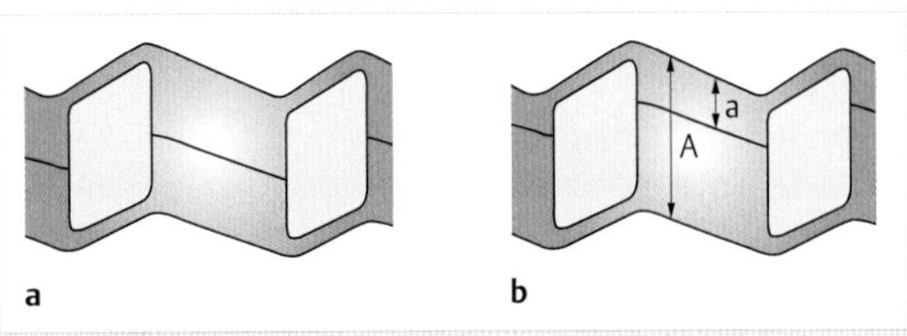

Fig. 15.74 Aortic valve in M mode in an unremarkable tricuspid aortic valve (**a**) and in a bicuspid valve (**b**). In the bicuspid valve, the coaptation line, which represents valve closure, is eccentric (distance a is not equal to half of distance A, as would be normal).

There is a distinct jump in pressure in the pull-back pressure curve from the left ventricle to the ascending aorta depending on the location of the stenosis.

The morphology of the aortic valve and the left ventricle can be visualized by angiography. In patients with Williams–Beuren syndrome, other vascular anomalies must be identified or ruled out by angiography (peripheral pulmonary stenoses, aortic arch anomalies, stenoses of the renal arteries).

MRI

MRI is not routinely needed, but it can help to visualize supravalvular stenoses better. In addition, the aortic valve opening size can be determined and left ventricular hypertrophy can be accurately visualized.

15.22.3 Treatment

Conservative Treatment

Neonates with a critical aortic stenosis require emergency treatment to maintain perfusion of the systemic circulation with prostaglandin E (initial dose 50 ng/kg/min). Catecholamines and diuretics are often needed to treat congestive heart failure. Other measures that may be needed are buffering with sodium bicarbonate and mechanical ventilation with a high PEEP for pulmonary edema. Rapid interventional or surgical treatment should be provided after the patient is stabilized.

Note

Subvalvular aortic stenoses should not be treated with digoxin or catecholamines because the pressure gradient in the left ventricular outflow tract can increase due to the medication-induced improvement in myocardial tone.

An attempt can be made to treat tunnel-like and primarily muscular subvalvular stenoses with calcium antagonists or beta blockers to bridge the time until surgery.

▸ **Indications for interventional catheterization or surgical treatment**

- Symptomatic patients
- Gradient over 50 to 60 mmHg (invasive measurement) or systolic gradient over 70 mmHg or mean pressure gradient over 40 mmHg (by Doppler ultrasound)
- Rapid progression of the gradient in a subvalvular aortic stenosis
- Impaired ventricular function
- Abnormal repolarization in the ECG
- Development of aortic insufficiency (affects mainly subvalvular aortic stenoses)

In small children, gradients higher than those indicated above are sometimes tolerated before the decision is made for interventional catheterization or surgical treatment. In cases of doubt, an exercise echocardiography may provide additional information on the increase in the gradient or the occurrence of symptom under stress.

Interventional Catheterization

Balloon valvuloplasty is now the treatment of choice for valvular aortic stenoses, but it is not a promising option for the less common subaortic stenoses and supravalvular aortic stenoses.

The results for balloon valvuloplasty in the treatment of valvular aortic stenosis are comparable with those of a commissurotomy, but not as good as results for balloon valvuloplasty of a pulmonary stenosis. The diameter of the balloon selected for the dilation is smaller or, at most, exactly as large as the aortic valve annulus, to minimize the (inevitable) postinterventional aortic insufficiency. By contrast, for balloon dilation of a pulmonary stenosis, a balloon is used that is larger than the valve annulus. Balloon valvuloplasty is contraindicated for more pronounced aortic insufficiency because of the risk of increasing insufficiency. Balloon valvuloplasty is not useful in a critical aortic stenosis with a hypoplastic left ventricle for which biventricular correction does not appear possible. In these cases, a Norwood procedure is performed as the first step toward univentricular palliation.

Surgical Treatment

▸ **Valvular aortic stenosis.** The preferred procedure for a valvular aortic stenosis is a *commissurotomy*, in which the fused valves in the area of the commissures are incised and the thickened valves are reconstructed (e.g., "shaving"). The results are comparable with those for balloon valvuloplasty.

In the event that there is more pronounced aortic insufficiency that cannot be reconstructed surgically, an artificial valve, a homograft, a bioprosthesis, or a Ross procedure are possible options.

In a *Ross procedure* the patient's own pulmonary valve is implanted in the aortic position and the pulmonary valve is replaced by a homograft (▸ Fig. 15.75). The procedure also involves transplanting the coronary arteries to the native pulmonary valve in the aortic position. The advantage of this method is that the neo-aortic valve generally has a long durability, grows with the patient, and unlike an artificial valve, does not require anticoagulation.

A *Ross–Konno procedure* is performed if there is a hypoplastic aortic valve annulus or an obstructed left ventricular outflow tract. First the valve annulus is split and widened. The left ventricular outflow tract must also be

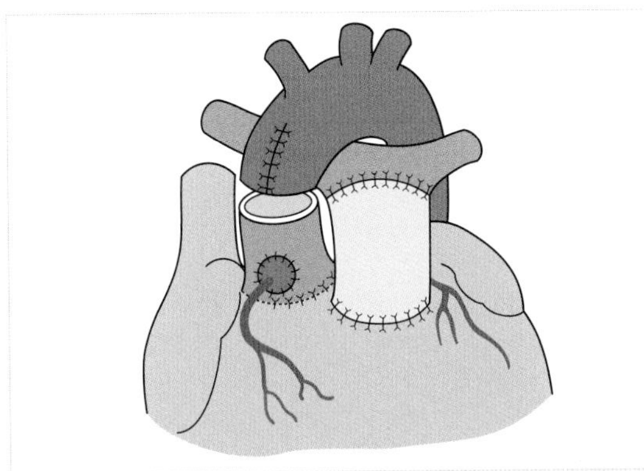

Fig. 15.75 Ross procedure. The patient's own pulmonary valve is implanted in the aortic position and replaced by a homograft. The procedure also involves transplanting the coronary arteries to the native pulmonary valve.

widened. To achieve this, the ventricular septum is split in the vicinity of the left ventricular outflow tract, creating a VSD, which is later closed with a patch. The outflow tract is widened by the patch.

The advantages of an *artificial valve replacement* are that it has a long usable life and is readily available. The valve does not grow with the patient, of course, and should therefore not be implanted until the patient has finished growing. In addition, lifelong anticoagulation is needed. For women who wish to have children, the teratogenic potential of Phenprocoumon or warfarin should be noted.

Bioprostheses are readily available and have the advantage that they do not require permanent anticoagulation. The usable life of the valve is limited considerably by degeneration and the fact that it does not grow with the patient, so a bioprosthesis must generally be replaced after a few years.

A human pulmonary or aortic valve, if possible with the same blood type, is usually used as a *homograft*. Lifelong anticoagulation is not necessary. However, homografts are available only to a limited extent and, like bioprostheses, must be replaced after a few years due to the failure to grow with the patients and degenerative processes.

▸ **Subvalvular aortic stenosis.** For a subaortic stenosis, the membrane or the fibromuscular collar is excised via a transaortic access. However, a recurrence develops later in almost one-third of cases. Postoperatively there is almost always a left bundle branch block. There is also a risk of complete AV block or an iatrogenic VSD. A Ross–Konno procedure may be necessary for severe and long, funnel-like stenoses. .

▸ **Supravalvular stenosis.** A patch enlargement of the ascending aorta is performed if there is a supravalvular stenosis.

▸ **Critical aortic stenosis with a transition to a hypoplastic left heart syndrome.** In these cases, the first step is univentricular palliation (Fontan procedure) by a Norwood I procedure within the first week of life (Chapter 15.20).

15.22.4 Prognosis and Clinical Course

▸ **Long-term outcome.** The postoperative mortality rate for neonates with a critical aortic stenosis with a sufficiently large left ventricle and no other cardiac anomalies is about 10%. For older children with a valvular aortic stenosis, the perioperative risk is about 1 to 2%. The early mortality of a Ross or Ross–Konno procedure is about 5%. The risk for a resection of a subaortic membrane is low, but up to 25% of the patients later develop a pressure gradient requiring treatment. Re-operations are necessary after bioprostheses and homografts are implanted due to valve degeneration and outgrowing the valve.

Note

An aortic stenosis is usually a progressive disease, in which the pressure gradient generally increases over time.

Balloon dilation and commissurotomy must be considered palliative procedures, as a remaining gradient remains and aortic insufficiency often develops. Re-operations (sometimes multiple) are the rule until definitive valve replacement (often mechanical) is performed.

▸ **Outpatient checkups.** Patients with an aortic stenosis must have regular cardiac examinations, as the extent of the stenosis usually increases over time and the gradient can sometimes become relevant even after years. In the echocardiography examination, particular attention must be paid to an increase in the gradient, the development of aortic insufficiency, and left ventricular function.

Even after a balloon valvuloplasty or commissurotomy, lifelong regular checkups, annually for older children and adults, are needed to detect the frequent occurrences of restenosis and aortic insufficiency.

Recurrences must be noted after resection of a subaortic stenosis, as they happen in 25% of patients.

After artificial valve replacement, patients require lifelong anticoagulation. After implantation of a valve prosthesis (mechanical, biological, homograft) endocarditis prophylaxis must be maintained. The same applies to reconstructed valves using foreign material or for the first 6 months after balloon dilation. If there are residual defects in the area of foreign material, these patients also require lifelong endocarditis prophylaxis.

▸ **Lifestyle and physical exercise capacity.** No limitation of physical activity is necessary in asymptomatic patients with a systolic gradient under 40 mmHg, an unremarkable ECG, and unremarkable exercise test. Isometric exercises and sports with a high dynamic component are not allowed for patients with a systolic gradient between 40 and 70 mmHg. No sports at all are allowed if the systolic gradient is over 70 mmHg (treatment indication).

▸ **Special aspects in adolescents and adults.** In adults, acquired aortic stenoses as a result of degenerative changes are more common. In patients over the age of 70, atherosclerotic changes are the most frequent cause of aortic stenosis. Aortic stenoses are less commonly due to postinflammatory/rheumatic causes. A bicuspid aortic valve predisposes a patient to aortic stenosis. It often does not become symptomatic until age 40 to 60 years.

In some adults with a high perioperative risk, interventional catheterization, in which an artificial aortic valve is implanted percutaneously (e.g., via the inguinal artery), may be an option.

15.23 Aortic Insufficiency

15.23.1 Basics

Definition

In aortic insufficiency, the aortic valve closes incompletely; this leads to reverse blood flow to the left ventricle during diastole. The failure to close can be a result of valve dysplasia, dilatation of the aortic root, prolapse of an aortic leaflet, or destruction of the valve (▸ Fig. 15.76). There may be acute or chronic aortic insufficiency depending on the etiology and course.

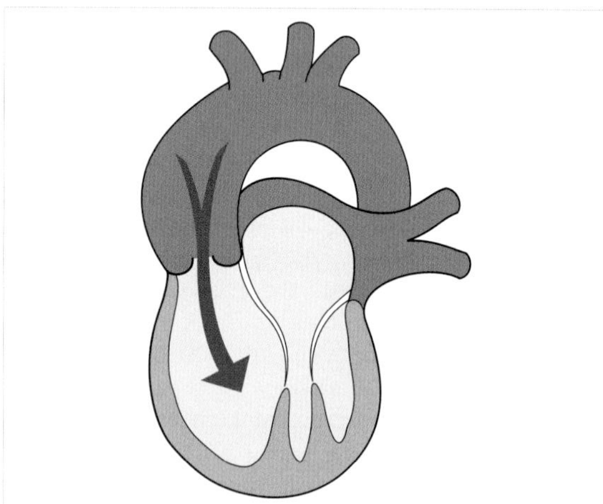

Fig. 15.76 Aortic insufficiency. Effect of chronic aortic insufficiency on the morphology of the heart and ascending aorta. In the long term this causes dilatation of the left ventricle and ascending aorta.

Epidemiology

An isolated aortic insufficiency is very rare in childhood. It usually occurs in association with other cardiac anomalies or after procedures performed at the aortic valve.

Classification

Aortic insufficiency is classified as acute or chronic. The two forms have different causes and the symptoms and clinical courses vary.

Etiology

- Acute aortic insufficiency:
  - Infectious endocarditis
  - Aortic dissection (e.g., in Marfan syndrome)
  - Acute result of a balloon valvuloplasty of the aortic valve
  - Trauma
- Chronic aortic insufficiency:
  - Bicuspid aortic valve: occurs in around 1% of individuals and is a predisposing factor for aortic stenosis and insufficiency (usually not becoming manifest until adulthood)
  - Aortic valve prolapse
  - Aneurysm of the ascending aorta (e.g., in association with Marfan syndrome)
  - VSD: In association with a perimembranous or infundibular VSD, a leaflet may prolapse into the VSD. The hemodynamic result is aortic insufficiency.
  - Rheumatic heart disease: Rheumatic fever is a frequent cause of aortic insufficiency, especially in developing countries.
  - Arterial hypertension
  - Residua after surgical or interventional catheter valvuloplasty

After a prosthetic aortic valve replacement, insufficiency can develop as a result of prosthesis dehiscence or paravalvular leakage. The degeneration of a bioprosthesis or homograft can also cause aortic insufficiency.

Associated Cardiac Defects

Aortic insufficiency can be associated with any other congenital heart defect. It occurs most frequently as a combined defect with aortic stenosis. The most common associated cardiac defects are:

- Bicuspid aortic valve
- Aortic stenosis
- Coarctation of the aorta (often associated with a bicuspid aortic valve)
- VSD
- d-TGA
- Tetralogy of Fallot
- truncus arteriosus

Pathology and Hemodynamics

The inability of an aortic valve to close leads to diastolic backflow to the left ventricle. The additional fluctuating volume causes volume overload in the left ventricle, resulting in compensatory left ventricular hypertrophy and dilatation of the left ventricle. The left ventricle can initially compensate the volume overload to a certain extent by an increase in compliance. *Mild chronic aortic insufficiency* can be tolerated for years.

Severe aortic insufficiency leads to reduced left ventricular function over time. Due to the diastolic blood flow into the left ventricle, the diastolic blood pressure is reduced and can, especially on exertion, lead to insufficient coronary perfusion. The increased ejection volume also leads to dilatation of the ascending aorta.

In *acute aortic insufficiency,* the left ventricle is not capable of adjusting to the sometimes massive volume overload. This can quickly lead to pulmonary congestion and edema.

15.23.2 Diagnostic Measures

Symptoms

Aortic insufficiency is usually only mild and causes few symptoms. The affected children may be unremarkable for years. In the clinical examination, wide pulse pressures are a result of the increased pulse volume and rapid drop in blood pressure due to regurgitation across the aortic valve. The pulses are accordingly strong ("water hammer pulse"). However, a water hammer pulse can also be observed in other situations in which there is an increased pulse volume or diastolic run-off, for example, fever or anemia, or in a large AV fistula or relevant PDA.

Symptomatic patients present with symptoms of heart failure such as exertional dyspnea or signs of reduced coronary perfusion (atypical angina pectoris).

In *acute aortic insufficiency,* there is sudden dyspnea, tachycardia, and sometimes severe chest pain (in this event, chest pain is usually a sign of aortic dissection).

Auscultation

The typical auscultation finding is a high frequency, blowing diastolic decrescendo murmur that can be heard along the left sternal border. The murmur is best auscultated when the patient is sitting or leaning forward. An *Austin–Flint murmur* is a low frequency mid-diastolic murmur with PMI over the cardiac apex which sounds similar to a mitral stenosis murmur. It is probably caused by reverse blood flow to the left ventricle due to aortic insufficiency, which competes with the blood flow across the mitral valve and impairs the opening of the mitral valve.

A paradoxical split second heart sound can be caused by the delayed closing of the aortic valve as a result of the increased left ventricular pulse volume. A gallop rhythm is a sign of already clearly reduced left ventricular function.

ECG

Typical signs of chronic aortic insufficiency are signs of left ventricular hypertrophy (left axis deviation, prominent Q waves, tall R waves, and ST segment changes in the left ventricular leads).

Chest X-ray

The X-ray image shows a dilated ascending aorta. The aortic knob appears prominent in the X-ray image. In a relevant aortic insufficiency, enlargement of the left ventricle leads to cardiomegaly, which corresponds to the extent of chronic insufficiency. The cardiac waist is prominent. In decompensated aortic insufficiency, the left atrium is also enlarged and there are signs of pulmonary congestion or edema.

Echocardiography

Echocardiography can be used to confirm the diagnosis, clarify the underlying cause, and determine the extent of aortic insufficiency.

In particular, the shape and thickness of the leaflets should be noted (thickened or fused? bicuspid or tricuspid? vegetation? prolapse of a leaflet?). The size and morphology of the aortic root and ascending aorta should also be assessed (aneurysm of the ascending aorta?). There is typically end-diastolic dilatation of the left ventricle in chronic aortic insufficiency. The fractional shortening of the left ventricle is increased.

Note

"Normal", impaired or deteriorating left ventricular function in aortic insufficiency is always a warning sign.

The extent of the regurgitation jet across the aortic valve can be visualized with color Doppler ultrasound. The color jet is limited to the outflow tract if the insufficiency is mild. Because of the rapid equalization of pressure between the left ventricle and the aorta in aortic insufficiency, the regurgitation velocity drops rapidly in the CW Doppler flow profile. A pressure half-time of 300 ms or less is a sign of severe insufficiency. Diastolic flutter movement of the anterior mitral leaflet caused by the regurgitation jet of the adjacent aortic valve is an indirect sign of aortic insufficiency.

In acute aortic insufficiency, the end-diastolic diameter of the left ventricle is not generally widened. Left ventricular function is typically limited or normal. Especially in acute severe aortic insufficiency, there is premature closure of the mitral valve appearing in the ECG even before the P wave.

Cardiac Catheterization

Cardiac catheterization is not routinely needed. In individual cases it can be used to identify associated cardiac anomalies or to measure left ventricular function and degree of insufficiency accurately. Preoperatively, it can also provide details on the course of the coronary arteries.

MRI

MRI may provide additional information on the morphology of the valve and on the thoracic aorta and quantification of left ventricular function and regurgitation volume.

15.23.3 Treatment

Conservative Treatment

Pharmacological afterload reduction is a major component of conservative treatment. The drugs of choice in childhood are ACE inhibitors, which are indicated for all patients who present with more than slight aortic insufficiency, are symptomatic, and/or suffer from arterial hypertension. Patients with Marfan syndrome should be administered angiotensin receptor antagonists or beta blockers routinely.

For acute or decompensated chronic aortic insufficiency, intravenous afterload reducers such as sodium nitroprusside and positive inotropic substances (dobutamine, milrinone) and intravenous diuretics are administered.

▸ **Indications for surgical valve reconstruction or replacement**

- Signs of heart failure
- Evidence of myocardial ischemia
- Decreasing left ventricular function

Surgical Treatment

Surgical valve reconstruction must be weighed against valve replacement. It should also be noted that dilatation of the aortic root or ascending aorta sometimes also has to be surgically corrected (e.g., annuloplasty, replacement of the ascending aorta including reimplantation of the coronary arteries), making the procedure considerably more complex. The disadvantage of replacing the aortic valve with an artificial valve is that lifelong anticoagulation is needed; the disadvantage of a biological prosthesis is its shorter lifespan.

The Ross procedure is an alternative to valve replacement (Chapter Fig. 15.22). The patient's own pulmonary valve is implanted in the aortic valve position and a homograft is implanted between the right ventricle and pulmonary artery as a pulmonary valve. This operation is technically complicated and involves reimplantation of the coronary arteries, but it is the only method that allows growth of the neo-aortic valve. A Ross procedure is contraindicated in patients with dilatation of the aortic root as a result of a connective tissue disease (e.g., Marfan syndrome), as similar changes can also be expected in the autologous pulmonary valve after it is implanted in an aortic position.

15.23.4 Prognosis and Clinical Course

▸ **Long-term outcome.** Many patients with chronic aortic insufficiency remain asymptomatic for years, as the left ventricle can adapt well to the chronic volume overload. However, acute aortic insufficiency usually quickly leads to left heart failure.

▸ **Outpatient checkups.** Regular outpatient checkups at least once a year are necessary even for mild aortic insufficiency. More frequent checkups are needed for all patients with moderate to severe aortic insufficiency to establish an indication for surgery in time. In particular, increase in size of the left ventricle, decrease in left ventricular function, evidence of myocardial ischemia in the ECG or patient's history, and signs of heart failure.

Long-term endocarditis prophylaxis is needed for all patients after implantation of a prosthetic valve (mechanical, biological, homograft). After reconstruction of a heart valve using foreign material, endocarditis prophylaxis is recommended for 6 months and lifelong if there are residual defects in the vicinity of patches or prosthetic material.

▸ **Physical exercise capacity and lifestyle.** Patients with mild to moderate aortic insufficiency and a normal-sized left ventricle have no restrictions regarding physical exercise capacity or engaging in sports, but patients with left ventricular hypertrophy, arrhythmias, or significant dilatation of the ascending aorta are subject to restrictions. Depending on the extent of the findings, these patients must avoid sports with a high level of static stress in particular. In severe cases, all sports must be avoided. Patients with Marfan syndrome who have aortic insufficiency should not engage in competitive sports.

▸ **Special features in adolescents and adults.** In adults, degenerative vascular and connective tissue diseases are the major causes of aortic insufficiency. A majority of patients with aortic insufficiency who were diagnosed in childhood do not become symptomatic and need treatment until adulthood. For women who wish to have children, the teratogenicity of vitamin K antagonists

(Phenprocoumon, warfarin) after artificial valve replacement must be noted.

15.24 Coarctation of the Aorta

15.24.1 Basics

Synonyms: coarctatio aortae, aortic coarctation

Definition

Coarctation of the aorta is a narrowing of the aorta at the junction between the distal aortic arch and the descending aorta.

Epidemiology

Coarctation of the aorta constitutes 8 to 10% of all congenital heart defects. Boys are affected about twice as often as girls.

Pathogenesis

There are two theories of the pathogenesis of aortic coarctation: The first is that it is probably due to decreased blood flow in the aortic isthmus in the embryonic period. This theory is most likely true especially if there are associated intrauterine cardiac defects that lead to decreased blood flow to the aortic arch and the isthmus region. Due to reduced perfusion, the isthmus region cannot develop properly and remains hypoplastic. In such cases there is often not only localized coarctation, but also tubular hypoplasia of the aortic arch proximal to the isthmus.

Another theory assumes that scattered ductal tissue is present in the posterior aortic wall that contracts postnatally and leads to stenosis. This idea is supported by the fact that coarctation often becomes clinically manifest when the ductus arteriosus closes postnatally, and during surgery additional ductal tissue can be removed in the area of coarctation.

Classification

The earlier classification in pre- and postductal coarctation of the aorta as infantile and adult coarctation is misleading and has largely been abandoned. In most cases, the stenosis is neither pre- nor postductal but rather, juxtaductal—directly opposite the ductal opening.

Pathology

In most patients there is a circumscribed juxtaductal coarctation of the aorta (▶ Fig. 15.77). Macroscopically there is a notch in the posterior aortic wall (posterior shelf).

A long segment of tubular hypoplasia of the transverse aortic arch proximal to the coarctation occurs mainly in patients with an additional obstruction of the left ventricular outflow tract or a VSD. In these cases, the decreased perfusion of the aortic arch during the embryonic period probably led to the underdevelopment of the aortic arch and isthmus.

In rare cases, coarctation can be found in other aortic segments such as the abdominal aorta. In such cases, there are often additional vascular stenoses (e.g., renal artery stenosis).

Hemodynamics

In the critical coarctation of the aorta in the neonate, adequate blood flow to the lower half of the body is dependent on the patency of the ductus arteriosus, through which the right ventricle supplies the lower half of the body with blood. Accordingly, oxygen saturation in the legs is reduced (the hemodynamic situation corresponds to the fetal circulation). When the ductus closes, the lower half of the body is no longer or only inadequately perfused. The acute increase in afterload leads to rapid ventricular decompensation (congestive heart failure, shock).

If coarctation is less pronounced, there is chronic pressure overload of the left ventricle. A pressure gradient is present between the upper and lower halves of the body; blood pressure in the upper half of the body is hypertonic (prestenotic component of the systemic circulation), but pressure in the lower half of the body is decreased or normal. Over time, collateral circulation develops (via the intercostal arteries and the internal thoracic artery) between the upper and lower halves of the body.

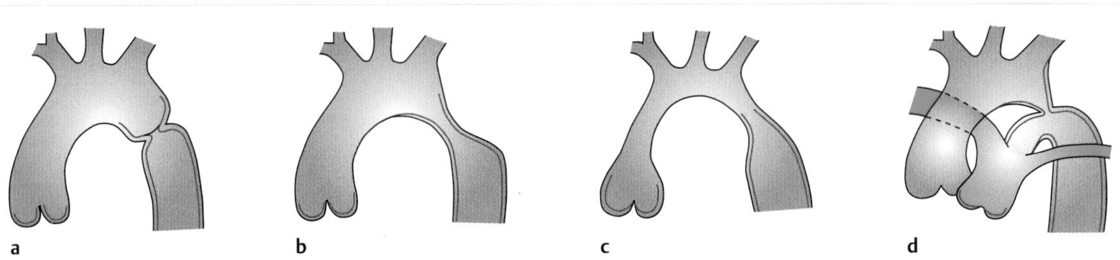

Fig. 15.77 Forms of coarctation of the aorta. **a** Circumscribed aortic coarctation. **b** Tubular aortic coarctation. **c** Aortic coarctation with hypoplasia of the entire aortic arch. **d** Critical coarctation of the aorta with ductal-dependent systemic perfusion.

> **Note**
>
> A blood pressure gradient between the upper and lower halves of the body may be absent in neonates with severe congestive heart failure or with a PDA.

Associated Cardiac Anomalies

Associated cardiac anomalies are common with coarctation of the aorta. Up to 85% of coarctations of the aorta are associated with a bicuspid aortic valve.

In a *complex coarctation of the aorta*, there are other associated cardiac anomalies in addition to a PDA. These cases often have dramatic clinical manifestations in the neonatal period. Common associated cardiac anomalies are left ventricular obstructions or a VSD, which lead to decreased intrauterine perfusion of the aortic arch and the isthmus region:

- Bicuspid aortic valve
- Aortic stenosis
- Shone complex (combination of different obstructions of the left heart)
- Hypoplastic left heart syndrome
- VSD
- AV canal
- d-TGA
- DORV with subpulmonary VSD (Taussig–Bing anomaly)

Vascular anomalies are also frequently observed:

- Stenosis at the origin of the left subclavian artery
- Arteria lusoria (in this case the right subclavian artery arises as the last branch from the aortic arch distal to the left subclavian artery and runs to the right behind the esophagus)
- Cerebral aneurysms

Associated Syndromes

Aortic coarctation occurs often in combination with Turner syndrome. Around 30% of these patients have aortic coarctation. Rarely, aortic coarctation is associated with the following syndromes: Ellis-van Creveld syndrome, Holt–Oram syndrome, Marfan syndrome, Down syndrome.

15.24.2 Diagnostic Measures

Symptoms

The clinical symptoms of aortic coarctation vary considerably depending on the severity of the stenosis and associated anomalies. On the one hand there is the critical coarctation of the aorta, which can manifest itself as early as in the neonatal period with the clinical features of cardiogenic shock (i.e., neonatal form). On the other hand, there are clinical courses in which patients do no become symptomatic until later in childhood or even adulthood (i.e., adult form).

Symptomatic coarctation of the aorta in the neonatal period:

- Rapidly progressive heart failure with poor feeding, tachypnea/dyspnea, hepatosplenomegaly, grayish-pallid skin tone.
- Weakened or absent femoral pulses.
- If there is severe congestive heart failure, the left ventricle is not able to build up adequate blood pressure. The lower body is perfused through the PDA.
- Ductal-dependent perfusion of the lower half of the body results in differential cyanosis. If there is critical aortic coarctation, the lower half of the body is supplied with venous blood via a right-to-left shunt at the ductal level. A relevant difference in pulse oximetry exists between the right arm (preductal) and the legs (postductal).
- Because of the diminished perfusion of the lower half of the body, there is a danger of renal failure, acidosis, and necrotic enterocolitis.
- No cardiac murmur can be auscultated in about half of cases. A systolic murmur can sometimes be heard if there is an associated VSD or other cardiac anomalies. If ventricular function is significantly impaired, there may be a gallop rhythm.

Manifestation in older children, adolescents and adults:

- Leading symptoms are weakened or absent foot/inguinal pulses and a systolic blood pressure gradient between upper and lower halves of the body.
- Hypertension of the upper half of the body with headache, dizziness and nosebleeds.
- Cold feet, calf pain during exercise, intermittent claudication (decreased perfusion of the lower extremity).

Auscultation

In a severe coarctation of the aorta that is already symptomatic in the neonatal period, a murmur is often absent. In older children, a late systolic spindle-shaped murmur with a PMI in the infraclavicular area and between the shoulder blades is typical. A systolic murmur can also be heard if there is a bicuspid aortic valve. A continuous vascular murmur in the back is a sign of collaterals between the upper and lower halves of the body.

ECG

In a critical coarctation of the aorta of a neonate, the ECG initially shows signs of right ventricular hypertrophy because the right ventricle has to supply the lower body through the PDA. Left ventricular hypertrophy does not develop until after the closure of the ductus.

The ECG of older children is often normal. Otherwise there are signs of left ventricular hypertrophy and possibly corresponding repolarization disturbances.

Chest X-ray

Critically ill neonates have cardiomegaly and possibly signs of pulmonary edema as an expression of congestive heart failure.

In older children, a dilated ascending aorta and a prominent aortic knob can be seen. The heart size is usually normal. Rib notching is pathognomonic: these notches at the caudal edge of the ribs are caused by the dilated intercostal arteries (collateral circulation). Such changes are not found until the children are older. The "figure of 3" sign is an indentation in the course of the descending aorta shaped like the number 3.

Echocardiography

In children, coarctation of the aorta can be reliably diagnosed by echocardiography. In adolescents and adults, other imaging techniques are sometimes needed.

The coarctation of the aorta can usually be best visualized in the suprasternal view with the neck hyperextended or in the right parasternal view. In neonates, the isthmus can also be readily visualized from the subcostal direction.

In a circumscribed coarctation of the aorta, there is typically a posterior infolding of the aortic wall ("posterior shelf") after the origin of the left subclavian artery with poststenotic dilatation. It must be assumed to be hemodynamically relevant if the stenosis diameter is less than 4 mm in a mature neonate.

The diagnosis can be difficult to make if the ductus arteriosus is still patent. In these cases, it can be difficult to clearly circumscribe the stenosis. The following characteristic findings may be indirect signs of coarctation of the aorta:

- The left subclavian artery often arises quite far distally from the aortic arch.
- The aortic arch may also appear angular in aortic coarctation (▶ Fig. 15.78).

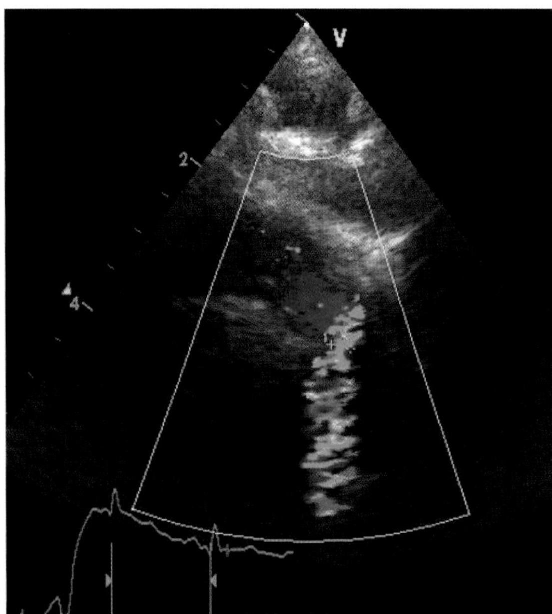

Fig. 15.78 Echocardiographic image of a circumscribed aortic coarctation. The image shows the typical finding of a circumscribed coarctation of the aorta in the suprasternal long axis. The "angular" aortic arch and the changes in color in the stenotic region can be seen.

- If there is critical coarctation of the aorta with ductal-dependent perfusion of the lower half of the body, a right-to-left shunt occurs via the ductus arteriosus.

The ascending aorta, the entire aortic arch, the isthmus region, and the descending aorta must be measured. Hypoplasia of the transverse arch is not uncommon, especially when there are other obstructions of the left heart or a VSD. The length of the stenotic aortic segment must be measured. The head and neck vessels and renal arteries should also be examined to rule out stenosis.

It is also important to determine the size and function of the left ventricle. In a critical coarctation of the aorta, there is usually dilatation of the left ventricle with impaired left ventricular function.

Additional anomalies must be excluded, in particular a bicuspid aortic valve, additional obstructions of the left heart, or a VSD.

The CW Doppler can determine the gradient above the stenosis. Typically there is a "saw-tooth curve" above the stenosis (▶ Fig. 15.79). The CW Doppler can also show the more rapid flow in the area of the stenosis that overlays the slower prestenotic flow; this can sometimes be seen in the form of flow profile overlay in the Doppler curve. An important sign and indirect evidence of a coarctation of the aorta is reduced flow in the abdominal aorta or the celiac trunk.

Cardiac Catheterization

In most cases, diagnostic cardiac catheterization is not necessary. Cardiac catheterization is indicated primarily if interventional therapy is planned. Additional anomalies or anatomy that cannot be clearly visualized in echocardiography can usually be visualized or ruled out using other imaging techniques.

MRI

The aortic isthmus and the entire aorta can be visualized very well by MRI. Associated anomalies and collateral vessels can be reliably visualized. The 3D reconstruction of the aorta including the isthmus is often quite

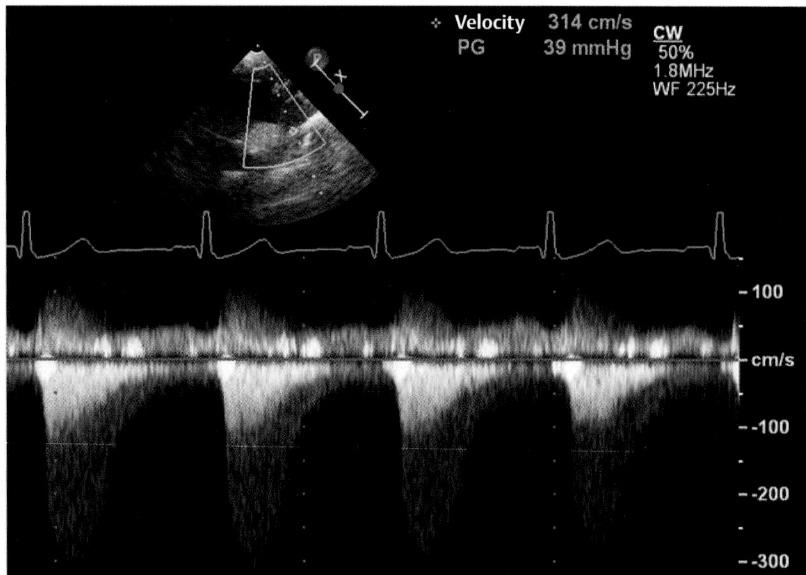

Fig. 15.79 Saw-tooth wave of an aortic coarctation in the CW Doppler sonogram. In CW Doppler, a typical saw-tooth profile can be seen across the stenosis. The overlay of the prestenotic and stenotic flow profile can also be seen clearly in this image.

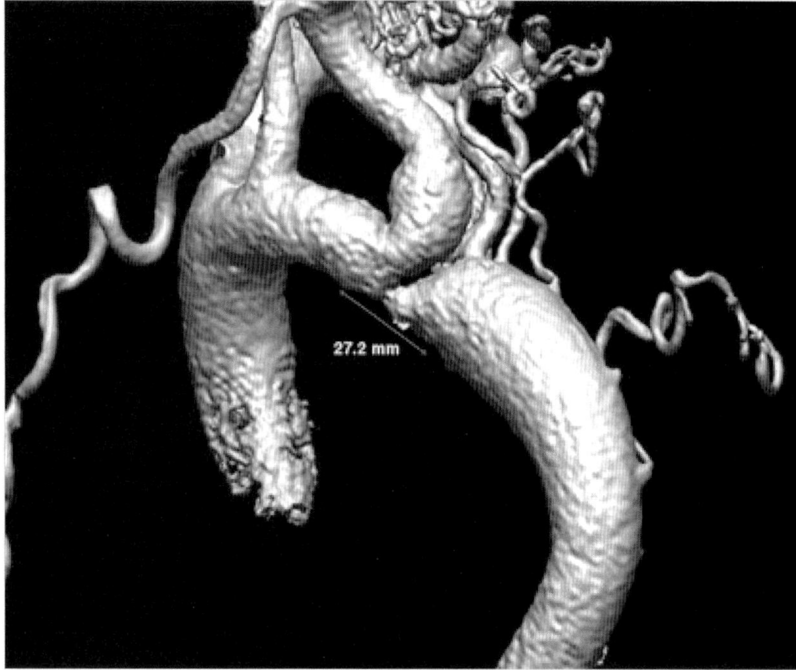

Fig. 15.80 MRI 3D reconstruction of an aortic coarctation. The 3D reconstruction clearly illustrates the anatomy of a circumscribed coarctation of the aorta.

impressive (▶ Fig. 15.80). After interventional or surgical treatment, aneurysms in the isthmus region can be visualized or ruled out. Disadvantages of MRI are that the pressure gradient cannot be directly determined as in cardiac catheterization and no interventions are possible.

15.24.3 Treatment

Conservative Treatment

If there is a critical coarctation of the aorta, a continuous prostaglandin E infusion (initially 50 ng/kg/min) can be administered to maintain or re-establish the patency of the ductus arteriosus until surgical treatment is possible.

Catecholamines and diuretics may be administered to treat congestive heart failure. Administration of additional oxygen should be avoided as it reduces the right-to-left shunt across the ductus by reducing pulmonary resistance. If ventilation is required, mild hypoventilation with a high PEEP should be attempted to increase pulmonary resistance. Afterload reduction (e.g., with sodium nitroprusside) may be useful for improving systemic perfusion.

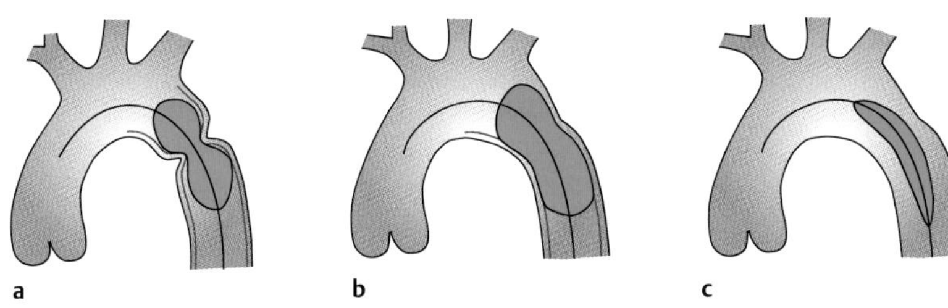

Fig. 15.81 Balloon dilation of coarctation of the aorta. The balloon catheter is advanced into the aorta from a retrograde arterial access (**a**). In the region of the coarctation of the aorta, the stenosis is dilated by pumping the balloon (**b**). After deflating the balloon, the success of the procedure can be assessed (**c**).

▶ **Indications for interventional catheterization or surgery**

- Critical coarctation of the aorta in neonates
- Systolic blood pressure gradient between the upper and lower halves of the body higher than 20 mmHg
- Hypertension of the upper half of the body above the 97th percentile

Interventional Catheterization

Interventional catheter balloon angioplasty of coarctation of the aorta is the treatment method of choice in older children, adolescents, and adults. In adolescents and adults, interventional catheter balloon angioplasty is generally combined with implantation of a stent in the isthmus. Interventional catheterization is also the method of choice for the treatment of (postoperative) restenoses.

In neonates, the rate of restenosis is too high, so balloon angioplasty is not the standard therapy for this age group. This method may be used as a palliative measure if surgery is not an option due to other reasons.

In balloon angioplasty, the isthmus stenosis is dilated gradually until the balloon diameter has reached 2.5 to 3 times the isthmus diameter (▶ Fig. 15.81). The maximum balloon diameter should not be larger than the prestenotic diameter of the aortic arch or the aorta at the level of the diaphragm. In adolescents and adults, when the final size of the aortic diameter has been (almost) reached, an additional stent may be implanted, which can be dilated at a later time.

Possible complications are aneurysms caused by intima lesions, restenosis, aortic rupture, stent dislocation, or thromboembolic complications in the region of the arterial catheter access.

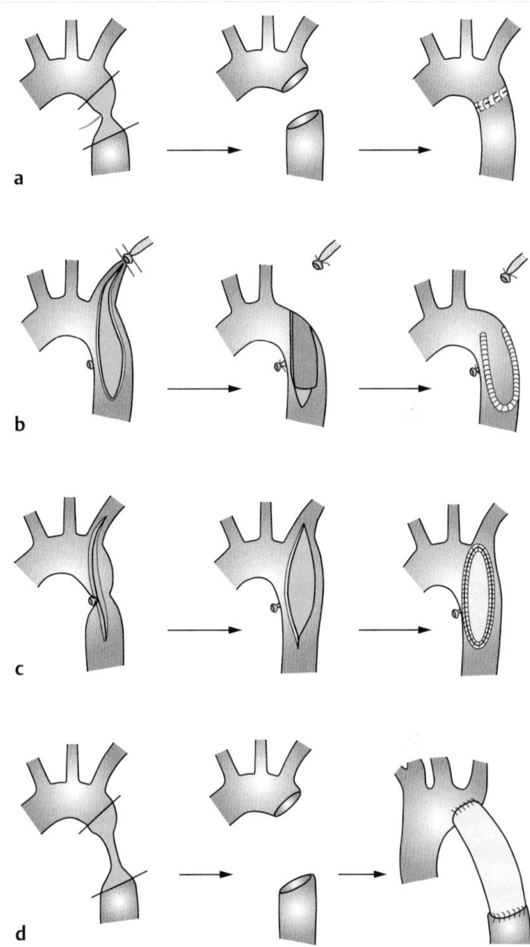

Fig. 15.82 Surgical procedures for treating coarctation of the aorta. **a** Resection and end-to-end anastomosis. **b** "Subclavian flap" aortoplasty. **c** Patch augmentation. **d** Conduit implantation (Adapted from Park 2008)[29].

Surgical Treatment

Surgery is the method of choice for an untreated coarctation of the aorta in neonates. Different procedures may be used, generally by means of a left lateral thoracotomy without cardiopulmonary bypass:

- *Resection of the coarctation of the aorta and end-to-end anastomosis* (▶ Fig. 15.82 **a**). In this procedure, the stenosis is resected and the proximal and distal ends of the aorta are anastomosed. If there is a longer stenotic segment or tubular hypoplasia of the aortic arch, extended oblique resection followed by an end-to-end anastomosis is necessary.
- *"Subclavian flap" aortoplasty* (▶ Fig. 15.82 **b**): In this procedure, which is only used in rare exceptions today, the isthmus is widened by turning down a segment of the left subclavian artery to patch it. Postoperatively,

the blood pressure in the left arm is low due to the surgery. The postoperative blood supply to the left arm is from collateral vessels.

- *Augmentation with a Dacron/Gore-Tex patch* (▶ Fig. 15.82 **c**): In this procedure, the aorta in the isthmus region is incised longitudinally and the isthmus is widened with an oval patch. This procedure is rarely performed today because it has the highest rate of restenosis at 50%, and one-third of cases develop aneurysms at the operation site.
- *Conduit implantation* (▶ Fig. 15.82 **d**): Implantation of a conduit for long segments of severe stenosis is only rarely needed. The disadvantage of this procedure is that as the patient grows, it may be necessary to replace the conduit.

If there is simultaneously a VSD, a decision must be made whether to correct both defects in a single operation by means of a median sternotomy with cardiopulmonary bypass, or whether to first correct the isthmus stenosis through a left lateral thoracotomy and then close the VSD at a later stage if necessary.

Potential specific postoperative complications are:

- Paradoxical postoperative hypertension due to a regulation disorder of the prestenotic baroreceptors that are accustomed to elevated blood pressure
- Spinal cord ischemia and paraplegia due to extended aortic clamping time and insufficient collateralization (extremely rare)
- Early restenosis: in residual, insufficiently resected ectopic ductal tissue, mostly after pretreatment with prostaglandins
- Recurrent/phrenic nerve paresis
- Chylothorax
- Secondary bleeding from collaterals and area of the sutures (especially if there is postoperative hypertension)
- Post-coarctation syndrome: nausea 4–8 days postoperatively, colicky abdominal pain, ileus, tarry stools due to postoperative “unaccustomed” volume of mesenteric blood, particularly if there is untreated hypertension postoperatively

15.24.4 Prognosis and Clinical Course

▶ **Long-term outcome.** The perioperative mortality rate after surgical correction of an isolated coarctation of the aorta in neonates is around 3.5%. If a VSD is closed simultaneously, the mortality rate is slightly higher, but below 10%. In older children, the mortality rate after surgery or catheter intervention is less than 1%.

Patients with untreated coarctation of the aorta have a limited life expectancy. There is an increased risk for aneurysm, rupture or dissection of the aorta, endarteritis, myocardial infarction, retinal damage, and strokes.

The restenosis rate and the rate of relevant residual stenosis is about 5 to 10% for operations in older children. In critical coarctation of the aorta, which may require early surgery, the rates are much higher.

The risk of postoperative persistent arterial hypertension, despite effective elimination of the stenosis, increases with the age at the time the correction was made.

Patients with mild forms of aortic coarctation have practically a normal life expectancy after surgery.

▶ **Outpatient checkups.** Even after correction of aortic coarctation, lifelong regular (e.g., annual) checkups are necessary. The checkups include blood pressure measurements on all limbs to rule out restenosis and hypertension. In echocardiography, in addition to restenosis, special attention should be paid to the possible development of an aneurysm in the area of the operation and dilatation of the ascending aorta. Particularly in elderly patients, there are sometimes limitations to echocardiography, so an MRI may be required for the reliable assessment of the area that was operated. An aneurysm should be repaired surgically immediately.

If left ventricular function was reduced preoperatively, frequent monitoring is necessary until function is recovered. If there is an associated bicuspid aortic valve, special attention must be given to the development of an aortic stenosis or regurgitation. Persistent arterial hypertension is an indication for antihypertensive drug therapy. Beta blockers are generally used for this purpose. If there is relevant hypertension, even trivial residual gradients should be treated with interventional catheterization. Exercise tests should be performed every 3 to 4 years.

Endocarditis prophylaxis for the first 6 months after surgery is recommended after an interventional catheter stenting or surgical correction using foreign material. Residual defects in the area of foreign material necessitate long-term endocarditis prophylaxis.

▶ **Physical exercise capacity and lifestyle.** If the systolic pressure gradient between the upper and lower limbs is over 20 mmHg or there is exercise-induced hypertension, sports are not permitted until definitive therapy is undertaken, except for sports with a low dynamic and no static stress.

Competitive sports are allowed 3 months after surgery or catheter intervention if the residual gradient is below 20 mmHg and the blood pressure at rest and during exercise is normal. Pronounced isometric stress should still be avoided. Of course, restrictions on sports apply if a significant aortic dilatation or aneurysm has developed in the surgical area.

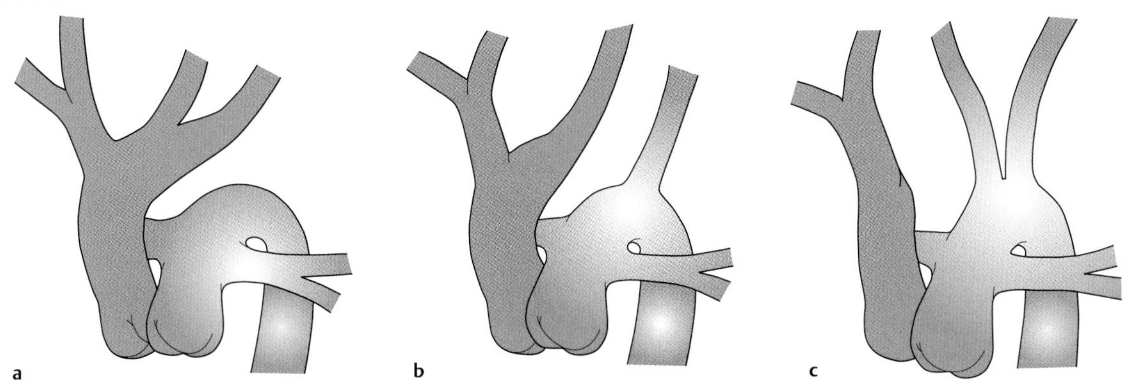

Fig. 15.84 Types of interrupted aortic arch. **a** Type A: Interruption of the aortic arch distal to the left subclavian artery. **b** Type B: Interruption of the aortic arch between the common carotid artery and the unilateral subclavian artery. **c** Type C: Interruption between the two common carotid arteries.

► **Special aspects in adolescents and adults.** Most patients who were not diagnosed with coarctation of the aorta until adolescence or adulthood are asymptomatic. The diagnosis is usually made when a heart murmur or arterial hypertension is noted and investigated in a physical examination.

The majority of adult patients, however, have been treated surgically or by interventional catheterization. In these patients, attention must be paid to aneurysms in the operated isthmus, which develop in up to 30% of patients, especially after patch augmentation, and need to be repaired surgically. Restenosis is also not uncommon. Because of the frequent association with a bicuspid aortic valve, valvular aortic stenosis or regurgitation occasionally develops in adulthood.

Primary catheter interventional stent implantation is increasingly the treatment of choice for patients who were first diagnosed with coarctation of the aorta in childhood, adolescence or adulthood. However, the later the surgical or interventional catheterization is performed, the higher the risk of persistent arterial hypertension—even if no residual gradient is present after treatment. In these cases, ACE inhibitors or beta blockers (e.g., carvedilol) are usually used to treat hypertension.

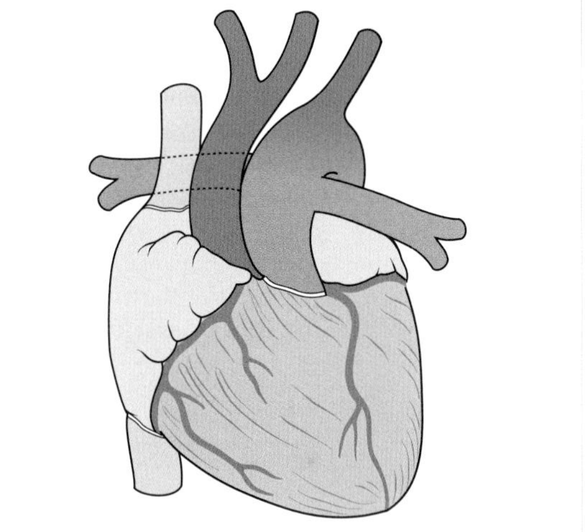

Fig. 15.83 External view of a heart with an interrupted aortic arch (type B).
The interruption of the aortic arch between the left subclavian artery and the left carotid artery can be seen clearly. The ductus arteriosus that supplies the systemic blood flow distal to the interruption is very prominent. The ascending aorta appears narrower than the pulmonary artery.

15.25 Interrupted Aortic Arch

15.25.1 Basics

Definition

In an interrupted aortic arch, the thoracic aorta is completely interrupted. Between the two parts there is at most a tissuelike connection but no lumen. Perfusion of the lower half of the body and the aortic arch distal to the interruption depends on the patency of the ductus arteriosus (► Fig. 15.83).

Epidemiology

An interrupted aortic arch is very rare and constitutes around 1% of all critical congenital cardiac malformations. Boys and girls are roughly equally affected.

Classification

Types A to C are distinguished according to the position of the interruption in relation to the outlet of the head and neck vessels (► Fig. 15.84):

- Type A: The interruption is distal to the left subclavian artery (location similar to coarctation of the aorta; 33%).
- Type B: The interruption is between the common carotid artery and the unilateral subclavian artery (66%).
- Type C: The interruption is between the two common carotid arteries (rare).

Pathogenesis

An interrupted aortic arch is a conotruncal anomaly of the aortic arch in the area of the 3rd/4th pharyngeal pouch. There are likely different etiologies for type A and type B. For example, 75% of type B interrupted aortic arches are associated with microdeletion of 22q11, which is much less frequently found in type A and type C. Type A is sometimes considered to be an extreme form of coarctation of the aorta.

Hemodynamics

The blood supply to the lower half of the body and the aorta distal to the interruption are completely dependent on the PDA. Only in extremely rare cases is the lower half of the body supplied by collaterals. When the ductus closes, the children become symptomatic. In the rare cases where no VSD is present, differential cyanosis develops between the upper and the lower halves of the body (the SaO_2 of the upper half of the body is greater than the lower half) due to a right-to-left shunt.

Associated Anomalies

Note

An interrupted aortic arch is almost always associated with other cardiac anomalies. In addition to a PDA, a VSD, a subaortic stenosis, and a bicuspid aortic valve are particularly common and relevant. Only 3 to 4% of cases involve an isolated interrupted aortic arch.

The most common associated cardiac anomalies are:

- PDA, which is almost always present; it ensures systemic perfusion distal to the stenosis
- VSD, which is present in 90% of cases; it is often a malalignment VSD that can lead functionally to a subaortic stenosis due to displacement of the left ventricular outflow tract
- Subaortic stenosis
- Aortic valve anomalies (e.g., bicuspid aortic valve)
- Mitral valve anomalies (e.g., mitral valve atresia)
- Aortopulmonary window
- Truncus arteriosus communis
- Double-outlet right ventricle
- Transposition of the great vessels
- Right aortic arch

In an interrupted aortic arch, occasionally an aberrant right subclavian artery arises as an arteria lusoria distal to the left subclavian artery and runs to the right behind the esophagus.

Associated Syndrome

In 75% of type B cases, microdeletion of 22q11 is present; this is rare in type A and very rare in type C.

Note

In an interrupted aortic arch, especially type B, microdeletion of 22q11 should always be taken into consideration.

15.25.2 Diagnostic Measures

Symptoms

Children become symptomatic within the first days of life after the closure of the ductus arteriosus. The main symptoms, similar to a critical coarctation of the aorta, are usually signs of acute heart failure or cardiogenic shock:

- Congestive heart failure with tachypnea/dyspnea, hepatomegaly, poor feeding, and lethargy up to cardiogenic shock
- Gray-cyanotic appearance of the lower half of the body as a result of hypoperfusion distal to the interruption of the aortic arch
- Difference in blood pressure between the upper and lower halves of the body. Caution: Blood pressure differences occur only when left ventricular function is still adequate or has recovered. In cardiogenic shock, the blood pressure in all extremities is dramatically reduced. It should also be noted that in the presence of an arteria lusoria, which arises distal to the interruption and supplies the right arm, there is no difference in blood pressure between the right arm and the legs.
- Difference in oxygen saturation between upper and lower halves of the body (i.e., differential cyanosis). This difference is usually not particularly prominent because a VSD is almost always present, leading to increased saturation of pulmonary arterial blood via a left-to-right shunt and pulmonary recirculation.
- Metabolic acidosis
- Renal failure with oliguria/anuria
- Increased risk of necrotic enterocolitis due to hypoperfusion of the lower half of the body

Auscultation

The auscultation findings are usually unspecific. If there is a VSD, there is a typical systolic murmur with PMI in the 3rd/4th left parasternal ICS. No murmur can generally be auscultated during the phase of an acute congestive heart failure. There may be a gallop rhythm as a sign of a congestive heart failure.

ECG

The ECG is usually not very indicative. There may be signs of right ventricular hypertrophy because the right ventricle must supply the systemic circulation via the ductus arteriosus.

Chest X-ray

Typical findings are cardiomegaly and increased pulmonary vascular markings (signs of excessive pulmonary blood flow with a relevant VSD, or of pulmonary congestion with left heart failure). The thymus (narrow mediastinal shadow) may be missing if there is microdeletion of 22q11.

Echocardiography

A lack of continuity between the ascending and descending aorta can be seen in echocardiography. A wide pulmonary artery, which appears to be much larger than the ascending aorta, is also typical. The strikingly narrow ascending aorta usually proceeds to the head and neck vessels at an unusually steep slope.

The exact location (interruption with respect to the individual carotids) and the extent of the interruption must be determined by echocardiography. In addition, the ductus arteriosus that merges into the descending aorta must be visualized. A right-to-left shunt across the ductus can be visualized by color Doppler sonography.

It is important to assess the left ventricular outflow tract; a malalignment VSD often leads to a functional subaortic stenosis by displacing the muscular outflow septum to the left. The location, size, and hemodynamic relevance of the VSD can also be assessed.

An aberrant subclavian artery and other associated anomalies (bicuspid aortic valve, transposition of the great vessels) must be either ruled out or visualized.

Cardiac Catheterization

Cardiac catheterization is sometimes indicated for the reliable visualization of the anatomy. To visualize the distal aorta, contrast medium is injected into the pulmonary artery and ductus arteriosus. To visualize the proximal segments of the aortic arch, the ascending aorta is probed in an antegrade direction. Associated anomalies must be ruled out or visualized.

MRI

MRI facilitates the good visualization and 3D reconstruction of the entire aorta. Associated anomalies can be ruled out or visualized. Postoperatively, the MRI is used mainly to assess restenosis or residual stenosis of the aortic arch.

15.25.3 Treatment

Conservative Treatment

Continuous infusion of prostaglandin E (initially 50 ng/kg/min, dosage should be reduced later) can maintain patency of the ductus arteriosus until surgery. Intubation and mechanical ventilation often become necessary in the preoperative phase. Oxygen should not be routinely administered if possible because it lowers the pulmonary resistance thus reducing the right-to-left shunt across the ductus arteriosus or may lead to excessive pulmonary blood overflow if there is a large VSD. Blind buffering should also be avoided for the same reasons. Catecholamines and diuretics may be used to treat heart failure.

Surgical Treatment

Surgery is performed within the first days of life after stabilizing the patient. A single-stage procedure is generally preferred. If there are complex associated cardiac anomalies, it may sometimes be better to first reconstruct the aortic arch and band the pulmonary artery to prevent excessive pulmonary blood flow if there is a relevant VSD. The associated anomalies are corrected in a second procedure.

The continuity between the ascending and descending aorta can be restored by direct anastomosis (▶ Fig. 15.85), but it may sometimes be necessary to implant a conduit. The correction of associated cardiac anomalies may complicate the procedure considerably.

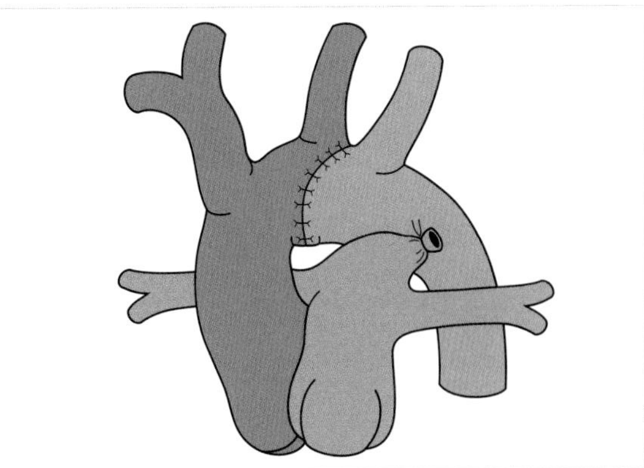

Fig. 15.85 Correction of an interrupted aortic arch (type B). The two segments of the aortic arch are directly anastomosed to each other. In addition, a patent ductus arteriosus is transected and ligated.

15.25.4 Prognosis and Clinical Course

▶ **Long-term outcome.** Without treatment, the majority of the children die within the first weeks of life. The postoperative mortality rate has been reduced considerably in recent years. The mortality rate of a single-stage procedure is reported to be 10%, and 30% in a two-stage procedure with complex associated cardiac anomalies.

If the patient survives the immediate postoperative period, the prognosis is usually very good. However, reoperations and interventional catheterization may be required for up to half of patients. The reasons for this are mainly restenosis and residual stenosis of the aortic arch or an increasing subaortic stenosis, which may have been only mild preoperatively.

▶ **Outpatient checkups.** Regular, lifelong cardiac checkups are necessary after correction of an interrupted aortic arch. In the checkups particular attention must be paid to restenosis and residual stenosis and the development of a relevant subaortic stenosis. A bicuspid aortic valve poses an increased risk of developing aortic stenosis and/or regurgitation.

Endocarditis prophylaxis is required for the first 6 postoperative months if foreign material was used. Long-term endocarditis prophylaxis is necessary if there are residual defects in the area of foreign material.

▶ **Physical capacity and lifestyle.** The quality of life for most patients after the surgical correction is good to very good. Similar conditions apply to physical capacity as for patients with a corrected coarctation of the aorta (Chapter 15.24). However, there may also be relevant associated anomalies such as a subaortic stenosis or valvular aortic stenosis in individual cases.

▶ **Special aspects in adolescents and adults.** Practically all adolescent and adult patients with an interrupted aortic arch underwent surgical correction as neonates. MRI is particularly useful as an imaging system for reliably assessing restenosis and residual stenosis when the diagnostic limits of echocardiography have been reached.

15.26 Congenital Vascular Rings

15.26.1 Basics

Synonym: "rings and slings"

Definition

Vascular rings are a group of vascular anomalies that lead to compression of the trachea and/or esophagus through the formation of complete or incomplete vascular rings. A number of different variant anomalies in the origin and course of the vessels of the aortic arch are known. Only a small group of these vascular anomalies causes symptoms, generally being variations that lead to the formation of vascular rings.

Epidemiology

Congenital vascular rings constitute 1 to 3% of all cardiovascular anomalies. Due to the many asymptomatic variants, the frequency is probably underestimated. Boys are affected somewhat more often than girls.

Pathogenesis

Vascular rings are formed when there is faulty obliteration of the symmetrical embryonic branchial arch arteries, from which the aortic arch develops along with the vessels that arise from it later.

Classification

A differentiation is made between complete and incomplete vascular rings. Complete vascular rings encircle the trachea and esophagus. Incomplete vascular rings do not completely encircle the trachea and esophagus, but can compress trachea, bronchi, and/or esophagus. Complete vascular rings often cause more severe symptoms than incomplete vascular rings.

Associated Anomalies

Associated cardiac and noncardiac anomalies occur in up to half of patients with congenital vascular rings.

- Associated cardiac anomalies:
  - VSD
  - Tetralogy of Fallot
  - Coarctation of the aorta
  - PDA
- Associated noncardiac anomalies:
  - Tracheo-esophageal fistula
  - Cleft lip and palate
  - Subglottal stenosis
  - Bronchotracheomalacia
  - Cricoid cartilage (especially with pulmonary slings)

Associated Syndromes

- Microdeletion of 22q11 (in up to 25% cases of a double aortic arch)
- Trisomy 21
- CHARGE syndrome

15.26.2 Complete Vascular Rings

Double Aortic Arch

Around one-third of all congenital vascular rings involve a double aortic arch. The aortic arch develops in pairs in

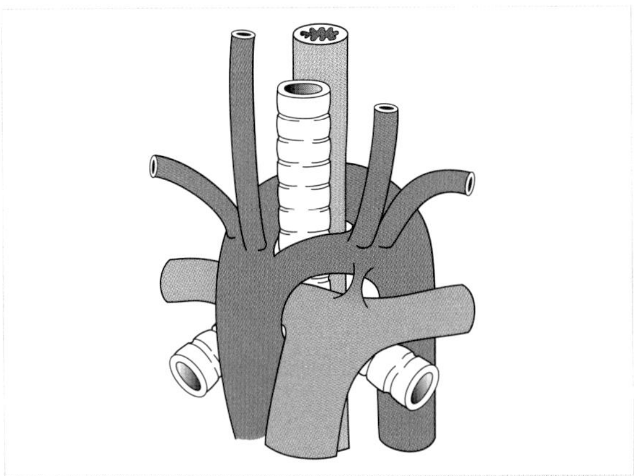

Fig. 15.86 Double aortic arch. A complete ring is formed. The right and left aortic arches completely encircle the trachea and esophagus. The right aortic arch runs behind the trachea and esophagus, the left aortic arch in front. In most cases, the right aortic arch is larger than the left.

the embryonic period from the 4th branchial arch arteries. Normally, the right aortic arch is obliterated. If both branchial arch arteries persist, a double aortic arch is formed.

In a double aortic arch, the ascending aorta separates into two vessels that completely encircle the trachea and esophagus, forming a loop (▶ Fig. 15.86). At the start of the descending aorta, the two aortic arches are rejoined. The left aortic arch runs in front of the esophagus and trachea, the right aortic arch behind them. Separate vessels arise from each of the two aortic arches—the respective carotid and subclavian arteries for that side. That is, the right carotid and right subclavian arteries arise from the right aortic arch and the left carotid and left subclavian arteries arise from the left aortic arch. The calibers of the two aortic arches are often unequal. In most cases, the right aortic arch has a larger caliber. A ligamentum arteriosum may increase the constriction of the trachea and esophagus.

Right Aortic Arch with Aberrant Left Subclavian Artery and Left Ductus Arteriosus or Ligamentum Arteriosum

This anomaly is responsible for at lease one-third of all congenital vascular rings. The right aortic arch crosses the right main bronchus and then runs behind the trachea and esophagus. The left ductus arteriosus or ligamentum arteriosum runs at the left of the trachea from the descending aorta to the pulmonary artery. The trachea and esophagus are thus completely encircled. The left common carotid artery arises as the first arch vessel from the aortic arch, the second is the right common carotid artery, and the third is the right subclavian artery. The left subclavian artery arises aberrantly as the last arch vessel together with the ductus arteriosus from the *diverticulum of Kommerell*. This is an evagination of the aortic arch that can additionally constrict the trachea and esophagus (▶ Fig. 15.87).

Excursus: Left Aortic Arch—Right Aortic Arch

A normal aortic arch is a left aortic arch. A left aortic arch runs *in front* of the trachea and esophagus and crosses the left main bronchus. A right aortic arch crosses the right main bronchus and then runs *behind* the trachea and esophagus.

In most cases, a right aortic arch runs down at the right of the spinal column (at the right of the descending aorta). Occasionally, the aorta may also cross to the left in front of the spinal column and then descend at the left of the spinal column (at the left of the descending aorta). In a right aortic arch, the origins of the head and neck vessels should be arranged in a mirror image compared with a left aortic arch, but there are many other variants. If the origins of the aortic arch vessels are a mirror image, the first aortic arch to arise is the left brachiocephalic trunk, which separates into the left common carotid artery and left subclavian artery. The second aortic arch vessel is the right common carotid artery, and the third is the right subclavian artery. No ring is formed in most cases because the ductus arteriosus / ligamentum arteriosum usually runs from the brachiocephalic trunk to the left pulmonary artery in front of the trachea and esophagus. However, a right aortic arch is frequently associated with a tetralogy of Fallot or other heart defects.

As a rule of thumb, the first vessel to arise from the aortic arch is the common carotid artery of the contralateral side or a vessel from which the carotid arises. The first vessel to arise from a left aortic arch is thus the right common carotid artery or brachiocephalic trunk, from which the right common carotid artery originates. Correspondingly, in a right aortic arch, the first aortic arch vessel to arise is the left common carotid artery or the brachiocephalic trunk, from which the left common carotid artery originates.

15.26.3 Incomplete Vascular Rings

Pulmonary Sling

A pulmonary sling is very rare. The left pulmonary artery arises from the right pulmonary artery on the right side of the aorta and trachea. It crosses to the left between the trachea and esophagus (▶ Fig. 15.88). This can lead to compression of the trachea and/or esophagus. This anomaly is often associated with cricoid cartilage of the distal trachea.

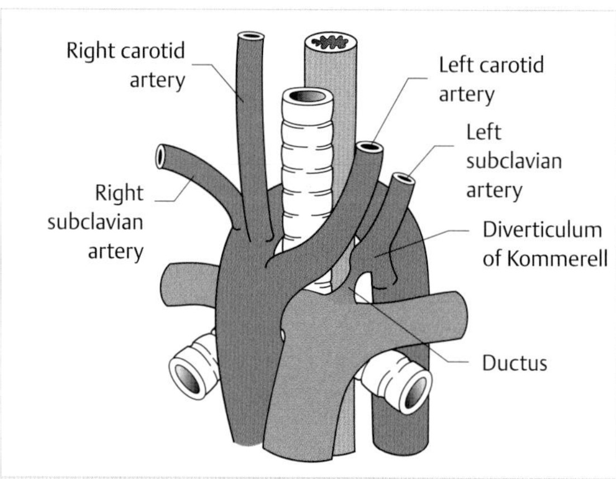

Fig. 15.87 Right-sided aortic arch with aberrant left subclavian artery and left ligamentum arteriosum. The right aortic arch runs behind the esophagus and trachea. The complete vascular ring formation arises because the ligament runs at the left of the trachea and esophagus to the bifurcation of the pulmonary artery. The ductus arteriosus arises jointly with the left subclavian artery from a diverticulum of Kommerell.

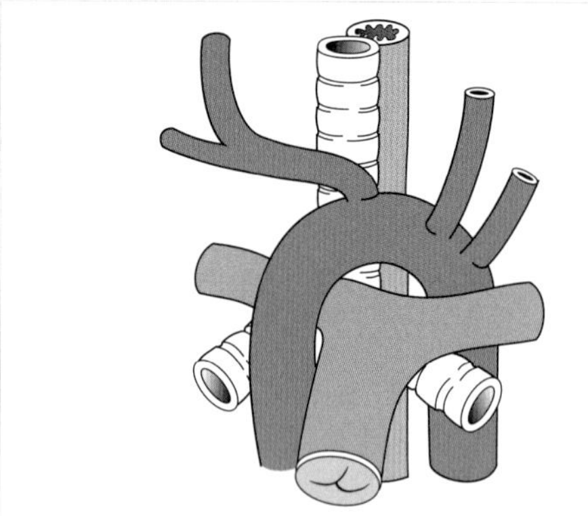

Fig. 15.89 Anomalous right brachiocephalic trunk. The right brachiocephalic trunk originates unusually far medially from the aortic arch and has a correspondingly long segment in front of the trachea, which can be compressed.

Anomalous Right Brachiocephalic Trunk

An anomalous right brachiocephalic trunk constitutes approximately 10% of all congenital vascular rings. The brachiocephalic trunk originates unusually medially from the aortic arch and has a correspondingly long segment in front of the trachea, which can be compressed (▶ Fig. 15.89).

Arteria Lusoria

In an arteria lusoria, the right 4th branchial arch artery is obliterated instead of the left. Normally the right subclavian artery arises from the brachiocephalic trunk (▶ Fig. 15.90). An anomalous origin of the right subclavian artery as the last vessel to arise distal to the aortic arch is called arteria lusoria. The arteria lusoria crosses from the left to the right side behind the esophagus and trachea. This can compress the esophagus and trachea, but patients are asymptomatic in most cases.

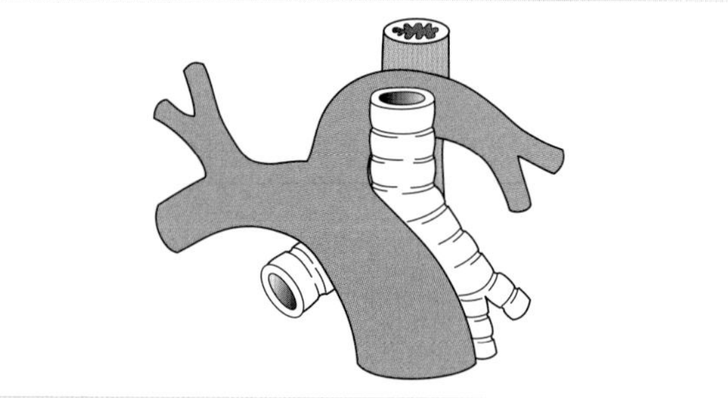

Fig. 15.88 Pulmonary sling. The left pulmonary artery originates at the right of the aorta and trachea from the right pulmonary artery and runs to the left between the trachea and esophagus.

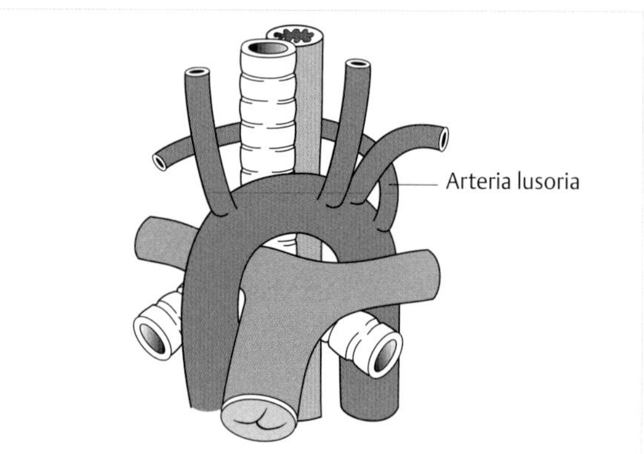

Fig. 15.90 Arteria lusoria. Anomalous origin of the right subclavian artery, which arises as the last vessel distal to the left subclavian artery from the aortic arch. The arteria lusoria crosses behind the esophagus and from left to right.

15.26.4 Diagnostic Measures

Symptoms

The leading symptoms of vascular rings are inspiratory stridor and dysphagia resulting from compression of the trachea and esophagus. Complete vascular rings generally cause more pronounced symptoms than do incomplete vascular rings.

Children with a double aortic arch or a pulmonary sling usually become symptomatic within the first months of life. The other vascular rings often do not cause symptoms until later in infancy or early childhood.

The typical symptoms are:

- Stridor, increased stridor on swallowing

- Wheezing, barking cough, dyspnea, suffocation, reflex apnea, cyanosis
- Dysphagia (usually when solid foods are added to diet), vomiting
- Chronic cough, susceptibility to infections, failure to thrive
- Apnea (often triggered by feeding or exertion)
- Possibly compensatory hyperextension of the neck to reduce the tracheal stenosis

▶ **Differential diagnoses.** Possible differential diagnoses that should be considered with inspiratory stridor and dysphagia: laryngomalacia, mediastinal tumor, foreign body, croup or laryngotracheitis, vocal cord paresis or dysfunction, choanal stenosis, tracheoesophageal fistula, stenoses and anomalies of the digestive tract.

Auscultation

If there are no concomitant cardiac anomalies, the cardiac auscultation finding is unremarkable.

ECG

The ECG is unremarkable if there are no concomitant cardiac anomalies.

Lung Function Test

The flow volume curve typically indicates an extrathoracic obstruction. Sometimes an expiratory obstruction can also be detected.

Chest X-ray

In the radiographs there may be a visible impression on the trachea resulting from the vascular ring. A protrusion of the trachea in an anterior direction in the lateral image is a sign of a vascular ring. In a right aortic arch, a soft tissue shadow is visible at the right in front of the trachea and the trachea is also typically displaced to the left. If necessary, the examination can be supplemented by a barium swallow to make impressions on the esophagus visible.

Echocardiography

Echocardiography provides important information for investigating possible vascular rings. If a normal left aortic arch with a normal origin and normal bifurcation of a right brachiocephalic trunk and normal bifurcation of the pulmonary artery are visualized, a vascular ring can very probably be ruled out. The vessels of the aortic arch are best visualized from a suprasternal view.

Echocardiography can also be used to rule out or detect associated heart defects. However, echocardiography is limited by the fact that the airways and atretic vascular segments are very difficult if not impossible to visualize.

Bronchoscopy

Bronchoscopy is not obligatory, but should be performed if primary anomalies of the trachea or bronchi are assumed. A typical finding of vascular rings is a saber-shaped, pulsating compression in the trachea or bronchi, possibly combined with tracheomalacia.

Cardiac Catheterization

Cardiac catheterization for investigation of vascular rings has largely been replaced by MRI.

MRI

MRI is the diagnostic method of choice for visualizing vascular rings. In MRI scans the heart, vessels, trachea, bronchi, and esophagus can be visualized in detail and their relative positions determined.

15.26.5 Treatment

Conservative Treatment

Conservative treatment is only an interim measure until definitive surgical treatment: raising the upper half of the body, reducing the swelling from infections, and possibly giving sedation.

Surgical Treatment

Surgery is the definitive treatment for vascular rings. It is indicated in all symptomatic patients. A left lateral thoracotomy is made for the access route. If the anatomy is complex (e.g., pulmonary sling), a medial sternotomy may be needed. The surgical procedure depends on the underlying vascular ring:

- *Double aortic arch:* In a double aortic arch, the smaller arch (usually the left) is transected. If there is also a ring formed by the ligamentum arteriosum, it is always transected.
- *Right aortic arch with aberrant left subclavian artery and left ligamentum arteriosum*: The ligament is transected. If there is a prominent diverticulum of Kommerell, it is usually excised and the aberrant subclavian artery is implanted in the left common carotid artery.
- *Pulmonary sling:* The left pulmonary artery is transected at the origin, mobilized, and implanted in front of the trachea in the main pulmonary artery. If there is also cricoid cartilage leading to a tracheal stenosis, the affected tracheal segment may have to be partially excised.
- *Anomalous right brachiocephalic trunk:* Aortopexy is recommended for patients with pronounced symptoms. The aortic arch and brachiocephalic trunk are fixated to the back of the sternum to prevent compression of the trachea and esophagus by displacement of the vessels.

- *Arteria lusoria:* The arteria lusoria is transected and reimplanted only rarely in symptomatic patients with dysphagia.

15.26.6 Prognosis and Clinical Course

▸ **Long-term outcome.** The prognosis after surgical correction of a vascular ring is generally very good. The perioperative mortality rate is now under 1%. The long-term results are usually good. However, stridor may persist for weeks or even months postoperatively, especially in small children, until the tracheal cartilage is stabilized. If there are concomitant tracheal or bronchial anomalies, the problems may persist.

▸ **Outpatient checkups.** Postoperatively, persistent symptoms such as stridor and difficulty swallowing should be checked in particular. These symptoms may be caused by insufficient excision of a diverticulum of Kommerell, incomplete transection of the vascular ring, or concomitant anomalies. Even after successful surgery, it may be weeks or even months before complete regression of symptoms occurs.

After correction of a pulmonary sling, the area of the implantation site in the left pulmonary artery should be checked for stenosis. Differences in blood pressure between the two arms after the reimplantation of an aberrant subclavian artery indicate a stenosis.

▸ **Physical exercise capacity and lifestyle.** After a relevant vascular ring has been diagnosed, patients should avoid physical exertion until surgery. Life-threatening hypoventilation or even apnea (Hering–Breuer reflex) can sometimes occur on exertion. After surgical correction, the majority of patients do not have any limitations of physical exercise capacity unless there are other anomalies. In some (even asymptomatic) patients, there may still be abnormal lung function postoperatively.

▸ **Special aspects in adolescents and adults.** A relevant vascular ring is very rarely diagnosed in adulthood. The patients are usually already symptomatic in infancy and early childhood. It is possible, however, that older patients were misdiagnosed as having asthma and treated for it for many years before the correct diagnosis was made.

15.27 Mitral Stenosis

15.27.1 Basics

Definition

Mitral stenosis is an anomaly in which an obstruction hinders diastolic blood flow from the left atrium to the left ventricle.

Epidemiology

An isolated congenital mitral stenosis is rare and constitutes only 0.5% of all congenital heart defects. A congenital mitral stenosis usually occurs in combination with other heart defects (e.g., as a Shone complex combined with other stenoses of the left heart).

In developing countries, by far the most cases of mitral stenosis are caused by rheumatic fever, but this form rarely becomes manifest in childhood.

Pathogenesis

The valve leaflets, mitral valve annulus, tendinous cords, and papillary muscles must all be intact for the mitral valve to function properly. Any problems in the development of these structures can lead to congenital mitral stenosis.

If there are other obstructions of the left heart (e.g., aortic stenosis or atresia), the mitral valve cannot develop properly because of the reduced blood flow, and remains hypoplastic.

In rheumatic fever, a streptococcal infection leads to an abnormal immune reaction that affects different organ systems. In the heart, cross-reactions of antibodies directed against cardiac proteins lead to pancarditis. In the long term, this results in scarring of the valves.

In addition, a mitral stenosis can arise postoperatively after a (Mustard/Senning) atrial baffle procedure.

Hemodynamics

As a result of the mitral stenosis, diastolic filling of the left ventricle is reduced and the pressure in the left atrium increases. Cardiac output is reduced correspondingly, initially only under exertion, later at rest as well.

Due to the increased pressure in the left atrium, there is congestion in the pulmonary veins—in an extreme case, pulmonary edema. Pulmonary hypertension also develops, which can lead to right ventricular load.

Classification

Classification is based on the location of the stenosis with respect to the mitral valve. There can be supravalvular, valvular, and subvalvular mitral stenoses. However, more than one location is usually affected in congenital mitral stenosis, resulting in differing degrees of mitral stenosis. In congenital mitral stenosis, the tendinous cords are typically shortened and thickened and the edges of the valve leaflets are also thickened. The papillary muscles are often deformed and located close together. The mitral valve annulus is frequently hypoplastic. Hypoplasia of the mitral valve annulus is closely correlated with hypoplasia of the left ventricle (see Chapter 15.20).

Special forms of congenital mitral stenosis are listed below.

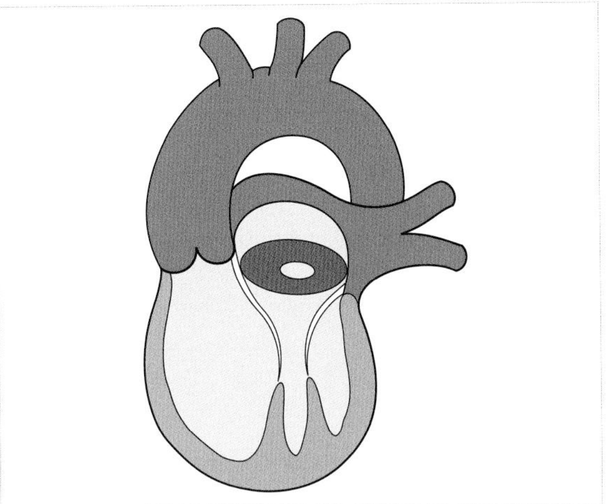

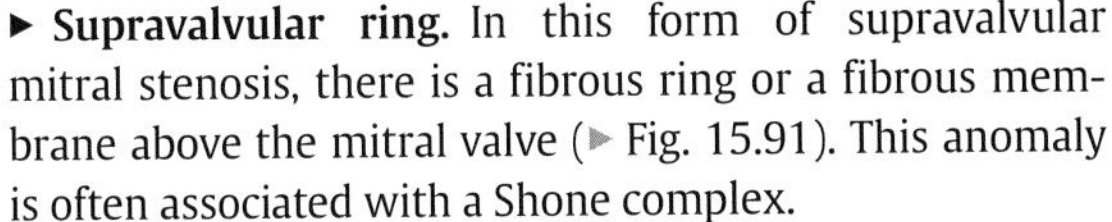

Fig. 15.91 Supravalvular ring of the mitral valve. Stenosis above the mitral valve caused by a fibrous ring or fibrous membrane. Unlike a cor triatrium, the membrane is below the foramen ovale.

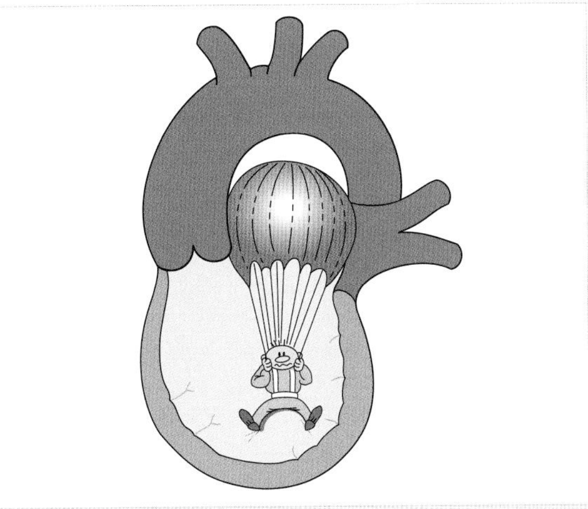

Fig. 15.92 Parachute mitral valve. The tendinous cords of the mitral valve are pulled together like a parachute to a single papillary muscle (monopapillary muscle).

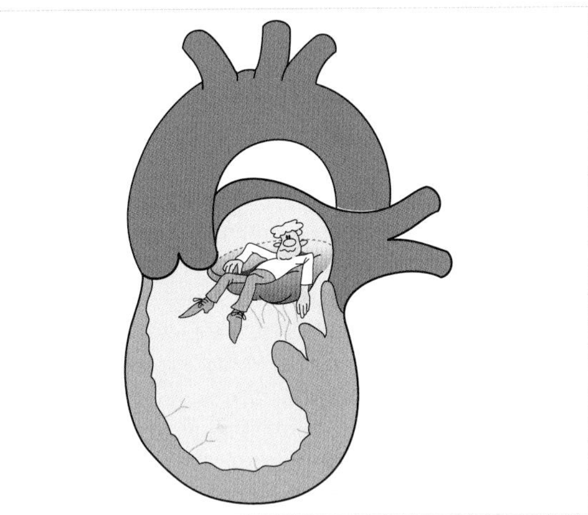

Fig. 15.93 Hammock mitral valve. The tendinous cords of the mitral valve are shortened or absent entirely. Sometimes the leaflets are attached directly to papillary muscles. Tendinous cords crossing the valve can additionally obstruct blood flow across the valve. The shape of the valve is similar to a hammock.

▸ **Supravalvular ring.** In this form of supravalvular mitral stenosis, there is a fibrous ring or a fibrous membrane above the mitral valve (▸ Fig. 15.91). This anomaly is often associated with a Shone complex.

▸ **Cor triatrium.** In a cor triatrium, the left atrium is divided into two segments by a membrane. Functionally, a cor triatrium is equivalent to a supravalvular mitral stenosis, but the genesis is different, viz. in a cor triatrium, the embryonic pulmonary venous confluence, which develops behind the left atrium, is only incompletely involved in the left atrium during embryonic development. Its hemodynamic relevance depends mainly on the size of the opening in the membrane. A cor triatrium usually occurs in isolation, but may also be associated with anomalous pulmonary venous connections, a PDA, or a persistent left superior vena cava.

A cor triatrium can be distinguished from a supravalvular ring by the location of the membrane: In a cor triatrium, the membrane is always above the foramen ovale and the left cardiac appendage; in a supravalvular ring, it is always below these structures.

▸ **Parachute mitral valve.** In a parachute mitral valve, there is only one papillary muscle (monopapillary muscle) in the left ventricle, so the tendinous cords of the two leaflets are pulled together like a parachute (▸ Fig. 15.92). A parachute valve is the most common form of congenital mitral stenosis and leads to an obstruction, especially a subvalvular obstruction.

▸ **Hammock valve.** In a hammock valve, the leaflets are typically thickened and rolled up at the edges. In addition, the tendinous cords are markedly shortened or absent entirely, so the leaflets are sometimes attached directly to the papillary muscles (▸ Fig. 15.93). These papillary muscles are deformed (papillary muscle stumps) and are attached high on the left ventricular posterior wall. Furthermore, bands of tissue may cross the mitral valve opening and displace it. From above, the mitral valve looks like a hammock. Hemodynamically, valve insufficiency is the most prominent feature, but there is often a stenosis as well. This anomaly is very rare overall. The term "mitral arcade" is often used synonymously.

▶ **Double-orifice mitral valve.** In this case, the mitral valve has two separate openings. This is caused by excessive tissue that crosses the actual mitral valve opening and divides it. In most cases, the two openings are not located centrally, but are eccentric.

Associated Cardiac Anomalies

A supravalvular mitral stenosis and a parachute mitral valve are components of the Shone complex, in which various obstructions of the left heart occur concomitantly —for example, supravalvular mitral stenosis, parachute mitral valve, subvalvular aortic stenosis, valvular aortic stenosis, and coarctation of the aorta.

A cor triatriatum is often associated with a persistent left superior vena cava and anomalous pulmonary venous connections. A severely hypoplastic mitral valve can occur in association with a hypoplastic left heart syndrome. In addition, a VSD often occurs with a congenital mitral stenosis. The combination of mitral stenosis and an ASD is called Lutembacher syndrome.

15.27.2 Diagnostic Measures

Symptoms

Depending on the extent of the stenosis and the concomitant anomalies, the most prominent signs will be lung congestion and reduced cardiac output. Mild mitral stenoses are usually asymptomatic. More severe stenoses have the following typical symptoms:

- Recurrent infections, dry (congestive) cough (especially when lying), tachypnea/dyspnea
- Pulmonary congestion, pulmonary edema, obstructive pulmonary vascular changes, pulmonary hypertension
- Poor feeding, failure to thrive, reduced physical capacity
- Hepatosplenomegaly and edema if there is right heart insufficiency
- Possible dysphagia on maximum dilatation of the left atrium with compression of the esophagus or atelectasis if there is pressure on the bronchi
- Supraventricular arrhythmias (e.g., atrial flutter/fibrillation) as a result of atrial dilatation

Auscultation

The first heart sound is prominent to loud. A mitral opening sound is sometimes heard after the second heart sound. The more severe the stenosis, the shorter the interval between the second heart sound and the mitral opening click.

A low-frequency "rumbling" diastolic murmur, usually beginning shortly after the second heart sound or after the mitral opening click, is typical for a mitral stenosis. The PMI is over the cardiac apex and the 4th left parasternal ICS. The murmur increases in the left lateral position.

ECG

In a relevant mitral stenosis, there is typically a P mitrale (notched P wave with a duration over 0.1 s), possibly signs of right ventricular pressure overload, and possibly repolarization disturbances over the right heart. Over time, this may lead to atrial flutter/fibrillation due to atrial overload.

Chest X-ray

The enlargement of the left atrium can be detected in the X-ray images: atrial dilatation leads to widening of the tracheal bifurcation located immediately above and behind the left atrium. The cardiac waist is typically flattened; sometimes the enlarged right atrium can be distinguished as a shadow within the cardiac silhouette. The lateral image shows narrowing of the retrocardiac space with impression of the esophagus.

Cloudiness in the lower lung fields and unclear margins of widened pulmonary vessels are indicative of pulmonary congestion. Kerley B lines, horizontal lines mainly seen in the lower and lateral fields, may also be detected. The pulmonary segment is prominent if there is hypertension.

Echocardiography

The diagnosis can be made reliably and the extent of stenosis assessed by echocardiography. The 2D image shows enlargement of the left atrium. The right ventricle and atrium are often enlarged as well.

The severity of the stenosis can be determined in a CW Doppler examination: peak diastolic flow across the mitral valve of over 2 m/s indicates a relevant mitral stenosis. However, the mean pressure gradient across the mitral valve and the velocity time interval (VTI) are better suited for quantification.

The severity can be determined using the mean pressure gradient:

- Mild stenosis: < 5 mmHg
- Moderate stenosis: 5–10 mmHg
- Severe stenosis: > 10 mmHg

The mitral valve opening area can be estimated using the pressure half-time (PHT, ▶ Fig. 15.94) and an empirically determined constant (220):

$$\text{Mitral opening area } (\text{cm}^2) = \frac{220}{\text{PHT (ms)}}$$

Right ventricular pressure across a tricuspid insufficiency can be estimated using the Bernoulli equation. A concomitant mitral valve insufficiency can also be visualized or ruled out by color Doppler.

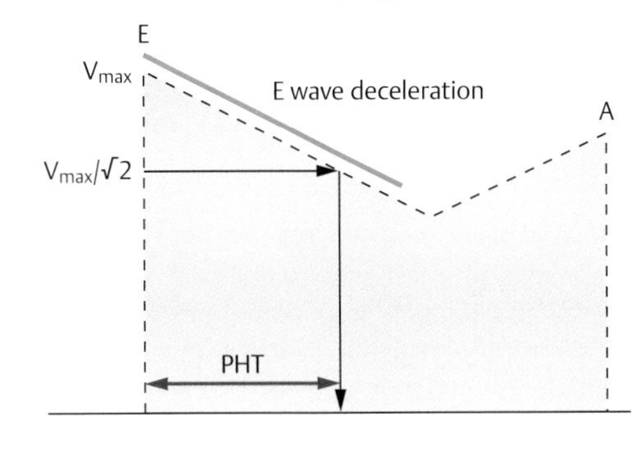

Fig. 15.94 Determining the pressure half time (PHT) in a mitral stenosis. The mitral inflow profile is visualized by CW Doppler. The typical E wave and A wave of the transmitral inflow are visible. The PHT is the time in which the initial maximum pressure gradient has fallen to half.

In addition, the following anatomical structures must be visualized in detail and assessed:

- Supravalvular region: Is there a supravalvular ring (polar light sign) or cor triatriatum? Pulmonary venous stenosis?
- Valve annulus: diameter of mitral and tricuspid valves.
- Leaflets: The leaflets are often thickened and fused if there is a valvular stenosis. In addition, the mobility of the leaflets must be assessed.
- Tendinous cords: The tendinous cords are often thickened or shortened.
- Papillary muscles: In a parachute mitral valve, there is a monopapillary muscle that the tendinous cords are attached to, like a parachute. In a hammock valve, the papillary muscles are short and thick.

Cardiac Catheterization

Cardiac catheterization is not necessary in most cases, but it can be helpful if there are difficulties quantifying the hemodynamics or to rule out associated anomalies reliably.

The hemodynamic measurements include determining the pressure in the pulmonary system and in the left atrium, and measuring the transmitral gradient (difference between the A wave in the left atrium and the left ventricular end-diastolic pressure). The atrial pressure is measured using the wedge pressure across a blocked pulmonary artery catheter or after probing the left atrium. In a mitral stenosis, the atrial pressure in the diastole is higher than the end-diastolic ventricular pressure. The atrial contraction wave (A wave) is increased; the early diastolic drop in pressure is flat.

15.27.3 Treatment

Conservative Treatment

Diuretics are indicated for pulmonary congestion or edema. Digoxin (or possibly a beta blocker) may be administered to lower the heart rate and increase the duration of the diastole. This helps to empty the left atrium.

However, caution should be exercised when giving digoxin. The rule of thumb used to be: "Never give digoxin with a mitral stenosis." Due to the improved inotropy from digoxin, the right ventricle develops a greater cardiac output, which may not "fit" through the stenotic mitral valve. This can result in pulmonary edema and acute decompensation.

For an associated mitral insufficiency, the afterload is reduced pharmacologically with ACE inhibitors to improve the ejection fraction. Anticoagulation as thromboembolism prophylaxis and possibly antiarrhythmic treatment should be considered for atrial fibrillation.

► **Indication for surgery or interventional catheterization**

- Symptomatic patients (NYHA class III or IV) with congenital mitral stenosis and a mean pressure gradient over 10 mmHg
- Moderately symptomatic patients with a congenital mitral stenosis and a mean pressure gradient over 10 mmHg
- Asymptomatic patients with a pulmonary pressure of 50 mmHg or more and a mean pressure gradient across the mitral valve of 10 mmHg or more
- Recurrent atrial fibrillation, thromboembolic events, hemoptysis
- Symptomatic children with failure to thrive, exertional dyspnea, or pulmonary edema

Interventional Catheterization

Balloon dilation is the treatment of choice for congenital mitral stenoses if the valve morphology is suitable for a balloon valvuloplasty. In some cases, it may be useful as an initial palliative step to delay surgery.

Although balloon valvuloplasty is the treatment of choice in rheumatic mitral stenosis, the results in congenital mitral stenoses are not satisfactory. The most frequent complication is a postinterventional mitral insufficiency. Balloon valvuloplasty is therefore contraindicated for an already more severe mitral insufficiency.

Surgical Treatment

The surgical procedure depends on the morphology of the mitral valve and the age of the patient. In infancy and childhood, valve-preserving surgery is always preferable to valve replacement. Mitral valve replacement can still be performed later if the results are unsatisfactory.

► **Isolated valvular mitral stenosis.** If balloon valvuloplasty is not possible in an isolated valvular mitral stenosis, an open or closed commissurotomy is performed. The operative risk is less than 1%.

► **Parachute mitral valve.** Valve reconstruction is generally attempted for a parachute mitral valve. It may include splitting the monopapillary muscle and excising excessive tissue between the tendinous cords. Sometimes replacement of the mitral valve cannot be avoided.

► **Supravalvular ring/cor triatriatum.** Resection of the ring or the membrane is an appropriate procedure. The prognosis is good.

► **Mitral valve replacement.** If surgical reconstruction of the mitral valve is not possible, it must be replaced. This can be performed on valves with a diameter of about 15 mm. Synthetic valves are available (e.g., St. Jude). Their advantage is their durability, but a distinct disadvantage in childhood is that the valve does not grow with the child, making re-operation necessary. In addition, lifelong anticoagulation with a coumarin derivative (phenprocoumon, warfarin) is needed. Bioprosthetic valves (porcine valves, heterografts) are a possible alternative. Long-term anticoagulation is not necessary in this case. The disadvantage is that early re-operations are often required due to degeneration of the bioprosthetic valve. In small children, an inverted aortic valve may be used.

15.27.4 Prognosis and Clinical Course

► **Long-term outcome.** Patients with mild mitral stenosis can sometimes remain asymptomatic for a surprisingly long time. Atrial flutter or fibrillation is relatively rare in childhood. Every interventional or surgical valve correction of a congenital mitral stenosis or parachute mitral valve is a palliative procedure, because even postoperatively, residual defects usually remain and re-operations are often needed (usually mitral valve replacement).

► **Outpatient checkups.** Patients with a mitral valve stenosis need lifelong checkups. It is important to correctly determine the time when an intervention or operation becomes necessary. In addition to determining the gradients across the valve by echocardiography, the clinical symptoms must be noted. An ECG is necessary to rule out atrial arrhythmias.

Postinterventionally or postoperatively, residual stenoses or restenoses should be noted. After valve replacement in childhood, the child can be expected to "outgrow" the valve. If a bioprosthesis was used, it must be checked for degeneration. After implantation of a mechanical valve, strict anticoagulation is important (target INR 2.5–3.5). For a bioprosthesis, ASA is recommended as platelet aggregation inhibitor for the first 3 months. If there is no atrial fibrillation, no further anticoagulation is needed after that. After a valve reconstruction using foreign material, endocarditis prophylaxis is necessary for the first 6 months following surgery, lifelong if there is a residual defect in the vicinity of foreign material. Long-term endocarditis prophylaxis is also required after the implantation of prosthetic valves (mechanical or biological).

► **Physical capacity and lifestyle.** In mild asymptomatic mitral stenosis, physical activity does not generally need to be restricted. Patients with a mild mitral stenosis and sinus rhythm may engage in sports with a low static and low to moderate dynamic load. Sport is contraindicated if there is a severe mitral stenosis or significant pulmonary hypertension. Contact sports are not suitable for patients who require anticoagulation due to a valve replacement or atrial fibrillation.

► **Special aspects in adolescents and adults.** In adults, rheumatic fever as a result of a streptococcal infection is the most common cause of a mitral stenosis. The treatment of choice for the majority of cases is a balloon valvuloplasty. Women who require anticoagulation after valve replacement should be aware of the teratogenicity of phenprocoumon or warfarin if they want to conceive.

15.28 Mitral Insufficiency

15.28.1 Basics

Definition

Mitral insufficiency is the incomplete closure of the mitral valve during the ventricular systole. This leads to the systolic regurgitation of blood into the left atrium (▸ Fig. 15.95). Mitral insufficiency can be a result of changes in the valve annulus, the mitral leaflets, the tendinous cords, or the papillary muscles.

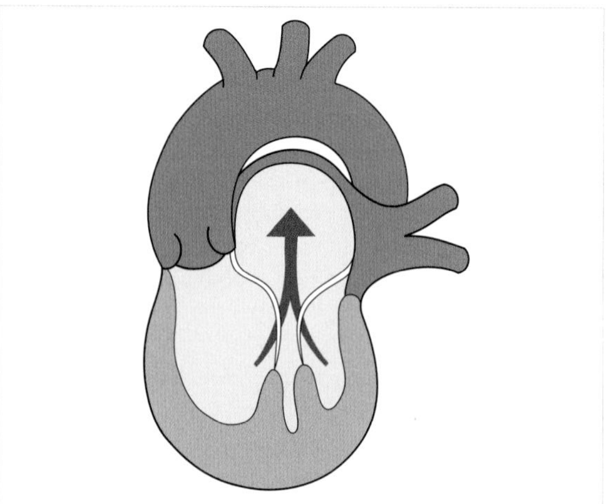

Fig. 15.95 Mitral insufficiency. Systolic regurgitation of blood from the left ventricle into the left atrium. The left atrium and ventricle are dilated due to the regurgitant flow volume.

Epidemiology

Congenital mitral insufficiency is rare in isolation. Mitral insufficiency is most often associated with other heart defects, connective tissue diseases, or metabolic disorders.

In developing countries, mitral insufficiency is a typical consequence of rheumatic fever. In industrial countries, this is now very rarely the cause.

Etiology

► **Congenital mitral insufficiency:**

- Cleft mitral valve: cleft in the anterior mitral leaflet. A mitral cleft is usually a component of an atrioventricular septal defect ("AV canal").
- Congenital mitral valve anomalies such as a parachute mitral valve, hammock mitral valve (Chapter 15.27)
- Association with other congenital heart defects

► **Acquired mitral insufficiency:**

- Valve perforation or scarring following endocarditis (rheumatic or infectious) or myocarditis
- Result of Kawasaki syndrome
- Myxomatous changes of the mitral valve in association with connective tissue diseases (e.g., Marfan syndrome, Ehlers–Danlos syndrome, pseudoxanthoma elasticum) or lysosomal storage diseases (mucopolysaccharidosis, homocystinuria)
- Impairment of mitral valve function due to a cardiac tumor
- Traumatic papillary muscle avulsion
- Necrosis, scarring, or papillary muscle avulsion as a result of myocardial ischemia
- Dilatation of the mitral valve annulus: Dilatation of the annulus can develop, for example, in a dilated cardiomyopathy, myocarditis, Bland–White–Garland syndrome, or an aortic defect and leads to incomplete valve closure.

Note

In adult and adolescent patients, mitral insufficiency is most often associated with a mitral valve prolapse.

Associated Heart Defects

A mitral cleft as the cause of mitral insufficiency typically occurs in association with an AV canal. Other heart defects that are commonly associated with mitral insufficiency are transposition of the great arteries (TGA) or an anomalous origin of the left coronary artery from the pulmonary artery (Bland–White–Garland syndrome). In these cases, however, mitral insufficiency is usually the result of ventricular dilatation.

Pathology and Hemodynamics

The failure of the mitral valve to close means that the left ventricle drains in two directions in the systole: into the aorta, and also through regurgitation into the left atrium (regurgitant blood flow). If the regurgitant flow volume is large, the left atrium is dilated. To maintain sufficient systemic cardiac output, the stroke volume of the left ventricle must be increased. This results in left ventricular dilatation. The clinical symptom of the reduction of the systemic cardiac output is congestive heart failure. In addition, there is pulmonary congestion (pulmonary hypertension, pulmonary edema).

A gradually developing chronic mitral insufficiency is usually well tolerated for a long time and compensated by hyperdynamic contractility of the left ventricle and tachycardia. Symptoms do not occur until the function of the left ventricle weakens. However, acute mitral insufficiency (papillary muscle avulsion, etc.) can rapidly lead to cardiac decompensation with pulmonary edema and cardiac shock.

15.28.2 Diagnostic Measures

Symptoms

Chronic *mild mitral insufficiency* does not cause any clinical symptoms. In a relevant chronic mitral insufficiency, there are signs of congestive heart failure such as reduced physical capacity, failure to thrive, increased sweating, pallor, and tachypnea. Palpitations can occur due to atrial arrhythmias.

In *severe mitral insufficiency*, cardiac asthma may develop as the result of pulmonary edema and possible compression of the bronchi by the dilated left atrium.

In *acute mitral insufficiency* (e.g., as the result of a papillary muscle avulsion), acute left heart failure with pulmonary edema is the main symptom.

Auscultation

The first heart sound is normal or weakened as a result of the incomplete valve closure. The second heart sound can be widely split due to the shortened left ventricular ejection time and early aortic valve closure. A prominent second heart sound occurs if there is pulmonary hypertension.

A high-frequency, "blowing" holosystolic murmur that can be best heard at the apex with radiation into the axilla is characteristic. There may also be a low-frequency diastolic murmur as a sign of a relative mitral stenosis.

ECG

The ECG of a mild mitral insufficiency is unremarkable. Otherwise there are signs of left atrial overload (P mitrale: wide, notched P wave) and of left ventricular hypertrophy. If pulmonary hypertension persists, signs of right ventricular hypertrophy also develop. Supraventricular tachycardias or atrial flutter/fibrillation can develop with chronic severe mitral insufficiency.

Chest X-ray

The enlarged left atrium and ventricle seen radiographically correlate with the extent of mitral insufficiency. Enlargement of the left atrium causes widening of the tracheal bifurcation. Engorgement of the pulmonary vasculature leads to signs of pulmonary congestion. Pulmonary edema occurs if there is acute or decompensated chronic mitral insufficiency.

Echocardiography

The extent and exact location of the regurgitation can be detected by color Doppler ultrasound. The dilatation of the left atrium and ventricle correlates with the severity of chronic mitral insufficiency. Left ventricular contractility is hyperdynamic in order to eject sufficient output to the system circulation. Normal fractional shortening may therefore be a first indication of imminent left ventricular decompensation. Pathological changes of the valve structure or associated anomalies such as a mitral valve prolapse can be ruled out or detected by echocardiography.

The severity of mitral insufficiency can be determined based on the regurgitation jet in the color Doppler sonogram (▸ Fig. 15.96). In a mild insufficiency, there is a limited color jet hitting the proximal one-third of the left atrium near the valve. In a moderate mitral insufficiency, the color jet reaches the dilated left atrium. In severe mitral insufficiency, the color jet can be detected up to the pulmonary veins. The left atrium and ventricle are generally enlarged.

Cardiac Catheterization

Cardiac catheterization is not routinely performed. If it is needed, the left atrial pressure can be determined using the pulmonary capillary wedge pressure. The pulmonary artery pressure should also be determined. The extent of regurgitation across the valve is visualized in the contrast medium ventriculography (▸ Table 15.9).

MRI

MRI may provide additional information on function (e.g., severity of regurgitation, exact determination of left atrial and left ventricular volume).

15.28.3 Treatment

Pharmacological Treatment

If there is no treatable cause of the mitral insufficiency such as acute Kawasaki syndrome or Bland–White–Garland syndrome, the aim of pharmacological treatment is to reduce the regurgitant flow and improve left ventricular stroke volume. ACE inhibitors are therefore usually administered to reduce afterload. If there are signs of congestive heart failure such as dyspnea or reduced physical capacity, diuretics and digoxin can also be given.

For acute or decompensated chronic mitral insufficiency, intravenous afterload reducers such as sodium

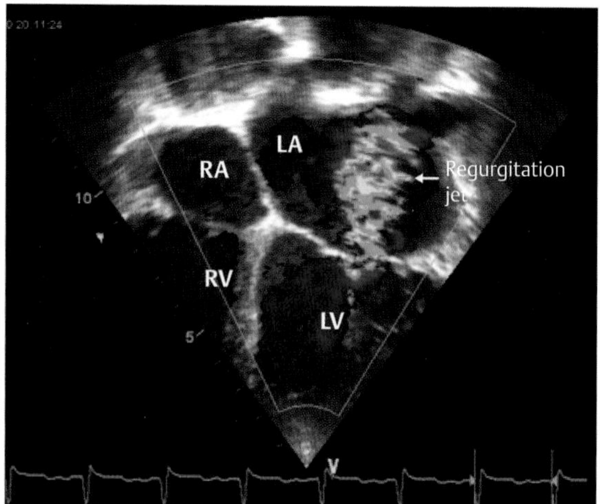

Fig. 15.96 Color Doppler finding of mitral insufficiency. In the four-chamber view, systolic regurgitation can be detected across the mitral valve into the left atrium (Arrow: regurgitation jet).
RA, right atrium; LA, left atrium; RV, right ventricle; LV, left ventricle.

Table 15.9 Classification of mitral insufficiency based on the contrast medium reflux in contrast medium ventriculography

Classification	Contrast medium reflux	Regurgitation fraction
Grade I	Minimal reflux, incomplete opacification of left atrium	< 20%
Grade II	Complete opacification of the left atrium after several beats, lower density of contrast medium in the left atrium than left ventricle	20–40%
Grade III	Complete dense opacification in the left atrium, identical density of contrast medium in the left atrium and ventricle	40–60%
Grade IV	Immediate complete opacification of the left atrium, higher density of contrast medium in the left atrium than left ventricle, contrast medium reflux up to the pulmonary veins	> 60%

nitroprusside and positive inotropic substances (dobutamine, milrinone) and intravenous diuretics are given.

Surgical Treatment

Surgery is usually needed for symptomatic patients (NYHA class III and IV). Mitral valve replacement (mechanical synthetic valve or bioprosthesis) should be weighed against valve reconstruction. Valve reconstruction is usually preferable in children.

15.28.4 Prognosis and Clinical Course

▸ **Long-term outcome.** The prognosis depends largely on the extent of mitral insufficiency, the cause, and associated heart defects. A cleft mitral valve can generally be successfully treated surgically, while complex anomalies of the mitral valve (parachute mitral valve, hammock mitral valve) are among the greatest challenges in cardiac surgery.

Chronic mild mitral insufficiency may be asymptomatic for many years, while acute mitral insufficiency can lead to cardiogenic shock within a very short time.

▸ **Outpatient checkups.** Regular outpatient checkups are necessary even for mild mitral insufficiency to note a possible change in the findings.

After valve replacement, the function of the valve must be monitored regularly. After implantation of a mechanical valve, long-term anticoagulation must be maintained (target INR 2.5–3.5). If a bioprosthetic valve is used, platelet aggregation inhibition with ASA is recommended for the first 3 months. No further anticoagulation is needed if there is no atrial fibrillation. After valve reconstruction using foreign material, endocarditis prophylaxis is needed for the first 6 postoperative months and lifelong if there are residual defects in the area of the foreign material. After the implantation of prosthetic valves (mechanical or biological), long-term endocarditis prophylaxis is also needed.

▸ **Physical exercise capacity and lifestyle.** Mild chronic mitral insufficiency is generally well tolerated and does not cause any symptoms. Patients with mild to at most moderate mitral regurgitation with a sinus rhythm can engage in sports with no limitations. Patients with moderate mitral insufficiency and normal left ventricular function with at most mild left ventricular enlargement should avoid sports with a high static load. Sports are not recommended for patients with severe mitral insufficiency. After surgical correction, contact sports should be avoided if there is an increased risk of bleeding due to anticoagulation.

▸ **Special aspects in adolescents and adults.** In adults, mitral insufficiency is usually acquired. It occurs in adults most often in association with a mitral valve prolapse (Chapter 15.29). In developing countries, mitral insufficiency is usually the result of rheumatic fever.

Atrial arrhythmias such as atrial flutter/fibrillation are considerably more common in adults than in children.

After a synthetic valve replacement, the teratogenicity of warfarin and phenprocoumon should be noted for women who wish to conceive.

15.29 Mitral Valve Prolapse

15.29.1 Basics

Synonyms: Barlow syndrome, floppy mitral valve, mitral click-murmur syndrome, systolic click-murmur syndrome

Definition

In a mitral valve prolapse (MVP), the mitral leaflet protrudes excessively into the left atrium during the systole (▸ Fig. 15.97). A mitral valve prolapse is sometimes associated with mitral insufficiency.

A *mitral valve prolapse syndrome* is when a mitral valve prolapse is associated with clinical symptoms.

Epidemiology

Mitral valve prolapse is rare in children, but its prevalence increases with age. Women are affected twice as often as men. According to recent studies, a mitral valve prolapse can be detected in around 2.4% of the population by echocardiography.

Etiology

In a mitral valve prolapse there is a discrepancy between the size of the mitral leaflets and the valve opening. Either there is excess leaflet tissue, excessively long

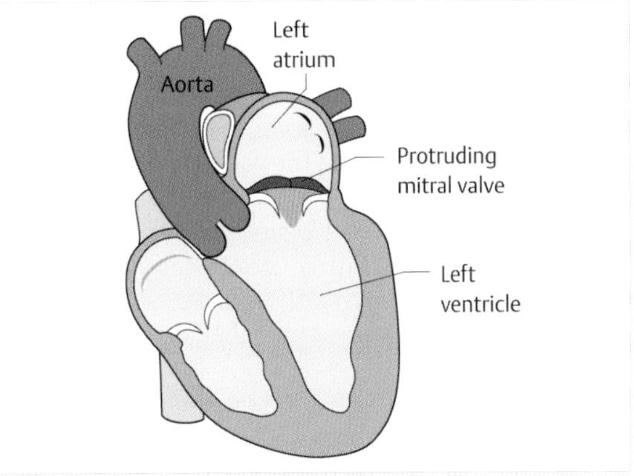

Fig. 15.97 Mitral valve prolapse. During the systole, one or both of the mitral leaflets protrudes excessively into the left atrium.

tendinous cords, or a relatively small left ventricle. The cause is unclear in more than half of cases. Sometimes there is myxomatous degeneration of parts of the mitral valve. Probably one form occurs in familial clusters and has an autosomal dominant inheritance pattern. A mitral valve prolapse often occurs in conjunction with connective tissue diseases. Rare causes are rheumatic heart diseases, coronary heart disease (papillary muscle dysfunction), a hypertrophic cardiomyopathy, or a tendinous cord avulsion.

Associated Anomalies

The following additional cardiac anomalies have been described in conjunction with mitral valve prolapse: ASD or atrial septum aneurysm, tricuspid valve prolapse, aortic valve prolapse, accessory conduction pathways, and coronary anomalies.

Associated Diseases and Syndromes

Mitral valve prolapse occurs frequently in conjunction with connective tissue diseases such as Marfan syndrome, Ehlers–Danlos syndrome, osteogenesis imperfecta, and pseudoxanthoma elasticum, or with the fragile X syndrome. A mitral valve prolapse can be detected in nearly all patients with Marfan syndrome.

Mitral valve prolapse also occurs with general diseases such as thyroid function disorders, sickle cell anemia, and muscular dystrophy.

15.29.2 Diagnostic Measures

Symptoms

Most patients with a mitral valve prolapse are completely asymptomatic. Symptoms are especially rare in children. Symptomatic patients often have a diffuse range of nonspecific problems. It is often difficult to tell whether the symptoms are caused by the mitral valve prolapse or occur independently of it.

Typical symptoms are reduced physical exercise capacity, dizziness, syncopes, dyspnea, chest pain, or palpitations. The hypothesis that the symptoms are caused by the sudden systolic pulling of the papillary muscles with consecutive ischemia of the papillary muscles seems very questionable.

Patients with a mitral valve prolapse, especially young women, often have an asthenic habitus. Chest deformities such as pectus excavatum, small chest diameter, flat back, kyphosis, or scoliosis are typical.

Complications

Most of the affected individuals do not develop any serious problems over time. Possible complications are an increase in mitral regurgitation, tendinous cord rupture, infectious endocarditis, serious arrhythmias (supraventricular and ventricular arrhythmias, pre-excitation), or thromboembolism.

Sudden cardiac deaths have even been described in association with a mitral valve prolapse. Risk factors for sudden cardiac death are thickened mitral leaflets, recurrent syncopes, sustained supraventricular tachycardia, and/or complex ventricular arrhythmias and cases of sudden death in the family. Young women are especially affected.

Auscultation

The leading finding is a systolic click with or without a mid-to-late systolic murmur. This can be best heard at the cardiac apex. The click is a brief, high-frequency sound caused by the sudden tension when the mitral leaflet prolapses. The mechanism can be compared with a sail on a boat that is suddenly filled with wind. The click can also merge with the first heart sound so that on auscultation, it sounds like a conspicuously loud first heart sound.

A holosystolic murmur can be a sign of mitral regurgitation, but is rare in childhood.

There are characteristic findings in the *dynamic auscultation*:

Maneuvers to reduce the filling of the left ventricle cause the mitral leaflet to prolapse sooner and the click then occurs earlier in the systole. Left ventricular filling can be reduced, for example, by a standing position or in the straining phase of a Valsalva maneuver.

An increase in left ventricular filling has the opposite effect and causes the click to be heard later in the systole. This can be achieved, for example, by squatting, isometric stress (e.g., strong handshake), or after a Valsalva maneuver.

ECG

The ECG is unremarkable in most asymptomatic patients. However, occasionally ST segment changes are found, typically in leads II, III, and aVF. They include nonspecific changes in the ST segment, conspicuous T waves, or T wave inversion. The significance of these changes and the pathological mechanism are not understood. There may also be supraventricular and ventricular arrhythmias or pre-excitation.

Chest X-ray

The cardiopulmonary finding is usually unremarkable in an X-ray examination. Dilatation of the left atrium is found only in severe mitral insufficiency, but there may be anomalies of the osseous thorax (e.g., scoliosis).

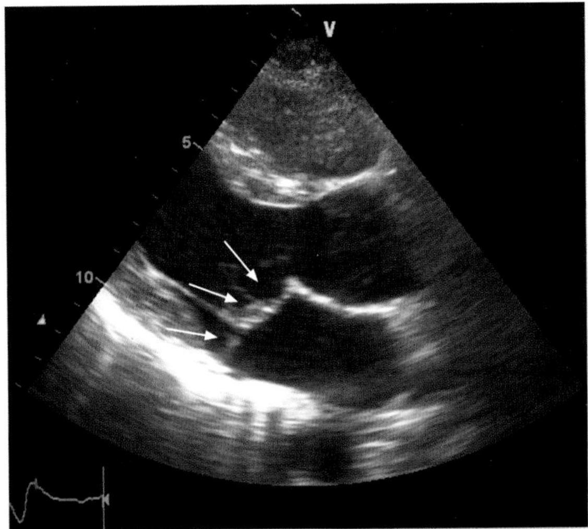

Fig. 15.98 Echocardiography finding of a mitral valve prolapse. The systolic protrusion of the mitral leaflets into the left atrium can be seen in the parasternal long axis.

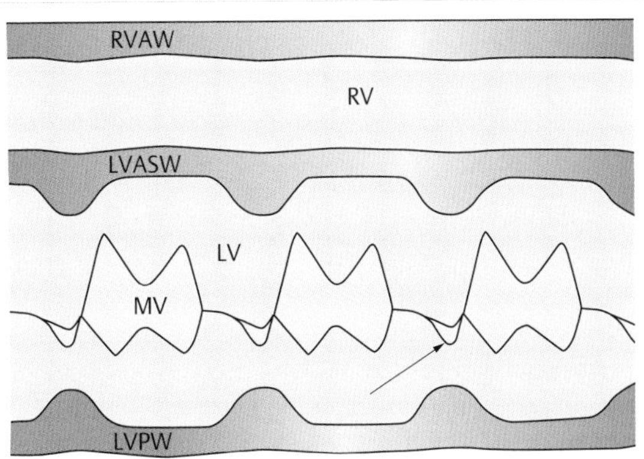

Fig. 15.99 Illustration of a mitral valve prolapse in the M mode. The posterior mitral leaflet moves to the rear in the late systole (arrow).[43]
RVAW, right ventricular anterior wall; RV, right ventricle; LV, left ventricle; MV, mitral valve; LVPW, left ventricular posterior wall.

Echocardiography

A mitral valve prolapse can be reliably visualized by echocardiography. One or both of the mitral leaflets protrude into the left atrium by more than 2 mm during systole ("hammock phenomenon"). The prolapse of the mitral leaflets can be visualized most reliably in the parasternal long axis (▸ Fig. 15.98) or in the apical two-chamber view. The diagnosis should not be made if slight sagging of leaflets with a normal thickness can be seen only in the four-chamber view.

There may be myxomatous proliferation of the mitral leaflets and the tendinous cords are sometimes elongated. The presence of mitral insufficiency should also be noted.

The late systolic prolapse of one or both mitral leaflets can be seen in the M mode (▸ Fig. 15.99).

Cardiac Catheterization

Cardiac catheterization is not usually needed. In adults with a mitral valve prolapse, possible symptoms such as chest pain or arrhythmias may be difficult to distinguish from the differential diagnosis of coronary heart disease and coronary angiography may sometimes be needed.

Electrophysiological Examination

An electrophysiological examination may be indicated if there is an accessory conduction pathway.

MRI

MRI is not usually indicated, but a mitral valve prolapse is often discovered as an incidental finding in an MRI.

15.29.3 Treatment

Conservative Treatment

Asymptomatic patients do not need treatment. For symptomatic patients with chest pain, palpitations, or dizziness, treatment with beta blockers can be attempted.

The risk of endocarditis is slightly higher if there is mitral regurgitation or if the mitral leaflets are thickened in a pronounced prolapse. However, according to the new guidelines, endocarditis prophylaxis is not necessary.

Surgical Treatment

Surgery (mitral valve reconstruction, only rarely mitral valve replacement) is indicated only for severe mitral insufficiency associated with left atrial or left ventricular dilatation or congestive heart failure.

15.29.4 Prognosis and Clinical Course

▸ **Long-term outcome.** The overall prognosis is very good. Most patients are completely asymptomatic and do not require treatment. Life expectancy is usually not affected.

Complications such as more pronounced arrhythmias, sudden death, endocarditis, increasing mitral regurgitation, or congestive heart failure are extremely rare in childhood, but may increase with age.

▸ **Outpatient checkups.** Checkups every 2 years are sufficient for asymptomatic patients. Symptomatic patients and patients with risk factors (see Symptoms, Chapter 15.29.2) should of course have more frequent checkups.

► **Physical exercise capacity and lifestyle.** No limitation of physical activity and sports is necessary in asymptomatic patients with no relevant mitral regurgitation.

Patients with recurrent syncopes, sudden cardiac death in the family, or relevant arrhythmias (atrial fibrillation, re-entrant tachycardia, ventricular arrhythmia) should not engage in competitive sports.

► **Special aspects in adolescents and adults.** Most adult patients are asymptomatic. However, if symptoms occur in association with a mitral valve prolapse, they generally begin in adolescence or adulthood. It is often difficult to distinguish the symptoms, which are usually nonspecific, such as dizziness, palpitations, or chest pain from other differential diagnoses (especially from coronary heart disease).

Complications such as severe mitral insufficiency, more pronounced arrhythmias, infectious endocarditis, thromboembolism, or sudden heart death are very rare overall (< 2% of all patients with a mitral valve prolapse), but can have a decisive effect on the prognosis. Patients with an increased risk include older men, who typically have a relevant mitral insufficiency. The risk of requiring mitral valve surgery by age 75 is estimated to be 4 to 5% for men and 1.5 to 2% for women.

15.30 Coronary Anomalies

15.30.1 Basics

A number of congenital anomalies of the coronary arteries occur, which affect the origin, course, or ostia. Most of these anomalies are not clinically significant and are incidental findings made during cardiac catheterizations or autopsies.

However, there are anomalies that can lead to hypoperfusion and the risk of sudden death. There are also anomalous origins and courses that occur in association with congenital heart defects (e.g., d-TGA, tetralogy of Fallot) that must be noted if surgical correction is planned.

Large coronary fistulas can lead to early congestive heart failure due to volume overload.

Embryology

At the beginning of development, the myocardium is supplied by blood from the ventricles through diffusion. As the myocardium thickens, this method of supply is no longer adequate and a trabecular network of sinusoids develops in the myocardium. This reduces the diffusion distance between blood and myocardial cells. During further development, the myocardium becomes denser and a vascular network arises that is connected with other mediastinal vessels. The persistence of these connections leads to coronary fistulas.

Endothelial sprouts also probably develop at the base of the truncus arteriosus, the common precursor of the aorta and pulmonary artery. These endothelial sprouts later connect with the myocardial vascular network and form the coronary vessels. It is not yet known whether only two sprouts arise or whether sprouts develop from each sinus that are later obliterated except for the two. An unusual obliteration, an abnormal position of the endothelial sprouts, or an anomalous septation of the truncus arteriosus in the aorta and pulmonary artery can result in coronary anomalies.

Normal Coronary Anatomy

The coronary arteries usually arise from the sinuses of Valsalva directly above the aortic valve (► Fig. 15.100). For the nomenclature of the coronary vessels, it is important to note that they are designated not according to their origin, but according to their branching pattern and the territory they supply.

- The *right coronary artery* (RCA) usually arises from the right sinus of Valsalva of the aorta. It runs in the right atrioventricular groove (AV groove). The first branch from the RCA is the conus branch, which supplies the right ventricular outflow tract. The RCA supplies the right atrium, large parts of the right ventricle, the posterior one-third of the ventricular septum, and the sinus and AV nodes.
- The *left coronary artery* (LCA) typically arises from the left sinus of Valsalva. Shortly after its origin, it divides into the anterior interventricular branch—in the English-speaking world known as the left anterior descending (LAD) branch—and the circumflex (RCX) branch.
  - The LAD runs in the anterior interventricular groove to the cardiac apex. It supplies the wall of the left ventricle, the anterior two-thirds of the ventricular septum, and the anterior wall of the right ventricle.
  - The RCX runs in the left AV groove and supplies the posterior lateral wall of the left ventricle.

However, the supply territories and forms of the coronary arteries are quite variable.

Epidemiology

Coronary anomalies are found in more than 5% of individuals who have coronary angiographies. Most of these anomalies are not clinically significant. Among the most common anomalies are three coronary ostia. In this case, the conus branch of the RCA usually arises separately from the right sinus of Valsalva.

Classification

The classification of coronary anomalies is not standardized. The following categories are based on a teaching perspective. The most common coronary anomalies are listed in ► Table 15.10.

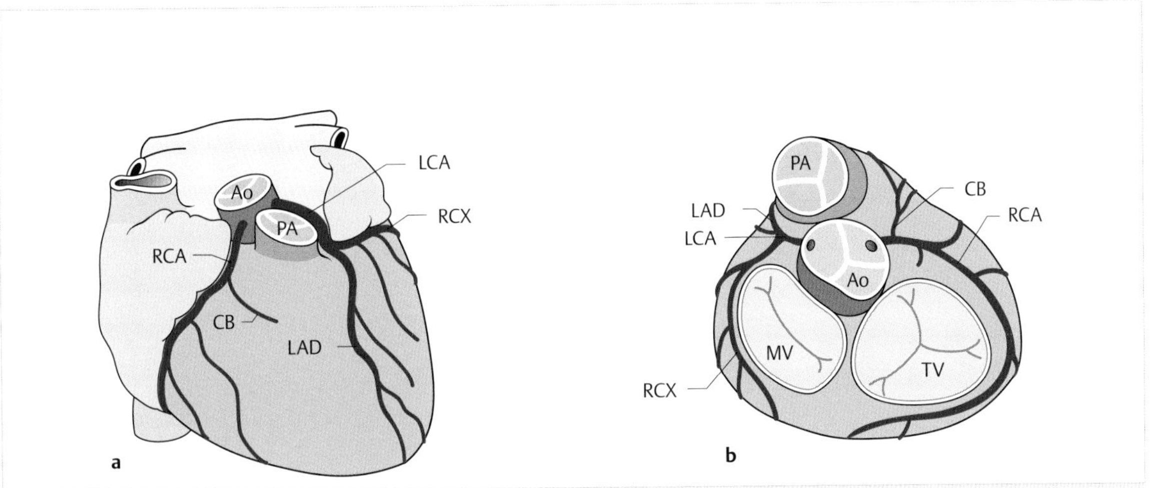

Fig. 15.100 Normal anatomy of the coronary arteries. In the view from the front (**a**) and the view from above (**b**), the origins of the right and left coronary artery from the corresponding sinuses of Valsalva of the aorta and their branches and courses can be seen. The left coronary artery arises from the left sinus of Valsalva. Shortly after its origin, it branches into the anterior interventricular branch (left anterior descending [LAD]) and the circumflex branch. The right coronary artery arises from the right sinus of Valsalva of the aorta. The first branch from the right coronary artery is the conus branch, which supplies the right ventricular outflow tract.
RCA, right coronary artery; LCA, left coronary artery; LAD, left anterior descending branch; RCX, (ramus) circumflex branch of the left coronary artery; CB, conus branch; Ao, aorta; PA, pulmonary artery; MV, mitral valve; TV, tricuspid valve.

15.30.2 Origins of Coronary Artery Anomalies

Association of Anomalous Origins with Congenital Heart Defects

Anomalous origins of the coronary arteries are found frequently with congenital heart defects. The two most important are tetralogy of Fallot and d-TGA.

▸ **Tetralogy of Fallot.** Anomalous origins are present in nearly 10% of Fallot patients. Particularly significant are coronary anomalies in which the coronary arteries cross the right ventricular outflow tract. Because the right ventricular outflow tract is often opened and augmented with a patch during surgical correction of tetralogy of Fallot, coronary anomalies must be noted. For example, a large-caliber conus branch that supplies the right ventricular outflow tract and an anomalous origin of the LAD from the right coronary artery are very common. In this case, the LAD crosses the right ventricular outflow tract (▸ Fig. 15.101).

▸ **Transposition of the great arteries.** In d-TGA, the coronary arteries arise from the two sinuses that are directly adjacent to the pulmonary artery ("facing sinuses"). The LCA usually arises from the left facing sinus and the RCA from the right facing sinus, but there are a number of anomalies (e.g., origin of the RCX from the RCA or intramural courses of the coronary arteries). Since transferring the coronary arteries is a major element of the arterial switch procedure, the origins and courses of the coronary artery must be clarified preoperatively. Anomalies may make a switch procedure impossible, in which case a Mustard/Senning atrial baffle procedure must be performed.

▸ **Other heart defects with coronary anomalies.** Coronary anomalies that need to be noted for surgical correction also occur frequently in the following heart defects: l-TGA, truncus arteriosus communis, double-outlet right ventricle (DORV), and double-inlet left ventricle (DILV).

Origin of the LCA from the Right Sinus of Valsalva or from the RCA

If the LCA arises from the right sinus of Valsalva or the RCA, it generally runs between the aorta and pulmonary artery (▸ Fig. 15.102). This may lead to compression of the LCA in this area. There is a risk of myocardial ischemia with angina pectoris, syncopes, and sudden cardiac death. These complications typically occur in association with physical exertion in adolescents or young adults. Due to the stress-related increase in cardiac output, the caliber of the aortic root and pulmonary artery increase and exert pressure on the coronary artery that is located between them. A reduction in the lumen of the coronary ostia also plays a certain role. In the anomalous origins described above, the ostia branch off from the sinus relatively obliquely so that the lumen of the ostia is additionally constricted by

Table 15.10 Summary of the most clinically significant coronary anomalies

Coronary anomaly	Clinical significance
Anomalous origins of the coronary arteries from the aorta	
• Origin of the LCA or LAD from the right sinus of Valsalva	Compression of the affected coronary artery between the aorta and pulmonary artery leads to myocardial ischemia (especially under exertion)
• Origin of a single coronary artery from the right sinus of Valsalva	Compression of the affected coronary artery between the aorta and pulmonary artery leads to myocardial ischemia (especially under exertion)
• Origin of the left RCX from the RCA	No clinical significance
Anomalous origins of the coronary arteries from the pulmonary artery	
• Origin of the LCA from the pulmonary artery (Bland–White–Garland syndrome)	Myocardial ischemia after the drop in pulmonary resistance (Chapter 15.31)
• Origin of the RCA from the pulmonary artery	Outcome is usually better than in Bland–White–Garland syndrome
Anomalous calibers of the coronary arteries	
• Coronary artery stenoses	Myocardial ischemia depending on the severity of the stenoses
• Atresia of a coronary artery ostium	Survival only if there is sufficient collateralization
• Coronary artery aneurysms	Thrombosis, rupture
Myocardial sinusoids	
• Persistence of the embryonic sinusoids as direct connection between the ventricles and coronary arteries	Association with pulmonary or aortic atresia with an intact ventricular septum. Caution: Coronary perfusion may be dependent on the sinusoids (Chapter 15.16)
Coronary artery fistulas	
• Coronary fistulas usually drain into the right heart or in the pulmonary circulation (RA, RV, PA)	Left-to-right shunt, heart failure if the fistulas are large, myocardial ischemia, rupture, endocarditis

LCA, left coronary artery; RCA, right coronary artery; RCX, (ramus) circumflex branch; RA, right atrium; RV, right ventricle; PA, pulmonary artery.

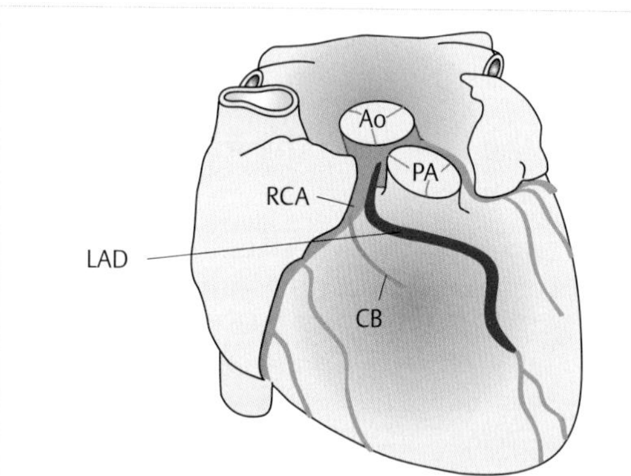

Fig. 15.101 Origin of the left anterior descending branch (LAD) from the right coronary artery (RCA). The figure illustrates that the course of the LAD crosses the right ventricular outflow tract if there is an anomalous origin from the RCA. This anomaly must be noted when surgically opening the right ventricular outflow tracts during a correction procedure for a tetralogy of Fallot.
Ao, aorta; CB, conus branch; PA, pulmonary artery.

tension or pressure due to increased filling of the heart (▶ Fig. 15.103).

▶ **Diagnostic measures.** Visualization of the course of the coronary arteries by echocardiography, MRI, and/or coronary angiography.

▶ **Treatment.** Surgical treatment may involve bypass surgery or reimplantation of the LCA in the left sinus of Valsalva to ensure perfusion of the supply territory of the left coronary artery. Isolated cases have also been described in which the affected coronary artery was effectively protected from external compression by an intraluminal stent.

Anomalous Origin of the Coronary Arteries from the Pulmonary Artery

This most often involves an anomalous origin of the left coronary artery from the pulmonary artery. This anomaly (Bland–White–Garland syndrome) is described in Chapter 15.31.

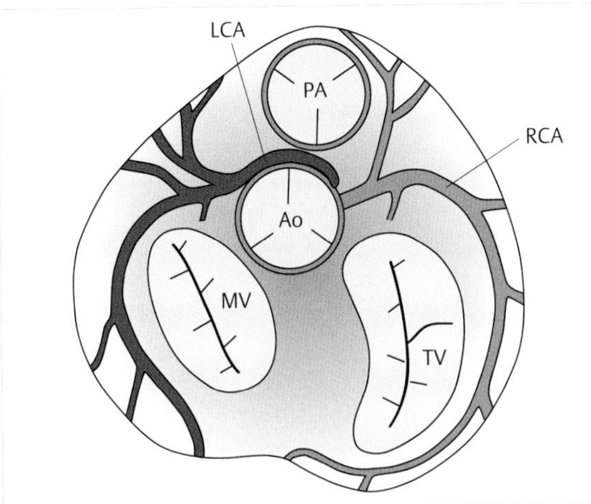

Fig. 15.102 Anomalous origin of the left coronary artery from the right sinus of Valsalva. The image illustrates that the left coronary artery runs between the aorta and the pulmonary artery in this anomaly. There may be compression of the coronary artery in this area, especially on exertion.
MV, mitral valve; TV, tricuspid valve; Ao, Aorta; PA, pulmonary artery; RCA, right coronary artery; LCA, left coronary artery.

15.30.3 Caliber Anomalies of the Coronary Arteries

Stenoses of the Coronary Arteries

Congenital or acquired coronary stenoses can involve the ostium or the further course of the vessels. They lead to hypoperfusion of the myocardium distal to the stenosis and may result in myocardial ischemia with angina pectoris and myocardial infarction.

▸ **Causes.** Causes of coronary artery stenoses are:

- Surgical procedures (e.g., coronary transfer in an arterial switch procedure, aortic valve procedures, bypass surgery)
- Myocardial bridging: A congenital tunnel-shaped course of the coronary arteries within the myocardium can lead to stenosis of the coronary vessels.
- Hyperlipoproteinemia
- Arteritis (e.g., Takayasu Arteritis, systemic lupus erythematosus, panarteritis, syphilis)
- Williams–Beuren syndrome: Intima hyperplasia of the coronary vessels can develop as a result of a supravalvular stenosis
- Thromboses or intima hyperplasia of coronary aneurysms (e.g., as a result of Kawasaki syndrome)
- Transplant vasculopathy after a heart transplant

▸ **Treatment.** Treatment in children follows the same principle as in adults:

- Reduction of risk factors such as hyperlipidemia or hypertension

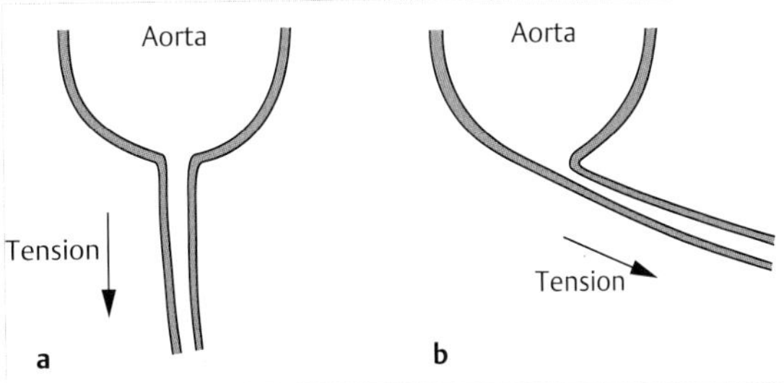

Fig. 15.103 Constriction of the coronary ostia due to tension from the acute angle of the coronary artery branching from the sinus of Valsalva. When the coronary artery arises from the sinus at an acute angle (**b**) the tension on the coronary artery causes a clear constriction of its lumen. When the coronary artery arises at a right angle (**a**), tension changes the lumen to a much lesser extent.

- Bypass surgery
- PTCA with or without stent implantation

Atresia of a Coronary Artery Ostium

This is a rare congenital anomaly that occurs mainly in association with aortic or pulmonary atresia. The affected coronary artery is extremely hypoplastic; the unaffected artery is widened to compensate for this. Survival is possible only if there are enough collaterals between the two coronary arteries. Coronary perfusion is sometimes dependent on myocardial sinusoids in such cases.

Coronary Artery Aneurysms

Coronary artery aneurysms in childhood occur most often as a result of Kawasaki syndrome. Less common causes are arteritis (Takayasu arteritis, syphilis), trauma, or a coronary artery dissection. It can be complicated by a rupture or thrombosis and stenosis of the aneurysm. Treatment options are bypass surgery or in some cases PTCA.

15.30.4 Myocardial Sinusoids

Persistence of the embryonic myocardial sinusoids occurs especially with defects such as pulmonary or aortic atresia with an intact ventricular septum. In the absence of AV valve insufficiency, the sinusoids are the only possible outflow for blood from the affected ventricle. It is essential to note that in these patients, coronary perfusion may depend on flow across the myocardial sinusoids from the ventricles. In these cases, the sinusoids naturally may not be closed. In addition, the pressure in the affected ventricle may not be lowered, for example, by opening the atretic pulmonary or aortic valve, as otherwise sufficient perfusion pressure for coronary perfusion would no longer be available.

The diagnosis can be suggested by echocardiography if an unusual flow from the ventricle to the epicardium can be visualized in the color Doppler ultrasound scan. The diagnosis is confirmed by coronary angiography.

15.30.5 Coronary Artery Fistulas

Coronary artery fistulas are pathological connections between the coronary arteries and the ventricles or other vessels (▶ Fig. 15.104). They are usually congenital, but can also arise after cardiac procedures such as myocardial biopsies, coronary angiographies, or cardiac surgery.

The fistulas arise somewhat more often from the RCA than from the LCA. More than 90% of the time, they open into the low-pressure system of the right heart or the pulmonary circulation. In descending order, they open into the right ventricle, the right atrium, and the pulmonary artery, less often into the superior vena cava or the coronary sinus, and in rare exceptions, into the left atrium or ventricle.

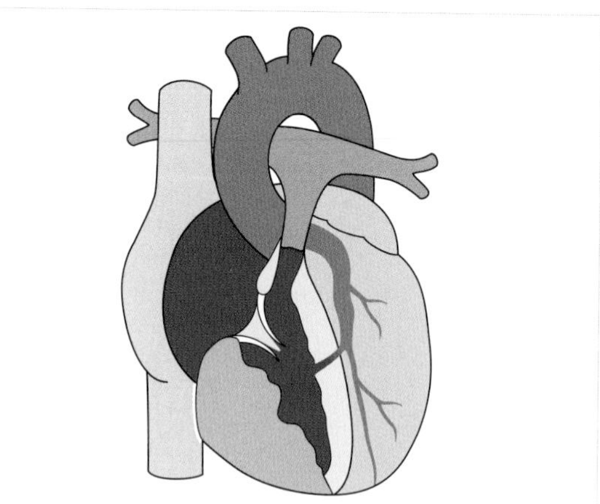

Fig. 15.104 Coronary fistula. Fistula between the left anterior descending branch of the left coronary artery and the right ventricle. Due to volume overload, the coronary artery is widened up to the origin of the fistula; distal to the fistula it narrows markedly.

▶ **Pathophysiology.** Drainage into the right heart results in a left-to-right shunt. The shunt volume depends on the size of the fistulas and the pressure ratios between the affected coronary artery and the orifice. If the fistula drains into the low-pressure area of the right heart, the direction of blood flow is from the coronary artery to the right heart.

Large fistulas may lead to a steal phenomenon so that myocardial ischemia develops distal to the fistula. Proximal to the fistula, the coronary artery is enlarged corresponding with volume overload.

▶ **Clinical symptoms.** Small fistulas are usually asymptomatic; there may be a continuous systolic–diastolic murmur. Large fistulas cause symptoms of congestive heart failure and pulmonary hypertension as early as infancy.

▶ **Complications.** Typical complications of relevant coronary artery fistulas are:

- Myocardial infarction as a result of steal
- Pulmonary hypertension as a result of volume overload in the lungs
- Endocarditis
- Vary rarely rupture of a fistula
- Thromboembolic events
- Cardiac arrhythmias, especially supraventricular arrhythmias if the right atrium is enlarged due to a fistula opening into the right atrium or coronary sinus

▶ **ECG.** The ECG is unremarkable for smaller fistulas. If there are larger fistulas with a left-to-right shunt, signs of left ventricular volume overload and right heart pressure overload may develop due to pulmonary hypertension.

▶ **Chest X-ray.** A small fistula usually has an unremarkable radiological finding. In large fistulas, there may be cardiomegaly with increased pulmonary vascular markings.

▶ **Echocardiography.** Most coronary artery fistulas can be diagnosed by echocardiography. The 2D image shows the enlargement of the affected coronary artery. An attempt can be made to visualize the flow in the coronary artery to the orifice using color Doppler ultrasonography.

▶ **Cardiac catheterization.** The fistula and orifice can be identified by angiography. The volume of the shunt can also be calculated. The fistula can sometimes be successfully closed by interventional catheterization.

▶ **MRI.** The fistula can often be visualized and the shunt volume calculated in an MRI.

▶ **Differential diagnosis.** Possible differential diagnoses are anomalies that cause a (systolic) diastolic murmur or display (systolic) diastolic flow in the color Doppler:

- PDA
- Small aortopulmonary fenestration
- Aortic insufficiency
- AV fistulas in the vicinity of the heart
- Aortopulmonary collaterals (MAPCAs)
- Perforated sinus of Valsalva aneurysm
- Aorto-left ventricular tunnel

15.30.6 Treatment

Conservative Treatment

If necessary, congestive heart failure is treated pharmacologically until the definitive treatment by interventional catheterization or surgery.

▶ **Indication for interventional catheter or surgical treatment.** Large, hemodynamically relevant fistulas should be closed by interventional catheterization or surgery as soon as possible after the diagnosis is made.

There is no standard procedure for fistulas that are not hemodynamically relevant, do not cause clinical symptoms, and are not associated with other cardiac anomalies. While "wait and see" is sometimes recommended, many authors are of the opinion that closure is indicated for even small, asymptomatic fistulas in order to avoid the complications listed (especially coronary ischemia under exertion).

Interventional Catheterization

Closure by interventional catheterization is the treatment of choice for most coronary fistulas. Spring coils, double umbrellas, or occluders (as in the closure of a PDA) can be used. The closure rate using these systems is high. Major risks involved are embolization of the closure system, fistula dissection, arrhythmias, and myocardial ischemia after closure of the fistula.

Surgical Treatment

Surgical treatment involves ligation of the fistula, while preserving the other coronary branches. Coronary arteries widened by an aneurysm may have to be excised or reduced in size. The risk of this procedure is low in infancy and childhood, but higher in adults.

15.30.7 Prognosis and Clinical Course

Spontaneous closures of coronary artery fistulas are rare. The rupture of a coronary artery fistula is also rare. Depending on the size of the fistula, congestive heart failure and pulmonary hypertension may develop as a result of the shunt. In adulthood, there is a risk of myocardial infarction due to atherosclerotic changes in the fistulas. After closure of the fistula, life expectancy is usually normal.

15.31 Bland–White–Garland Syndrome

15.31.1 Basics

Synonym: Anomalous origin of the left coronary artery from the pulmonary artery (ALCAPA)

Definition

In Bland–White–Garland syndrome, the left coronary artery arises from the main pulmonary artery or the left pulmonary artery instead of from the aorta (▶ Fig. 15.105).

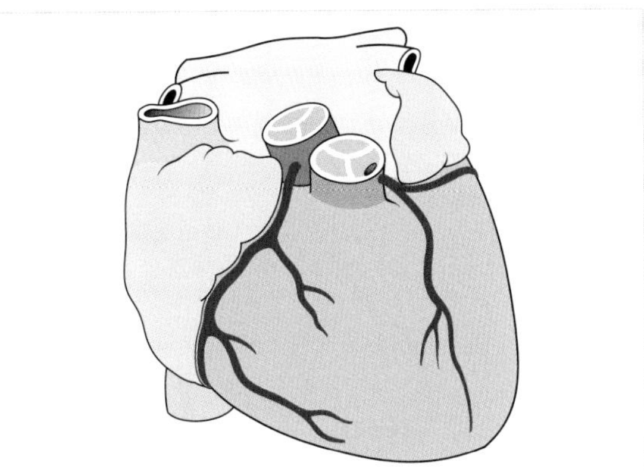

Fig. 15.105 Bland–White–Garland syndrome. The left coronary artery arises from the pulmonary artery. The right coronary artery usually arises from the right sinus of Valsalva of the aorta as normal.

Epidemiology

This is a rare anomaly that constitutes about 0.25 to 0.5% of all congenital heart defects. The incidence is 1-in-20,000 to 30,000 live births.

Pathogenesis

The underlying cause is probably the anomalous development of the coronary ostia. The anomalous septation of the embryonic truncus arteriosus in the aorta and pulmonary artery has also been discussed as a cause.

Pathology and Hemodynamics

In the Bland–White–Garland syndrome, the left coronary artery is supplied with deoxygenated blood from the pulmonary artery in the neonatal period. The perfusion pressure that the pulmonary artery develops for myocardial perfusion is lower than the aortic pressure. This leads to hypoperfusion of the left ventricular myocardium. In the neonatal period, the perfusion pressure is still high enough to ensure adequate perfusion of the myocardium due to the high pulmonary resistance and resulting high pulmonary pressure. When the pulmonary resistance drops, the extent of collateral circulation between the anomalous left and the normal right coronary artery determines the individual's fate. If collateralization is insufficient, infarction of the left ventricular myocardium occurs rapidly. If collateral blood flow is high, a steal phenomenon develops: The blood from the right coronary artery then flows into the pulmonary artery through the collateral vessels and the left coronary artery (retrograde flow in the left coronary artery) instead of into the

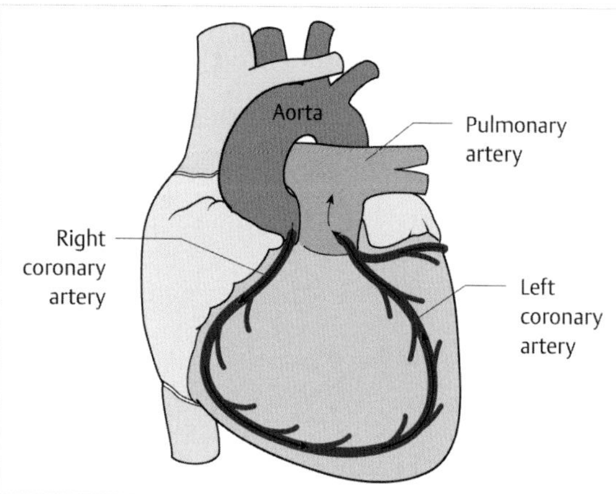

Fig. 15.106 Steal phenomenon in Bland–White–Garland syndrome. There is retrograde perfusion of the left coronary artery from collaterals. The blood from the left coronary artery flows into the pulmonary artery.

myocardium (▶ Fig. 15.106). The result is chronic myocardial ischemia.

Since the right coronary artery also has to supply the territory of the left coronary artery via collateral blood flow, the right coronary artery usually has a larger diameter. The ostium of the anomalous left coronary artery is usually located clearly superior to the pulmonary valve.

The left ventricle has areas of infarction due to ischemia and its function is usually considerably impaired. Dysfunction of the mitral valve (regurgitation) due to the ischemic lesions of the papillary muscles is also typical.

Note

Left ventricular infarction in Bland–White–Garland syndrome occurs not because the left coronary artery is supplied with venous blood from the pulmonary artery, but because of reduced perfusion pressure or a steal phenomenon between the left and right coronary arteries.

15.31.2 Diagnostic Measures

Symptoms

Affected children usually become symptomatic between 2 and 6 months of age when pulmonary resistance drops. The main symptoms are myocardial ischemia (unexplained crying due to angina pectoris) and congestive heart failure (increased sweating, pallor, poor feeding, dyspnea). The diagnosis is often not made until acute decompensation occurs, for example, during a pulmonary infection.

If there is sufficient collateralization (15–20% of cases), the children may not develop any major symptoms for a long time. Symptoms of coronary insufficiency do not develop until later in these cases.

Note

An anomalous origin of the coronary arteries must always be ruled out in every case of unclear congestive heart failure, reduced left ventricular function, or cardiomegaly, especially accompanied by mitral regurgitation.

Auscultation

Auscultation is not very useful. If there is severe heart failure, a gallop rhythm may be heard. Sometimes the "blowing" murmur of mitral regurgitation can be heard at the cardiac apex. If collateral blood flow is pronounced, a continuous murmur can be auscultated at the upper left sternal margin (PMI somewhat lower than in a PDA).

ECG

Signs of left ventricular (anterolateral) myocardial ischemia in leads I, aVL, and V_4 to V_6 are typical: deep Q waves, loss of R wave progression, and ST segment changes. Later there are signs of left ventricular volume overload.

Note

Depending on collateral blood flow and the supply type, the ECG may also be unremarkable in Bland–White–Garland syndrome.

Chest X-ray

The most conspicuous findings are cardiomegaly and signs of pulmonary congestion depending on the extent of collateralization and the size of the left-to-right shunt across the coronary arteries.

Echocardiography

Typical findings—depending on collateral blood flow—are an enlarged right coronary artery and absence of a left coronary artery arising from the aorta. An experienced examiner can sometimes visualize the origin of the left coronary artery from the pulmonary artery. Using color Doppler ultrasonography, it may be possible to detect the blood flow out of the left coronary artery to the pulmonary artery. If there is sufficient collateralization, this retrograde blood flow in the left coronary artery occurs continuously in systole and diastole; if collateralization is less pronounced, only in the diastole.

The left ventricle typically has thin walls and impaired contractility. There is often mitral regurgitation. The image suggests dilated cardiomyopathy. There may be increased echogenicity of the papillary muscles and/or the endocardium as a result of myocardial ischemia.

MRI

In larger patients, the anomalous origin of the left coronary artery can be reliably visualized in an MRI. Myocardial perfusion can be assessed after injecting contrast medium. Blood flow in the left coronary artery can also be quantified.

Cardiac Catheterization

A definitive diagnosis can be made by aortogram and selective coronary angiography as follows. After injection of contrast medium into the (usually dilated) right coronary artery, there is retrograde opacification of the left coronary artery via collaterals in Bland–White–Garland syndrome. The contrast medium then flows into the pulmonary artery. Collateralization can also be assessed. Hemodynamic measurements usually show an increase in the left ventricular end-diastolic and left atrial pressure, indicating poor left ventricular function.

Note

Cardiac catheterization can definitively rule out a Bland–White–Garland syndrome.

15.31.3 Treatment

Conservative Treatment

Treatment of congestive heart failure including catecholamines, diuretics, and afterload reduction may be necessary to bridge the period until the patient is stabilized and definitive surgery can be performed.

Surgical Treatment

Surgery is the definitive treatment. It is always indicated (even for asymptomatic patients) as soon as possible after the diagnosis is made. Implantation of the left coronary artery into the aortic root is usually preferred. Depending on the anatomical situation and the clinical condition, other methods may also be used.

► **Direct implantation of the left coronary artery into the aorta.** Implantation of the anomalous left coronary artery into the aortic root is the surgical procedure of choice. The left coronary artery is excised with a cuff from the pulmonary arterial wall around it and implanted into

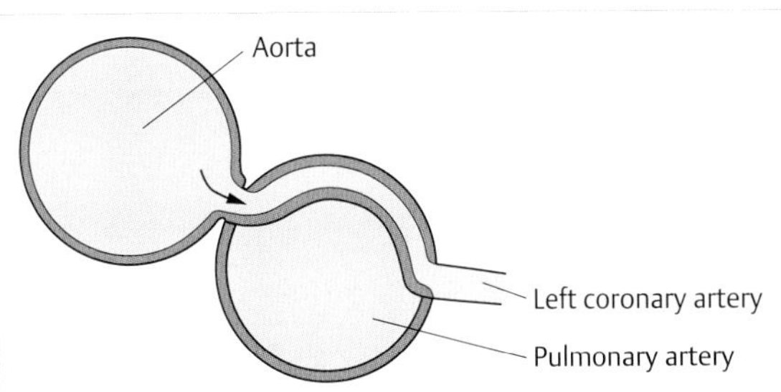

Fig. 15.107 Principle of the Takeuchi procedure. The anomalous left coronary artery is redirected to the aortic root through a tunnel. The tunnel is sutured into the posterior wall of the pulmonary artery.[29]

the aortic root in a procedure similar to an arterial switch procedure. However, if the anatomical situation is unfavorable, tension or kinking of the coronary artery can lead to occlusion, so this method is not suitable for all patients.

► **Takeuchi procedure.** The Takeuchi procedure (► Fig. 15.107) is the surgical procedure that was often used for Bland–White–Garland syndrome. In this technique, a millimeter-sized aortopulmonary window is made. The connection between the two vessels is created by making a tunnel at the posterior wall of the pulmonary artery connected to the ostium of the left coronary artery. Aortic blood then flows through the tunnel to the left coronary artery. The disadvantage of this method is that the lumen of the pulmonary artery is constricted by the tunnel, resulting in supravalvular pulmonary stenosis.

► **Tashiro procedure.** In this more recent variation, the anomalous left coronary artery is excised with a pulmonary arterial cuff. The upper and lower segments of the cuff are then sutured together to form a vascular tube. The left coronary artery is anastomosed with the aortic root via this "extension." The advantage of this technique is that, in contrast to the Takeuchi procedure, it does not cause obstruction of the pulmonary valve.

► **Ligation of the left coronary artery at the origin from the pulmonary artery.** Ligation of the left coronary artery eliminates the outflow of coronary arterial blood to the pulmonary artery (coronary steal). However, this procedure is possible only if there is sufficient collateralization. It is not usually performed today.

► **Aortocoronary bypass.** Bypass surgery is an alternative for severely ill or elderly patients.

► **Mitral valve surgery.** In addition to the procedures described above, reconstruction or even replacement of the mitral valve is sometimes necessary if there is severe mitral regurgitation.

▸ **Cardiac transplant.** A heart transplant is the last treatment option if there is severe infarction of the left ventricle.

15.31.4 Prognosis and Clinical Course

▸ **Long-term outcome.** The long-term outcome depends mainly on the extent of the myocardial infarction and preoperative left ventricular function. The "stunned myocardium" often displays a remarkable recovery, but it can sometimes take months to years. The early mortality rate after surgery has been reduced considerably in recent years and is reported to be less than 8% after reimplantation of the left coronary artery. Specific problems in the long term, depending on the surgical procedure, are closure of a bypass, development of a stenosis in the main pulmonary artery after a Takeuchi procedure, and development of a coronary stenosis after reimplantation of the left coronary artery. Mitral regurgitation persists in around half of patients even after corrective surgery.

▸ **Outpatient checkups.** After correction of Bland–White–Garland syndrome, regular lifelong cardiac checkups are needed. The recovery of left ventricular function must be assessed and signs of coronary insufficiency and cardiac arrhythmias (ventricular arrhythmias) must be noted. In addition to the patient history, an exercise ECG can provide information on coronary stenoses. Cardiac catheterization is often recommended 1 year after surgery and again 5 to 10 years after surgery.

After a Takeuchi procedure, the supravalvular pulmonary stenosis caused by the surgical technique must be monitored. Persistent severe mitral regurgitation can necessitate re-operation.

▸ **Physical capacity and lifestyle.** Patients with Bland–White–Garland syndrome have a clearly increased risk of sudden cardiac death. After corrective surgery, left ventricular function usually recovers and the risk of sudden cardiac death is reduced. Most patients then have good physical capacity. Recovery of left ventricular function, the extent of mitral regurgitation, and possible ventricular arrhythmias are decisive for physical capacity and the ability to engage in sports.

▸ **Special aspects in adolescents and adults.** Around 5 to 10% of patients do not become symptomatic until adulthood. These patients usually have sufficient collateralization of the coronary vessels. Bland–White–Garland syndrome must therefore be considered as a differential diagnosis when investigating coronary insufficiency, especially in young adults.

15.32 Anomalies of the Systemic Veins

15.32.1 Basics

The embryonic vena cava system develops initially bilaterally and is symmetrical. In situs solitus, the venae cavae on the left side are usually obliterated, leaving the right superior and right inferior venae cavae which drain the systemic venous blood from the upper and lower halves of the body. In a situs inversus, the two left venae cavae persist. Anomalies of the venae cavae often occur with anomalous positions of the heart or complex heart defects. A number of possible anomalies of the systemic veins have been reported, the most important of which are described below.

15.32.2 Persistent Left Superior Vena Cava

In this anomaly, which occurs in 5 to 25% of all congenital heart defects, the left superior vena cava is not obliterated.

In the most frequent type, the left superior vena cava (LSVC) is connected with the coronary sinus, which drains the systemic venous blood into the right atrium (▸ Fig. 15.108). This occurs because the coronary sinus and the LSVC arise from the same embryonic vessel. If the LSVC drains into the coronary sinus, the sinus will be conspicuously large in echocardiography. Since the systemic venous blood of the LSVC reaches the right atrium in this manner, the patients are not clinically affected and not cyanotic. The LSVC may be visible in an X-ray image at the left mediastinal border. In most cases, there is also the normal right superior venae cava. In somewhat more than half the cases, the two superior venae cavae are connected by an innominate vein.

The LSVC very rarely drains directly into the left atrium. Due to the mixing of systemic venous blood in the systemic circulation, these patients present with cyanosis. This anomaly is almost always associated with complex heart defects. There is no coronary sinus. Possible treatment options include ligation or surgical connection of the vessel with the right atrium.

Note

Attention must always be paid to an LSVC for operations using cardiopulmonary bypass with respect to the cannulation site and it must therefore be diagnosed or ruled out prior to surgery.

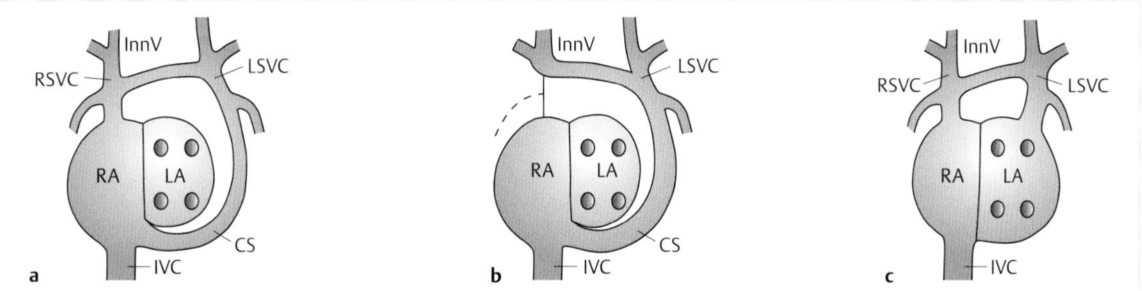

Fig. 15.108 The most important variants of a persistent left superior vena cava (LSVC).[29]
a LSVC draining into the coronary sinus (most common variant). There is a right superior vena cava. The two venae cavae are connected via an innominate vein. **b** LSVC draining into the coronary sinus. The right superior vena cava is atretic. The blood from the entire upper half of the body drains through the clearly dilated coronary sinus into the right atrium. **c** LSVC draining into the left atrium. There is no coronary sinus. The two venae cavae are connected by an innominate vein.
RA, right atrium; LA, left atrium; IVC, inferior vena cava; CS, coronary sinus; RSVC, persistent right superior vena cava; InnV, innominate vein.

15.32.3 Interrupted Inferior Vena Cava with Azygos Continuation

The embryonic inferior vena cava develops from four segments: a suprahepatic, an infrahepatic, a renal, and an inferior segment. In an interrupted inferior vena cava, the infrahepatic segment is absent. The inferior vena cava is thus interrupted cranial to the orifice of the renal veins. The venous blood from the lower half of the body flows out through a dilated azygos vein to the superior vena cava ("azygos continuation"). The hepatic veins drain directly into the right atrium (▶ Fig. 15.109). In the absence of another heart defect, the patients are clinically unremarkable, but the anomaly can complicate cardiac catheterization or surgery.

An interrupted inferior vena cava with azygos continuation usually occurs in association with complex heart defects and in heterotaxy syndromes.

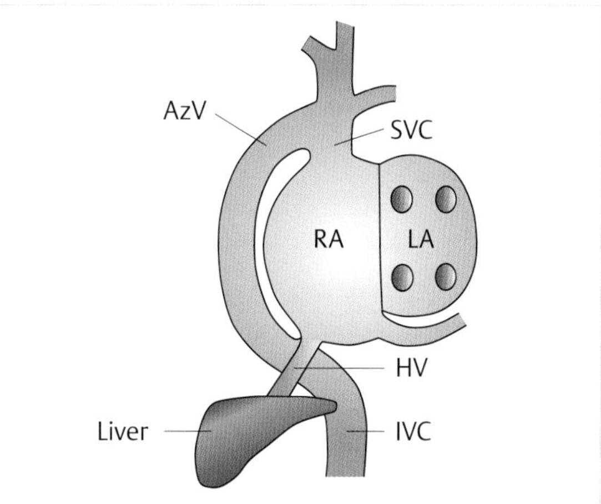

Fig. 15.109 Interrupted inferior vena cava with no connection to the right atrium. The venous blood from the lower half of the body flows out through a dilated azygos vein to the superior vena cava ("azygos continuation"). The hepatic veins drain directly into the right atrium.[29]
RA, right atrium; LA, left atrium; AzV, azygos vein; IVC, inferior vena cava; SVC, superior vena cava; HV, hepatic veins.

15.33 Dextrocardia

15.33.1 Basics

Definition

Dextrocardia is a defect in which the heart is located in the right half of the thorax.

Classification

The major types are mirror-image dextrocardia, dextroversion of the heart, and dextroposition of the heart.

▶ **Mirror-image dextrocardia.** In mirror-image dextrocardia, all cardiac structures are arranged in an exact mirror image of the normal position—that is, the cardiac apex points to the right, but the right ventricle is located normally in front directly behind the sternum. The left ventricle is in a posterior position (▶ Fig. 15.110 **d**).

A mirror-image dextrocardia is usually associated with a total situs inversus. Around 25% of these patients have a Kartagener syndrome (combination of situs inversus with ciliary dyskinesia, bronchiectasis, and hypoplastic or aplastic frontal sinuses and nasal polyps).

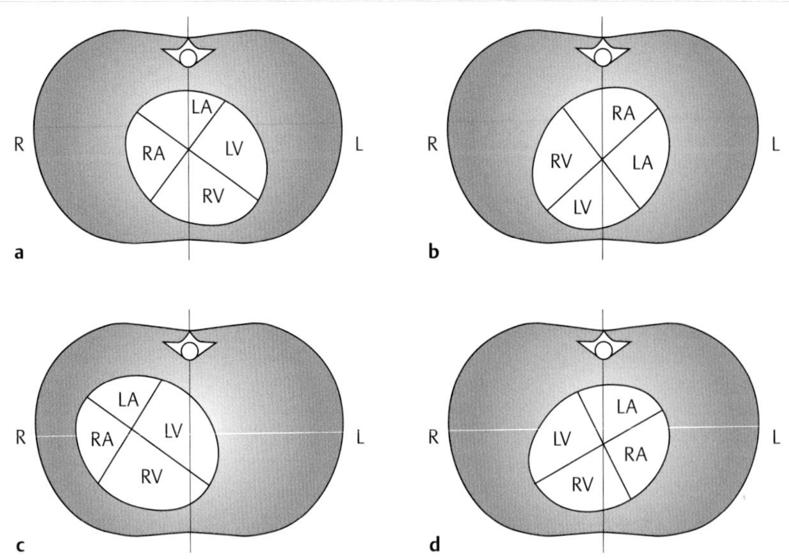

Fig. 15.110 Forms of dextrocardia. **a** Normal position of the heart. **b** Dextroversion of the heart. **c** Dextroposition of the heart. **d** Mirror-image dextrocardia.
RA, right atrium; LA, left atrium; RV, right ventricle; LV, left ventricle.

Additional cardiac anomalies are rare in patients with total situs inversus, but common in patients with mirror-image dextrocardia and situs solitus.

▶ **Dextroversion of the heart.** In dextroversion, the heart is rotated to the right (▶ Fig. 15.110 **b**). The heart has more or less been shifted from its normal position to the right. This results in the cardiac apex pointing to the right. The right ventricle, which is normally anterior directly behind the sternum, is posterior in dextroversion. The left ventricle is anterior behind the sternum. Dextroversion is often associated with complex heart defects, for example, with anomalous pulmonary venous connections.

▶ **Dextroposition of the heart.** In dextroposition of the heart, the heart is displaced to the right as a result of a shift of the mediastinum to the right (▶ Fig. 15.110 **c**). In this case, the cardiac apex still points to the left and the right ventricle is anterior behind the sternum. Dextroposition can occur in a scimitar syndrome, for example, in which the heart is displaced to the right due to a hypoplastic right lung.

15.33.2 Diagnostic Measures

The clinical symptoms of dextrocardia are determined by the accompanying cardiac anomalies. The diagnosis is made by clinical examination (location of the cardiac apex, auscultation of the heart sounds, palpation of the liver), echocardiography, ECG, chest X-ray (position of the heart in the thorax, position of the gastric bubble and liver), and, if needed, abdominal ultrasound (position of the abdominal organs and vessels).

Note

In patients with dextrocardia, when making an ECG, it is useful to switch the electrodes for the right and left arms and attach the precordial leads on the right side.

If the ECG electrodes are put in the normal positions, in mirror-image dextrocardia, the P waves, QRS complexes and T waves are negative in lead I.

15.34 Heterotaxy Syndromes

15.34.1 Basics

Definition

Heterotaxy syndromes are a group of anomalies involving the abnormal arrangement of the thorax and abdominal organs.

Heterotaxy syndromes are associated with the lateral displacement of the thorax organs. This means that both lungs are structured either as two left or as two right lungs. The two main bronchi have the typical features of a hyparterial left main bronchus or an eparterial right main bronchus. Accordingly, a patient has two left lungs with two lobes each or two right lungs with three lobes each.

The heart may be located in the left half of the thorax as normal (levocardia), in the middle (mesocardia), or in the right half of the thorax (dextrocardia). A left or right atrial isomerism is almost always present, that is, both atria have the typical features of a left or a right atrium. Heterotaxy syndromes are often associated with complex heart defects.

Note

In simple terms, in right isomerism the normal right half of the body is formed twice: There are two morphologic right atria and two morphologic right lungs. The spleen, normally found on the left side of the body, is absent (asplenia).

In left isomerism, the left half of the body is formed twice with two morphologic left atria, two morphologic left lungs, and accessory spleens (polysplenia).

There are many possible arrangements of the abdominal organs in heterotaxy syndromes (▶ Table 15.11). Intestinal malrotation is common. The unpaired abdominal organs can be in normal position (situs solitus), mirror-image reversed (situs inversus), or indifferent (situs ambiguus). The spleen is almost always affected in heterotaxy syndromes: There is either asplenia or polysplenia. There is only rarely a normal-sized spleen in an atypical location. Asplenia is often associated with right atrial isomerism, so sometimes the term asplenia syndrome is used synonymously. Polysplenia is correspondingly common in left atrial isomerism (synonym: polysplenia syndrome).

The clinically most important heterotaxy syndromes are right atrial and left atrial isomerism.

Table 15.11 Characteristic morphological features of thorax organs and upper abdominal vessels

Organ	Characteristic features
Right atrium	Orifice of the venae cavae; broad-based, pyramid-shaped atrial appendage
Left atrium	Finger-shaped atrial appendage
Right lung	Three lobes, eparterial main bronchus
Left lung	Two lobes, hyparterial main bronchus
Upper abdominal vessels	Aorta on the left of the spine, inferior vena cava on the right of the spine

15.34.2 Right Atrial Isomerism

Synonyms: formerly called asplenia syndrome, Ivemark syndrome

Basics

▶ **Definition.** In right atrial isomerism (right isomerism) both atria have the morphologic features of a right atrium. There is an overall tendency toward "bilateral right-sidedness." The spleen as a left-sided organ is usually absent (asplenia). Typically, both lungs have the structure of a right lung and have three lobes each. The main bronchi on either side are eparterial. Anomalies of the abdominal organs are common and include, for example, a midline liver and intestinal malrotation. The stomach may be located on the left or the right side (▶ Fig. 15.111 and ▶ Table 15.12).

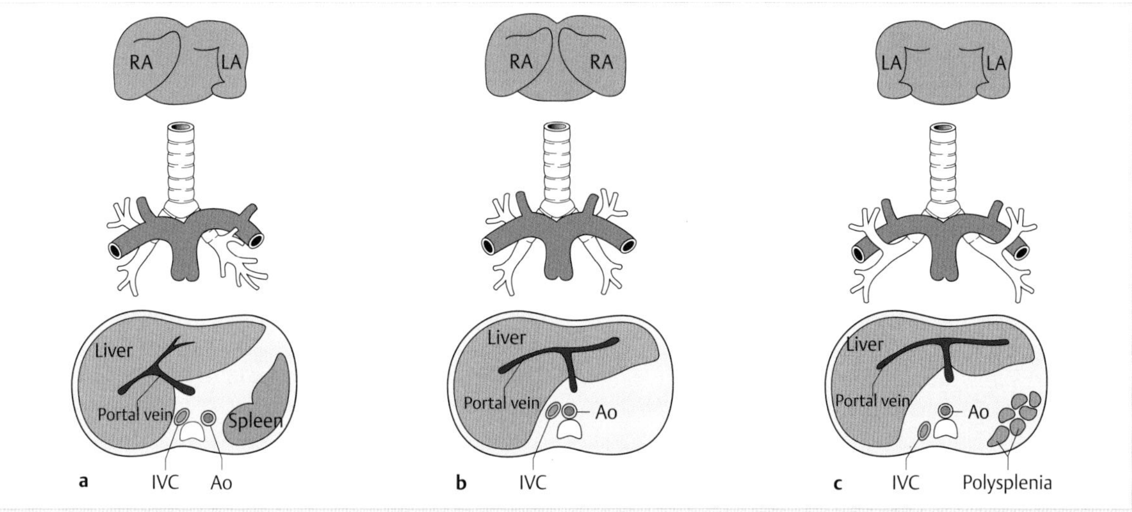

Fig. 15.111 Anatomical features of right atrial and left atrial isomerism.[18] **a** Situs solitus. **b** Right isomerism: Both atria are shaped like right atria, each lung has three lobes, the main bronchi are eparterial on both sides, aorta and inferior vena cava are on the same side of the spinal column, the liver is usually in the midline, and there is asplenia. **c** Left isomerism: Both atria are shaped like left atria, each lung has two lobes, the main bronchi are hyparterial on both sides, there is azygos continuation. The liver can be either on the right or the left side, less often in the middle, and there is asplenia.
RA, right atrium; LA, left atrium; Ao, aorta; IVC, inferior vena cava.

Table 15.12 Overview of the typical cardiac findings in right and left atrial isomerism (from Parks 2002)

Structure	Right atrial isomerism (asplenia syndrome)	Left atrial isomerism (polysplenia syndrome)
Systemic veins	• Bilateral superior vena cava • Normal inferior vena cava • Inferior vena cava and aorta are on the same side of the spinal column (juxtaposition)	• Interrupted inferior vena cava (missing intrahepatic segment) • Azygos continuation
Pulmonary veins	• Total anomalous pulmonary venous connection (often with obstruction)	• Normal pulmonary venous connection (50%) • Partial anomalous pulmonary venous connection (50%)
Atria	• Morphologic right atria on both sides • Coronary sinus absent • ASD I	• Morphologic left atria on both sides • Coronary sinus absent
AV valves	• Common AV valve (atrioventricular septal defect)	• Normal AV valves (50%) • Common AV valve (50%)
Ventricles	• Functionally univentricular heart (70%)	• Usually two ventricles, often VSD or double-outlet right ventricle
Great vessels	• Transposition of the great vessels (d-TGA or l-TGA) • Pulmonary stenosis or atresia	• Normal position of the great vessels • Unremarkable pulmonary valve (60%)
Conduction system	• Two sinus nodes • Two AV nodes • Re-entrant tachycardia (origin: between the AV nodes)	• No sinus node • Usually single AV node • Bradycardia • Occasionally AV block

▶ **Epidemiology.** Right isomerism occurs in approximately 1% of all neonates with symptomatic heart defects. Boys are affected somewhat more often than girls.

▶ **Cardiac manifestation.** Both atria have the morphological features of a right atrium. Accordingly, two sinus nodes may be present. There is often a double superior vena cava and a right aortic arch. The inferior vena cava can be either on the right or on the left side, but is typically on the same side of the spinal column as the abdominal aorta and located anterior to it.

The associated heart defects are complex: Almost always, only one AV valve is present; there is a single ventricle in more than half of cases. Transposition of the great vessels is typical. The aorta runs either parallel to and at the right of the pulmonary artery (d-TGA) or parallel to and at the left of the pulmonary artery (l-TGA).

The pulmonary artery is usually stenotic or even atretic. In most cases, there is also a total anomalous pulmonary venous connection. The pulmonary veins normally drain into the left atrium, which is not present in right isomerism.

▶ **Hemodynamics.** There is usually complete mixing of pulmonary and systemic blood as a result of the associated heart defects. Pulmonary stenosis or atresia leads to severe cyanosis shortly after birth.

Diagnostic Measures

▶ **Symptoms.** Typical symptoms are cyanosis and a liver that can be palpated at the midline.

▶ **Laboratory tests.** Evidence of Howell–Jolly or Heinz bodies in the blood smear indicates asplenia.

▶ **Auscultation.** The auscultation is not very specific. A VSD or pulmonary stenosis murmur can often be heard.

▶ **ECG.** As a result of the single AV valve (atrioventricular septal defect, AVSD), there is typically marked left axis deviation. The axis and shape of the P wave can vary as there may be two sinus nodes.

▶ **Chest X-ray.** The heart is usually of normal size or slightly enlarged. If there is a pulmonary stenosis or atresia, the pulmonary vascular markings are typically decreased. There can be levocardia, mesocardia, or dextrocardia. There are main bronchi on both sides which arise relatively steeply from the trachea, like two right bronchi, and branch into three lobar bronchi on each side. The liver is usually centrally located; the gastric bubble can be on the right or the left side.

▶ **Echocardiography.** In echocardiography, the exact anatomy should be systematically visualized. The aorta and inferior vena cava typically run on one side of the spinal column. Particular attention should be paid to the associated heart defects:

- Single AV valve/AVSD (almost always present)
- Total anomalous pulmonary venous connection (80%, often difficult to visualize with certainty)
- Single ventricle (50%)

- Transposition of the great arteries (d-TGA or l-TGA in more than half of cases)
- Right aortic arch
- Pulmonary stenosis or atresia (around 75% of cases)
- Less often: "common atrium," hypoplastic left heart syndrome, double-outlet right ventricle (DORV), tricuspid atresia

▶ **Cardiac catheterization and MRI.** Both examinations can detect specific anatomical details that cannot be explained by echocardiography.

▶ **Abdominal ultrasonography.** Abdominal ultrasound can be used to clarify the anatomy and positions of the abdominal organs. In unclear cases, it can be supplemented by MRI.

Treatment

▶ **Conservative treatment.** If there is a critical pulmonary stenosis or atresia, the ductus arteriosus must be kept patent with prostaglandin E to ensure pulmonary perfusion.

Antibiotic prophylaxis with oral penicillin V (200,000–400,000 units twice a day) is indicated for asplenia until (at least) adulthood.

In addition to the usual immunizations (including Haemophilus influenza), early immunization against pneumococcus and meningococcus is recommended (Chapter 30).

▶ **Surgical treatment.** Surgical treatment depends on the associated cardiac anomalies. If there is critical hypoperfusion, insertion of an aortopulmonary shunt is indicated in the neonatal period. A total anomalous pulmonary venous connection with obstruction of the pulmonary veins is a cardiac surgery emergency and must be acted on immediately after the diagnosis is made. The postoperative course can sometimes be complicated considerably by insufficiency of the single AV valve. In the long term, univentricular palliation in a Fontan procedure is almost always necessary.

Prognosis and Clinical Course

Without palliative surgery and antibiotic prophylaxis, most of the children die within the first year of life. A total anomalous pulmonary venous connection is a risk factor.

Lifelong cardiac follow-up is always indicated after palliative surgery. The long-term problems are similar to those of other patients with Fontan circulation (including disposition for edema, protein-loss enteropathy, supraventricular arrhythmia, insufficiency of the systemic ventricle, and reduced physical capacity).

15.34.3 Left Atrial Isomerism

Synonym: formerly called polysplenia syndrome

Basics

▶ **Definition.** In left atrial isomerism (left isomerism), both atria have the features of a left atrium (▶ Fig. 15.111 c, ▶ Table 15.12). There is an overall tendency to "bilateral left-sidedness." Both lungs typically have the structure of a left lung and have two lobes each. The main bronchi are hyparterial on both sides. Visceral anomalies are common. The liver is usually on the left or the right side; only 25% of cases have a midline liver. The bile ducts may be atretic. The stomach and liver are usually on opposite sides. Polysplenia is typical, but functional asplenia may be present.

▶ **Epidemiology.** Left atrial isomerism is even less common than right isomerism and constitutes much less than 1% of all congenital cardiac anomalies. Girls are probably affected somewhat more often than boys.

▶ **Cardiac manifestations.** Unlike right isomerism, two ventricles are usually present in left atrial isomerism. In most cases, there is an ASD or an AVSD. Often a VSD is present, sometimes a double-outlet right ventricle as well. TGA and pulmonary stenosis or atresia are much less common than in right isomerism. A total anomalous pulmonary venous connection is also less common. There may be a partial anomalous pulmonary venous connection. Up to 25% of patients have no or only insignificant cardiac defects. An interrupted inferior vena cava is typical. In these cases, the intrahepatic segment of the inferior vena cava is atretic and the venous blood from the lower half of the body drains into the superior vena cava through the azygos vein (azygos continuation). If the vena cava is on the left side, the venous blood from the lower half of the body drains into the superior vena cava through the hemiazygos vein. The hepatic veins drain directly into the atrium with azygos continuation.

Since both atria are morphologic left atria, no sinus node is present. There is usually an ectopic atrial or junctional rhythm.

▶ **Hemodynamics.** Since there is rarely pulmonary stenosis, excessive pulmonary blood flow and congestive heart failure develop more often in left atrial isomerism (e.g., associated with a VSD or AVSD). Cyanosis is less common or less pronounced than in right isomerism.

Diagnostic Measures

▶ **Symptoms.** Signs of congestive heart failure (tachypnea, dyspnea, failure to thrive, increased sweating) develop in the neonatal period if there is excessive pulmonary blood flow. Cyanosis is not usually present or is mild.

► **Laboratory tests.** If there is functional asplenia, Howell–Jolly and Heinz bodies can be detected in the blood smear. Long-term antibiotic prophylaxis is indicated for functional asplenia, just as for anatomical asplenia.

► **ECG.** Since no sinus node is present, there is generally an unusual P axis (often –30 to –90°) as a sign of an ectopic atrial rhythm. Sometimes there is also a junctional rhythm. Bradycardia arrhythmias are frequent; sometimes there is a congenital AV block. In case of an AVSD, there is typically marked left axis deviation.

► **Chest X-ray.** Depending on the underlying cardiac defects, there is usually mild cardiomegaly and increased pulmonary vascular markings. Both main bronchi have the features of morphologic left main bronchi. The location of liver and stomach should also be noted.

► **Echocardiography.** Echocardiography is used to systematically visualize the visceroatrial situs and search specifically for associated cardiac anomalies. There is typically azygos continuation with an absent intrahepatic segment of the inferior vena cava. A thick venous vessel (azygos vein) can be seen posterior to the aorta. The hepatic veins drain directly into the atrium. The following cardiac anomalies are common:

- Transposition of the great vessels
- Two superior venae cavae
- Partial anomalous pulmonary venous connection
- Common AV valve
- Functionally univentricular heart
- VSD, DORV
- Pulmonary stenosis

► **Cardiac catheterization and MRI.** Both examinations can detect special anatomical details that cannot be explained by echocardiography.

► **Abdominal ultrasonography.** Abdominal ultrasound can be used to clarify the anatomy and positions of the abdominal organs. In unclear cases, it can be supplemented by MRI.

Treatment

► **Conservative Treatment.** Symptomatic treatment of congestive heart failure is given to bridge the time until surgery.

► **Surgical Treatment.** Depending on the associated cardiac anomalies, biventricular correction is possible in about half of cases. Univentricular Fontan palliation is needed for the remainder. In patients with azygos continuation, the entire systemic venous blood except for the blood from the hepatic veins is conducted to the pulmonary arteries from the time the upper cavopulmonary anastomosis is made. Excessive pulmonary blood flow may make it necessary very early on to transect the pulmonary artery and create a dosed aortopulmonary shunt as the first palliation. The pulmonary artery is now only rarely banded. For symptomatic bradycardia, a pacemaker must also be implanted.

Prognosis and Clinical Course

Left untreated, around 60% of affected children die within the first year of life. Children with a congenital AV block have a poor prognosis. The long-term problems in patients treated with Fontan palliation are described above for right isomerism.

16 Acquired Cardiac Diseases

16.1 Myocarditis

16.1.1 Basics

Synonym: inflammatory cardiomyopathy

Definition

Myocarditis is an inflammatory disease of the myocardium that can have greatly varying clinically courses and a variety of causes. The World Health Organization grouped these diseases under the term "inflammatory cardiomyopathy." The most common form of myocarditis in childhood is viral myocarditis.

Epidemiology

The incidence in children is unknown. Since many children are asymptomatic, the frequency is probably underestimated. Histological evidence of myocarditis is found in autopsies in up to 40% of children who died suddenly and were not killed by trauma. The clinical significance of these findings is unclear. There is myocardial involvement in 1 to 4% of enterovirus infections (especially Coxsackie virus type B).

Pathogenesis

In myocarditis, interstitial inflammation or myocardial damage leads to decreased myocardial function. The damage to the myocardium that is associated with myocardial cell death is probably due not only to direct damage to the myocardium from the pathogens, but also to immunological mechanisms. The result is dilatation of the ventricles with an increase in end-diastolic volume. Normally, the heart responds to an increase in end-diastolic volume with an increase in contractility (Frank–Starling mechanism), but this is not possible in myocarditis due to damage to the myocardium.

Histology

The histopathological classification is based on the *Dallas criteria*:

- Active myocarditis: inflammatory infiltration of the myocardium and myocytolysis; the infiltrates are mostly monocytic, less often neutrophilic, occasionally also eosinophilic
- Borderline myocarditis: lymphocytic infiltration of the myocardium without myocytolysis

Etiology

Infectious, immunological, and toxic triggers are possible causes of myocarditis (▶ Table 16.1). Infections, especially viral infections, are the most common causes in childhood. The most important pathogens are enteroviruses (especially Coxsackie virus type B) and adenoviruses.

Table 16.1 Causes of myocarditis (modified from Allen et al. 2008)[1]

Infections
• Viruses: Coxsackie B, adenovirus, echovirus, EBV, HSV, HIV, cytomegalovirus, rubella, measles, mumps, varicella, influenza, parvovirus B19, hepatitis C virus, polio, rabies • Bacteria: diphtheria, tuberculosis, mycoplasma, haemophilus, meningococcus, pneumococcus, Staphylococcus, Streptococcus, gonococcus, Salmonella, Clostridium, brucellosis, psittacosis, tetanus, Legionella • Protozoa: *Trypanosoma cruzi* (Chagas disease, common in Central/South America), Toxoplasma, Plasmodium, Leishmania • Rickettsia: *Rickettsia rickettsii*, *Coxiella burnetii* • Spirochetes: Borrelia, Leptospira, *Treponema pallidum* • Parasites: Ascaris, Echinococcus, Trichinella, schistosomes, *Taenia solium* • Fungi (especially in immunosuppressed patients): Candida, Cryptococcus, Aspergillus
Immune mediated
• Allergies: various drugs (e.g., antibiotics, diuretics, clozapine), insect/snake bites • Autoimmune/immunological diseases: lupus erythematosus, sarcoidosis, dermatomyositis, scleroderma, inflammatory bowel disease, vasculitis, Kawasaki disease, hypereosinophilic syndrome • Transplant rejection
Toxic
• Drugs: catecholamines, anthracyclines, cocaine, alcohol, carbon monoxide • Metals: copper, lead, iron, arsenic • Physical toxicants: radiation, hyperthermia, electric shock • Poisons: including scorpion poison

16.1.2 Diagnostic Measures

Symptoms

The clinical course of acute myocarditis ranges from asymptomatic cases to fulminant, fatal courses with severe dyspnea, pulmonary edema, cardiogenic shock, and even death. Signs of acute heart failure are usually the major symptoms. Arrhythmias can also be the leading symptom of myocarditis.

In myocarditis following a viral infection, the patient typically develops fatigue, reduced physical capacity, tachycardia, and tachypnea.

The symptoms vary in different age groups. Especially in neonates and infants, the symptoms can be very nonspecific (restlessness, vomiting, cough, increased crying or whimpering). In older children, the major symptoms are reduced physical capacity and a general malaise.

Typical symptoms are:

- Tachycardia, extrasystoles: In principle, any type of arrhythmia is possible in connection with myocarditis, including AV conduction disturbance and ventricular tachycardia
- Tachypnea/dyspnea
- Chest pain: This can be the result of myocardial ischemia or concomitant pericarditis
- Gray-cyanotic skin tone, pallor, cool extremities, slow recapillarization
- Hepatomegaly, edema
- Hypotension, oliguria
- Lethargy, somnolence, increased irritability, cerebral seizures
- Fever, hypothermia

Laboratory

The following are the typical laboratory findings in myocarditis. It should be noted, however, that there are no laboratory parameters that can prove or rule out myocarditis. This also applies to the myocardial enzymes. Detection of pathogens in a culture, which is best done in an endomyocardial biopsy, is crucial.

- Inflammatory markers (CRP, ESR): The inflammatory markers are usually elevated in myocarditis, but inconspicuous inflammatory parameters do not rule out myocarditis.
- Lymphocytosis and neutropenia indicate a viral genesis.
- Anemia
- Elevated myocardial enzymes: Increases in CK-MB, LDH and especially troponin I are signs of myocardial damage. But normal myocardial enzyme levels do not rule out myocarditis.
- Metabolic acidosis: Metabolic acidosis can be a sign of congestive heart failure.
- Elevated transaminases: An increase in transaminases may be the result of a viral-induced hepatopathy, liver congestion, or liver failure associated with congestive heart failure.
- Increase in urinary metabolites (creatinine, urea) with oliguria/renal failure
- Autoantibodies: ANA, double-stranded DNA antibodies, Sm antibodies, RNP antibodies, SSA antibodies, SSB antibodies, and antimitochondrial antibodies can indicate an autoimmune cause.
- Antimyocardial antibodies: Antimyolemmal antibodies (AMLA) and/or antisarcolemmal antibodies (ASA) can often be detected after 4 weeks and are typical but not specific for viral myocarditis.
- Virus serology: The virus serology is indicative only if there is a substantial increase in the titer over time, making a follow-up about 3 weeks after the onset of the disease useful. Serology tests are therefore not suitable for making a rapid diagnosis.
- Virus isolation in smears and cultures (e.g., throat urine, stool)
- PCR / in situ hybridization: Direct evidence of the virus genome or RNA in a myocardial biopsy is the method of choice for virus detection.

Auscultation

It may be possible to hear a mitral regurgitation murmur —blowing systolic murmur with point of maximum impulse (PMI) at the cardiac apex. A gallop rhythm occurs in congestive heart failure. In pulmonary edema, there are fine crackles over the lungs.

ECG

In some patients, changes in the ECG are the only evidence suggestive of myocarditis. In theory, all types of arrhythmias may be associated with myocarditis. Especially feared are ventricular tachycardias. A new onset of cardiac arrhythmia always suggests myocarditis. Typical ECG findings of myocarditis include:

- Sinus tachycardia: Sinus tachycardia is the most common ECG finding in myocarditis. If fever is present simultaneously, the tachycardia is usually more rapid than expected from the fever alone.
- Ventricular tachycardia: Ventricular tachycardia may be the first symptom of myocarditis.
- Extrasystoles
- AV block grade I to III, bundle branch block, prolonged QT interval.
- ST segment depression. However, if there is simultaneous pericardial effusion, ST segment elevation is more likely.
- T wave flattening or inversion, often with small or absent Q waves in V_5/V_6
- Occasionally low voltage

Echocardiography

An indicative finding in echocardiography is an enlarged, poorly contractile left ventricle. However, the echocardiography cannot distinguish reliably between acute myocarditis and dilated cardiomyopathy. Typical findings are:

- end-diastolic and diastolic enlargement of the left ventricle (and possibly enlarged right ventricle),
- poor ventricular function with reduced fractional shortening and ejection fraction,
- regional wall motion abnormalities,
- mitral and/or tricuspid regurgitation as a result of a dilatation of the valve annulus,
- possibly pericardial effusion.

The coronary anatomy should be visualized if possible to rule out a coronary anomaly, especially Bland–White–Garland syndrome, which should be considered as a differential diagnosis.

Chest X-ray

Cardiomegaly is a typical radiological finding. There may be signs of pulmonary congestion up to pulmonary edema.

Cardiac Catheterization

The hemodynamic measurements show a decreased cardiac index, increased left ventricular end-diastolic pressure, and increased left atrial pressure. Left ventricular function is reduced. A coronary anomaly should be ruled out by a coronary angiography.

The main indication for cardiac catheterization is to conduct an endomyocardial biopsy, which is the gold standard for diagnosing myocarditis. The biopsy is usually taken from the right ventricular septum. Aside from confirming the diagnosis, it can aid in the classification according to the Dallas criteria (see Histology, Chapter 16.1.1). The immunohistological examination of the specimens reduces the incidence of false negative results. Molecular biological methods (PCR, in situ hybridization) can be used to identify the pathogen. The risk of myocardial perforation during the biopsy is increased in critically ill and younger children.

MRI

Using contrast medium and the late-enhancement technique in addition to other imaging methods, the location and the extent of inflammation can be determined, but the changes are not specific for myocarditis.

Differential Diagnoses

Differential diagnoses of myocarditis are:

- Decompensated heart failure
- Coronary anomaly (in particular Bland–White–Garland syndrome)
- Dilated cardiomyopathy
- Endocardial fibroelastosis
- Myocardial infarction
- Metabolic disorders associated with cardiac involvement (e.g., carnitine deficiency, glycogenosis)

16.1.3 Treatment

General Measures

Patients with suspected myocarditis should be admitted to hospital and be monitored by ECG. Bed rest during the acute phase of the disease probably reduces viral replication.

► **Treatment of congestive heart failure.** The following measures are used in the treatment of congestive heart failure:

- Diuretics: Diuretics should initially be dosed with caution, because sufficient preload is often necessary to ensure adequate cardiac output.
- Digoxin: Due to increased digoxin toxicity in myocarditis, patients should be started at half the dosage.
- Beta blockers: If blood pressure is sufficiently high, start at a low dosage (not for severe heart failure).
- ACE inhibitors: For afterload reduction if blood pressure high enough.
- Catecholamines (e.g., dobutamine) and phosphodiesterase inhibitors (e.g., milrinone): For severe heart failure under intensive care monitoring.
- Sedation, intubation and mechanical ventilation for cardiogenic shock or pulmonary edema.
- Mechanical circulatory support for circulatory failure not manageable by conventional methods: Extracorporeal membrane oxygenation (ECMO) or left ventricular assist device (VAD), possibly as an interim measure until heart transplant.

Antiarrhythmic Treatment

Cardiac arrhythmias can lead to a significant deterioration of symptoms. However, it should be noted that most antiarrhythmic drugs have negative inotropic effects. Amiodarone is often used.

Supraventricular and ventricular tachycardias, which can lead to hemodynamic instability, should be treated rapidly with cardioversion. If there is a complete AV block and low ventricular rate, a temporary transvenous pacemaker may have to be placed. In most cases, AV conduction recovers.

Hemodynamically relevant, treatment-refractory arrhythmias can be an indication for temporary mechanical circulatory support with ECMO or VAD.

Immunosuppressive Treatment

The use of immunosuppressive drugs is still controversial. A large United States multicenter study showed no benefit of immunosuppressive therapy with prednisone in combination with azathioprine or cyclosporine A in comparison with purely symptomatic treatment. Steroids are therefore used in most centers only for myocarditis based on a confirmed autoimmune disease.

▸ **Immunoglobulins.** There is evidence that immunoglobulins administered at a dosage of 2 g/kg IV over 24 hours improve left ventricular function in acute myocarditis.

▸ **Interferon α.** Interferon is currently being investigated in studies to verify whether it is useful in viral myocarditis. No reliable evidence is available to date. On the other hand, interferon itself can lead to drug-induced myocarditis.

Specific Treatment

Specific treatment is possible for a few forms of myocarditis. A selection is listed below:

- Bacterial myocarditis: antibiotics, depending on the pathogen
- Fungal myocarditis: antifungals depending on the pathogen
- Kawasaki disease: ASA, immunoglobulins, possibly steroids
- Rheumatic carditis: penicillin, NSAIDs, possibly steroids
- Diphtheria: fastest possible treatment with diphtheria antitoxin and high-dose penicillin
- Borrelia: intravenous ceftriaxone for 4 weeks
- Giant cell myocarditis: This rare but severe disease that affects mainly young people is verified by histological evidence of giant cells in the myocardium. An association with inflammatory bowel disease or autoimmune disease is suspected. Some studies have shown a positive effect of immunosuppression in giant cell myocarditis (cyclosporine in combination with steroids, azathioprine, or muromonab-CD3).
- Eosinophilic myocarditis: steroids

Heart Transplant

If there is no improvement of left ventricular function or if there is a transition to dilated cardiomyopathy, a heart transplant is the last treatment option.

16.1.4 Prognosis

Most cases (60–70%) of myocarditis heal completely without consequences. The mortality rate is highest in neonates at 75%. In older children, the mortality rate for serious progressive forms is reported to be 10 to 25%. The transition to chronic myocarditis or dilated cardiomyopathy is greatly feared. It is not known how many cases of myocarditis develop into dilated cardiomyopathy, but it is assumed that 27 to 40% of dilated cardiomyopathies in childhood are caused by myocarditis

16.2 Endocarditis

16.2.1 Basics

Definition

Endocarditis is an acute or subacute infection of the endocardial structures of the heart—the heart valves, the mural endocardium, or the endothelium of major vessels in the vicinity of the heart. Endocarditis may also involve foreign material such as a surgical patch, shunt connections (e.g., aortopulmonary shunts) or artificial vascular conduits, and artificial heart valves. Endocarditis can destroy the valves and lead to septic emboli.

Epidemiology

The lifetime risk for endocarditis in the general population is 5 to 7:100,000 patient-years, but increases significantly if there are risk factors such as congenital heart disease, prosthetic valves, or previous endocarditis. Some 90% of affected children have a congenital heart defect. Overall, the incidence is increasing among children, but neonates are rarely affected. In 80 to 90% of cases, endocarditis affects the valves of systemic circulation (aortic/mitral valve). Endocarditis of the pulmonary and tricuspid valves is more frequent in intravenous drug users.

Pathogenesis

In many congenital or acquired heart defects, turbulent blood flow causes a lesion of the adjacent endothelium or endocardium, where deposits of platelets and fibrin form. If there is transient bacteremia (e.g., simple infectious diseases, surgical or dental procedures), this thrombotic vegetation is colonized with bacteria, which have a tendency to adhere to the thrombotic deposits where they are well protected from the body's immune system and from antibiotics. As a result of fibrin and platelet aggregation as well as due to bacterial growth, a typical endocarditis vegetation develops. Direct progression of the process can lead to the development of abscesses, for example, in the myocardium or in the valve annulus.

Embolization of vegetation can cause tissue infarction and septic colonization in the rest of the body. In addition, extracardiac manifestations may be caused by immune complex deposits (e.g., glomerulonephritis, vasculitis).

Highly virulent pathogens (e.g., staphylococci) can invade previously undamaged valves and usually lead to a fulminant course of the disease (acute endocarditis). Less virulent pathogens (e.g., viridans group streptococci, enterococci) settle on previously damaged valves and lead to a more gradual course of the disease (subacute endocarditis, endocarditis lenta).

Etiology

Bacteria in particular, less often fungi, are decisive in causing infectious endocarditis (▶ Table 16.2). Viridans group streptococci and enterococci are the most common pathogens of *subacute* endocarditis. *Staphylococcus aureus*, enterobacteria, pneumococci, and hemolytic streptococci are typical pathogens of *acute* endocarditis. In 5 to 25% of cases, the pathogen is not identified.

16.2.2 Diagnostic Measures

Medical History

The medical history must include risk factors for bacteremia such as surgery, dental procedures, infections, toothaches, and previous endocarditis.

Forms

▶ **Acute endocarditis.** Dramatic history of fever, chills, congestive heart failure, decreased consciousness up to multiple organ failure. Acute endocarditis is usually caused by highly virulent pathogens (e.g., staphylococci, beta-hemolytic streptococci, pneumococci) that can destroy even previously intact heart valves.

▶ **Subacute endocarditis (endocarditis lenta).** This form occurs practically only in patients with an existing cardiac defect. It is caused by less virulent pathogens (viridans streptococci, enterococci, gram-negative bacteria of the intestinal flora, fungi) and almost always affects previously damaged heart valves. The course is often very non-specific, particularly in the early stages, with intermittent fever or low-grade fever and fatigue.

Symptoms

There are various clinical symptoms of endocarditis including not only general symptoms such as fever and fatigue, but also cardiac symptoms and immunological phenomena and the consequences of bacterial microemboli. Typical symptoms are:

- Fever with tachycardia, and possibly chills (caution: In patients previously treated with antibiotics these symptoms may be partially obscured), in subacute endocarditis also low-grade fever
- General symptoms:
  - Headache, fatigue, decrease in physical capacity
  - Weight loss, loss of appetite
  - Night sweats
  - Myalgia, arthralgia
- Cardiac symptoms:
  - Murmur: new occurrence or increase of an already existing murmur (in infections of prosthetic valves often a sign of perivalvular spread)
  - Valve perforation, avulsion
  - Myocardial abscesses
- Skin symptoms:
  - Petechiae
  - Osler nodes: lentil-sized, painful, reddish nodules, mainly on the fingers and toes (sign of immune complex vasculitis)
  - Janeway lesions: hemorrhagic, painless skin lesions on the hands and feet
  - Splinter hemorrhages: subungual hemorrhages at the tips of the fingers and toes
- Bacterial microemboli:
  - CNS: acute loss of consciousness, focal neurological deficits
  - Spleen infarction
  - Pulmonary infarction involving the right heart
- Renal involvement:
  - Hematuria, proteinuria
  - Glomerulonephritis
  - Renal infarction
- Eye involvement:
  - Roth spots: retinal hemorrhages
- Splenomegaly

▶ **Duke criteria.** The Duke criteria (▶ Table 16.3) are based on clinical findings and are divided into major and minor criteria.

Laboratory

The detection of pathogens in a culture and resistance testing are of major importance. Other typical laboratory findings in endocarditis are:

- Elevated inflammation markers (CRP, ESR): a normal ESR value practically rules out endocarditis.
- Anemia
- Leukocytosis with left shift
- Thrombocytopenia
- Detection of the pathogen in culture and resistance testing: Prior to initiating antibiotic therapy, several (preferably 6–8) blood samples each are taken for aerobic and anaerobic blood cultures. Blood cultures should be taken from different veins if possible. The samples may be taken independently of the fever profile (continuous bacteremia). During the acute course, blood cultures should be taken within 1 to 2 hours if possible so antibiotic therapy can be initiated quickly. In subacute courses, additional cultures can be taken within 1 to 2 days. The cultures are incubated for at least 3 weeks.
- Immunological markers: Rheumatoid factors, ANA, circulating immune complexes, or cryoglobulins can sometimes be detected in endocarditis.
- Urine: Hematuria or proteinuria can be signs of renal infarction or glomerulonephritis.

ECG

The ECG changes found in endocarditis are non-specific and can be interpreted only retrospectively. Possible abnormalities are:

Table 16.2 Endocarditis pathogens, their treatment, and special features during the course of the disease

Pathogen	Origin	Special features	Treatment principles
Gram-positive pathogens			
Streptococcus viridans (*S. sanguinis*, *S. mutans*, *S. mitis*, *S. anginosus*, *S. salivaris*, *S. oralis*), *Streptococcus bovis*	Oropharynx	Colonization of previously damaged valves, usually subacute course	Usually very sensitive to penicillin; possible combination therapy with gentamicin (shorter treatment duration)
Enterococci (*Enterococcus faecalis*, rarely *E. faecium*, *E. durans*)	Urogenital/gastrointestinal tract	Usually subacute course, increasingly nosocomial infections caused by multidrug-resistant enterococci	Often penicillin-resistant; monotherapy with ampicillin, penicillin or vancomycin is insufficient; bactericidal effect only in combination with gentamicin
Beta-hemolytic streptococci	Oropharynx	Frequent colonization of normal heart valves and metastatic abscesses in other organs	Usually very sensitive to penicillin; possible combination therapy with gentamicin (shorter treatment duration)
Pneumococci		Often fulminant course, myocardial abscesses, purulent pericarditis, purulent meningitis	Usually very sensitive to penicillin; possible combination therapy with gentamicin (shorter treatment duration)
Staphylococcus aureus	Skin, soft tissue, catheter infections	Often acute endocarditis, even in not previously damaged valves. Complications: valve annulus abscesses, myocardial abscesses, purulent pericarditis; increasingly methicillin-resistant strains (MRSA)	"Staphylococcal penicillins" (oxacillin, flucloxacillin) in combination with gentamicin; vancomycin and gentamicin for MRSA; rifampicin in addition for prosthetic valves
Coagulase-negative staphylococci (*Staphylococcus epidermidis*, *Staphylococcus lugdunensis*)		Colonization of artificial heart valves and implants. Frequent cause of early endocarditis within the 1st year after valve replacement, usually subacute form	"Staphylococcal penicillins" (oxacillin, flucloxacillin) in combination with gentamicin; vancomycin and gentamicin for MRSA; rifampicin in addition for prosthetic valves
Gram-negative pathogens			
HACEK group (Haemophilus, Actinobacillus, Cardiobacterium, Eikenella, Kingella)		Low virulence (previously damaged and prosthetic valves especially affected), difficult to detect in culture (incubation for at least 3 weeks)	Treatment of choice: ceftriaxone
Pseudomonas aeruginosa		Especially in intravenous drug users, prosthetic valves, catheter infections	Piperacillin and beta-lactamase inhibitors or ceftazidime and tobramycin, surgical revision often required
Fungi			
Candida, Aspergillus		Risk factors: immunosuppression, long-term antibiotic therapy, foreign body (long-term central venous catheters, surgical implants), difficult to detect by culture, often large vegetations	Prompt surgical treatment usually necessary; amphotericin B (possibly liposomal amphotericin B), flucytosine, in individual cases, newer antifungal agents (caspofungin, voriconazole)
Rare pathogens: enterobacteriaceae, corynebacteria, Rickettsia, Coxiella burnetii, Brucella spp, Bartonella spp, Chlamydia			

Table 16.3 Modified Duke criteria

Major criteria	
Positive blood cultures	• Typical endocarditis pathogens detected in at least two blood cultures taken separately: *Streptococcus viridans*, *Streptococcus bovis*, HACEK group bacteria, *Staphylococcus aureus*, or enterococci • Permanent positive blood cultures with evidence of pathogens that can cause endocarditis: ◦ Two or more positive blood cultures at a sampling interval of about 12 h or ◦ Three positive of three cultures or positive majority of four or more blood cultures taken separately (interval of at least 1 h between the first and last sample)
Evidence of endocardial involvement	• Echocardiographic evidence of vegetation, paravalvular abscess, or dehiscence of an artificial valve • New valve regurgitation
Minor criteria	
Predisposition	Intravenous drug use, congenital heart defect
Fever ≥ 38°C	
Vascular phenomena	Arterial embolism, septic pulmonary infarctions, intracranial hemorrhage, conjunctival bleeding, Janeway lesions
Immunological findings	Glomerulonephritis, Osler nodes, Roth spots, positive rheumatoid factor
Positive blood cultures that do not meet the main criterion	
Positive serology for a pathogen consistent with endocarditis	
Echocardiographic findings that are consistent with endocarditis but do not meet the main criterion	

Note: The diagnosis of infective endocarditis is considered likely if two major criteria, one major criterion and three minor criteria, or five minor criteria are present.

- AV block
- Bundle branch blocks
- Repolarization disturbances

Echocardiography

Echocardiography is very valuable for diagnosing endocarditis. If the findings from transthoracic echocardiography are not sufficient, transesophageal echocardiography is required. Echocardiography can be used for the following:

- Detection of bacterial vegetation: Bacterial vegetations with a size of 2 to 3 mm can be detected. Detection is difficult in previously severely damaged valves and artificial valves. There is a particularly high risk of emboli if there is mobile vegetation on the mitral valve larger than 10 mm.
- Assessment of valve regurgitation
- Detection of complications such as abscesses, paravalvular leak, prosthetic dehiscence, leaflet perforations, tendinous cord avulsions, "kissing lesions"
- Assessment of ventricular function
- Assessment of treatment: verification of the regression of vegetation under antibiotic therapy

The following structures may resemble vegetation in echocardiography and must therefore be considered as a differential diagnosis: valve calcifications, healed vegetations, cardiac tumors, thrombotic deposits (especially at the edge of prostheses or at sutures), avulsions of tendinous cords or papillary muscles, prominent Eustachian valve.

Note

An unremarkable echocardiography does not rule out endocarditis.

Differential Diagnoses

Endocarditis should always be considered as the differential diagnosis of unexplained fever. The following are possible differential diagnoses:

- Sepsis
- Pneumonia
- Kawasaki syndrome
- Rheumatic fever
- Collagenosis and rheumatic diseases
- Chronic inflammatory diseases (Crohn disease)
- Noninfectious endocarditis, such as rheumatic endocarditis in rheumatic fever, Libman–Sacks endocarditis in systemic lupus erythematosus, Loeffler syndrome (eosinophilic endomyocarditis)
- Cardiac tumors (e.g., atrial myxoma)
- Myocarditis
- Malignant diseases (e.g., leukemia)
- Vasculitis

In febrile patients with cyanotic heart defects and neurological deficits, brain abscesses should also be considered.

16.2.3 Treatment

The treatment of endocarditis requires several weeks of bactericidal antibiotic therapy, usually as combination therapy to take advantage of synergistic effects. Depending on the clinical picture, antibiotic therapy is initialized before the completion of the antibiogram, taking the most likely pathogens into account (▶ Table 16.4). After the antibiogram is received, which must include information on the minimum inhibitory concentration and minimum bactericidal concentration, the antibiotic regimen is optimized. The treatment duration is usually 4 to 6 weeks. In patients with a prosthetic valve, the total duration of treatment is extended to at least 6 weeks.

The treatment recommendations are constantly being updated and should always be discussed with the responsible microbiologists. In vancomycin and gentamicin therapy, the drug levels have to be determined regularly and the dosage should be adjusted accordingly.

In severe cases, surgical treatment may be indicated in combination with antibiotic treatment. In fungal endocarditis, early surgical treatment is usually required. Because of the high recurrence rate, secondary prophylaxis with fluconazole (Candida endocarditis) or itraconazole (Aspergillus endocarditis) is recommended for at least 2 years.

Surgical Treatment

In severe cases, antibiotic therapy alone is not sufficient and surgical intervention is required, usually in the form of a valve replacement.

Table 16.4 Antibiotic treatment of endocarditis depending on the expected range of pathogens

Acute endocarditis of unknown pathogens		
Vancomycin	40 mg/kg/d in 4 individual doses (max. 2 g/d)	4–6 weeks
+ Gentamicin	3–5 mg/kg/d in 1 individual dose (max. 240 mg/d)	4–6 weeks
Viridans group streptococci		
Penicillin G	0.5 mill. IU/kg/d in 4 individual doses (max. 20 mill. IU/d)	4 weeks
+ Gentamicin	3–5 mg/kg/d in 1 individual dose (max. 240 mg/d)	2 weeks
If there are no complications, a 2-week course is sufficient		
Staphylococci (methicillin sensitive)		
Flucloxacillin	200 mg/kg/d in 4 individual doses (max. 8–12 g/d)	4–6 weeks
+ Gentamicin	3–5 mg/kg/d in 1 individual dose (max. 240 mg/d)	3–5 days
In prosthetic valve endocarditis: + rifampicin	10 mg/kg/d in 3 individual doses (max. 900 mg/d)	≥ 6 weeks
Enterococci and other penicillin-resistant streptococci		
Ampicillin	200–300 mg/kg/d in 4 individual doses (max. 12–15 g/d)	4–6 weeks
+ Gentamicin	3–5 mg/kg/d in 1 individual dose (max. 240 mg/d)	4–6 weeks
HACEK organisms		
Ceftriaxone	100 mg/kg in 1 individual dose	4 weeks
Candida		
Amphotericin B	0.5–1 mg/kg/d in 1 individual dose	≥ 6 weeks
+ 5-flucytosine	150 mg/kg/d in 3 individual doses	≥ 6 weeks
Aspergillus		
Amphotericin B	0.5–1 mg/kg/d in 1 individual dose	≥ 6 weeks

Indications for surgical treatment are:

- Acute aortic or mitral regurgitation with cardiac pump failure / pulmonary edema
- Perivalvular abscess, fistula
- Difficult to treat pathogens (e.g., MRSA, fungi)
- Severe sepsis and septic shock for more than 48 hours
- Persistent fever despite adequate antibiotic treatment after 5 to 10 days (caution: drug-induced fever)
- Persistent bacteremia/fungemia despite adequate antibiotic therapy
- New mobile vegetation over 10 mm in diameter at the mitral valve
- Increase in size of vegetation or spread to previously normal valves
- Local destructive course of vegetation
- Acute cerebral embolism (after ruling out a cerebral hemorrhage)
- Prosthetic valve endocarditis (initially conservative treatment if penicillin-sensitive streptococci are detected)

16.2.4 Prophylaxis

Patients who have a particularly high risk for bacterial endocarditis should be given antibiotic endocarditis prophylaxis before diagnostic or therapeutic procedures that can lead to bacteremia. The choice of antibiotic depends on the location of surgery and the expected range of pathogens. The German Society of Pediatric Cardiology and the Paul Ehrlich Society issue appropriate patient ID cards that contain the current recommendations. However, prophylactic administration of antibiotics is not useful for the prevention of viral infections. Systematic antibiotic treatment is essential for manifest bacterial infections.

Since endocarditis is often caused by pathogens from the oropharynx, *good oral* and *dental hygiene* must be maintained.

► **Endocarditis risk.** There is a *particularly high* risk of endocarditis in the following situations:

- Artificial cardiac valves, including mechanical valves, bioprostheses, and homografts
- Reconstructed cardiac valves using foreign material for a period of 6 months after the operation
- Previous bacterial endocarditis
- Congenital heart disease:
  - Unoperated cyanotic heart defects, including palliative shunts and conduits
  - Fully corrected heart defects with implanted foreign material during the first 6 months after surgery
  - Corrected heart defects with residual defects at or in the vicinity of prosthetic patches or prostheses
- Heart transplant recipients with cardiac valvular disease

► **Endocarditis prophylaxis.** In 2007, the recommendations of the German Society of Pediatric Cardiology were adapted to the US guidelines in coordination with the German Society of Cardiology. Endocarditis prophylaxis is currently recommended only for patients with a particularly high risk. Previously, all patients with congenital heart disease were advised to take antibiotic prophylaxis for endocarditis, with a few exceptions (e.g., isolated ASD II). The benefit of such an approach was not proven and the current recommendations therefore include only patients who are at a particularly high risk for endocarditis (see above) or where the risk of complications in infective endocarditis is very high. However, it is still true that the risk of endocarditis is generally increased in nearly all congenital heart defects.

The following procedures are examples of situations where there is a risk of developing bacteremia and endocarditis and antibiotic prophylaxis is therefore needed (▶ Table 16.5).

- *Dental procedures where there is a risk of bleeding*: scaling, periodontal curettage and surgery, root canal treatment, dental and orthodontic surgery including tooth extractions
- *ENT procedures*: tonsillectomy, adenoidectomy, other operations involving the mucosa, bronchoscopy with biopsies

Endocarditis prophylaxis in not necessary for interventions in the gastrointestinal tract, the urinary tract, or the skin if no infection is present in these areas. If an infection is present on the organs that were operated on, endocarditis prophylaxis should take into account the relevant pathogens that can be expected in the area of the operation, for example, streptococci and staphylococci on infected skin or enterococci in the gastrointestinal tract.

16.2.5 Prognosis

The cure rate of endocarditis is 80 to 85%. In infections with streptococci and viridans group streptococci, the cure rate is higher; for problematic pathogens (e.g., MRSA) it is significantly lower. Fungal endocarditis has the lowest cure rate. Patients with a previous endocarditis have an increased risk of developing endocarditis again.

Table 16.5 Endocarditis prophylaxis for oral, pharyngeal, and upper respiratory tract surgery

Situation	Drug and dosage
Standard regimen	Amoxicillin 50 mg/kg orally (max. 2 g)
Alternative	Penicillin V 50,000 U/kg orally (max. 2 mill. U)
Penicillin or ampicillin allergy	Clindamycin 20 mg/kg orally (max. 600 mg)
Application: single dose 30 to 60 minutes before the procedure. If oral intake is not possible, the same dose is administered intravenously.	

16.3 Pericarditis

16.3.1 Basics

Definition

Pericarditis is an inflammatory disease of the pericardium usually associated with a pericardial effusion. The myocardium is often affected in addition to the pericardium (perimyocarditis). The causes can be infectious or noninfectious. In childhood, most cases of pericarditis are either idiopathic or are caused by viruses. In extremely rare cases, cardiac tamponade can occur as a complication of pericardial effusion. Constrictive pericarditis is a possible later complication.

Epidemiology

The incidence in children is not known.

Pathogenesis and Pathology

As a result of an inflammatory reaction, serofibrinous, hemorrhagic, or purulent fluid secretions collect in the pericardium. The accumulation of fluid in the pericardium leads to impaired diastolic filling and decreased cardiac output. If the effusion increases slowly, the pericardium can expand greatly, but the pericardium cannot respond adequately to a rapid increase of effusion. Therefore, slowly developing effusions can often be surprisingly well compensated, while a rapid increase in pericardial effusion quickly leads to cardiac tamponade. The heart attempts to compensate the impaired diastolic function and reduced cardiac output by means of an increase in the heart rate, increase in the peripheral systemic resistance, and an increase of the venous constriction.

Etiology

The causes of pericarditis include infectious, immunologic, neoplastic, and traumatic pathogens (▶ Table 16.6).

In childhood, infectious causes are most common, especially viral infections (usually Coxsackie viruses). The range of pathogens is similar to that of myocarditis. Many cases that are classified as idiopathic pericarditis are probably due to a viral infection in which no particular pathogen can be isolated.

16.3.2 Diagnostic Measures

Medical History

In viral pericarditis, there are often signs in the patient's previous history pointing to a viral infection such as cough, runny nose, or diarrhea.

Symptoms

Indicative clinical findings are:

- Chest pain: The pain is usually breathing dependent. Pain can often be relieved by sitting down and leaning forward. Because every movement of the chest increases the pain, patients are usually remarkably still.
- Fever

Table 16.6 Causes of pericarditis

Infections	• Viruses: Coxsackie B, adenovirus, echo virus, EBV, HHV 6, HIV, measles, mumps, varicella, influenza, parvovirus B19, hepatitis B virus • Bacteria: Staphylococcus aureus, pneumococci, Haemophilus influenza, meningococci, streptococci, mycoplasma, Mycobacterium tuberculosis, gonorrhea, Chlamydia, or anaerobic gram-negative pathogens (especially in immunosuppressed). • Parasites: Echinococci, Toxoplasma • Fungi (especially in immunosuppressed): Aspergillus, Candida, Histoplasma
Immune-mediated	• Autoimmune and immunological diseases: acute rheumatic fever, lupus erythematosus, juvenile rheumatoid arthritis, sarcoidosis, dermatomyositis, scleroderma, Kawasaki disease, inflammatory bowel disease, Wegener granulomatosis • Postpericardiotomy syndrome, post-infarction syndrome (Dressler syndrome) • Transplant rejection • Allergic: serum disease
Toxic	• Uremia • Pharmaceuticals: including minoxidil, hydralazine, amiodarone, immunosuppressants, chemotherapeutics • Physical toxicant: radiation
Neoplastic	• Metastases (e.g., bronchial or breast cancer), leukemia, lymphoma, paraneoplastic, very rarely primary tumors (mesothelioma, rhabdomyosarcoma, teratoma, fibroma, leiomyoma)
Other rare causes	• Hypothyroidism • Trauma • Hemorrhage (e.g., under anticoagulation) • Dissecting aortic aneurysm

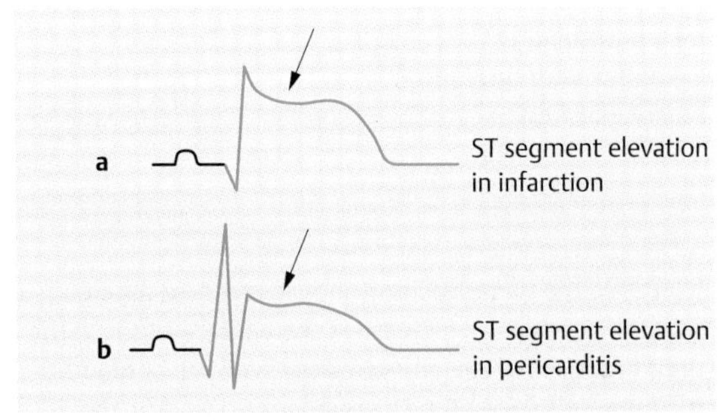

Fig. 16.1 Typical ECG changes in pericarditis. In acute pericarditis there is usually ST segment elevation of the ascending limb of the S wave (**b**). In myocardial infarction, however, there is ST segment elevation of the descending limb of the R wave (**a**). In addition, the ST segment changes in myocardial infarction affect the supply territory of one coronary artery, while in pericarditis, the changes are found in all leads or almost all leads.[38]

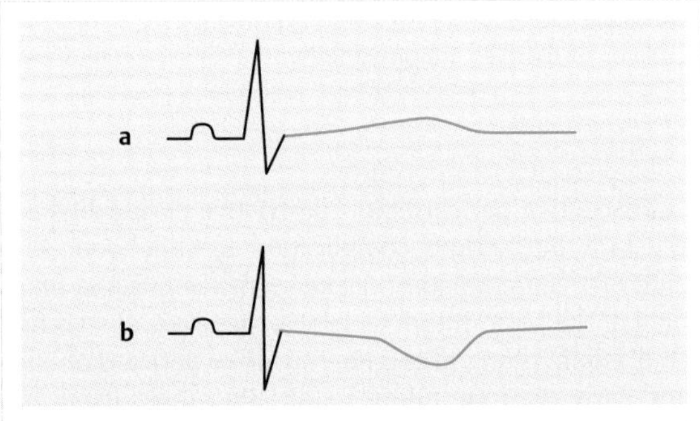

Fig. 16.3 ECG changes in stage 2 and stage 3 of pericarditis. **a** Stage 2: T-wave flattening. **b** Stage 3: terminal T wave inversion.[38]

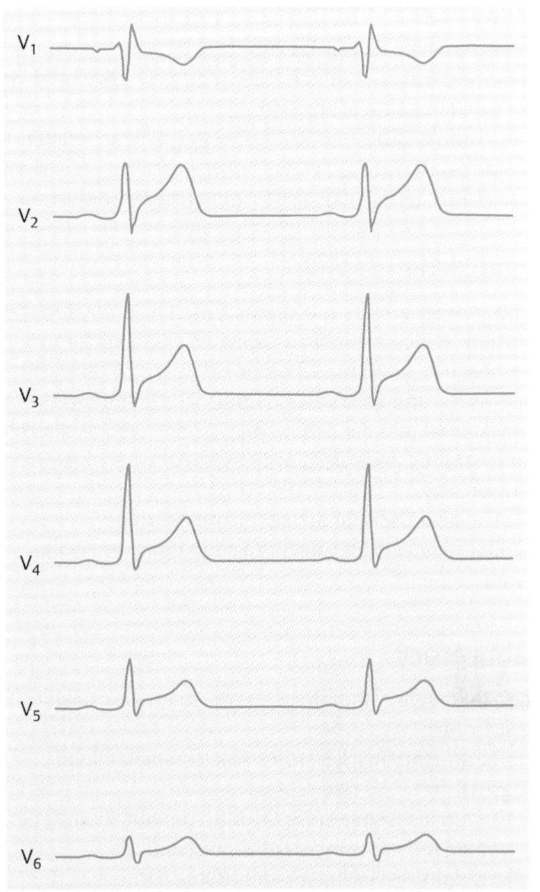

Fig. 16.2 Example of an ECG of pericarditis with pericardial effusion. ST segment elevation of the ascending limb of the R wave.

- Congestive heart failure: In an acute pericardial effusion that leads to pericardial tamponade, the main sign is acute heart failure.

Auscultation

- Pericardial friction rub: This a typical auscultation finding that is very specific for pericarditis and can be auscultated in the majority of patients—at least intermittently. The murmur sounds close to the ear and resembles the squeak of leather shoes or the sound made when walking in fresh snow.
- Soft heart sounds: As effusion increases, the heart sounds become increasingly softer.

ECG

The ECG changes typically occur in stages. They meet the criteria for epicardial damage.

- Stage 1 (within the first hours and days): concave ST segment elevation in all or at least in most leads (DD: myocardial infarction, ▶ Fig. 16.1, ▶ Fig. 16.2)
- Stage 2 (usually after a few days): normalization of the ST segment, flattening of the T wave (▶ Fig. 16.3)
- Stage 3 (typically 2–4 weeks after onset of disease): T wave inversion in all or at least in many leads (▶ Fig. 16.3)
- Stage 4: normalization of T waves, in chronic cases, there is often no normalization of T waves

If there is pronounced pericardial effusion, the following changes may occur:

- Low voltage
- Electrical alternans (height and orientation of the QRS complexes change from beat to beat, as the heart moves "back and forth" in the effusion)

Chest X-ray

Often no changes can be detected in acute pericarditis, even if pericardial tamponade has already developed due to a rapid increase of effusion.

In chronic cases, the X-ray shows the heart dilated on all sides, described as "water-bottle heart." In constrictive pericarditis, pericardial calcifications may be detected.

Echocardiography

Echocardiography is the method of choice for detecting effusion, which presents as a hypoechoic border around the heart. A small fluid border between the epicardium and pericardium, however, is normal. Under certain circumstances, internal echoes may be detected as a sign of fibrin strands. Indicators of hemodynamically significant effusion are:

- Collapse of the right atrium in late diastole
- Collapse or compression of the free right ventricular wall

Laboratory

The following laboratory tests may be useful for pericarditis:

- Inflammatory markers (CRP, ESR, complete blood count)
- Myocardial enzymes (CK, CK-MB, troponin I): may be elevated if there is myocardial involvement
- Blood cultures: useful for identifying pathogens in febrile patients
- Virus serology (e.g., Coxsackie B, echoviruses, adenoviruses), possibly streptococcal titers, tuberculin test
- TSH, free T3, free T4: to rule out hypothyroidism
- Auto-antibodies (e.g., ANA, anti-DNA antibodies, c-ANCA) in suspected autoimmune disease for the evaluation of chronic pericardial effusion
- Analysis of the pericardial fluid including protein, LDH, glucose, cholesterol, culture (bacteria, tuberculosis, fungi), Gram and Ziehl–Neelsen staining, cytology, possibly viral culture or PCR
- Pericardial biopsy: necessary only in extremely rare cases, such as with unexplained chronic course and low effusion volume that precludes pericardiocentesis.

16.3.3 Complications

▸ **Pericardial tamponade.** Pericardial tamponade occurs especially if there is a rapid increase of effusion. It leads to impairment of diastolic filling. Typical signs of pericardial tamponade are:

- Low cardiac output with centralization up to cardiogenic shock
- Tachycardia
- Dyspnea
- Signs of right heart failure:
    - Increased central venous pressure
    - Hepatomegaly
    - Jugular vein distention
- Pulsus paradoxus

Excursus: Pulsus paradoxus

Normally, the negative intrathoracic pressure during inspiration leads to an increase in the venous return to the right heart. However, an even larger volume of blood simultaneously "pools" in the pulmonary vascular bed. This explains why left ventricular stroke volume is reduced, despite the larger venous blood supply during inspiration. In case of pericardial tamponade, diastolic filling of the heart is obstructed, further decreasing the stroke volume during inspiration. There is pronounced weakening of the pulses and of blood pressure (> 10 mmHg) during inspiration. The term pulsus paradoxus is misleading. The blood pressure response in pulsus paradoxus is not actually paradoxical, but is more pronounced than under normal circumstances. Other possible causes of pulsus paradoxus include hypovolemia or restrictive cardiomyopathy.

▸ **Constrictive pericarditis.** Constrictive pericarditis is a very rare, but serious complication in childhood. As a result of an inflammatory response, thickening and hardening of the pericardium develops, massively obstructing the diastolic filling of the heart. Unlike pericardial effusion, early diastolic filling is initially unrestricted, but then ends abruptly. A typical cause of constrictive pericarditis is tuberculosis. In industrialized nations, constrictive pericarditis is usually idiopathic or occurs, for example, after infective pericarditis, cardiac surgery, autoimmune diseases, or malignancies.

The most important differential diagnosis for constrictive pericarditis is restrictive cardiomyopathy.

Typical symptoms of constrictive pericarditis are:

- Signs of right heart failure: hepatomegaly, ascites, edema, pleural effusion, jugular vein distention
- Signs of left heart failure (less often): pulmonary congestion, dyspnea
- Pulsus paradoxus
- Auscultation: early diastolic murmur in the left parasternal region. The murmur is probably caused by the abrupt end of ventricular filling.
- Echocardiography: thickened pericardium and possibly calcification, distended jugular veins, and dilated venae cavae. An abrupt movement of the interventricular septum ("septal bounce") may be seen in the early diastole.
- Chest X-ray: The heart size is usually normal; there is possibly evidence of pericardial calcification, possibly pleural effusion or pulmonary congestion.

- Ventricular pressure measurement: "square root sign" (the ventricular pressure curve resembles the mathematical sign for square root). After a normal systolic pressure curve, there is a rapid drop in pressure in the ventricle in the early diastole as a result of initially unimpeded diastolic relaxation. A diastolic plateau develops for the remainder of the diastole due to the subsequent "diastolic restraint."
- MRI/CT scans: These modalities give good assessment of pericardial thickness.

16.3.4 Treatment

Specific Treatment

There is no specific treatment for most cases of pericarditis that are idiopathic or caused by a viral infection.

In bacterially induced pericarditis, high-dose antibiotics are indicated, which are selected according to the pathogen identified in the pericardial fluid and administered intravenously for about 4 to 6 weeks. Appropriate initial therapy may consist of a combination of a third-generation cephalosporin and penicillinase-resistant penicillin, possibly supplemented by an aminoglycoside. Surgical drainage of the pericardium is often required for bacterial pericarditis.

A combination of antituberculosis therapy for at least 9 months is needed for tuberculous pericarditis.

Fungal pericarditis is treated with antifungal drugs (e.g., amphotericin B and flucytosine).

Treatment of the underlying disease is the priority if pericarditis is caused by a malignant pericardial effusion, uremia, or autoimmune disease.

Symptomatic Treatment

Essential components of the treatment are bed rest, anti-inflammatory treatment, and adequate pain management. Diuretics are usually not very suitable for reducing the effusion.

Anti-inflammatory Treatment

► **Nonsteroidal anti-inflammatory drugs.** NSAIDs—such as ibuprofen (30–40 mg/kg/d), naproxen (10–15 mg/kg/d), aspirin, or indomethacin—are the treatment of choice. Treatment is often required for several months because relapses after discontinuation of treatment are common.

► **Corticosteroids.** Steroids (e.g., prednisolone 1–2 mg/kg/d) are indicated if the patient does not respond to NSAIDs, but bacterial pericarditis must be ruled out beforehand. Locally instilled steroids may have a favorable effect on preventing constrictive pericarditis in bacterial pericarditis.

Pericardiocentesis and Drainage

Pericardiocentesis is required urgently or as an emergency procedure in a hemodynamically significant effusion or in pericardial tamponade. It is performed electively for diagnostic purposes to obtain pericardial fluid in suspected bacterial pericarditis or in chronic cases with unknown causes.

The puncture is carried out under echocardiography guidance, usually from a subxiphoid window in a half-sitting position under analgesia and continuous hemodynamic monitoring. Under certain circumstances, a pigtail catheter is advanced into the pericardium using the Seldinger technique for continuous drainage.

Complications include perforation of a heart cavity, damage to a coronary vessel, pneumothorax, arrhythmias, or infections.

Surgical Treatment

► **Pericardial drainage.** In purulent pericarditis, a pericardial drain introduced using the Seldinger technique is usually not sufficient and surgical pericardial drainage is required. Antiseptic irrigation can also be performed via this drain. Recurrent effusions may require a pericardial fenestration to drain the effusion into the pleural space.

► **Pericardiectomy.** Pericardiectomy is the treatment of choice for constrictive pericarditis.

16.3.5 Prognosis

The prognosis is good for idiopathic and viral pericarditis. Both almost always heal completely without consequences. Bacterial pericarditis, however, is a dangerous disease that is fatal if untreated. Optimal therapy can reduce the mortality rate to below 20%. Constrictive pericarditis requiring a pericardiectomy rarely develops.

16.4 Rheumatic Fever

16.4.1 Basics

Definition

Rheumatic fever is an immunological disease that occurs following an infection with group A beta-hemolytic streptococci (*Streptococcus pyogenes*), usually a throat infection. Rheumatic fever occurs 2 to 5 weeks after the streptococcal infection and is feared because of complications involving the cardiac valves that can lead to permanent valve damage years later.

Epidemiology

Rheumatic fever has become rare since the introduction of antibiotics in industrialized countries, but it is still the leading cause of acquired cardiac valve disease worldwide. It is estimated that 5 to 30 million children and young adults suffer from chronic rheumatic heart disease globally, the vast majority of them in developing countries. Approximately 90,000 people die from the consequences of this disease every year. The prevalence in industrialized countries is currently less than 5 per 100,000 schoolchildren; however, some increase has been reported in recent years. Primarily children between the ages of 5 and 15 years are affected by acute rheumatic fever. An untreated pharyngeal infection with group A beta-hemolytic streptococci leads to rheumatic fever in 0.3–3% of cases.

Pathogenesis

Rheumatic fever is an autoimmune disease caused by beta-hemolytic streptococci. The pathogenesis is not fully understood, but it is assumed that antibodies against the M protein of streptococci are formed during the course of a streptococcal infection. These antibodies exhibit cross-reactivity with autologous tissue such as the sarcolemmal antigens tropomyosin and myosin (molecular mimicry). These antibodies and cytotoxic lymphocytes attack endogenous tissue of the heart, joints, subcutaneous tissues, and the central nervous system (CNS) in genetically predisposed patients (e.g., in association with HLA DR3, DR4, and DR7).

In addition, there is immune complex-induced capillary damage with immune complexes in the myocardium (Aschoff nodules) and in the region of the cardiac valves.

16.4.2 Diagnostic Measures

Symptoms

There is typically a renewed acute fever 10 to 20 days after pharyngitis or tonsillitis caused by group A beta-hemolytic streptococci or scarlet fever. In addition to general symptoms (fever, headache, fatigue, abdominal and joint pain), there may also be arthritis, skin lesions, cardiac involvement, and involvement of the CNS (chorea minor).

► **Jones criteria.** Rheumatic fever is diagnosed based on clinical criteria (Jones criteria, ► Table 16.7).

The gold standard for detecting group A beta-hemolytic streptococci is a throat swab (however, no pathogens are usually detected in the throat swab at the onset of rheumatic fever). An elevated or rising streptococcal titer (see Laboratory, Serology (p.247)) is also an indication of a resolved infection. The streptococcal antigen test is less specific.

Rheumatic fever can be diagnosed in patients with Sydenham chorea without the criteria listed above, provided that other causes of chorea have been excluded.

Table 16.7 Jones criteria for rheumatic fever of the American Heart Association (1992)

Major criterion	Minor criterion
• Carditis	• Fever
• Migratory polyarthritis	• Arthralgia
• Sydenham's chorea	• Elevated laboratory inflammatory markers (ESR, CRP)
• Subcutaneous nodules	• Prolonged PQ interval in the ECG
• Erythema marginatum	

Note: The diagnosis is likely if two major criteria or one major criterion and two minor criteria are present. There must also have been a preceding infection with group A beta-hemolytic streptococci.

To diagnosis a relapse, it is sufficient to have one major criteria or arthralgia, unexplained fever, or elevated CRP level with evidence of a streptococcal infection.

► **Polyarthritis.** Polyarthritis is the most common major symptom and usually the earliest manifestation of rheumatic fever. Clinical signs include redness, swelling, and warmth of the affected joints. It mainly affects the large joints and "jumps" from joint to joint over time ("migratory polyarthritis"). There is a very good response to aspirin. The disease practically never leads to chronic arthritis.

► **Poststreptococcal arthritis.** A distinction is made between polyarthritis associated with rheumatic fever and poststreptococcal arthritis. Poststreptococcal arthritis usually occurs earlier (typically within 10 days) after a streptococcal infection while polyarthritis takes longer, responds poorly to aspirin, and does not "jump" from joint to joint. Other major criteria for rheumatic fever are not present.

Erythema nodosum or erythema multiforme may occur concomitantly. Cardiac involvement may develop in about 10% of cases.

► **Carditis.** Cardiac involvement is largely responsible for late morbidity and mortality. Typically, there is pancarditis with varying involvement of the different layers of the heart. The endocardium is almost always involved. Involvement of the mitral valve (mitral regurgitation) is typical, less often the aortic valve, and sometimes both.

► **Sydenham chorea.** Sydenham chorea (chorea minor, St. Vitus dance) is a late manifestation of rheumatic fever. It usually occurs several months after the manifestation in other organs and is characterized by uncontrolled movements of different muscle groups, which increase when the patient is excited and subside or disappear completely at rest or during sleep. Children appear clumsy. The disease heals completely with treatment.

► **Erythema marginatum.** This is a ring-shaped, reddish-blue, nonitchy rash that blanches under pressure and increases with heat. It occurs mainly on the trunk and proximal limbs (DD: erythema annulare centrifugum in a Borrelia infection).

► **Subcutaneous nodules.** Subcutaneous nodules are caused by granulomas. They are between lentil and walnut sized and are located primarily on the tendon insertions of elbows, wrists, and knees or in the occipital area and in the region of the vertebral processes.

► **Differential Diagnosis.** There are many differential diagnoses, including fever of unknown origin, and pediatric arthralgia. The most important differential diagnoses are:

- Juvenile chronic rheumatoid arthritis
- Reactive arthritis (e.g., after EBV, Borrelia, Yersinia, Salmonella infection)
- Collagenosis (e.g., systemic lupus erythematosus)
- Hematologic disorders (e.g., sickle cell anemia, leukemia)

Auscultation

A new heart murmur during rheumatic fever is an important indicator of cardiac involvement. Typical auscultation findings depend on the structural heart disease:

- Mitral regurgitation: apical "pouring" systolic murmur that gets louder in the left lateral position
- Aortic regurgitation: early diastolic murmur with PMI in the 2nd/3rd left parasternal intercostal space
- Pericardial effusion: soft heart sounds
- Pericardial rub: sign of pericarditis
- Gallop rhythm in congestive heart failure

Laboratory

► **Inflammatory markers.** ESR and CRP are elevated. A normal ESR rules out rheumatic fever. There may be mild normochromic, normocytic anemia.

► **Serology.** An antistreptolysin 0 (ASL) titer of over 300 or a rising titer indicates an acute streptococcal infection. The ASL titer rises especially after throat infections with streptococci. After a streptococcal infection, the titer usually reaches its maximum after 4 to 5 weeks, or during the second or third week of rheumatic fever. It is therefore advisable to check the titer (e.g., when the diagnosis is suspected and about 2 weeks later). Overall, however, the titer increases in only 80% of patients with rheumatic fever, so other streptococcal titers should also be investigated.

The anti-deoxyribonuclease-B titer (anti-DNAse B) rises especially in streptococcal skin infections. In some cases, evidence of anti-hyaluronidase may be useful for the diagnosis.

► **Throat swab.** The gold standard for the detection of group A beta-hemolytic streptococcus is the bacteriological culture from the throat swab. However, at the onset of rheumatic fever, group A streptococci can usually no longer be detected. The antigen test has a sensitivity of about 70%.

ECG

Typical findings are:

- Prolonged PQ interval, atrioventricular block
- ST segment or T wave changes as an indication of pericarditis
- Extrasystoles, junctional tachycardia

Chest X-ray

Cardiomegaly may be seen in the radiograph. A prominent left atrium is usually indicative of relevant mitral regurgitation.

Echocardiography

Echocardiography is the primary imaging technique for assessing the following parameters:

- Myocardial function as a measure of the severity of myocarditis
- Pericardial effusion as a sign of pericarditis
- Assessment of the heart valves, particularly noting mitral or aortic regurgitation (acute disease) or stenosis (chronic course)

16.4.3 Complications

The major complications of rheumatic fever are *rheumatic valve diseases*. As a result of rheumatic fever, insufficiency initially occurs, which eventually develops into stenosis due to scarring. This affects mainly the mitral and aortic valve. Globally, rheumatic fever is by far the most common cause of mitral stenosis in adulthood.

Rheumatic endocarditis determines the long-term prognosis of the disease. In English, the term "chronic rheumatic heart disease" (RHD) is used. As Lasègue succinctly stated: "Rheumatic fever licks at the joints and brain, but bites the heart."

16.4.4 Treatment

The main therapeutic measures in addition to antibiotic treatment to eliminate the streptococci are anti-inflammatory therapy with aspirin and possibly steroids and symptomatic treatment (bed rest, treatment of possible cardiac failure).

General Measures

Bed rest is recommended. The duration depends on the extent of the disease (1–2 weeks for uncomplicated arthritis; with carditis, as long as heart failure persists).

Greater physical stress should be avoided for 2 to 3 months after carditis.

Antibiotic Treatment

To eradicate streptococci, oral penicillin is administered for 10 days, followed by long-term antibiotic prophylaxis (see Prophylaxis below) to prevent recurrences.

Penicillin V is the treatment of choice:

- Dosage: 100 000 U/kg/d orally in 3 single doses (max. 3 × 1.2 mill U)
- Duration: 10 days

Alternatives:

- If compliance is poor, depot penicillin (benzylpenicillin) IM Dosage: 600,000 U for children over 27 kg body weight, 200,000 U for children under 27 kg
- For penicillin allergy, erythromycin 30–40 mg/kg/d orally in 2 to 3 single doses

Anti-inflammatory Treatment

The aim of anti-inflammatory treatment is to suppress the inflammatory reaction in order to prevent heart damage. Non-steroidal anti-inflammatory drugs (NSAIDs) are usually sufficient. In severe carditis, treatment is supplemented by steroids.

ASA (aspirin) is the treatment of choice:

- Dosage: in the acute phase 80 to 100 mg/kg/d in 4 single doses (target serum level 20–30 mg/dL)
- Duration: until complete disappearance of symptoms and normalization of inflammatory markers

Alternatives:

- Naproxen 10 to 20 mg/kg orally in 2 single doses
- Ibuprofen 20 to 40 mg/kg orally in 3 single doses

Steroids

Steroids are indicated for severe carditis (pronounced cardiomegaly, congestive heart failure, complete AV block).

Dosage: prednisolone 2 mg/kg/day (max. 80 mg/d) for 1 to 2 weeks, then gradually reduced over 2 weeks. Parallel to the gradual discontinuation of prednisolone, ASA medication should be started.

Treatment of Heart Failure

Digoxin was formerly given to treat heart failure (caution: increased digitalis toxicity), but today diuretics and ACE inhibitors are usually administered.

Surgical Treatment

Surgical valve repair or valve replacement may be necessary even in the acute stage if there is cardiac decompensation due to hemodynamically significant valve regurgitation.

Treatment of Unusual Courses

► **Sydenham chorea.** Anti-inflammatory therapy is not necessary, but antibiotic treatment as for other manifestations of rheumatic fever is needed.

Also recommended are bed rest, shielding from external stimuli, and padding the bed to prevent injury. Symptoms can be improved in part through sedation with phenobarbital, haloperidol, or benzodiazepines. In some cases, treatment with valproate or carbamazepine is successful.

► **Poststreptococcal arthritis.** NSAIDs and possibly intra-articular steroid injections as with other reactive arthritis. Antibiotic prophylaxis for 1 year is recommended for cases without cardiac involvement. If there is cardiac involvement, the same criteria for antibiotic prophylaxis apply as for rheumatic fever (see Prophylaxis below).

Prophylaxis

After rheumatic fever, long-term antibiotic prophylaxis is necessary to avoid relapses. The duration depends on the severity of the disease and may have to be maintained for life (► Table 16.8).

- Penicillin 2 × 200,000 U/d orally regardless of body weight
- If compliance is poor: benzylpenicillin 1.2 mill. U IM every 3 weeks
- For penicillin allergy, erythromycin 250 mg orally per day

► **Endocarditis prophylaxis.** Endocarditis prophylaxis is no longer recommended for most patients with rheumatic heart disease. Exceptions include for example patients with prosthetic valves or valves repaired with prosthetic material and patients with previous endocarditis.

16.4.5 Prognosis

Even after the introduction of penicillin, the probability of heart valve disease in rheumatic fever is still around 10 to 40%. The most frequent problem is mitral stenosis. The likelihood of permanent damage to the heart

Table 16.8 Secondary prophylaxis of rheumatic fever

Course of rheumatic fever	Duration of antibiotic prophylaxis
Without cardiac involvement	5 years, but at least until age 21
With cardiac involvement but without valve damage	10 years, but at least until adulthood
With cardiac involvement and valve damage	At least 10 years, but at least until the age of 40, sometimes life-long

Table 16.9 Diagnostic criteria for Kawasaki syndrome

Fever	• At least 5 days of recurring, antibiotic-resistant, high fever up to 40°C • Duration of fever usually 10 days without treatment • Fever responds only briefly to antipyretics
Conjunctivitis	• Usually bilateral, non-purulent conjunctivitis • Begins shortly after the fever • Duration about 10 days
Changes in the limbs	• Acute: palmar or plantar erythema, edema of the hands or feet • Subacute: peri-ungual desquamation of the fingers or toes in the 2nd–3rd week of illness
Polymorphous exanthema	• Polymorphous exanthema mainly on the trunk • Usually begins within 5 days after the onset of fever • Usually maculopapular, also scarlatiform eruption, may be similar to purpura or reminiscent of erythema multiforme
Changes in the lips and oral cavity	• Red, dry, cracked and swollen lips • Raspberry tongue, pronounced mucosal redness
Cervical lymph adenopathy	• Usually unilateral swelling of the cervical lymph nodes (> 1.5 cm) • Least common of the classical criteria

depends on the severity of the initial cardiac involvement.

Relapses occur most frequently in the first year after the disease. The risk of cardiac involvement increases with each recurrence.

Since the introduction of antibiotics, the mortality rate of acute rheumatic fever in industrialized countries is nearly 0%, but in developing countries it can still be as high as 10%.

16.5 Kawasaki Syndrome

16.5.1 Basics

Synonym: mucocutaneous lymph node syndrome

Definition

Kawasaki syndrome is an acute febrile systemic disease that is associated with necrotizing vasculitis of small and medium-sized arteries. One feared complication is the development of coronary artery aneurysms or ectasia with subsequent stenosis.

Epidemiology

Children between 1 and 2 years of age are most often affected. About 75% of the children are younger than 5 years, and about 25% are infants. The disease is most common in Japan (180 per 100,000 children under 5 years); the incidence is 30 per 100,000 in Caucasian children. Overall, the incidence is increasing in all ethnic groups. Boys are affected slightly more often than girls. There is a seasonal increase in winter and spring.

Etiology

The cause is unknown. Different infectious causes on the basis of a genetic or immunological predisposition are suspected. Superantigens and cytotoxic T cells also appear to play a role.

Pathology

There is generalized vasculitis with preference for small and medium-sized arteries, but all vessels can be affected. A systemic inflammatory reaction with activation of the immune system in various organs also occurs.

16.5.2 Diagnostic Measures

Symptoms

▸ **Diagnostic criteria.** A typical Kawasaki syndrome is present if fever persists for 5 days and at least four of the diagnostic criteria listed in ▸ Table 16.9 are present.

In patients who have fewer than four of the criteria listed, Kawasaki disease can be diagnosed if there is evidence of changes in the coronary arteries. If the patient has a high fever and least four of the classical criteria, the diagnosis can be made as soon as the fourth day of fever.

▸ **Other affected organs.** In addition to the changes mentioned in the diagnostic criteria, the following organ systems are often affected.

- *Cardiovascular*: abnormalities of the coronary arteries (aneurysms, ectasia, later stenosis, frequency 15–25%), myocarditis (in more than 50% of cases), pericarditis, valvular regurgitation (especially aortic and mitral valve regurgitation), congestive heart failure, arrhythmias, aneurysms of noncoronary arteries (iliac, femoral,

axillary or renal vessels), Raynaud phenomenon symptoms
- *Gastrointestinal tract*: often vomiting, diarrhea, and abdominal pain, gallbladder hydrops, rarely acute abdomen (paralytic ileus), hepatosplenomegaly
- *Respiratory tract*: cough, hoarseness, rhinitis
- *CNS*: often pronounced irritability, aseptic meningitis, rarely peripheral facial palsy or hearing loss
- *Urinary tract*: dysuria, sterile leukocyturia, very rarely kidney failure
- *Muscles/joints*: in the first week of illness, often arthritis/arthralgia of multiple joints (e.g., finger joints); after the 10th day of illness, arthritis/arthralgia usually of the large joints (such as knees or ankles)
- *Eyes*: anterior uveitis, spontaneous recovery without specific therapy

► **Coronary artery aneurysms.** The most feared complication in Kawasaki disease is a coronary artery aneurysm, which occurs in 15 to 25% of untreated children. As a rule of thumb, a coronary artery aneurysm is present when the coronary artery diameter in children under 5 years of age exceeds 3 mm or the lumen is more than 1.5 times as large as in the immediate vicinity. In a Kawasaki syndrome, coronary artery aneurysms almost always involve the proximal segments of the coronary arteries, which in general can be readily visualized by echocardiography. Coronary artery aneurysms in childhood associated with febrile illness are very specific for Kawasaki disease.

Even years after the acute illness, coronary artery aneurysms can develop thrombosis or stenosis and lead to myocardial infarction, arrhythmias, and sudden cardiac death. The risk of myocardial infarction is highest after around 4 weeks and can become manifest with atypical symptoms.

Risk factors for the development of coronary artery aneurysms include:
- Age < 1 year and > 6 years
- Male gender
- Fever ≥ 14 days
- Na < 135 mmol/L
- Hematocrit < 35%
- Leukocytes > 12,000/µL

► **Incomplete Kawasaki syndrome.** An incomplete Kawasaki syndrome is when, aside from fever, fewer than four of the classic symptoms are present. It is more common in children under 1 year old and can often be fatal because coronary artery aneurysms are frequent in this age group. Significantly elevated inflammatory parameters and fever of unknown origin, particularly in infants, always suggest an incomplete Kawasaki syndrome.

Differential Diagnoses

The differential diagnoses of Kawasaki syndrome include mainly immunological and infectious febrile diseases:
- Viral infections: measles, rubella, three-day-fever, cytomegalovirus, parvovirus B19, adenovirus, enteroviruses
- Bacterial diseases: scarlet fever, toxic shock syndrome, "staphylococcal scalded skin syndrome," leptospirosis
- Autoimmune diseases: systemic form of juvenile idiopathic arthritis (Still disease), rheumatic fever, polyarteritis nodosa
- Drugs: Stevens–Johnson syndrome
- Other diseases: e.g., mercury poisoning

Laboratory

Leukocytosis (> 15,000/µL) and an elevated ESR or CRP value is present in the acute phase in almost all patients. Thrombocytosis with level above 500,000/µL is characteristic of the later phase.

The typical laboratory findings are summarized here:
- Leukocytosis with a left shift
- Elevated ESR and CRP
- Anemia
- Pronounced thrombocytosis (often after the second to third week of illness)
- Elevated transaminases, elevated bilirubin (sign of liver involvement)
- Hypoalbuminemia (especially in a long and severe course of the disease)
- Hyponatremia (possibly an expression of inappropriate ADH secretion)
- Abnormal plasma lipids (decreased cholesterol and HDL during the acute phase)
- Cerebrospinal fluid (CSF) pleocytosis (in 33–50% of patients, often without elevated protein in the CSF)
- Sterile leukocyturia
- Sterile joint fluid with leukocytosis

Laboratory tests for investigating differential diagnoses or complications:
- Blood cultures, throat swab, stool cultures, antistreptococcal titer
- ANA
- Serology (measles, EBV, rubella, cytomegalovirus, parvovirus, adenoviruses, enteroviruses)
- Urea, creatinine
- For suspected myocarditis or myocardial infarction: cardiac enzymes (CK, CK-MB, LDH, troponin I)
- For suspected disseminated intravascular coagulation: Quick, INR, PTT, fibrinogen

ECG

The ECG changes in Kawasaki syndrome are usually nonspecific. Arrhythmia may occur with prolonged PQ interval and nonspecific repolarization disturbances (changes in ST segment or T wave).

A myocardial infarction is often difficult to diagnose in children. A deep and wide Q wave (> 0.35 mV and 35 ms) is suggestive of myocardial infarction. In the first 2 weeks of illness, this change can also suggest myocarditis. But especially after this time it is essential to consider a myocardial infarction. Another indicator of an infarction is an ST segment elevation of about 2 mm and a prolonged QTc interval of about 440 ms in combination with other criteria.

Echocardiography

There is an indication for echocardiography as soon as Kawasaki syndrome is suspected. Follow-up after 2 weeks and again after 6 to 8 weeks is useful for uncomplicated cases. More frequent tests should be performed in children with an increased risk for developing coronary anomalies. Examinations at least once a year, even after the acute illness is healed, are necessary if there is evidence of coronary aneurysms.

The echocardiography assessment should investigate the following:

- Echogenicity of the coronary arteries (echogenicity is often increased even before other coronary changes occur)
- Coronary anomalies such as coronary aneurysms, ectasia, or stenoses
- Left ventricular function
- Dilatation of the aortic root
- Valve insufficiency (especially mitral or aortic regurgitation)
- Rule out regional dyskinesia (suggestive of ischemia)
- Detect or rule out pericardial effusion
- Rule out noncoronary aneurysms (especially abdominal vessels and subclavian arteries)

Cardiac Catheterization

Coronary angiography is generally not recommended even if mild coronary ectasia or fusiform coronary aneurysms have been detected. If it is necessary for more severe findings, it is usually carried out 6 to 12 months after the onset of illness. If ischemia is suspected, immediate catheterization is indicated. Coronary angiography should be combined with angiography of the abdominal arteries and the subclavian arteries.

MRI

Changes in the coronary arteries can be assessed just as well by MRI as by using coronary angiography.

Exercise Tests

Exercise tests are necessary for detecting myocardial ischemia under exertion but should not be performed in the acute phase of the disease.

16.5.3 Treatment

To reduce the risk of coronary artery aneurysms, treatment should begin before the 10th day of illness, but if it is not diagnosed until later, it is still useful to start treatment after the 10th day.

The standard treatment is a combination of intravenous immunoglobulins and aspirin (ASA). The duration of treatment depends on the disease and the occurrence of coronary changes.

Acute Treatment

► **Aspirin (ASA).** *Dosage*: In the acute phase 80 to 100 mg/kg/d in 4 single doses (a lower dose of 20–50 mg/kg/d is likely just as effective), 48 to 72 hours after defervescence dose reduction to 3 to 5 mg/kg/d as a single dose.

Duration of therapy: In absence of coronary artery aneurysms, ASA can be discontinued after 6 to 8 weeks; if there is evidence of coronary artery aneurysms, treatment is continued at least until the complete disappearance of coronary pathology.

Risks: There is a risk of Reye syndrome, especially in association with varicella or influenza infection. If there is a clinical suspicion of one of these diseases, the ASA therapy should be terminated. In addition, an annual influenza vaccination is recommended for children older than 6 months undergoing long-term aspirin therapy. If possible, aspirin should not be given within 6 weeks after varicella vaccination.

► **Intravenous immunoglobulins.** *Dosage:* 2 g/kg as an infusion over 12 hours as a single dose.

Note on vaccinations: MMR and varicella vaccinations should not be given sooner than 11 months after immunoglobulin therapy because of potential interference with the transmitted passive antibodies, which can prevent the long-term success of vaccination. Children may be vaccinated earlier, but the booster should not be given until after at least 11 months.

► **Steroids.** There is no clear evidence yet of the benefit of steroids in the acute phase of the disease. However, they may be used in patients at risk for disease progression who do not respond to intravenous immunoglobulins.

Approximately 10 to 20% of patients do not respond to a one-time administration of intravenous immunoglobulins. In such cases, 2 g/kg immunoglobulin as an infusion over 12 hours should be administered. If there is no improvement despite repeated immunoglobulin therapy, methylprednisolone at a dose of 30 mg/kg intravenously over 2 hours for 1 to 3 days is indicated.

► **Additional treatment options.** Additional treatment options based on individual case reports are plasma exchange, monoclonal antibodies against cytokines, and the cytotoxic agents abciximab and cyclophosphamide.

► **Giant aneurysms (more than 8 mm).** In giant aneurysms, anticoagulation with phenprocoumon or warfarin is recommended to reduce the risk of thrombosis with subsequent stenosis of the aneurysms.

► **Treatment of myocardial infarction or relevant coronary stenosis.** Lysis therapy and often bypass surgery are necessary for myocardial infarction or relevant coronary stenosis. Percutaneous transluminal coronary angioplasty (PTCA) is often difficult and risky because of the calcifications that are usually present in the coronary arteries.

► **Long-term treatment and follow-up.** The long-term treatment and follow-up depend on the occurrence of coronary anomalies (► Table 16.10).

16.5.4 Prognosis

The prognosis of coronary artery aneurysms depends on the size and shape of the aneurysm. Fusiform aneurysms with a diameter of less than 8 mm have the best prognosis. Up to 30% of giant aneurysms more than 8 mm in diameter develop stenosis due to intima proliferation and vascular fibrosis, which can lead to myocardial infarction, arrhythmias, and sudden cardiac death.

Timely treatment with immunoglobulins can prevent the development of such giant aneurysms in about 95% of cases. With rapid treatment, the prognosis is good.

The overall mortality rate is between 0.1% and 2%. Most deaths occur within 15 to 45 days after onset of illness.

16.6 Cardiac Tumors

16.6.1 Basics

Epidemiology

Primary cardiac tumors are rare in childhood. By far the most common cardiac tumors in children are rhabdomyomas, which are associated with tuberous sclerosis in more than half of cases.

Almost all primary cardiac tumors in childhood are benign according to histological criteria. Malignant cardiac teratomas or sarcomas are a rarity. Secondary malignant cardiac tumors are also rare and occur in association with lymphomas, leukemia, neuroblastomas or sarcomas, for example.

Pathology

The following are the most common cardiac tumors in childhood:

► **Rhabdomyomas.** Rhabdomyomas are by far the most common cardiac tumors in childhood. They make up more than half of all cardiac tumors in children and 50%

Table 16.10 Long-term treatment and follow-up after Kawasaki syndrome (from Newburger et al. 2004)[90]

Risk level	Treatment	Physical activity	Checkups	Angiography
I: No coronary anomalies ever detected	No treatment after the first 6–8 weeks	No limitation after 6–8 weeks	Cardiac checkup every 2–5 years, possibly echocardiography after 1 year	Not recommended
II: Temporary coronary ectasia (no longer detected after 6–8 weeks)	No treatment after the first 6–8 weeks	No limitation after 6–8 weeks	Cardiac checkup every 2–5 years, possibly echocardiography after 1 year	Not recommended
III: One small to medium-sized aneurysm (3–6 mm) of a main coronary artery	ASA 3–5 mg/kg/d until the documented disappearance of the aneurysm	Under age 11: no restrictions after the first 6–8 weeks Age 11–20: depending on results of exercise tests	Annual cardiac examination including ECG, echocardiography, if necessary exercise test in patients over 11 years	Recommended if evidence of ischemia
IV: More than one large aneurysm (about 8 mm) or several aneurysms in a coronary artery without obstruction	Long-term therapy with ASA 3–5 mg/kg/d; In giant aneurysms combined with warfarin/phenprocoumon or low molecular weight heparin	No contact sports (risk of bleeding), other activities depending on the exercise test	Semi-annual cardiac examination including ECG, echocardiography, if necessary exercise test	First angiography after 6–12 months, earlier if clinically indicated; repetition if evidence of ischemia
V: Coronary artery obstruction	Long-term therapy with ASA 3–5 mg/kg/day, in persistent giant aneurysms possibly combined with warfarin/phenprocoumon or low molecular weight heparin	No contact sports (risk of bleeding), other activities, depending on the exercise test	Semi-annual cardiac examination including ECG, echocardiography, if necessary exercise test	Angiography also to assess treatment options

of cases are associated with tuberous sclerosis. The most common site is the ventricular septum, but rhabdomyomas usually occur at several locations in the heart. The size may vary from few millimeters to a few centimeters. Rhabdomyomas can lead to obstruction of blood flow and arrhythmias and must then be removed surgically. However, spontaneous regression is the rule.

Note

Rhabdomyomas are the most common cardiac tumors in childhood. They occur frequently in multiples and are usually associated with tuberous sclerosis.

Other typical symptoms of tuberous sclerosis are tumors of the CNS and the kidneys, adenoma sebaceum, hypopigmentation ("white spots"), cerebral seizures, and mental retardation.

▶ **Fibromas.** Cardiac fibromas are usually single solid tumors that can theoretically affect all segments of the heart, but are usually located on the free ventricular walls or the ventricular septum. The tumor can measure up to several centimeters. Occasionally, the tumors tend to develop calcification. Fibromas can lead to an obstruction of the blood flow to the heart and to arrhythmia. Surgical excision is usually possible, but a residual tumor may be left to avoid damaging the surrounding myocardium.

▶ **Teratomas.** Teratomas are embryonic tumors that contain tissue from all three germ layers. They are found mainly in fetuses and neonates. They are usually located at the base of the heart near the great vessels and are surrounded by pericardial tissue. They can compress the aorta and the pulmonary artery and lead to pericardial effusion. Surgical removal is usually possible.

▶ **Myxomas.** Myxomas are the most common cardiac tumors in adolescence and adulthood. In younger children, they are a rarity. Typically, myxomas are located in the left atrium, rarely in the right atrium, and almost never in the ventricles. Myxomas are pedunculated and often cause problems by "beating into" the left atrium up to the mitral valve. They are also the starting point for thrombi that then result in thromboembolic complications in the systemic circulation. Myxomas of the right atrium cause problems of the tricuspid valve and thromboembolism in the pulmonary circulation. The treatment of choice is surgical excision of the myxoma.

16.6.2 Diagnostic Measures

Symptoms

The clinical symptoms of cardiac tumors are often nonspecific and depend mainly on the location and the size of the tumor. Cardiac tumors are sometimes discovered as an incidental finding in fetal ultrasonography or echocardiography.

Syncopes and chest pain are nonspecific symptoms. Tumors that extend into the cavity of a ventricle can lead to obstruction of the inflow and outflow tract. The main clinical feature is low cardiac output. Arrhythmias and conduction disorders also occur. Pre-excitation syndromes have been described with rhabdomyomas; the tumor tissue is used as an accessory conduction pathway. Tumors in the vicinity of heart valves may result in valve stenosis or regurgitation and cause the corresponding murmur. Pedunculated tumors (especially myxomas) may also affect the valve function and constitute a starting point for embolism.

Tumors that affect the pericardium usually cause symptoms of pericardial effusion.

General symptoms such as fever, fatigue, weight loss, and myalgia are typical for myxomas.

Thromboembolisms develop through fragmentation of the tumor or from thrombi on the surface of the tumors.

ECG

Signs of atrial or ventricular hypertrophy may be noted in the ECG. Changes in the ST segment occur in larger tumors. These repolarization disturbances can also suggest myocardial ischemia. Supraventricular and ventricular extrasystoles and tachycardia may occur depending on the location of the tumor. Conduction disturbances (AV block, bundle branch block) are also typical. Pre-excitation syndromes have been described for rhabdomyomas.

Chest X-ray

Cardiomegaly, an unusual cardiac silhouette, or calcifications in the heart shadow may be signs of a cardiac tumor.

Echocardiography

Echocardiography is the diagnostic method of choice. It can be used to detect a tumor and determine its size and location. Doppler ultrasound can be used to assess whether the tumor leads to obstruction of the inflow and outflow tract or damage to the cardiac valves, and systolic and diastolic function can also be assessed. A pericardial effusion indicates intraperitoneal tumors, which are usually metastases of noncardiac primary malignant tumors.

Typical echocardiography findings are summarized in ▶ Table 16.11.

MRI

MRI can provide detailed information on the tumor location, consistency, and borders to surrounding tissue. Contrast agent uptake can provide information on the histology of the tumor.

Table 16.11 Typical echocardiography findings of the most common primary cardiac tumors in childhood and adolescence

Tumor	Typical finding
Rhabdomyoma	Multiple intramural tumors of varying sizes
Fibroma	Single intramural tumor originating from the ventricular septum or free ventricular wall, variable size
Myxoma	Pedunculated tumor in the left atrium, originating from the atrial septum
Teratoma	Cystic tumor, originating in the vicinity of the great vessels, surrounded by pericardial tissue, pericardial effusion

Cardiac Catheterization

Cardiac catheterization is indicated only in exceptional cases. Tumor biopsy is contraindicated because of the risk of tumor seeding.

16.6.3 Treatment

Surgical excision is thus far the only treatment option for cardiac tumors requiring treatment.

Indications for surgical resection include:

- tumors that cause congestive heart failure
- ventricular arrhythmia that does not respond to drug therapy
- tumors that cause obstruction of the inflow or outflow tract or relevant valve dysfunction

For asymptomatic patients with multiple rhabdomyomas, it is preferable to wait for spontaneous regression. Fibromas can usually be removed in toto. Myxomas can also usually be easily excised. To avoid a recurrence, care should be taken to remove the entire stem of a myxoma.

Surgical excision is not possible in very rare cases of very massive tumors and a heart transplant is the last treatment option.

16.6.4 Prognosis

Rhabdomyomas associated with tuberous sclerosis regress spontaneously within the first year of life in up to 80% of patients. Fibromas that are not excised must be checked regularly, since they have a tendency to grow. After surgical resection, regular follow-up is necessary. Recurrences may occur, especially with myxomas or incomplete excision of the tumor.

17 Cardiomyopathies

17.1 Dilated Cardiomyopathy

17.1.1 Basics

Definition

Dilated cardiomyopathy (DCM) is a myocardial disease characterized by enlargement of all cardiac chambers (▶ Fig. 17.1). The dilatation of the left ventricle is usually most pronounced. DCM is associated with impairment of systolic and diastolic function.

Epidemiology

DCM is rare in childhood, but is still the most common form of cardiomyopathy in children. The incidence is 0.5 to 2.6 per 100,000 children. All age groups can be affected. In children, the disease often becomes manifest within the first 2 years of life. Boys are affected slightly more often than girls.

Etiology

For the majority of patients, the cause is unknown (idiopathic DCM). The cases in which triggers are detected were formerly referred to as secondary cardiomyopathies (▶ Table 17.1). The most common cause of secondary cardiomyopathy is *myocarditis*. The most important triggers of secondary DCM include *metabolic disorders*, *chemotherapy* with anthracyclines, and *neuromuscular diseases* (e.g., Duchenne muscular dystrophy). Long-term strain on the heart caused by an arrhythmia may also lead to the clinical features of DCM. *Ischemic myocardial damage* must always be ruled out as a cause of DCM. Examples for the cause of myocardial ischemia are, for example, myocardial infarction (Kawasaki syndrome), or an anomalous origin of the left coronary artery from the pulmonary artery (Bland–White–Garland syndrome).

Genetic, familial forms account for over one-third of all DCM diseases. The most common is autosomal dominant inheritance. But autosomal recessive, X-chromosomal, and mitochondrial inheritance patterns have also been described. This mainly affects genes encoding myocardial proteins such as actin, desmin, dystrophin, and tafazzin.

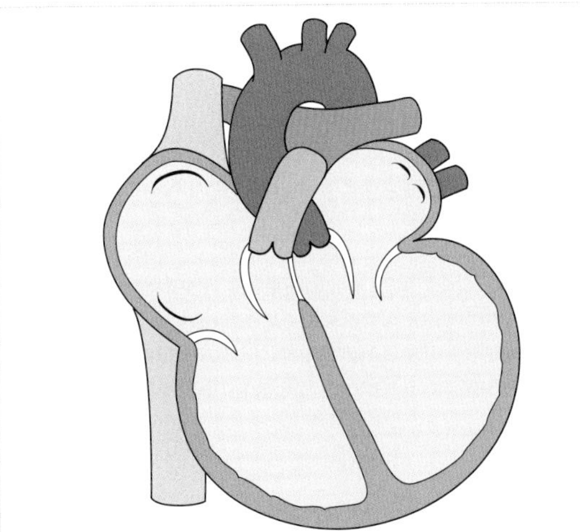

Fig. 17.1 Dilated cardiomyopathy (DCM). The characteristic feature of DCM is the enlargement of all cardiac chambers. Dilatation of the left ventricle is usually most pronounced.

> **Note**
>
> Due to the high proportion of familial DCM, family members of affected patients must undergo investigative echocardiography. The tests must be repeated regularly since late manifestations are also possible.

Pathology

Systolic dysfunction is the main functional symptom. Dilatation of the cardiac chambers and elevated end-diastolic pressure lead to increased ventricular wall tension. The dilatation is due to structural dilation, the remodeling of the actin–myosin scaffold of the sarcomeres. There is histological evidence of hypertrophy and hyperplasia of the myocytes and of fibrosis. Progressive fibrosis causes decreased compliance of the heart and thus leads to diastolic dysfunction.

17.1.2 Diagnostic Measures

Symptoms

The main clinical symptoms are signs of congestive heart failure: fatigue, failure to thrive, increased sweating, cool, pale skin, prolonged capillary refilling time, tachypnea, dyspnea, tachycardia, exertional cyanosis, hepatomegaly, and edema. Abdominal pain (due to liver congestion) and nausea may be nonspecific signs of heart failure. Palpitations suggest supraventricular or ventricular arrhythmias. A bulge in the chest (voussure) may be visible with pronounced cardiomegaly.

Auscultation

A gallop rhythm may often be auscultated, suggesting heart failure. The first heart sound is usually soft. Pulmonary hypertension may develop as a result of pulmonary congestion. In this case, the second heart sound is pronounced. A systolic murmur can be heard at the cardiac

Table 17.1 Causes of dilated cardiomyopathy (DCM)

Viral infections (myocarditis)	Coxsackie B, adenovirus, echo virus, EBV, CMV, HSV, HIV, rubella, measles, mumps, varicella, influenza, parvovirus B19, hepatitis C virus, polio, rabies
Bacterial infections	Diphtheria, mycoplasma, tuberculosis, Lyme disease, sepsis
Parasites	Toxoplasma gondii, Ascaris
Fungal infections	Histoplasma, Aspergillus, Candida, Cryptococcus
Neuromuscular diseases	Becker, Duchenne, Emery–Dreifuss, limb-girdle muscular dystrophy; myotonic dystrophy, Friedreich ataxia, Kearns–Sayre syndrome, congenital myopathy, Barth syndrome
Deficiencies	Anorexia nervosa, copper, iron, selenium, or thiamine deficiency
Immunological diseases	Rheumatic fever, rheumatoid arthritis, systemic lupus erythematosus, dermatomyositis, Kawasaki syndrome
Hematological diseases	Thalassemia, sickle cell anemia
Drugs or toxins	Anthracyclines, cyclophosphamide, chloroquine, cocaine, tricyclic antidepressants, interferon, alcohol, anabolic steroids
Endocrine disorders	Hypo/hyperthyroidism, hypoparathyroidism, pheochromocytoma, hypoglycemia
Metabolic diseases	Glycogen storage diseases, carnitine deficiency, impaired beta-oxidation or fatty acid transport, Refsum disease, mucopolysaccharidosis, oligosaccharidosis, mitochondropathies, defects in glucose/ pyruvate metabolism and defects in the citric acid cycle, hemosiderosis
Myocardial ischemia	Bland–White–Garland-Syndrome, myocardial infarction
Arrhythmias	Supraventricular/ventricular tachycardia
Malformation syndromes	Cri-du-chat (cat's cry) syndrome
Familial DCM	Different modes of inheritance, most often autosomal dominant, affecting mainly genes that encode myocardial proteins (actin, desmin, dystrophin)

apex if there is mitral regurgitation. Moist crackles over the lungs suggest pulmonary edema.

Laboratory

BNP (B-type natriuretic peptide) can be used as a marker of heart failure. The laboratory inflammation markers and cardiac enzymes such as troponin I or CK-MB can be elevated in myocarditis.

The basic diagnostic tools to rule out specific and secondary cardiomyopathies are the following laboratory tests:

- Blood/plasma:
  - Differential blood count
  - Viral titers: Coxsackie B, adenovirus, echo virus, EBV, HSV, HIV, cytomegalovirus, rubella, measles, mumps, varicella, influenza, parvovirus B19, hepatitis C virus, polio
  - Iron, ferritin (hemochromatosis)
  - Blood gas analysis, lactate, pyruvate, beta-OH butyrate, acetoacetate (fasting and postprandial), ammonia, glucose (mitochondropathy, organ acidopathy, disorder of fatty acid transport/oxidation)
  - Carnitine (disorder of fatty acid transport/oxidation)
  - Free fatty acids, beta-OH butyrate (in hypoglycemia; disorder of fatty acid transport/oxidation)
  - CK (myopathy), CK-MB, troponin
  - BNP
  - AST, ALT, creatinine, urea (hepatopathy, multisystem disease)
  - Tandem mass spectrometry (TMS; including disorders of fatty acid oxidation)
  - Acidic α-glucosidosis in leukocytes (Pompe disease in infants)
- Urine:
  - Organic acids (organ acidopathy, respiratory chain defect, defect of fatty acid oxidation)
  - Glycosaminoglycans, oligosaccharides in the urine (mucopolysaccharidosis, glycoproteinosis)

ECG

The ECG is usually remarkable, but the changes are nonspecific. Common ECG findings in DCM are:

- Sinus tachycardia
- Signs of left ventricular hypertrophy

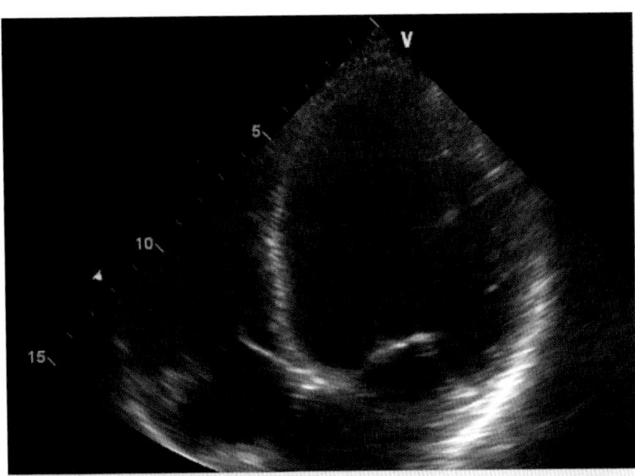

Fig. 17.2 Echocardiographic findings of dilated cardiomyopathy (DCM). The pronounced dilatation of the left ventricle can be visualized in the apical four-chamber view.

- Low voltage
- Repolarization disturbances
- Intraventricular conduction disturbances, left bundle branch block, first degree atrioventricular block
- Pathological Q waves suggestive of ischemia (In Bland–White–Garland syndrome there is typically a pattern of anterolateral myocardial ischemia with deep Q waves and ST-segment elevation and a T inversion in leads I, aVL, V_5 and V_6)
- Arrhythmias: ventricular arrhythmias, but also atrial flutter/fibrillation

Chest X-ray

Cardiomegaly is present, usually the result of left atrial and left ventricular enlargement. There is widening of the tracheal bifurcation and elevation of the left main bronchus due to left atrial enlargement. There may also be signs of pulmonary congestion or pulmonary edema and in some cases pleural effusion as well.

Echocardiography

Indicative findings are enlargement of the cardiac chambers, especially of the left atrium and the left ventricle, and impaired contractility (▶ Fig. 17.2). The enlarged left ventricle contracts poorly. The fractional shortening, stroke volume, and ejection fraction are substantially reduced as a sign of left ventricular dysfunction. These parameters are also used to monitor the course of the disease. In addition, there is diastolic dysfunction with decelerated relaxation. The hepatic veins and the inferior vena cava are enlarged as a sign of right heart failure. Pericardial and pleural effusions should be noted and thrombi in the ventricles and atria must be ruled out.

The origins of the coronary arteries must be visualized to be sure Bland–White–Garland syndrome (anomalous origin of the left coronary artery from the pulmonary artery) is not overlooked. Coronary artery aneurysms must also be noted and Kawasaki syndrome ruled out.

With color Doppler ultrasound, mitral or tricuspid regurgitation can often be detected, which is the result of dilatation of the valve annulus. Right ventricular pressure can be estimated based on tricuspid regurgitation using the Bernoulli equation.

> **Note**
>
> In dilated cardiomyopathy, an anomalous origin of the coronary arteries must always be ruled out.

Cardiac Catheterization

Indications for cardiac catheterization are primarily to rule out coronary anomalies and perform a myocardial biopsy. A myocardial biopsy may provide information on whether the cardiomyopathy is a postmyocarditis cardiomyopathy or other specific cardiomyopathy. But it is not without risks, especially if there is significantly impaired cardiac function. Myocarditis is associated with infiltration with lymphocytes and macrophages as well as with evidence of a viral genome.

Hemodynamic measurements show elevated left ventricular and right ventricular end-diastolic pressure, elevated pressure in the atria, and reduced cardiac output and sometimes pulmonary hypertension.

MRI

MRI is sometimes used in addition to echocardiography.

Differential Diagnosis

The following diseases must be ruled out:

- Coronary anomalies, particularly Bland–White–Garland syndrome
- Structural heart defects that can lead to an increasing (left) ventricular dysfunction or dilatation of the cardiac chambers (e.g., severe aortic stenosis, coarctation of the aorta, mitral regurgitation)
- Specific forms of DCM (▶ Table 17.1)

17.1.3 Treatment

No specific therapy is possible for idiopathic DCM. Diuretics, aldosterone antagonists, cardiac glycosides, ACE inhibitors, and beta blockers are used to treat heart failure (see Chapter 19).

Diuretics improve the symptoms of heart failure. ACE inhibitors reduce afterload and counteract remodeling. The role of cardiac glycosides is currently not definitively known. Beta blockers, particularly carvedilol, are gaining importance in the treatment of DCM. They protect the heart from chronic adrenergic stimulation, but they must be very carefully dosed and gradually increased because they can also cause dramatic deterioration of cardiac function.

In case of acute cardiac decompensation, catecholamines and other vasoactive substances are required. Dobutamine is usually used, which not only improves contractility but also decreases afterload. A combination with a phosphodiesterase inhibitor such as milrinone is useful. Milrinone also has positive inotropic characteristics and decreases afterload. In severe cases, treatment with a calcium sensitizer (levosimendan) or a combination of adrenaline and an afterload reducer (sodium nitroprusside) can also be attempted.

To prevent thromboembolic events, anticoagulation is required for poor cardiac function and/or atrial fibrillation.

Antiarrhythmic treatment is necessary in symptomatic arrhythmias. It should be noted, however, that most antiarrhythmic drugs have negative inotropic characteristics. Therefore, amiodarone is often needed. If there is treatment-refractory ventricular tachycardia, AICD implantation should be considered, even in children.

A biventricular pacemaker may be an option to improve ventricular function in patients with a left bundle branch block. The biventricular pacing may optimize synchronicity between right and left ventricle. In children, however, this therapeutic approach is still the subject of clinical trials.

Heart transplant is the last treatment option. A DCM in children is the most common indication for heart transplantation. An "assist device" (left ventricular assist device) may be required to bridge the time until the transplant.

One of the few secondary cardiomyopathies that are treatable with medication is a DCM due to a carnitine deficiency. Administration of carnitine usually leads to a significant improvement of cardiac function (100 mg/kg carnitine for 30 min as a short infusion, then 100 mg/kg/d as a continuous infusion over 24 to 72 h, then 50 to 100 mg/kg/d in 2 single doses).

Newer therapies with growth hormones or stem cells have not yet been established in clinical practice.

17.1.4 Prognosis

The prognosis is unfavorable due to the various causes and forms of the disease but difficult to predict for an individual case. The prognosis is best when the underlying cause is treatable (e.g., carnitine deficiency). Patients who had a recent viral infection associated with the development of DCM have a better prognosis. The prognosis in idiopathic DCM depends on cardiac function, left ventricular end-diastolic pressure, and the heart size, among other factors.

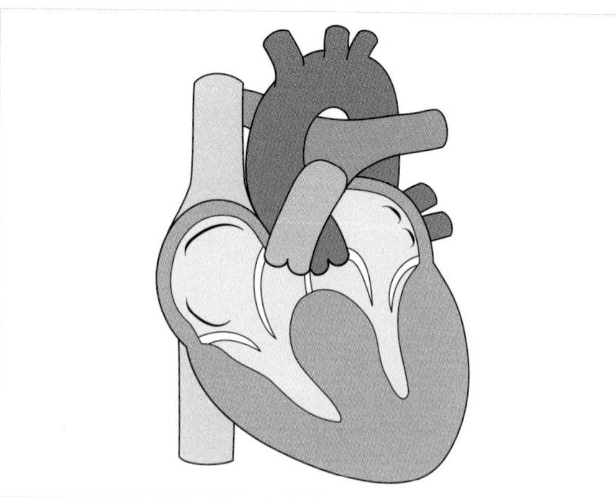

Fig. 17.3 Hypertrophic cardiomyopathy (HCM). This cardiomyopathy is characterized by myocardial hypertrophy that cannot be explained by other causes. In most cases, the interventricular septum is especially affected. The cavity of the left ventricle is narrowed as a result.

17.2 Hypertrophic and Hypertrophic Obstructive Cardiomyopathy

17.2.1 Basics

Synonyms: Hypertrophic obstructive cardiomyopathy (HOCM) was formerly known as idiopathic hypertrophic subaortic stenosis or asymmetric septal hypertrophy

Definition

Hypertrophic cardiomyopathy (HCM) is a genetic myocardial hypertrophy that cannot be explained by another cause such as valve stenosis. In principle, any region in the left ventricle can be affected, but it usually affects the interventricular septum. It is often asymmetric—that is, more pronounced on the left side—and subaortic (▶ Fig. 17.3).

If myocardial hypertrophy results in an obstruction of the left ventricular outflow tract it is called hypertrophic obstructive cardiomyopathy (HOCM).

Epidemiology

The incidence in the general population is about 1 in 500. It is one of the most common causes of sudden cardiac death in children and adults under age 35 years.

▶ **Genetics.** About half of cases are due to autosomal dominant inheritance pattern with variable penetration. More than 200 mutations have now been detected which encode almost all proteins of the sarcomere (e.g., beta MHC, myosin binding protein C, troponin T). New mutations are likely involved in at least some isolated cases. Certain mutations appear to be associated with a particularly high risk for sudden cardiac death.

Pathology and Hemodynamics

Myocardial hypertrophy, usually involving the interventricular septum, is noted on macroscopic inspection. The cavity of the left ventricle is narrowed as a result, leading to varying degrees of obstruction of the left ventricular outflow tract. The obstruction is caused on the one hand by hypertrophy of the septum, which bulges into the left ventricular outflow tract, and on the other hand, the outflow tract is often additionally constricted by an unusual anterior position of the mitral valve. The mitral valve also moves toward the hypertrophied septum during the systole (systolic anterior movement, SAM). This phenomenon is probably the result of the Venturi effect: Due to the increased flow velocity and turbulence in the left ventricular outflow tract, a maelstrom is created that "sucks" the mitral valve leaflets into the outflow tract during the systole.

The obstruction of the left ventricular outflow tract can be aggravated by an increase in contractility (e.g., by positive inotropic agents). A reduced preload and/or afterload (e.g., volume depletion, afterload reducers, Valsalva maneuver) can increase the gradient across the outflow tract.

As a result of the rigidity of the left ventricle, diastolic left ventricular dysfunction develops, which may lead to dilatation of the left atrium and to pulmonary venous congestion.

Subendocardial ischemia may be due to a relative coronary insufficiency. There is an imbalance between the oxygen demand of the hypertrophied myocardium and the oxygen supply through the coronary arteries. There is often "myocardial bridging" of the coronary arteries as well. This term refers to the finding where the coronary arteries are surrounded by myocardial bridges that may compress them. Intima and media hyperplasia or hypertrophy of the intra-myocardial coronary arteries may also develop.

In the final stage of HCM, dilated cardiomyopathy may develop as a result of the systolic dysfunction. A histological feature of HCM is myocyte and myofibrillar disorder (myocardial fiber disarray).

17.2.2 Diagnostic Measures

Symptoms

Most patients are asymptomatic, so in most cases the disease is not diagnosed. If HCM is suspected, in addition to the typical symptoms, the patients should be asked about sudden cardiac deaths and unexplained deaths in the family (30–60% of affected adolescents or young adults have a positive family history).

Typical symptoms of HCM are:

- Sudden cardiac death: The highest incidence of sudden cardiac death in HCM is among (young) adolescents. It typically occurs during sport or physical exertion. Ventricular fibrillation is usually the cause triggering death. Sudden cardiac death may be the first symptom of HCM.
- Dyspnea: Dyspnea is the most common complaint in symptomatic patients. Usually it is the result of diastolic dysfunction of the left ventricle with elevated filling pressures and pulmonary venous reflux into the lungs.
- Syncope: Syncope may be caused by arrhythmias or a decreased cardiac output under stress. Syncopes are associated with a significantly higher risk of sudden cardiac death.
- Angina pectoris: imbalance between oxygen demand of the hypertrophied muscle and coronary supply.
- Palpitations occur as a result of cardiac arrhythmias.
- Arrhythmias: Examples of arrhythmias in HCM are supraventricular and ventricular extrasystoles, sinus pauses, atrioventricular block, atrial fibrillation and flutter, and supraventricular and ventricular tachycardias. Ventricular tachycardia is a risk factor for sudden cardiac death.
- Heart failure: Symptoms of heart failure rarely occur in childhood. In severe cases heart failure is usually a result of diastolic dysfunction and subendocardial ischemia.

Auscultation

The first heart sound is normal. A paradoxical split may be heard in the second heart sound if there is extreme obstruction of the left ventricular outflow tract, since in these cases the pulmonary valve closes before the aortic valve. There is sometimes a gallop rhythm as a sign of diastolic dysfunction or heart failure.

If the left ventricular outflow tract is obstructed, there is a harsh systolic ejection murmur with point of maximum impulse (PMI) in the 4th left parasternal intercostal space. The systolic murmur is increased by exercise or a Valsalva maneuver, because this increases the gradient across the outflow tract.

In a mitral regurgitation there is a blowing, band-shaped systolic murmur with PMI above the apex of the heart and in the mid-axillary line.

ECG

Most affected patients have abnormalities in the ECG. However, the ECG changes are not specific.

- Signs of left ventricular hypertrophy, ST segment changes, deep Q waves with reduced or absent R waves in the left precordial leads, possibly a broad biphasic P wave (P mitrale)

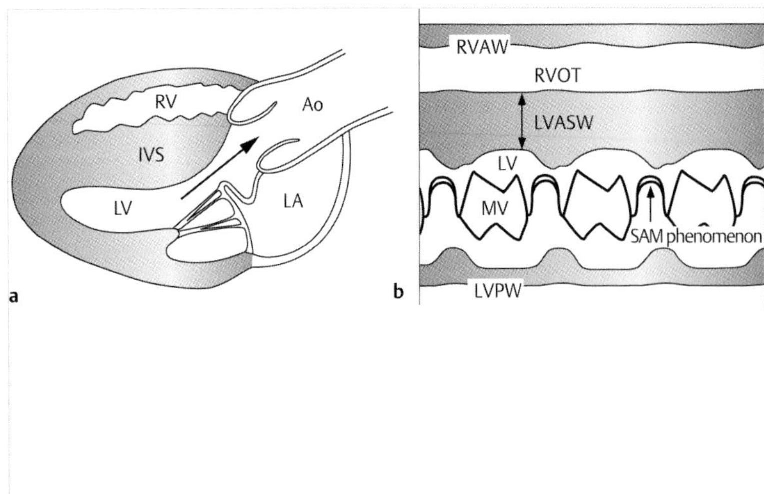

Fig. 17.4 Systolic anterior movement in hypertrophic obstructive cardiomyopathy. If there is obstruction of the left ventricular outflow tract, the anterior leaflet of the mitral valve protrudes into the outflow tract during systole (**a**). This phenomenon is probably due to the Venturi effect: as a result of the turbulent flow in the outflow tract, the anterior mitral leaflet is "sucked" into the outflow tract. This phenomenon can be readily visualized in M mode (**b**).[43] RV, right ventricle; LV, left ventricle; LA, left atrium; IVS, ventricular septum; Ao, aorta; MV, mitral valve; RVOT, right ventricular outflow tract; RVAW, right ventricular anterior wall; LVASW, left ventricular anterior septal wall; LVPW, left ventricular posterior wall; SAM, systolic anterior movement.

- Arrhythmias: extrasystoles, AV block, sinus pause, ectopic atrial rhythm, left bundle branch block, atrial fibrillation/flutter, supraventricular/ventricular tachycardia, rarely pre-excitation in a WPW syndrome

► **Holter monitor.** Checkups at least once a year are recommended for affected patients. It is particular important to note any ventricular tachycardias, which have an unfavorable prognosis and are associated with an increased risk of sudden cardiac death.

Echocardiography

Echocardiography is the method of choice for confirming the diagnosis. The following findings are typical:

- Hypertrophy of the interventricular septum and/or left ventricular free wall
- Narrow lumen of the left ventricle
- Obstruction of the left ventricular outflow tract (increase of the gradient due to measures that reduce the preload, such as the Valsalva maneuver)
- Assessment of the mitral valve: Frequently, abnormalities of the attachment apparatus (papillary muscles, tendinous cords) can be detected. Mitral regurgitation should be investigated.
- Systolic anterior movement (SAM): If there is an obstruction of the left ventricular outflow tract, the anterior leaflet of the mitral valve moves toward the septum during systole. This phenomenon can be readily visualized in M mode (► Fig. 17.4 b).
- Diastolic dysfunction: There is typically a reduced E wave, and thus reduced E/A ratio in the Doppler curve of transmitral inflow, however, tissue Doppler usually allows a better assessment of diastolic function.

Note

Patients with confirmed HCM should have an echocardiography examination at least once a year. Family members of HCM patients should be closely monitored even if the echocardiogram is unremarkable, as late manifestations have been described (recommendation: family members under 18 years of age annually, family members over 18 every 5 years).

Chest X-ray

X-rays are not very sensitive for HCM. The cardiac silhouette may vary in size (normal to slightly enlarged). The left atrium may appear enlarged as a result of mitral regurgitation or poor diastolic function.

Cardiac Catheterization

Cardiac catheterization has become less important because the diagnosis can usually be reliably made by echocardiography. If cardiac catheterization is performed, it is primarily used for the following:

- Assessment of left ventricular outflow tract obstruction (possibly under pharmacological stress)
- Classification of mitral regurgitation
- Assessment of diastolic function
- Visualization of the coronary (stenosis, myocardial bridging)
- Myocardial biopsy: If findings are unclear, a myocardial biopsy may be indicated.

MRI

MRI is increasingly important for the detailed visualization and measurement of the myocardium. In addition, myocardial damage (scarring) can be assessed using the late enhancement technique.

Exercise Test

Exercise tests are an important tool for risk assessment. An excessive rise in blood pressure during exercise or a low increase or even drop in systolic blood pressure is associated with an increased risk of sudden cardiac death. Normal blood pressure behavior is a favorable sign for the prognosis. Oxygen uptake capacity correlates with the patient's symptoms and diastolic dysfunction. Whether an exercise test is actually performed must be decided on a case-by-case basis because of the not-insignificant risk of the investigation.

Differential Diagnoses

Secondary cardiomyopathies can occur in many diseases that frequently become manifest with the clinical symptoms of HCM and must be distinguished from the genetic form (▶ Table 17.2).

The following laboratory tests are useful diagnostic measures for ruling out specific cardiomyopathies:

- Blood:
  - Differential blood count
  - Iron, ferritin (hemochromatosis)
  - Blood gas analysis, lactate, pyruvate, beta-OH butyrate, acetoacetate (fasting and postprandial), ammonia, glucose (mitochondropathy, organic acidopathy, disorder of fatty acid transport/oxidation)
  - Carnitine (disorder of fatty acid transport/oxidation)
  - Free fatty acids, beta-OH butyrate (for hypoglycemia; disorder of fatty acid transport/oxidation)
  - CK (myopathy), CK-MB, troponin, BNP
  - AST, ALT, creatinine, urea (hepatopathy, multisystem disease)
  - Tandem mass spectrometry (TMS, including disorders of fatty acid oxidation)
  - Acid alpha-glucosidase in leukocytes (in infants; Pompe disease)
  - Transferrin electrophoresis and isoelectric focusing (CDG syndrome)
- Urine
  - Organic acids (organic acidopathy, respiratory chain defect, defect of fatty acid oxidation)
  - Glycosaminoglycans, oligosaccharides in urine (mucopolysaccharidosis, glycoproteinosis)

In addition, secondary forms of left ventricular hypertrophy must be distinguished from HCM. Left ventricular hypertrophy may be present in aortic stenosis, coarctation of the aorta, or arterial hypertension, for example.

Associated Syndromes

HCM occurs frequently in association with the following syndromes:

- LEOPARD syndrome (lentigines syndrome)
- Noonan syndrome (short stature, chest deformity, craniofacial abnormalities)
- Wiedemann–Beckwith syndrome (macroglossia, microcephaly, hypoglycemia, ear abnormalities)
- Neurofibromatosis (café-au-lait spots, neurofibromas)
- Costello syndrome (short stature, cutis laxa, plantar skin furrows, coarse facial features)
- Cardio-facio-cutaneous syndrome (facial dysmorphism, wiry hair, palmar keratosis)
- Alström syndrome (hypogonadism)

17.2.3 Treatment

Treatment goals are:

- Minimize the risk of sudden cardiac death
- Slow the development of hypertrophy
- Eliminate symptoms

General Measures

Patients with HCM have *strict limitations on physical exertion*: competitive sport is prohibited. In particular, isometric stress must be avoided. Sports with low dynamic and low static load (e.g., billiards, fishing, or golf) may be possible. Volume depletion should be avoided, as this increases obstruction of the left ventricular outflow tract.

Pharmacological Treatment

▶ **Indication.** Pharmacological treatment is indicated in all symptomatic patients regardless of the extent of the left ventricular obstruction. In asymptomatic patients with no obstruction of the left ventricular outflow tract, the indication for pharmacological treatment is controversial.

▶ **Medication.** Beta blockers and calcium antagonists are used primarily. Propranolol or metoprolol are frequently prescribed as beta blockers; of the calcium antagonists, most experience has been gained with verapamil. Mainly vasodilatory calcium antagonists such as nifedipine are contraindicated because they increase the gradient across the left ventricular outflow tract due to afterload reduction.

- Beta blockers, for example, propranolol (dosage: 2–6 mg/kg/d in 3–4 single doses): Beta blockers are the drugs of choice, especially for obstructive forms. Their mechanism is based on a reduction of exercise-induced obstruction, an improvement of angina pectoris complaints, and antiarrhythmic potency.
- Verapamil (dosage: 4–8 mg/kg/d in 2–3 doses): Verapamil leads to a reduction of obstruction and probably improves diastolic function.

Table 17.2 Differential diagnoses and secondary forms of hypertrophic cardiomyopathy	
Disease	**Leading symptoms/diagnostics**
Storage diseases / metabolic diseases	
Glycogen storage diseases, especially Pompe disease (glycogen storage disease type II)	Hepatomegaly, "floppy infant," Pompe disease: alpha-1,4-glucosidase deficiency, lymphocyte vacuoles
Mucopolysaccharidosis	Skeletal deformities, coarse facial features, hepatomegaly, psychomotor retardation
Oligosaccharidoses	Skeletal deformities, facial dysmorphic features, psychomotor retardation, sometimes cherry-red macular spot
Gangliosidoses	Progressive psychomotor retardation, epilepsy, ataxia, spasticity, hepatosplenomegaly, macular spot
Gaucher disease	Hepatosplenomegaly, anemia, thrombocytopenia, Gaucher cells in bone marrow, acid phosphatase ↑
Fabry disease	Angiokeratoma of the skin, kidney failure, pain/paresthesia of the extremities, activity of alpha-galactosidase ↓
Disorders in pyruvate metabolism, citric acid cycle, and respiratory chain	Determination of lactate acetate (repeated measures), pyruvate, 3-OH butyrate, acetoacetate
Disorders of the beta-oxidation of fatty acids	Hypoketotic hypoglycemic coma (caused by catabolic metabolism), hepatopathy, muscle weakness, secondary carnitine deficiency
Disorders of fatty acid transport	Hepatopathy, reduced carnitine in plasma
Refsum disease	Retinitis pigmentosa, ataxia, deafness, normal intelligence, phytanic acid ↑, protein in cerebrospinal fluid ↑
CDG syndrome	Variable dysmorphic features, inverted nipples, failure to thrive, psychomotor retardation, transferrin electrophoresis and isoelectric focusing (screening test)
Tyrosinemia	Liver failure, hepatomegaly
Hemochromatosis	Hepatopathy, serum iron ↑, ferritin in plasma ↑
Familial hypereosinophilia	Massive eosinophilia, eosinophilic myocardial infiltration
Neuromuscular diseases	
Friedreich ataxia	Ataxia, pes cavus, absent deep tendon reflexes
Emery–Dreifuss muscular dystrophy	X-chromosomal linked inheritance (affecting men), red–green color blindness, elbow abnormalities, SA block, AV block
Myotonic dystrophy	Generalized hypotonia, facial diplegia, triangular mouth, clubfeet
Other diseases	
Intramural cardiac tumors (especially rhabdomyoma, fibroma)	Different echogenicity compared to the myocardium; association of rhabdomyoma with tuberous sclerosis
Steroid/ACTH therapy	History is indicative, deteriorating cardiac findings over time
Neonates of diabetic mothers	(Gestational) diabetes of the mother, deteriorating cardiac findings over time
Feto-fetal transfusion syndrome	Monochorionic twins, recipient affected
Nesidioblastosis (insulin-producing tumors)	Hypoglycemia, hyperinsulinism, deteriorating cardiac findings over time
Catecholamine therapy	Particularly in preterm infants, deteriorating cardiac findings over time

Note

Caution: Verapamil should not be used for symptomatic obstruction of the left ventricular outflow tract, as deaths in such patients have been described with verapamil.

Although beta blockers or verapamil improve the symptoms, they do not reduce the risk of sudden cardiac death.

Amiodarone is frequently used (dosage: 10 mg/kg/d in 2 single doses for the first week, then 3–5 mg/kg/d) for relevant arrhythmias (ventricular arrhythmias, recurrent atrial fibrillation). But the systemic side effects (corneal deposits, hypothyroidism, pulmonary fibrosis, increase in photosensitivity of the skin) should be noted.

Note

Positive inotropic agents such as digitalis or catecholamines are contraindicated in HCM, since they increase the obstruction. Afterload reducers such as nitrates and diuretics should be avoided because they increase the gradient across the left ventricular outflow tract.

Automated Implantable Cardioverter-Defibrillator (AICD)

The implantation of an AICD is indicated for secondary prevention after surviving cardiac arrest or for spontaneous sustained ventricular tachycardia. An AICD is also used for primary prevention in patients with multiple risk factors (high-risk patients).

Cardiac Pacemaker

This treatment approach uses special pacemaker stimulation to reduce the obstruction in the left ventricular outflow tract. For this purpose, a DDD pacemaker system is implanted and a very short AV interval, much shorter than the patient's own AV interval, is selected. The stimulation electrode is placed in the right ventricular apex. This probe position and the short AV interval cause the hypertrophied septum to move paradoxically: During systole, it moves away from the left ventricular outflow tract, so that the obstruction in the outflow tract decreases. No clear benefit of this therapy has yet been proven in studies.

Percutaneous Transluminal Septal Myocardial Ablation (PTSMA) and Transcoronary Ablation of Septal Hypertrophy (TASH)

In this interventional catheterization method, an infarction of the hypertrophied myocardium is provoked by injecting high-proof alcohol into a septal branch of the coronary artery. The subsequent scarring decreases muscular hypertrophy.

This method has so far been used only in adults and adolescents and is currently not a routine option for children. Complications include inducing potentially life-threatening arrhythmias, a complete AV block, and septal perforation.

Surgical Treatment

Unsuccessful conservative treatment of symptomatic patients with a gradient in the left ventricular outflow tract of over 50 mmHg at rest or 80 mmHg during exercise is currently considered to be an indication for surgical treatment.

Note

Asymptomatic obstruction of the left ventricular outflow tract is not an indication for surgery.

Surgical treatment consists of a transaortic myotomy or myectomy of basal segments of the hypertrophied septum (Morrow procedure). If there are associated mitral valve anomalies, additional surgical measures are required, such as resection of abnormal tendinous cords, splitting fused papillary muscles, or in exceptional cases, mitral valve replacement.

An incomplete or complete left bundle branch block is virtually always present postoperatively. There is often mild aortic regurgitation. In addition, there is a risk of requiring a pacemaker due to complete AV block. The mortality rate is reported to be 1 to 3%.

▸ **Heart transplant.** A heart transplant is the last treatment option. This is often considered for treatment-refractory patients with nonobstructive HCM who would not profit from a myotomy or myectomy of the left ventricular outflow tract.

17.2.4 Prognosis

The annual mortality rate for high-risk patients is 2 to 4%. The peak incidence of sudden cardiac death is between

14 and 30 years. Sudden cardiac death is usually associated with physical exertion. Rare complications of HCM are heart failure, atrial fibrillation, embolism, and the transition to dilated cardiomyopathy.

Surgical and pharmacological treatment can reduce symptoms considerably and significantly improve physical capacity. Surgery also reduces the risk of sudden cardiac death (probably most effective when verapamil is also taken postoperatively).

However, general statements on the prognosis are difficult to make because HCM is a very heterogeneous disease. The risk assessment must be made on a case-by-case basis depending on various risk factors. The following findings constitute a particularly high risk for sudden cardiac death (high-risk patients):

- Status post cardiac arrest or spontaneous, sustained ventricular tachycardia
- Positive family history of sudden cardiac death as a result of HCM
- Evidence of a high-risk mutation
- Abnormal blood pressure response to stress (exercise test)
- Ventricular tachycardia in Holter monitor
- Pronounced ventricular hypertrophy (left ventricular wall thickness over 30 mm; however, the significance of this parameter is controversial)

17.3 Restrictive Cardiomyopathy

17.3.1 Basics

Definition

Restrictive cardiomyopathy (RCM) is a rare disorder in which diastolic dysfunction as a result of reduced ventricular compliance is the major finding. Systolic function is usually good. The disease can affect one or both ventricles. Typical clinical features are signs of heart failure with good systolic function. As a result of the diastolic filling disorder of the ventricles, the atria are dilated. The ventricles are often of normal size.

Epidemiology

Restrictive cardiomyopathy is a very rare disease in childhood and accounts for less than 5% of all cardiomyopathies in children. It also occurs only rarely in adults in Western countries. It is more common in tropical latitudes as the subtype endomyocardial fibrosis.

► **Genetics.** Familial clustering has been described. There is some evidence that there may be an autosomal dominant inheritance pattern in familial cases.

Pathology and Hemodynamics

A characteristic finding is impaired ventricular diastolic filling as a result of rigidity of the ventricular walls. The systolic function of the ventricles is usually normal. The size of the ventricles is usually normal, but the atria are typically clearly dilated.

Histologically, varying degrees of fibrosis and myocyte hypertrophy are found in idiopathic RCM.

17.3.2 Diagnostic Measures

Symptoms

The initial symptoms are usually exercise-induced dyspnea or diminished physical capacity.

The physical examination may show signs of heart failure such as ascites, hepatomegaly, distention of the jugular veins, or edema.

Auscultation

A gallop rhythm can often be auscultated. The second heart sound may be pronounced. There may be a systolic murmur as a sign of AV valve regurgitation.

ECG

Abnormalities are almost always found in the ECG, but they are nonspecific. The most common are signs of right and/or left atrial overload (peaked and/or broad P waves). Signs of ventricular hypertrophy and ST changes may also be found. Supraventricular arrhythmias such as atrial flutter or conduction disturbances (AV block) may appear as a result of atrial overload.

Chest X-ray

Cardiomegaly can be seen radiographically as a result of atrial dilatation. Signs of pulmonary congestion should also be noted.

Echocardiography

Indicative findings in echocardiography are clearly dilated atria and normal-sized ventricles, usually with normal systolic function, but some patients also have some impairment of systolic function and mild ventricular hypertrophy. Ventricular thrombi can be seen quite often. In the four chamber view the atria seem very large and distended, while the ventricles are small (ice-cone-sign). An elevated E/A ratio in the flow across the mitral valve is often seen in Doppler ultrasound scanning as a sign of diastolic dysfunction.

MRI

An MRI is performed primarily due to suspicion of a secondary cardiomyopathy. A change in contrast agent and

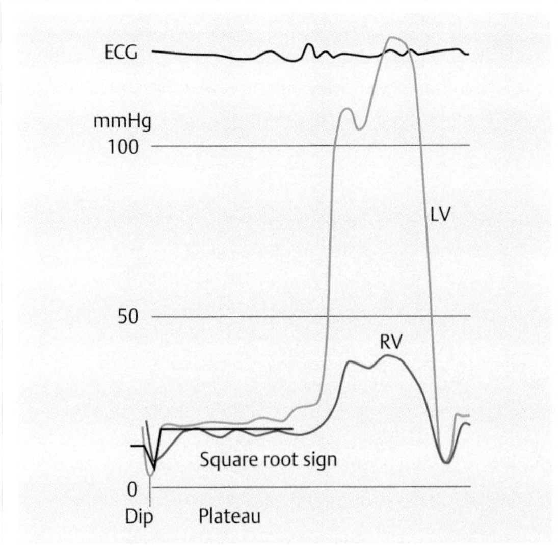

Fig. 17.5 Typical pressure curve in the left and right ventricle in restrictive cardiomyopathy (RCM). As a result of restriction after an early drop in diastolic pressure, there is a subsequent diastolic pressure plateau ("dip-plateau pattern" or square root sign).[39]

signal behavior can be a sign of a storage disease, for example.

Cardiac Catheterization

Cardiac catheterization is indicated if RCM is suspected. The hemodynamic measurements are used among other things to distinguish between restriction and constriction (e.g., constrictive pericarditis). In the simultaneous pressure measurement in the right and left ventricle, there is an increased end-diastolic pressure in the two chambers. In RCM, the end-diastolic pressure in the left ventricle is higher than in the right ventricle, while it is approximately equal in both ventricles in constrictive pericarditis.

A typical finding for both diseases is the "dip-plateau pattern," also known as the "square root sign" in the right and left ventricular pressure curve: An early drop in diastolic pressure ("dip") is followed by a diastolic pressure plateau (▶ Fig. 17.5). Pulmonary hypertension is often already present at the time a diagnosis is made.

Myocardial Biopsy

A myocardial biopsy is performed to rule out secondary forms (e.g., in amyloidosis or sarcoidosis), but a myocardial biopsy rarely contributes to detecting specific causes of RCM.

Differential Diagnoses

The diagnosis of idiopathic RCM is made by a process of exclusion. In particular, it must be distinguished from constrictive pericarditis and secondary forms of inflammatory or storage diseases. The most common differential diagnoses and causes of secondary forms are listed in ▶ Table 17.3.

17.3.3 Treatment

Pharmacological treatment has so far been limited to symptomatic treatment. Diuretics are used for signs of heart failure. Overdosing should be avoided because patients often react sensitively to an excessive reduction of preload. ACE inhibitors or calcium channel blockers are sometimes recommended. Due to the high incidence of thromboembolic complications, anticoagulation or platelet aggregation inhibition is recommended. The only definitive treatment is currently a heart transplant.

17.3.4 Prognosis

The prognosis of RCM in childhood is poor. About half of the children die within 2 years of the diagnosis. The outcome of the disease is thus worse than for hypertrophic or dilated cardiomyopathy. The majority of the children die as a result of heart failure.

17.4 Arrhythmogenic Right Ventricular Cardiomyopathy

17.4.1 Basics

Synonym: arrhythmogenic right ventricular dysplasia

Definition

Arrhythmogenic right ventricular cardiomyopathy (ARVC) is a genetic cardiomyopathy, characterized by increasing noninflammatory destruction of myocytes and replacement with fat and connective tissue. These changes can be the starting point for ventricular tachycardia.

Epidemiology

The estimated prevalence of this disease is 1:5,000, with pronounced regional differences. ARVC is especially common in northern Italy. It is considered to be the cause of 10 to 20% of all sudden cardiac deaths, mainly affecting young men and athletes.

▶ **Genetics.** The increased familial incidence of ARVC has long been known. In most cases, there is autosomal dominant inheritance. The known mutations affect the genes that encode desmosomal proteins. Among the identified genes that play a role in the autosomal dominant forms are cardiac ryanodine receptor, desmoplakin, and plakophilin 2. Mutations of the plakophilin 2 genes are probably the most common cause of ARVC. Autosomal

Table 17.3 Differential diagnoses and secondary forms of restrictive cardiomyopathy (RCM)

Disease	Typical findings/remarks
Constrictive pericarditis	Equal pressure in the left and right ventricles, history of recurrent pericarditis, trauma, or cardiac surgery
Pericardial tamponade	Pericardial effusion
Ebstein anomaly	Enlarged right atrium due to the apical displacement of the tricuspid valve
Amyloidosis	Deposits of amorphous protein substance in various organs
Hemochromatosis	Iron deposits in various parenchymal organs
Sarcoidosis	Noncaseating granulomas
Fabry disease	Lipid storage disease
Gaucher disease	Lipid storage disease
Hurler disease	Mucopolysaccharidosis
Glycogenosis	Glycogen storage diseases
Scleroderma	Systemic sclerosis with cardiac involvement
Pseudoxanthoma elasticum	Connective tissue disease, thickening of the endocardium
Result of chemotherapy or radiation	
Carcinoid	Skin flush, diarrhea, bronchial obstructions
Endomyocardial fibrosis	Especially in Africa, most common form of RCM in children in the tropics
Hypereosinophilic syndromes / Loeffler endocarditis	Eosinophilia for more than 6 months—cause of the eosinophilia usually unclear, may be eosinophilic leukemia or parasitic eosinophilia. Eosinophilic myocarditis of various degrees, involvement of other organs (lungs, bone marrow, central nervous system). Treatment of eosinophilia with steroids or cytotoxic agents

recessive forms have also been reported, including Naxos disease, which is associated with hyperkeratosis on the palms and soles and conspicuously woolly hair.

Pathology

Increased fatty-fibrous infiltration of the right ventricular myocardium (fibrolipomatosis) can be identified both macroscopically and histologically. The process usually begins in the right ventricle and then spreads. Involvement of the left ventricle is not uncommon. The septum is usually not involved. The result is dilatation affecting especially the right ventricle that leads to functional impairment.

17.4.2 Diagnostic Measures

Symptoms

ARVC usually manifests between the ages of 10 and 50 years, typically around the age of 30. The diagnosis is based on clinical symptoms and examination findings, which are divided into major and minor criteria (▶ Table 17.4).

Typical symptoms include:

- Palpitations
- Syncopes
- Ventricular tachycardia or extrasystoles, usually originating in the right ventricle
- Supraventricular arrhythmias
- Sudden cardiac death

Although functional impairment and dilatation of the right ventricle can be detected, symptoms of heart failure are rare. The symptoms are sometimes triggered by physical stress (e.g., during sports).

ECG

Almost half of patients have a normal ECG. Characteristic abnormalities are QRS complexes widened to more than 110 ms and evidence of epsilon waves at the end of the QRS complex in the right precordial leads (▶ Fig. 17.6). T wave inversion in the right ventricular leads is another typical finding, but this finding is not very useful in children, where negative T waves in the right precordial leads are normal. If ventricular tachycardia or extrasystoles are detected, they generally originate from the right ventricle and are deformed, as in a left bundle branch block.

Table 17.4 Clinical diagnostic criteria for ARVC (Adapted from Marcus et al. 2010)

Major criteria	Minor criteria
I Global and regional dysfunction and structural alterations	
• Regional RV akinesia, dyskinesia, or aneurysm *and* severe RV dilatation or severe reduction of RV function	• Regional RV akinesia or dyskinesia *and* mild RV dilatation or mild reduction of RV function
II Tissue characterisation of the wall	
• Extensive fibrous replacement of the RV free wall myocardium with or without fatty replacement of tissue on endomyocardial biopsy	• Less extensive fibrous replacement of the RV free wall myocardium with or without fatty replacement of tissue on endomyocardial biopsy
III Repolarization abnormalities	
• Inverted T waves in right precordial leads (V_1, V_2, and V_3) or beyond in individuals > 14 years of age (in the absence of complete RBBB QRS ≥ 120 ms)	• Inverted T waves in leads V_1 and V_2 in individuals > 14 years of age (in the absence of complete RBBB) or in V_4, V_5, or V_6 • Inverted T waves in leads V_1, V_2, V_3, and V_4 in individuals > 14 years of age in the presence of complete RBBB
IV Depolarisation/conduction abnormalities	
• Epsilon wave in the right precordial leads (V_1 to V_3)	• Late potentials detected by signal-averaged ECG • Delayed conduction in the RV myocardium
V Arrhythmias	
• Nonsustained or sustained ventricular tachycardia of LBBB morphology with superior axis	• Nonsustained or sustained ventricular tachycardia of RVOT configuration, LBBB morphology with inferior axis or of unknown axis • > 500 ventricular extrasystoles per 24 hours (Holter)
VI Family history	
• ARVC/D confirmed in a first-degree relative who meets current Task Force criteria • ARVC/D confirmed pathologically at autopsy or surgery in a first-degree relative • Identification of a pathogenic mutation categorized as associated or probably associated with ARVC/D in the patient under evaluation	• History of ARVC/D in a first-degree relative in whom it is not possible or practical to determine whether the family member meets current Task Force criteria • Premature sudden death (< 35 years of age) due to suspected ARVC/D in a first-degree relative • ARVC/D confirmed pathologically or by current Task Force criteria in second-degree relative
• Definite diagnosis: two major or one major and two minor or four minor criteria from different diagnostic categories. • Borderline diagnosis: one major and one minor or three minor criteria from different diagnostic categories. • Possible diagnosis: one major or two minor criteria from different diagnostic categories.	

ARVC/D arrhythmogenic right ventricular cardiomyopathy/dysplasia, RV right ventricular, RBBB right bundle-branch block, LBBB left bundle-branch block

Marcus FI, McKenna WJ, Sherrill D, et al. Diagnosis of arrhythmogenic right ventricular cardiomyopathy/dysplasia: proposed modification of the Task Force criteria. Eur Heart J. 2010; 31:806-14.

Echocardiography

Typical echocardiography findings include dilatation of the right ventricle and a thin ventricular wall. Localized akinesia or dyskinesia, right ventricular aneurysms, and trabecular hypertrophy should also be noted.

MRI

Note

Unremarkable findings in imaging technology do not rule out ARVC.

MRI is of great diagnostic importance. In addition to the morphological findings described above for echocardiography, MRI can detect fatty dysplasia as hyperintense zones in T1-weighted images. After administration of contrast medium, fibrous dysplasia can be visualized.

Myocardial Biopsy

If the decision is made to perform an endomyocardial biopsy, an open biopsy is usually necessary. A biopsy through a catheter is difficult because the changes are localized and the septum, which is otherwise used for biopsies, is usually not affected.

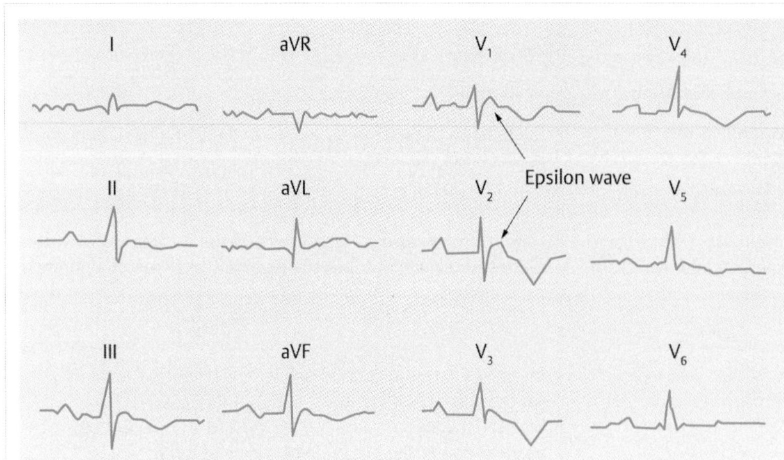

Fig. 17.6 Typical ECG findings in an arrhythmogenic right ventricular cardiomyopathy (ARVC). The ECG features T wave inversions and an epsilon wave in the right precordial leads.[110] (Jaoude, Leclercq, Coumel 1996)

Differential Diagnoses

For the differential diagnosis, other diseases that could be the cause of ventricular extrasystoles and tachycardia or right ventricular dilatation must be considered.

Causes of arrhythmia:

- Idiopathic tachycardia from the right ventricular outflow tract
- Long QT syndromes
- Catecholamine-sensitive polymorphic ventricular tachycardia
- Myocarditis
- Coronary heart disease
- Scarring after cardiac surgery (e.g., after tetralogy of Fallot correction)

Diseases associated with right ventricular dilatation:

- Uhl disease (a rare disorder with aplasia of the right ventricular myocardium and right ventricular free wall consisting almost entirely of epicardium and endocardium. Macroscopically, the right ventricular free wall appears paper-thin or parchmentlike)
- Dilated cardiomyopathy
- Atrial septal defects
- Ebstein anomaly

A fatty-fibrous myocardium is not specific for ARVC, but can also be the result of other disorders (e.g., myocarditis, myocardial infarction).

17.4.3 Treatment

Only symptomatic treatment is possible to date. The various treatment options are sometimes controversial, particularly the implantation of an implantable cardioverter defibrillator (ICD).

The following procedure is currently recommended by international professional associations:

- No competitive or intensive recreational sports
- Indications for ICD implantation:
  - Secondary prevention in patients with sustained ventricular tachycardia or ventricular fibrillation
  - Primary prevention in high-risk patients (pronounced right ventricular finding, involvement of the left ventricle, sudden cardiac death in a family member, unexplained syncope that may be associated with tachyarrhythmia)
- Antiarrhythmic therapy in patients who are not eligible for an ICD implantation or who experienced frequent electric shock discharges after ICD implantation. Beta blockers, amiodarone, or sotalol are often given as antiarrhythmic agents.
- Interventional catheter ablation of an arrhythmia focus is recommended in patients who despite ICD implantation and antiarrhythmic therapy frequently experience ventricular tachycardia and ICD discharges. This is not a definitive treatment due to the progressive nature of the disease.
- A heart transplant is the last treatment option.

17.4.4 Prognosis

A 10-year mortality rate of up to 30% has been reported for untreated patients. Antiarrhythmic treatment and/or ICD implantation improve the prognosis significantly. High-risk patients benefit particularly from these measures.

17.5 Endocardial Fibroelastosis

17.5.1 Basics

Definition

Endocardial fibroelastosis (EFE) is a diffuse thickening of the ventricular endocardium, affecting mainly the left ventricle. It is a primary disease of unknown origin or due to secondary changes associated with obstruction of the left heart (hypoplastic left heart syndrome, aortic stenosis, etc.) or metabolic diseases.

Epidemiology

EFE is an extremely rare disease whose prevalence has decreased significantly in recent years. The causes of this decline are unclear, but possibly are related to the decreasing incidence of mumps. The mumps virus has been repeatedly discussed as a possible cause of EFE.

► **Genetics.** The disease usually occurs sporadically, but familial clustering has also been reported.

Pathology/Hemodynamics

EFE is characterized by a thickening of the endocardium and is associated with myocardial dysfunction. Morphologically, there are two types of EFE: dilated and contracted. The dilated form occurs much more frequently; the heart is enlarged globally, mainly affecting the left atrium and ventricle. The left ventricle is lined with porcelainlike thickened endocardium. The papillary muscles can also be changed. The aortic and mitral valves are involved in about half of cases.

The contracted form is much less common. In this form, the left ventricle is of normal size or hypoplastic. Both atria and the right ventricle are markedly enlarged and hypertrophied, but have only slight or no fibrosis. The dilated form can transition to the contracted form.

Fetal endomyocarditis due to mumps or Coxsackie viruses has been discussed, but it is also believed that subendocardial hypoxia as a result of increased wall tension in obstructive heart disease may be a possible cause.

Associated Diseases

Secondary EFE may occur in association with left heart obstructions such as:

- Hypoplastic left heart syndrome
- Aortic stenosis
- Aortic atresia
- Coarctation of the aorta

In addition, metabolic disorders, autoimmune diseases, inflammatory processes, cardiomyopathy, or anomalies of the coronary arteries have been discussed as a cause of secondary EFE:

- Systemic carnitine deficiency
- Glycogenoses
- Mucopolysaccharidoses
- Myocarditis
- Neonatal or juvenile lupus erythematosus
- Bland–White–Garland syndrome
- Dilated cardiomyopathy, restrictive cardiomyopathy

17.5.2 Diagnostic Measures

Symptoms

Most cases become manifest within the first year of life. EFE usually presents with symptoms of heart failure such as poor feeding, failure to thrive, tachypnea, tachycardia, increased sweating, and pallor. A gallop rhythm may be detected on auscultation. A systolic murmur at the left sternal border may suggest mitral regurgitation.

ECG

Typical ECG findings are signs of left ventricular hypertrophy, including a strain pattern (negative ST segment and discordant negative T waves in the left precordial leads). Conduction abnormalities (left bundle branch block, atrioventricular block) and WPW syndrome have been described. Occasionally, ischemic changes similar to those of myocardial infarction may be detected.

Chest X-ray

Global cardiomegaly with or without signs of pulmonary congestion is a typical radiographic finding.

Echocardiography

The left atrium and ventricle are enlarged in primary EFE (in the rare form of contracted EFE, the left ventricle is of normal size or hypoplastic). There is markedly increased echogenicity of the left ventricular endocardium. Left ventricular function is impaired. Mitral regurgitation is often seen in the color Doppler ultrasound scan.

To rule out secondary EFE, left heart obstructions must be noted in particular. In some circumstances, EFE can be detected in utero by fetal echocardiography.

Cardiac Catheterization

The hemodynamic measurements show an increase in the left ventricular end-diastolic pressure, left atrial pressure, pulmonary artery pressure, and right ventricular pressure. Myocardial ischemia can sometimes be detected by angiography.

MRI

The extent of the disease can be readily visualized by MRI.

Endomyocardial Biopsy

Histological examination shows an accumulation of thickened endocardium with collagen and elastic fibers. The myocardium itself appears unremarkable.

17.5.3 Treatment

In secondary forms, the underlying condition is treated. Treatment of primary forms is limited to symptomatic measures. If there are thromboembolic complications, anticoagulation is indicated. In individual cases, surgical resection of the endocardial fibroelastosis has been reported. In the end stage of heart failure, a heart transplant is the last treatment option.

17.5.4 Prognosis

The overall prognosis is poor but individual cases of complete resolution of symptoms have been described. The earlier heart failure occurs, the worse the prognosis is likely to be.

17.6 Isolated Left Ventricular Noncompaction Cardiomyopathy

17.6.1 Basics

Synonyms: spongy myocardium, myocardial noncompaction

Definition

Isolated left ventricular noncompaction cardiomyopathy (NCC) is a very rare cardiomyopathy in which the embryonic myocardium persists, characterized by trabeculations and deep intertrabecular recesses. Noncompaction of the myocardium rarely occurs in isolation; it is usually associated with other cardiac defects.

Epidemiology

This is a very rare form of cardiomyopathy.

▶ **Genetics.** NCC is considered to be a genetic cardiomyopathy. NCC can occur sporadically or present in families. Mutations of the G4.5 genes that code for the tafazzin protein have been described in association with noncompaction of the myocardium. Other genetic mutations affect genes that code for proteins of the cytoskeleton such as *alpha*-dystrobrevin or Cypher/ZASP (Z-band alternatively spliced PDZ-motif protein).

Pathology and Hemodynamics

In myocardial noncompaction, the normal consolidation (compaction) of the embryonic myocardium does not take place. The embryonic myocardium with numerous trabeculations and recesses persists and normal myocardial development is not completed. The myocardium appears as a spongelike meshwork of interwoven myocardial fibers, resulting in reduced ventricular contractility.

Associated Diseases

Aside from isolated left ventricular noncompaction, similar or comparable changes in the myocardium may also present in association with various cardiac anomalies:

- Dilated cardiomyopathy
- Pulmonary atresia with intact ventricular septum
- Ebstein anomaly
- Bicuspid aortic valve
- Hypoplastic left heart syndrome
- Aortico-left ventricular tunnel
- l-TGA
- Ventricular septal defect
- WPW syndrome

In addition, noncompaction of the myocardium also occurs with neuromuscular diseases (e.g., Barth syndrome, Charcot–Marie–Tooth disease, mitochondriopathies).

17.6.2 Diagnostic Measures

Symptoms

Symptoms of patients with NCC may range widely depending on the severity of the disease. In many patients, NCC may remain asymptomatic for a long time. If noncompaction occurs without an associated cardiac defect, the disease sometimes does not become symptomatic until late adulthood. Typical symptoms are increasing heart failure, arrhythmia, or thromboembolism. Unfortunately, sudden cardiac death can be the first manifestation of the disease.

ECG

The ECG usually shows no characteristic changes. Bundle branch blocks, atrial fibrillation, and ventricular tachycardia may occur. Sinus bradycardia or WPW syndrome has also been reported.

Chest X-ray

The heart and lungs are initially unremarkable. Later there are signs of heart failure such as cardiomegaly.

Echocardiography

The diagnosis is generally made by echocardiography. The ventricular myocardium has a typical spongy appearance. The ventricular wall consists of a compact epicardium and endocardium, between which numerous trabeculations and deep recesses can be identified. There may also be similar changes in the papillary muscles. In general, the left ventricle is most affected, but both ventricles may be involved. Echocardiography is also needed to evaluate ventricular function and detect cardiac thrombi. Adults are more likely to suffer from signs of heart failure and children from depression of systolic function. Associated cardiac defects can be identified or ruled out by echocardiography.

Cardiac Catheterization

A cardiac catheter examination may be indicated to determine hemodynamic parameters or perform a biopsy of the myocardium.

MRI

An MRI scan can be used to evaluate the cardiac morphology and ventricular function.

17.6.3 Treatment

Until now, no curative, only symptomatic, treatment has been possible. Heart failure is treated according to the standard guidelines. Anticoagulation is recommended for atrial fibrillation or impaired ventricular function. The indication for inserting an ICD for arrhythmia is based on the recommendations for patients with dilated cardiomyopathy. In the terminal stages of heart failure, a cardiac transplant is the last treatment option.

17.6.4 Prognosis

In general, NCC has a poor prognosis. Increasing heart failure, ventricular tachycardia, thromboembolic complications, and the increased risk of sudden cardiac death contribute considerably to the high morbidity and mortality rate.

18 Cardiac Arrhythmias

18.1 Antiarrhythmic Drugs

18.1.1 Basics

Antiarrhythmic drugs play a central role in the treatment of cardiac arrhythmias in childhood. But their use must be weighed critically. There are numerous studies in adults showing that class I antiarrhythmic drugs do not reduce mortality, but even increase it in patients with ventricular tachycardia and myocardial ischemia. It is unclear, however, whether these results can be transferred to children, since coronary perfusion problems are not usually present in children. In addition, all antiarrhythmic drugs themselves have proarrhythmogenic effects. Furthermore, the majority of the antiarrhythmic drugs have a negative inotropic effect. Adverse effects on the central nervous system are not uncommon.

Classification

Antiarrhythmic drugs are classified according to their mechanism of action and influence on the action potential. They act by influencing the ion channels (Na, K, Ca) and beta receptors. ▶ Table 18.1 presents an overview of indications and properties and dosages are summarized in ▶ Table 18.2.

Class I Antiarrhythmic Drugs (Sodium Channel Blockers)

Class I antiarrhythmic drugs impair sodium transport into the cell. They are subdivided into the subclasses a, b, and c depending on their effect on the action potential:

- Class Ia prolongs the action potential: quinidine, procainamide
- Class Ib shortens the action potential: lidocaine, mexiletine
- Class Ic has no effect on the duration of the action potential: propafenone, flecainide

▶ **Class Ia antiarrhythmic drugs.** After administration of class Ia antiarrhythmic drugs, the sodium channels reactivate slowly. Accordingly, the QRS duration is prolonged. In addition, these antiarrhythmic drugs prolong the QTc interval. It is also important to note that they have a parasympatholytic (anticholinergic) effect on the sinus and AV nodes. The heart rate is increased and AV conduction is accelerated. Due to the shortened AV conduction, ventricular tachycardia may be induced in patients with atrial flutter. Class Ia antiarrhythmic drugs are rarely used in children.

▶ **Class Ib antiarrhythmic drugs.** Class Ib antiarrhythmic drugs act primarily on the ventricles. The effect on the atrial and AV node is low. The negative inotropic properties are not very pronounced. Lidocaine is administered only intravenously; mexiletine is administered orally. These antiarrhythmic drugs are rarely used in children.

▶ **Class Ic antiarrhythmic drugs.** Class Ic antiarrhythmic drugs cause a reduction of the atrial and ventricular rates. They also act on the conduction system. There is a decrease in the frequency of the sinus node as well as a conduction delay in the AV node and ventricles. In the ECG, the duration of the QRS complex increases. If QRS widening is 130% or more of the initial value, the dose should be reduced. These antiarrhythmic drugs are often used in children.

Class II Antiarrhythmic Drugs (Beta Blockers)

Examples of beta blockers are propranolol, metoprolol, and esmolol. They reduce the sympatico-adrenergic stimulation of the heart. Beta blockers have the following effects on the heart:

- Negative bathmotropic effect: reduce the excitability of the heart
- Negative chronotropic effect: reduce the heart rate
- Negative dromotropic effect: reduce the conduction speed
- Negative inotropic effect: reduce cardiac contractility

Typical indications for beta blockers are sinus tachycardia, supraventricular re-entrant tachycardia, long QT syndromes, symptomatic supraventricular extrasystoles, ventricular extrasystoles, and bursts. The use of beta blockers is limited by the deterioration of ventricular function, bradycardia, the risk of AV block, and exacerbation of bronchospasm, as well as the induction of hypoglycemia.

Class III Antiarrhythmic Drugs (Potassium Channel Blockers)

The class III antiarrhythmic drugs include sotalol and amiodarone. They block the rapid potassium efflux from the cell, but additionally also block the sodium and the calcium channels and the beta receptors. The action potential duration is prolonged. Class III antiarrhythmic drugs affect all cell types in the heart from the sinus node to the ventricular myocardium and are among the most potent antiarrhythmic drugs, especially amiodarone. They have both a supraventricular and a ventricular effect. The negative inotropic properties of amiodarone are also less pronounced, so it can be used even with a poor ventricular function if proper precautions are taken. However, application is limited by numerous serious side effects including corneal deposits, photosensitivity (sun screen

Table 18.1 Antiarrhythmic drugs (overview)

Class	Antiarrhythmic drug	Indication	ECG	Side effects	Common interactions	Contraindication	Remarks
Ia	Quinidine	Atrial flutter/fibrillation, with digitalis administered additionally to prevent rapid AV conduction	QRS ↑, QT ↑	• Gastrointestinal • Central nervous system • Hypotension • Negative inotropy • Proarrhythmogenic (torsades de pointes)	Increases digoxin level	• Long QT syndrome • Higher degree AV block • Sinus node dysfunction • Quinidine hypersensitivity	• Reduce dose in case of QRS prolongation to over 125% of the initial value or significant prolongation of the QTc interval • Administer a test dose first to determine possible hypersensitivity reaction • Has become less important because of numerous side effects
	Disopyramide	Like quinidine, in addition ventricular arrhythmia	QRS ↑, QT ↑	• Comparable with quinidine • Pronounced anticholinergic and negative inotropy		• Higher degree AV block • Sinus node dysfunction • Heart failure	Is commonly used in North America
Ib	Lidocaine	VT, ventricular flutter/fibrillation	QRS ↔, QT (↓)	Central nervous system		• Higher degree AV block • Severe intraventricular conduction disorder	• Only intravenous • Only slight negative inotropy
	Mexiletine	VT, VES	QRS, QT (↓)	Central nervous system		Severe intraventricular conduction disorder	• Intravenous and oral • Only slight negative inotropy
Ic	Propafenone	• SVT (in particular AVRT, AVNRT) • Ventricular arrhythmias	HR ↓, PQ ↑, QRS ↑	• Central nervous system • Gastrointestinal • Hypotension • Negative inotropy	Increase of the digoxin level	• Sinus node dysfunction • Higher degree AV block	• Risk of accumulation in patients with liver failure • Reduce dose if QRS interval is prolonged to over 130% of the initial value or the QTc interval is significantly prolonged
Ic	Flecainide	Ventricular arrhythmias (esp. VT) SVT (AVRT, AVNRT)	HR ↓, PQ ↑, QRS ↑	Similar to propafenone, also significantly proarrhythmogenic (particularly in adults)	Moderate increase of digoxin level	• Sinus node dysfunction • Higher degree AV block • Heart failure	
II	Propranolol	• Sinus tachycardia • SVES, VES • SVT (AVRT, AVNRT) • Long QT syndrome • Catecholamine-induced VT	HR ↓, PQ ↑, QT ↓	• Bradycardia • AV block • Negative inotropy • Fatigue • Nausea • Bronchospasm • Hypoglycemia		• Sinus node dysfunction • AV block • Bronchial asthma • Diabetes mellitus • Uncompensated heart failure	• Nonselective beta blockers (inhibition of β1 and β2 receptors) • Do not combine with calcium antagonists

Table 18.1 continued

Class	Antiarrhythmic drug	Indication	ECG	Side effects	Common interactions	Contraindication	Remarks
	Metoprolol	Similar to propranolol	HR ↓, PQ ↑, QT ↓	Similar to propranolol, but fewer systematic side effects		Similar to propranolol	Cardioselective beta blocker
	Esmolol	SVT, atrial flutter/fibrillation, VT	HR ↓, PQ ↑, QT ↓	Similar to propranolol, but fewer systematic side effects		Similar to propranolol	Particularly short-acting beta blocker for intravenous therapy
III	Amiodarone	Severe SVT (including atrial flutter/fibrillation, JET, VT	HR ↓, QT ↑	• Thyroid dysfunction • Pulmonary fibrosis • Photosensitivity, corneal deposits • Hypotension if rapid IV administration (alpha blockade)	Increase of the digoxin level	• Higher degree AV block • Sinus node dysfunction	• Very potent antiarrhythmic drug with serious extracardiac side effects • Only slight negative inotropy • Very long half-life • Should not be combined with class Ia antiarrhythmics • Reduce dose if QTc interval ≥ 0.53
III	Sotalol	SVT, VT	HR ↓, QT ↑	• Sinus bradycardia • Hypotension, bronchospasm • Proarrhythmogenic (torsades de pointes)		• Higher degree AV block • Sinus node dysfunction • Bronchial asthma • Diabetes mellitus • QT prolongation	• Potassium channel blocker and nonselective beta blocker • More often proarrhythmogenic than amiodarone
IV	Verapamil	• SVT, atrial fibrillation/flutter • Left ventricular fascicular VT	PQ ↑	• Blood pressure drop • Respiratory depression • Bradycardia • AV block • Negative inotropy		• IV bolus contraindicated in neonates and infants (pronounced negative inotropy) • Higher degree AV block • Sinus node dysfunction • Heart failure • Accessory conduction pathway (conduction via the accessory pathway can be encouraged)	• Do not combine with beta blockers and class Ia antiarrhythmics • Have IV calcium at hand as an antidote
Others	Orciprenaline	• Acute bradycardia • 2nd/3rd degree AV block	HR ↑	• Tachycardia • SVES, VES • Nausea • Agitation		• Tachycardia • Tachyarrhythmia • Digitalis-induced AV block (increased proarrhythmogenic risk)	Beta-sympathomimetic for acute IV therapy

Table 18.1 continued

Class	Antiarrhythmic drug	Indication	ECG	Side effects	Common interactions	Contraindication	Remarks
	Atropine	• Acute bradycardia • 2nd/3rd degree AV block	HR ↑, PQ ↓	• Proarrhythmogenic • Tachycardia • Dry mouth • Skin redness • CNS side effects		• Tachycardia • Glaucoma	• Parasympatholytic • Practically no effect on the ventricular myocardium
	Adenosine	Paroxysmal SVT (AVRT, AVNRT)	• Short-term AV block • Short-term sinus bradycardia	• Short-term: sinus bradycardia • AV block with escape rhythms • Bronchospasm • Apnea • Nausea		Bronchial asthma (but because of the very short half-life only relative contraindication)	Extremely short half-life, rapid bolus injection into a vein as near as possible to the heart
	Digoxin	• Fetal tachycardia • Reduction of the ventricular rate in atrial flutter/fibrillation	PQ ↑	Proarrhythmogenic		• Higher degree AV block, severe bradycardia • Accessory pathway (digoxin shortens the refractory period of the accessory pathways and may induce rapid conduction to the ventricles, e.g., in atrial fibrillation/flutter)	
	Magnesium	• Torsades de pointes tachycardia • VT with magnesium deficiency	HR ↓, PQ ↑	• Rapid IV administration: flush • Bradycardia • Blood pressure drop • AV conduction disturbances		• Bradycardia • Higher degree AV block • LV dysfunction • Severe renal impairment • Myasthenia	• Physiological calcium antagonist • Do not administer IV undiluted

HR, heart rate; PQ, PQ interval; QRS, width of ventricular complex; VT, ventricular tachycardia; SVT, supraventricular tachycardia; VES, ventricular extrasystoles; SVES, supraventricular extrasystoles; LV, left ventricular.
↑ elevated, ↓ reduced, ↔ unchanged.

Table 18.2 Antiarrhythmic drugs (dosage)

Class	Antiarrhythmic	IV dosage	Oral dosage
Ia	Quinidine	2–10 mg/kg every 3–6 h (IV treatment not recommended)	15–60 mg/kg/d in 4–5 single doses (sulfate formulation). Test dose before starting treatment 2 mg/kg
	Disopyramide		Infants: 10–30 mg/kg/d Toddlers: 10–20 mg/kg/d Children: 10–15 mg/kg/d Adolescents: 6–15 mg/kg/d In 4 single doses (standard formulation) or 2 single doses (retard formulation)
Ib	Lidocaine	1 mg/kg as bolus (can be repeated twice at 5-min intervals), then continuous infusion with 20–50 µg/kg/min	
	Mexiletine	3 mg/kg for 15 min, then continuous infusion with 1 mg/kg/h	5–15 mg/kg/d in 3 single doses
Ic	Propafenone	0.5–1 mg/kg	4–7 mg/kg/d in 3 single doses, can be increased to 15–20 mg/kg/d
	Flecainide		Initially 1–3 mg/kg/d in 3 single doses, gradually increase to 3–8 mg/kg/d in 3 single doses
II	Propranolol	0.01–0.1 mg/kg for 10 min, the same dose can be repeated every 6–8 h (start with a 0.01 mg/kg single dose for neonates), maximum 1 mg for toddlers and 3 mg for older children	Begin with 0.5–1 mg/kg/d (0.25 mg/kg/d for neonates) in 3–4 single doses, gradually increase up to the usual maintenance dosage of 2–6 mg/kg/d in 3–4 single doses
	Metoprolol	0.1 mg/kg as slow bolus	1–2 mg/kg 2 to 4 times daily
	Esmolol	200 µg/kg as slow bolus, then continuous infusion with 50–200 µg/kg/min	
III	Amiodarone	Saturation dose: 5 mg/kg as a rapid bolus in VT without pulse or ventricular fibrillation and for 30–60 min for hemodynamically stable patients (total of 2 to 3 times a week), then continuous infusion with 10 (to 20) mg/kg/d (dissolved in 5% glucose)	Saturation dose: toddlers 10–20 mg/kg/d in 2 single doses for 5–14 days, children and adolescents 10 mg/kg/d in 2 single doses for 5–14 days Maintenance dosage: 5–7 mg/kg/d in 1 single dose, gradually reduce to the lowest effective dosage
	Sotalol		80–200 mg/m^2 BSA/d (equivalent to approx. 4 mg/kg/d) in 3 single doses (toddlers) and 2 single doses (older children), 30 min before meals, do not take with milk
IV	Verapamil	0.1–0.2–0.3 mg/kg for 2 min (max. 5 mg), if unsuccessful, can be repeated after 30 min	4–8 mg/kg/d in 3 single doses (standard formulation) or 1 single dose (retard formulation)
Others	Orciprenaline	0.01–0.03 mg/kg as bolus, 0.1 µg/kg/min as continuous infusion	0.5–1 mg/kg/d in 4–6 single doses
	Atropine	0.02–0.04 mg/kg as bolus (minimum dose 0.1 mg, maximum dose 1 mg)	
	Adenosine	0.1 mg/kg (max. 6 mg) as rapid bolus, then flush quickly with NaCl 0.9%, repeat with 0.2 (to 0.3–0.5) mg/kg (max. 18 mg) if necessary	
	Magnesium	Begin with 0.3–0.5 mmol/kg for 30–60 min, can be repeated if necessary	

is necessary while staying in the sun), thyroid dysfunction (high iodine content in amiodarone), and irreversible lung fibrosis (rare). Regular eye examinations and tests of the thyroid and lung function parameters are therefore required. Class III antiarrhythmic drugs have a very long half-life of 2 to 7 weeks. After oral administration, the onset of its effect begins after 4 to 10 days; following intravenous bolus injection, the onset of effect begins within minutes.

Furthermore, class III antiarrhythmic drugs prolong the QTc interval in the ECG, sometimes considerably, and thus carry the risk of torsades de pointes tachycardia. Regular ECG monitoring is required.

Class IV Antiarrhythmic Drugs (Calcium Channel Blockers)

Class IV antiarrhythmic drugs include verapamil and diltiazem. Of all calcium antagonists, only verapamil has an antiarrhythmic effect. The effect of class IV antiarrhythmic drugs is mediated through inhibition of the slow calcium influx. They act in the heart especially at the sinus and AV nodes.

Calcium channel blockers should not be used in patients with accessory pathways because they facilitate conduction via the accessory pathway and can thus lead to unchecked conduction to the ventricles (triggering ventricular fibrillation) in patients with atrial flutter or fibrillation. Moreover, the intravenous bolus administration in neonates and infants is contraindicated because of the negative inotropic effect, which is especially pronounced in this age group.

Other Antiarrhythmic Drugs

► **Adenosine (purine nucleoside).** Adenosine causes a complete short-term blockage of AV conduction. It also has a negative chronotropic effect on the sinus node. It has an extremely short half-life (< 10 seconds), requiring rapid intravenous bolus administration. Adenosine is used mainly in supraventricular re-entrant tachycardia, where it can interrupt the re-entrant circuit by an AV block. It is also used diagnostically in supraventricular tachycardia to facilitate the classification of the tachycardia and in ambiguous cases to distinguish between supraventricular and ventricular tachycardia, for example. Ventricular tachycardias are not affected by adenosine. A relevant extracardiac side effect is the induction of bronchospasms.

► **Atropine (parasympatholytic).** Atropine acts through a competitive inhibition of acetylcholine. In the heart, it increases the sinus node rate and promotes AV conduction.

► **Orciprenaline (beta-sympathomimetic).** Orciprenaline increases the sinus node rate and impulse conduction in the atrium, the AV node, and the His–Purkinje system. It has a positive inotropic and a vasodilative effect. It also increases the excitability of heterotopic automaticity centers and increases myocardial oxygen consumption.

► **Digoxin.** Digoxin inhibits Na-K-ATPase. It acts on the cardiac rhythm by decreasing the sinus rate and inhibiting AV conduction. At the same time, it also increases the excitability of the atrial and ventricular myocardium and leads to an increase of ectopic impulse formation (risk of arrhythmias). In patients with accessory pathways, digoxin probably facilitates conduction via the accessory pathway. In patients with atrial flutter or fibrillation and an accessory pathway, there may be unchecked conduction of the atrial impulses into the ventricles that trigger ventricular fibrillation.

► **Magnesium.** Magnesium is a physiological calcium antagonist. As an antiarrhythmic agent, it is the drug of choice for torsades de pointes tachycardia.

► **Antiarrhythmic combination treatment.** Because of the risk of additive adverse effects, antiarrhythmic drugs may not be combined with those of the same class or subclass.

In addition, the following may not be combined or may be used together only if special precautions are taken (► Table 18.3):

- Class Ia and class III antiarrhythmic drugs: additive prolongation of the QTc interval
- Class Ia and class Ic antiarrhythmic drugs: additive prolongation of the QRS duration
- Class Ia antiarrhythmic drugs and calcium antagonists: additive negative inotropic and vasodilative effects
- Beta blockers and calcium antagonists: risk of sinus bradycardia and AV block
- Beta blockers and class III antiarrhythmic drugs: both amiodarone and sotalol have a beta-sympatholytic effect.
- Amiodarone and calcium antagonists: additive vasodilative effect

Table 18.3 Suitable combinations for antiarrhythmic combination treatment

Class	Ia	Ib	Ic	II	III	IV
Ia	–	+	–	+	–	–
Ib	+	–	+	+	+	n/a
Ic	–	+	–	+	+	n/a
II	+	+	+	–	–	–
III	–	+	+	–	–	–
IV	–	n/a	n/a	–	–	–

+, possible; –, not possible or possible only if special precautionary measures are taken; n/a, no references available.

Suitable combinations (▶ Table 18.3):

- Class Ia and Ib antiarrhythmic drugs
- Class Ic and Ib antiarrhythmic drugs
- Class I and II antiarrhythmic drugs
- Class Ib and III antiarrhythmic drugs
- Class Ic and III antiarrhythmic drugs

18.1.2 Pacemaker Therapy

Basics

A pacemaker is a system for primary electrical treatment of bradycardia arrhythmias. It consists of a generator unit and an electrode system. The generator unit generates the impulse that is conducted by the electrodes to the endocardium, myocardium, or epicardium and leads to depolarization of the myocardial cells.

Parameters of the pacing impulse are the amplitude (expressed in volts or milliamps) and pulse width (expressed in milliseconds; ▶ Fig. 18.1).

The amplitude required for effective stimulation is usually between 1 and 5 V with a pulse width of 0.2 to 0.6 ms. As amplitude and pulse width increase, energy consumption increases and the life of the battery decreases. Pacemaker batteries last an average of about 5 to 6 years.

▶ **Threshold.** The threshold is the minimum electrical stimulus that is required to stimulate the heart. Of particular importance is that the threshold increases significantly within the first days after pacemaker implantation as a result of inflammatory processes in the area of the electrodes. Over the next few weeks, the threshold decreases again and usually nearly approaches the baseline after 3 to 4 months. Modern electrodes that continually release steroids to the surrounding area can lower the threshold.

▶ **Rheobase.** The rheobase is defined as the smallest amplitude that can cause just one stimulation in an infinitely long pulse width. In practice, instead of an "infinitely long" pulse width, a pulse width of 1 ms is usually used to determine the rheobase.

▶ **Chronaxie.** Chronaxie is the term for the pulse width that can trigger effective stimulation when the rheobase amplitude is doubled. With these two values, modern pacemakers can independently calculate a chronaxie–rheobase curve (▶ Fig. 18.2). A combination of amplitude and pulse width located above the curve results in effective stimulation. For safety reasons, the stimulation amplitude is usually selected twice as high as the threshold in the range of the chronaxie. The pulse width is then selected to be approximately as long as the chronaxie.

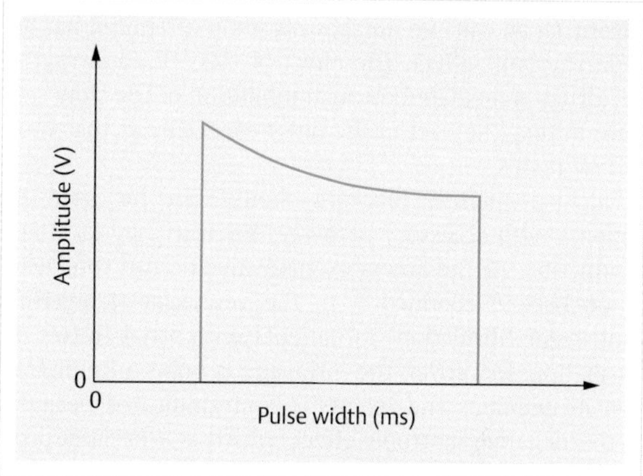

Fig. 18.1 Pacemaker impulse. The pacemaker impulse is defined by the amplitude of voltage (V) or current (mA), and the pulse width (ms).

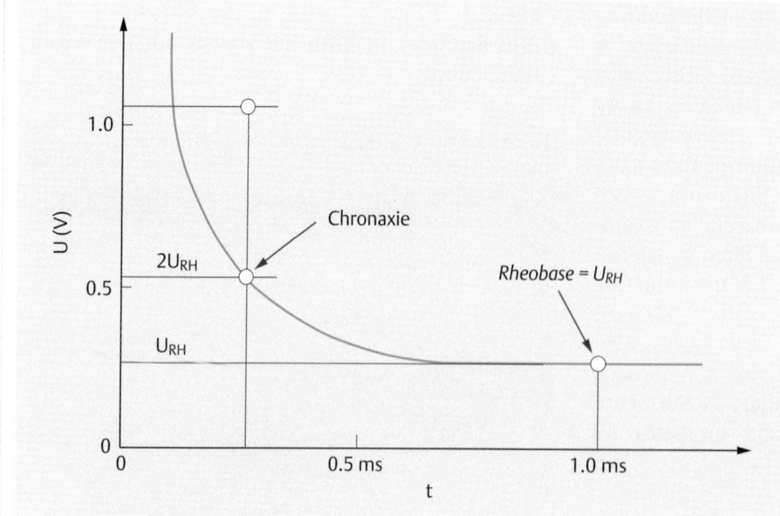

Fig. 18.2 Chronaxie–rheobase curve. The rheobase is the smallest amplitude that can generate one stimulation in an infinitely long pulse width. Chronaxie is defined as the pulse width at twice the rheobase amplitude. A combination of amplitude and pulse width located above the curve results in effective stimulation.

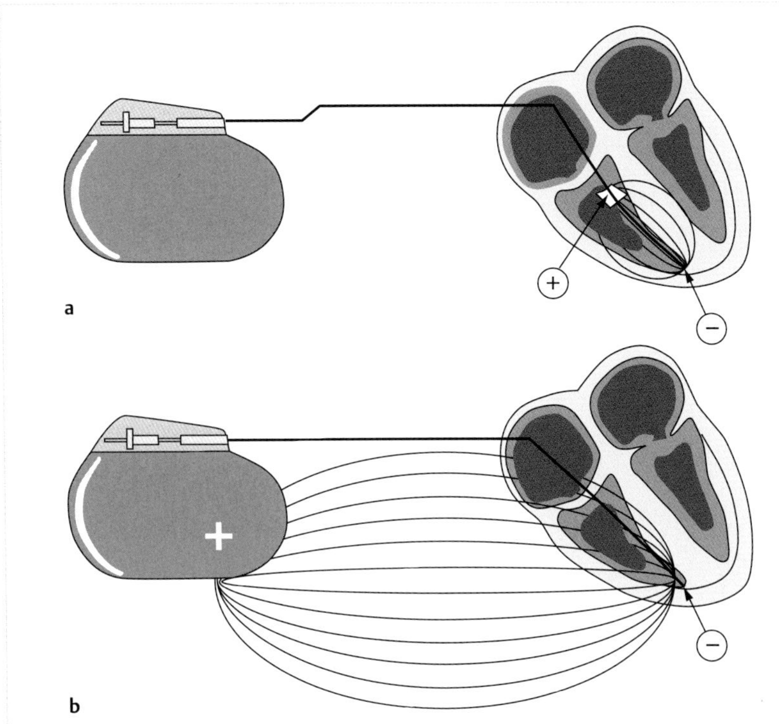

Fig. 18.3 Structure of unipolar and bipolar pacemaker electrodes. **a** In bipolar electrodes, both anode and cathode are in the electrode tip. Advantages are the low susceptibility to interference from external sources (muscle potentials) and frequently better sensing of intrinsic cardiac activity. However, the pacemaker spike in the ECG is small with bipolar electrodes. **b** In unipolar electrodes, the cathode is the electrode tip and the pacemaker case serves as the anode. The sensing field is correspondingly larger, thus permitting interference from external sources. An advantage is that unipolar electrodes are thinner and the pacemaker spike in the surface ECG is clearly visible.

Another possibility is to prolong the pulse width by three to four times.

► **Sensing threshold.** To ensure that even in intrinsic cardiac activity, the heart's signals are detected by the pacemaker, the sensing threshold of the electrode must be determined. This value describes which amplitude of intrinsic cardiac activity can be just detected by the electrode. A high value indicates a high threshold, thus low sensitivity. The more sensitive the detection threshold setting, the greater is the risk that noise signals such as muscle potentials will be incorrectly classified as cardiac activity (oversensing) and pacemaker stimulation will be suppressed. On the other hand, if the sensing threshold is too insensitive, the pacemaker will not recognize intrinsic cardiac activity and there will be interference between the cardiac activity and the pacemaker impulses (undersensing, pacemaker is asynchronous).

► **Pacemaker electrodes.** A distinction is made between unipolar and bipolar electrodes (► Fig. 18.3). In *unipolar* electrodes, the electrode tip is the cathode and the pacemaker box is the anode. In *bipolar* electrodes, both the anode and the cathode are located in the electrode tip. The main characteristics of the electrodes are as follows:

- Unipolar electrodes:
  - Low energy consumption
  - Significant pacemaker spikes in the surface ECG (readily assessable)
  - Small electrode thickness, good handling during transvenous implantation
  - Susceptible to interference from muscle potentials
- Bipolar electrodes:
  - Rarely cause muscle or diaphragmatic twitching
  - Better sensing behavior
  - Only small pacemaker spikes in the surface ECG (often difficult to assess pacemaker activity in the surface ECG)

Pacemaker Systems

Pacemakers are classified according to the stimulation site and sensing of intrinsic activity. A maximum five-character code describes the operation of the pacemaker (► Table 18.4).

The response of the pacemaker to sensed intrinsic activity of the heart can be inhibition or triggering. In inhibition, the pacemaker is inhibited by sensed activity and emits no electrical stimulus. In triggering, a pacing impulse is triggered by a sensed event.

Rate modulation systems can adapt the pacing frequency to physical stress. To assess physical activity, there are various sensors that measure factors such as muscle activity, QT interval, and temperature and respiratory excursions. This system is useful for sinus node dysfunction, for example, when the heart does not respond under stress with a corresponding increase in heart rate (chronotropic incompetence).

Table 18.4 NASPE/BPG pacemaker codes (North American Society of Pacing and Electrophysiology/British Pacing Guidelines)

I	II	III	IV	V
Chamber paced	Chamber sensed	Pacemaker response to sensed event	Rate modulation	Multi-site pacing
0 = None V = Ventricle A = Atrium D = Dual (A + V) S = Single	0 = None V = Ventricle A = Atrium D = Dual (A + V) S = Single	I = Inhibited T = Triggered D = Dual (I + T)	0 = None R = Rate modulation	0 = None V = Ventricle A = Atrium D = Dual (A + V)

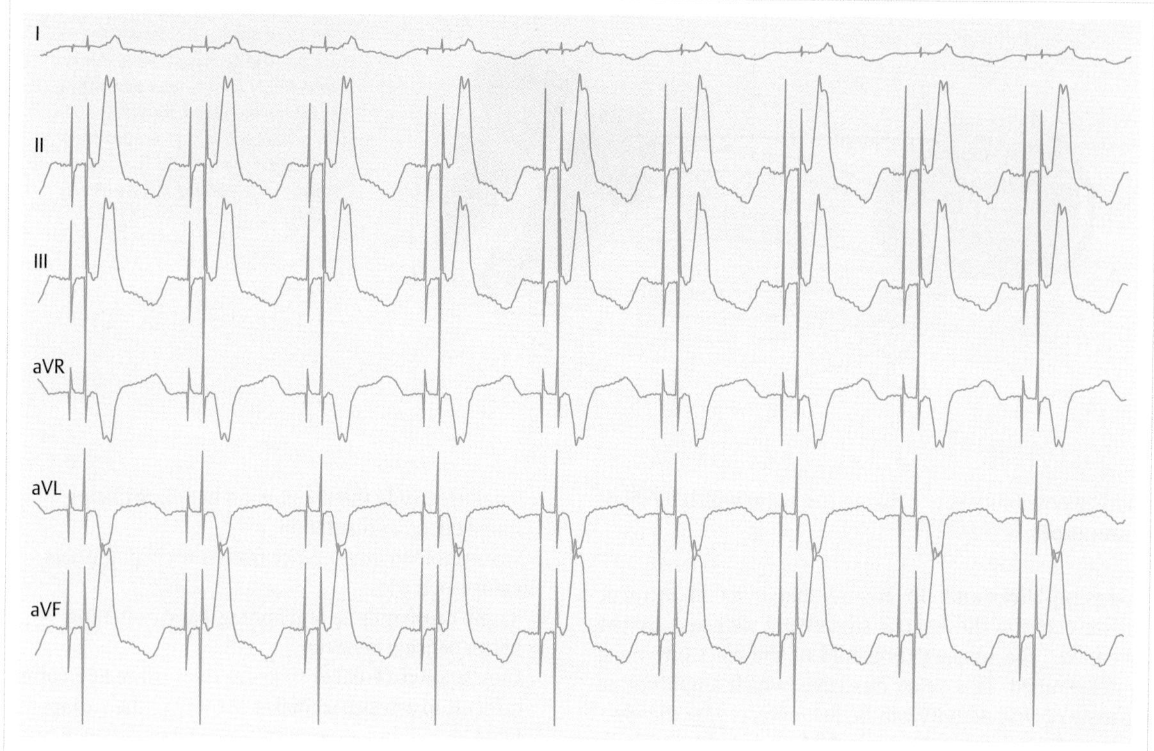

Fig. 18.4 Pacemaker ECG after the implantation of a DDD system. This pacemaker ECG was recorded in a patient in whom a temporary pacemaker in DDD mode with epicardial electrodes was implanted postoperatively. The spikes of atrial and ventricular stimulation are clearly visible. The QRS complexes have a bundle branch block pattern.

The fifth position in the pacemaker code is for the stimulation of a third ventricle, for example, in a biventricular pacemaker system.

The most common pacemaker systems used in children are explained below:

▸ **AAI.** The pacemaker stimulates the atrium when the intrinsic heart rate falls below the programmed intervention rate. Intrinsic activity inhibits the pacemaker. A prerequisite for implanting such a system is that AV conduction is not disturbed. Typical indication is sinus node dysfunction. For chronotropic incompetence, a system with rate modulation (AAIR) should be selected.

▸ **VVI.** The pacemaker stimulates the ventricle when the ventricle's intrinsic frequency falls below the programmed intervention rate. A disadvantage of this system is that contraction of the atria and ventricles is uncoordinated because the pacemaker does not take atrial activity into account. In childhood, this type is still sometimes implanted in neonates, as very small generator units are available. Rate modulation (VVIR) is usually also possible in these systems.

▸ **DDD.** This is a dual chamber system that stimulates the atrium and the ventricle in physiological sequence (AV sequential) when the intrinsic frequency falls below the programmed intervention rate. The atrial pacemaker impulse is suppressed if there is intrinsic atrial activity. If the atrial rate is lower than the programmed intervention rate, the atrium is stimulated. If the conduction of atrial activity to the ventricles is prevented by an AV block, the ventricle is stimulated according to a programmed AV interval (▶ Fig. 18.4). DDD systems are used in AV blocks. A great advantage is that the coordinates of the atria and the ventricles are preserved. DDD systems require an atrial and a ventricular electrode. The atrial electrode may be particularly difficult to anchor in young children. If necessary, reprogramming can allow a switch to an AAI or VVI system. A DDDR system is used for chronotropic incompetence.

Excursus: Additional technical terms for pacemaker technology

Intervention rate
In the absence of intrinsic activity, if the heart rate falls below the intervention rate, the pacemaker begins stimulation.

Maximum rate limit
The maximum achievable rate in a dual chamber system. If this rate is exceeded, the pacemaker switches to a 2:1 conduction from the atrium to the ventricle.

Escape interval
The period between the last intrinsic action and the first pacemaker stimulus.

Hysteresis (Greek for "lag")
If a pacemaker senses intrinsic activity, the escape interval is prolonged until the next pacemaker impulse, so that the heart "has more time" to create new intrinsic activity before the next pacemaker impulse is delivered.

To avoid over-pacing, the pacemaker is therefore "allowed" to stimulate only when the heart rate falls below the programmed intervention rate (e.g., intervention rate 60 bpm, hysteresis 50 bpm).

That means that the pacemaker stimulates at a frequency of 60 bpm when the patient's intrinsic rate drops below 50 bpm. Accordingly, some heart rates are lower than the programmed intervention rate. This prevents unnecessary intervention and encourages intrinsic activity of the heart.

AV interval
The time interval between atrial and ventricular stimulation or between sensing intrinsic activity in the atrium and ventricle stimulation.

Refractory period
The time interval after stimulation or sensing in which neither stimulation nor sensing is possible.

Postventricular atrial refractory period (PVARP)
The period following a ventricular pacemaker action at the atrial level when neither stimulation nor sensing is possible.

"Crosstalk"
An atrial stimulus is mistakenly sensed by the ventricle electrode to be a ventricular signal. Because of the misperception, the pacemaker gives no ventricular stimulus. The other possibility is that a ventricular impulse is mistakenly sensed by the atrial electrode to be atrial activity.

Blanking
The period in which all signals in the respective ventricle or atrium are ignored by the pacemaker. This is done to blank all signals coming from another ventricle or atrium. The blanking time is to prevent "cross talk." Thus, for example, if the atrial blanking period is sufficient, a ventricular R wave detected in the atrium is not misinterpreted as atrial activity.

Mode switch
Automatic change of stimulation mode when atrial tachyarrhythmia occurs, for example, switching from DDD (R) to DDI(R) or VDI(R). This prevents atrial tachycardia from being conducted 1:1 to the ventricle and inducing ventricular tachycardia.

Undersensing
Intrinsic activity is not detected by the pacemaker. ECG: pacemaker stimulation is independent of the P wave or the QRS complex. Cause: electrode defect or dislocation, sensing threshold too high.

Oversensing
Erroneous assessment of extracardiac signals (e.g., muscle potentials) or intracardiac signals as intrinsic cardiac activity (e.g., perception of the R wave in the atrium). ECG: no stimulation by the pacemaker. In DDD systems, rapid stimulation of the ventricle is also possible if rapid inappropriate signals are sensed in the atrium. Cause: almost exclusively in unipolar electrodes (poorer sensing properties), insulation defects, sensing threshold too low.

Exit block
Ineffective stimulation of the heart by the pacemaker impulse. ECG: pacemaker spike without subsequent QRS complex or without subsequent P wave. Cause: increased threshold, battery exhaustion, defective electrodes. Caution: risk of bradycardia or asystole.

Epidemiology

Permanent pacemaker therapy in childhood is most frequently needed in children with AV block after surgery for a congenital heart defect or for a congenital complete AV block, which occurs mainly in the context of a maternal autoimmune disease in about 1 in 15,000 neonates. Up to 5% of all cardiac surgeries result in a postoperative

Table 18.5 Indications for permanent pacemaker therapy in childhood (according to ACC, AHA, NASPE 2002 recommendations)

Class I (general agreement that pacemaker implantation is indicated)
• Higher degree and complete AV block with symptomatic bradycardia, progressive ventricular enlargement, heart failure, or reduced cardiac output
• Sinus node dysfunction with inadequate-for-age symptomatic bradycardia
• High degree or complete AV block after cardiac surgery, considered irreversible or persisting at least 7 days
• Congenital complete AV block with an escape rhythm with widened ventricular complexes, complex ventricular ectopy, or ventricular dysfunction
• Congenital complete AV block in a neonate with a structurally normal heart and a ventricular rate of less than 50–55 bpm or in conjunction with a congenital heart defect and a ventricular rate of less than 70 bpm (averaged over 7 beats)
• Persistent, bradycardia-induced ventricular tachycardia (with or without QT prolongation) with proven benefit of pacemaker therapy
Class IIa (conflicting opinions but tendency in favor of usefulness of pacemaker implantation)
• Bradycardia–tachycardia syndrome with concomitant antiarrhythmic therapy except digoxin
• Congenital complete AV block after age 1 year with an mean ventricular rate of less than 50 bpm or sudden asystole of more than two to three times the basic cycle duration or symptomatic chronotropic incompetence.
• Long QT syndrome with 2:1 AV block or complete AV block
• Asymptomatic sinus bradycardia in a child with a complex congenital heart defect and a ventricular rate of less than 35 bpm at rest or asystole of more than 3 s
Class IIb (conflicting opinions, less evidence of the efficacy of a pacemaker implantation)
• Temporary complete postoperative AV block with restitution of sinus rhythm with residual bi-fascicular block
• Congenital complete AV block in an asymptomatic neonate, child or adolescent with an acceptable ventricular rate, a narrow QRS complex, and normal left ventricular function
• Asymptomatic sinus bradycardia in an adolescent with congenital heart disease and a ventricular rate at rest below 40 bpm or asystole of more than 3 s.
• Neuromuscular disease with all grades of AV blocks (including 1st degree) with or without symptoms due to the incalculable risk of progression of functional impairment of the specific conduction tissue
Class III (general agreement that pacemaker implantation is not indicated)
• Temporary postoperative complete AV block with restitution of sinus rhythm
• Asymptomatic child with a postoperative bi-fascicular block with or without 1st degree AV block
• Asymptomatic 2nd degree AV block type I (Wenckebach)
• Asymptomatic sinus bradycardia in an adolescent with a minimum ventricular rate of about 40 bpm or asystole of less than 3 s.

complete AV block that persists in about half the cases. Typical operations with a risk for the occurrence of an AV block are interventions in the vicinity of the AV node in the cranial part of the ventricular septum (VSD closure, AV canal correction, aortic valve surgery, correction of Ebstein anomaly, etc.).

Sinus node dysfunction that develops in children and adolescents, especially in the long term after surgery in the atrium area (e.g., atrial baffle or Fontan operation), is another significant indication for permanent pacemaker therapy.

Indications

The detailed indications according to current guidelines are summarized in ▶ Table 18.5. The most important are:

- Symptomatic congenital complete AV block
- Complete AV block that persists longer than 7 to 14 days after cardiac surgery
- Sinus node dysfunction with symptomatic bradycardia

Pacemaker Implantation

▶ **Transvenous endocardial access.** In the usual procedure, the electrodes are advanced into the right atrium or the right ventricle under fluoroscopic guidance via the subclavian or jugular vein. The electrodes are then anchored in the atrium or ventricle with a screw or anchor mechanism. The pacemaker generator unit is implanted under the pectoral muscle or subcutaneously below the clavicle.

The transvenous access is usually possible in children weighing more than 10 kg. It is not possible in patients after Fontan surgery in whom the atrium or the ventricle cannot be accessed transvenously.

► **Subxiphoid access and epimyocardial electrodes.** In neonates or infants, epimyocardial electrodes are usually used that are placed directly on the atrium or ventricle. The pacemaker generator unit is then usually implanted in the preperitoneal region under the abdominal muscles.

► **Surgical complications**

- (Late) bleeding
- Pneumothorax
- Air embolism in transvenous implantation of the pacemaker
- Infection of the pacemaker pocket or of the system
- Vascular or myocardial perforation, pericardial effusion

► **Specific pacemaker complications**

- Probe dysfunction (dislocation, insulation failures, broken probe; in the ECG: exit block, undersensing, or oversensing)
- Incorrect sensing of muscle potentials
- Muscle/diaphragmatic twitching
- Increased thresholds with stimulation loss ("exit block"), especially during the healing phase
- Failure of the pacemaker unit or the battery
- Phantom programming through external interference frequencies (e.g., MRI, defibrillator)
- Venous thrombosis or vascular occlusion during the transvenous implantation

18.1.3 Special Pacemaker Applications

► **Temporary pacemaker.** Temporary pacemakers are used mainly in children after cardiac surgery associated with an increased risk of an AV block or arrhythmia, where a benefit from pacemaker therapy (e.g., JET, sinus bradycardia) is expected. Epimyocardial electrodes are applied intraoperatively and are led outward through the skin. The stimulation comes from an external pacemaker generator unit. The electrodes can later be easily removed by simply pulling them out or possibly cutting them off just below the skin level.

Temporary pacemaker electrodes can also be advanced into the right atrium or right ventricle via a sheath through the femoral vein, the subclavian vein, or the internal jugular vein.

► **Overdrive stimulation.** Supraventricular tachycardias including atrial flutter may possibly be terminated by overdrive stimulation (high atrial stimulation rate, e.g., 300–500 bpm). Transesophageal overdrive stimulation can also be carried out due to the close anatomical proximity of the left atrium and the esophagus.

► **External stimulation.** In an emergency, external stimulation via large adhesive electrodes is possible. Most modern defibrillators provide this feature today. However, external stimulation is painful and should be performed only on unconscious or deeply sedated patients.

► **Transesophageal stimulation.** Temporary transesophageal pacemaker stimulation is also possible in emergencies using special electrodes that are advanced into the esophagus.

18.1.4 Aftercare

The programming and the first test of the pacemaker are performed in the operating room. The next checkup is performed a few days after surgery because of the initially rising threshold, then usually after 1 and 3 months. Biannual checkups are sufficient later. When battery exhaustion is imminent, checkups should be more frequent, of course.

At each pacemaker checkup, the programmed parameters are monitored telemetrically. This monitoring includes the intervention rate, electrical amplitude, and width. Threshold tests are also performed and, if necessary, the parameters are adjusted. In children and adolescents, the probe location is also regularly monitored (e.g., annually) by chest X-ray. A pacemaker ID card is issued to all pacemaker patients, containing information on the generator unit, the electrodes, and the current settings.

18.1.5 Behavior in Everyday Life

Most electronic devices are safe for pacemaker patients. Unproblematic devices include radios, televisions, computers, infrared remote controls, wireless headphones, microwaves, ceramic hobs, airbags, landline telephones including wireless devices, ultrasonic devices (due to possible thermal effects a distance of 10 cm from the implant should be maintained), and X-ray equipment.

Mobile phone users should keep a distance of not less than 15 to 20 cm between phone and pacemaker generator unit (hold the cell phone to the ear on the opposite side and never carry it in the breast pocket over the device). Anti-theft systems in department stores should be passed quickly. When using a drill, avoid holding it close to the chest. Using electrical welding equipment is risky and being in the vicinity of transformer stations is strictly prohibited.

The vicinity of very large loudspeakers (disco, concert) should be avoided due to the strong magnetic field. In addition, bass vibration can cause rate modulation.

MRI is contraindicated. If an MRI is urgently indicated, supervision by a physician experienced in dealing with pacemakers is absolutely necessary. There are MRI compatable defibrillators available now (1,5 tesla, not 3 tesla), these devices however make MRI investigation of the chest impossible due to significant artifacts. Pacemaker wearers should be encouraged to engage in physical activity unless contraindicated by a heart defect. Recreational sports are unproblematic. Contact sports and horseback riding are not recommended. Martial arts, gymnastics on the uneven bars, platform diving, and scuba diving are absolutely prohibited.

18.1.6 Antitachycardia Pacemakers and Implantable Cardioverter Defibrillators

▶ **Antitachycardia pacemakers.** Antitachycardia pacemakers can detect supraventricular and ventricular tachycardias and terminate them through overstimulation.

▶ **Implantable cardioverter defibrillators.** Implantable cardioverter defibrillators (ICDs) are now available for children with malignant arrhythmias. The ICD can be implanted subpectorally like a pacemaker generator unit and the shock electrodes are inserted transvenously. These systems usually make it possible to terminate ventricular tachycardia through over-stimulation, cardioversion, or defibrillation. They also usually have the possibility of antibradycardia stimulation. The most common indications for implantation of an ICD in childhood are prior cardiac arrhythmias that necessitated resuscitation, ventricular tachycardia that cannot be controlled by other measures such as antiarrhythmic drugs or catheter ablation, cardiomyopathy, or long QT syndrome.

18.2 Sinus Arrhythmia

18.2.1 Basics

Definition

In a sinus arrhythmia there are phasic fluctuations in the heart rate. The electrical excitation originates in the sinus node, which is regulated by the autonomic nervous system. In childhood, a sinus arrhythmia is physiological. A loss of this heart rate variability in children is pathological and can be found in the context of neuropathy, for example.

Epidemiology

In childhood, a sinus arrhythmia is physiological and diminishes with increasing age. The most common cause by far is respiratory arrhythmia.

Etiology

In respiratory arrhythmia, there is an increase of the heart rate during inspiration and a decrease during expiration. The cause is probably an increased vagal tone during expiration.

18.2.2 Diagnostic Measures

Symptoms

A sinus arrhythmia is almost always asymptomatic. Palpitations occur very rarely.

Note

Significant symptoms such as dizziness or syncopes cannot be explained by respiratory arrhythmia.

ECG

In the ECG, there are variations of the RR intervals and possibly discrete changes in the P wave morphology (▶ Fig. 18.5). A phasic increase in heart rate during inspiration and a decrease during expiration are typical findings (mnemonic tip: Inspiration → Increase in heart rate).

Differential Diagnosis

Second degree sinoatrial (SA) block type II (Mobitz): In a 2nd degree SA block type II (Mobitz), there is an abrupt change of the PP intervals. The PP intervals in the SA block are a multiple of the normal PP intervals.

No further diagnostic procedures such as echocardiography, electrophysiology study, or laboratory tests are required for a sinus arrhythmia.

18.2.3 Treatment

No treatment is necessary.

18.2.4 Prognosis

This condition is not pathological.

18.3 Sinus Bradycardia

18.3.1 Basics

Definition

Sinus bradycardia is present when the heart rate of a sinus rhythm falls below the normal level for the age for a prolonged period (indicative values: in neonates < 100 bpm, in older children < 80 bpm, in adolescents < 60 bpm).

Epidemiology

Sinus bradycardia occurs frequently and can be considered physiological in many cases (e.g., physically fit athletes).

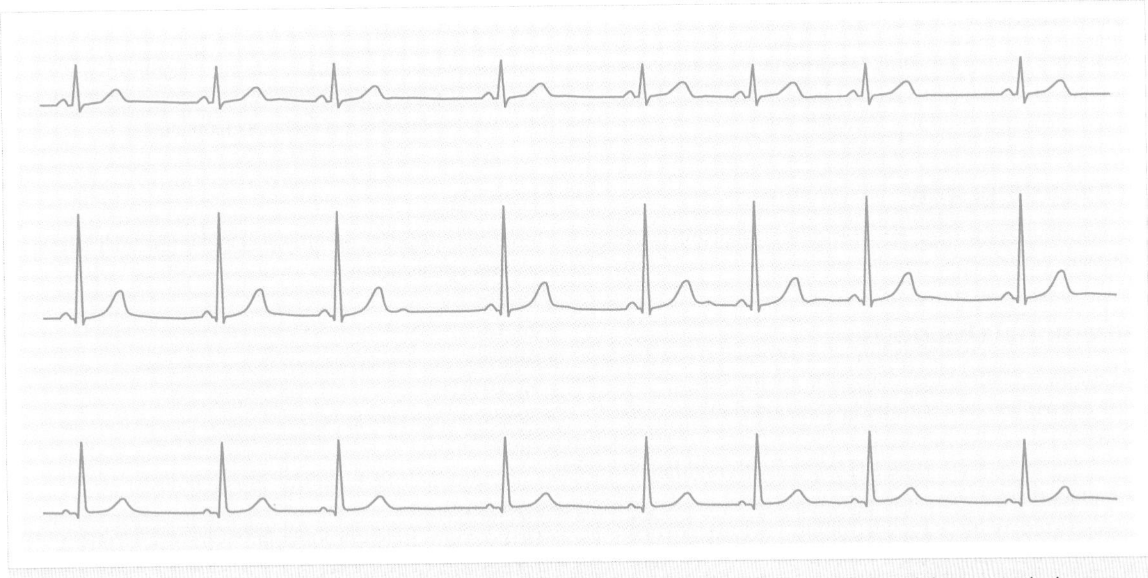

Fig. 18.5 Respiratory arrhythmia. Fluctuations of R-R intervals and the phasic change between increase and decrease in the heart rate can be seen in the ECG.

Etiology

Physiological and pathological causes of a sinus bradycardia must be distinguished. Sinus bradycardia is physiological in physically fit older children and adolescents (high vagal tone) and during sleep.

Pathological causes:

- Vasovagal reactions (vasovagal syncopes, severe anxiety/fright reactions)
- Premature birth (typical apnea and bradycardia syndrome in premature infants)
- Hypothyroidism
- Hypoxia (e.g., hypoxic neonates)
- Hypothermia
- Increased intracranial pressure
- Mechanical vagus nerve stimulation (Valsalva maneuver, bulbar pressure)
- Jaundice
- Drugs (e.g., beta blockers, digoxin, antidepressants)
- Hyperkalemia
- Sinus node dysfunction

Pathogenesis

Sinus bradycardia is caused by slowed impulse formation in the sinus node.

18.3.2 Diagnostic Measures

Symptoms

Sinus bradycardia is usually asymptomatic. Dizziness, palpitations, or syncope occur rarely. If, in severe cases, the heart rate is no longer sufficient to produce adequate cardiac output, symptoms of heart failure may develop. In pathological bradycardia, the heart rate does not increase sufficiently during exercise.

ECG

There is a regular sinus rhythm (each QRS complex is preceded by a P wave, P wave vector between 0 and 90°). The P waves are often flattened (especially visible in lead II, sometimes even negative in lead III). The PQ interval is often prolonged, but usually returns to normal under stress. If vagal tone is high, the T waves, especially in the precordial leads, are often pointed and high (over two-thirds of the amplitude of the QRS complex).

If the sinus rhythm is slow, escape systoles may be detected. In such cases, a secondary center kicks in to replace the pacemaker function of the slow sinus node. Typical junctional escape systoles that arise in the area of the AV node have narrow QRS complexes. The P wave is usually hidden in the QRS complex or is found shortly before or after the complex. If the rate of the escape mechanism is higher than that of the sinus node for a longer period, AV dissociation occurs, that is, the atria and ventricles beat independently of one another. In this case the atrial rate is slightly lower than the ventricular rate.

▸ **Holter ECG.** A 24-hour Holter ECG is sometimes indicated for documenting bradycardia episodes and the correlating them with the symptoms.

▸ **Exercise ECG.** In physiological bradycardia, there is an adequate increase of the heart rate under stress, whereas in pathological bradycardia, no increase occurs.

Laboratory

Laboratory tests are only occasionally indicated—for example, if electrolyte disorders, hypothyroidism, jaundice, or drug intoxication are suspected.

Echocardiography

Echocardiography may be useful for assessing cardiac function.

Differential Diagnosis

The following differential diagnoses are possible:

- 1st degree SA block (cannot be diagnosed in the surface ECG)
- 2nd degree SA block type II (Mobitz) with regular conduction
- 2nd degree AV block type II (Mobitz) with regular conduction: In a 2nd degree AV block, some P waves are not followed by QRS complexes, whereas in sinus bradycardia, each P wave is followed by a QRS complex.

18.3.3 Treatment

Asymptomatic patients do not require treatment. If there is secondary sinus bradycardia, the underlying cause should be treated first. Intravenous tropine, orciprenaline, isoprenaline, or epinephrine is used for the acute treatment of symptomatic patients. Rarely, a temporary external or internal pacemaker may be needed.

Symptomatic patients are treated with a pacemaker (e.g., AAI or AAI-R system) after a treatable cause is ruled out. In general, these are patients where sinus bradycardia develops in the context of a sinus node dysfunction.

18.3.4 Prognosis

In most cases, sinus bradycardia has no pathological significance. Secondary sinus bradycardia can usually be successfully treated by targeting the underlying cause. The treatment itself is often more difficult if the bradycardia is related to sinus node dysfunction.

18.4 Sinus Tachycardia

18.4.1 Basics

Definition

In sinus tachycardia, the heart rate is above the normal level for the age for a prolonged period (indicative values: > 180 bpm in neonates and infants, > 160 bpm in toddlers, > 140 bpm in older children). The site of the impulse formation is the SA node, that is, the vector of the P wave is between 0 and 90°. The rate of sinus tachycardia is almost never over 230 bpm.

Epidemiology

Sinus tachycardia is usually physiological, brought on by physical or emotional stress. Pathological causes are rare, but must be ruled out if tachycardia persists.

Etiology

Physiological causes are physical and emotional stress.

Pathological causes:

- Fever
- Pain
- Anemia
- Hyperthyroidism
- Hemorrhage, shock
- Heart failure
- Cor pulmonale (e.g., pulmonary embolism)
- Hypotension
- Orthostatic circulatory regulation disorders, postural orthostatic tachycardia syndrome (POTS)
- Myocarditis
- Drugs (e.g., beta-sympathomimetic drugs, anticholinergic drugs, catecholamines)
- Stimulants (e.g., nicotine, caffeine)

Pathogenesis

The sinus node is stimulated to more rapid depolarization by the autonomic nervous system. The increase in the heart rate sometimes serves as a compensatory mechanism to increase cardiac output (e.g., during exercise or in the context of heart failure).

18.4.2 Diagnostic Measures

Symptoms

Sinus tachycardia is usually asymptomatic and is well tolerated. Some patients complain of palpitations.

ECG

The heart rate is higher than normal for the age. Each QRS complex is preceded by a P wave. The vector of the P wave is between 0 and 90°. There are usually high and pointed P waves in leads II, III, and aVF. The PQ interval is shortened. The ST segment may start below the zero line and ascend. The T waves are frequently flattened. Sometimes the T and P waves merge. Unlike re-entrant tachycardia, which begins and ends abruptly, in sinus tachycardia the heart rate increases continuously and decreases gradually.

Differential Diagnosis

- Sinus node re-entrant tachycardia: The cause of the tachycardia is a re-entrant mechanism in the sinus node or in close proximity to the sinus node. Start and end are abrupt. The heart rate is usually between 150 and 250 bpm.

- AV re-entrant tachycardia with or without accessory pathway (AVRT, AVNRT): Abrupt start and end. In AV re-entrant tachycardia, the P waves are hidden in the QRS complex or located immediately after the QRS complex. The P wave is negative in leads II, III, and aVF. The heart rate is usually higher than in sinus tachycardia.
- Permanent junctional reciprocating tachycardia (PJRT): Negative P waves in leads II, III, and aVF are typical for PJRT. The P wave follows the QRS complex at a relatively great distance.
- Ectopic atrial tachycardia (EAT): In an EAT, the P wave vector is different from the sinus rhythm vector. If the ectopic focus is near the sinus node, the differential diagnosis can be difficult and may require an electrophysiology study.
- Chaotic atrial tachycardia (CAT): This form of supraventricular tachycardia is also referred to as a multifocal atrial tachycardia (MAT). Here, many different atrial foci are found as the origin of the electrical excitation. Correspondingly, there are different P wave morphologies and different P wave vectors in the ECG.

Laboratory

Laboratory tests are rarely required. In individual cases, the following tests are useful: serum electrolytes including K, Mg, Ca, possibly CK/CK-MB, troponin I, drug levels, TSH.

Echocardiography

Echocardiography is required in isolated cases. It can be used to rule out or detect congenital heart defects and assess cardiac function.

Electrophysiology Study

An electrophysiology study is only rarely indicated to narrow down the differential diagnoses such as ectopic atrial tachycardia or sinus nodal re-entrant tachycardia with the option of ablation treatment.

18.4.3 Treatment

Usually the underlying cause is treated. In some cases, treatment with a beta blocker may be useful.

18.4.4 Prognosis

Most sinus tachycardias are physiological reactions that have no pathological significance. Otherwise, the prognosis depends on the underlying disease.

18.5 Sinus Node Dysfunction

18.5.1 Basics

Synonyms: sick sinus syndrome (SSS), tachycardia–bradycardia syndrome

Definition

In sinus node dysfunction, the sinus node as the dominant pacemaker of the heart is dysfunctional. Furthermore, regulation of the sinus node by the autonomic nervous system is disrupted and sinoatrial conduction is impaired. This can cause various atrial arrhythmias such as sinus bradycardia, sinoatrial blocks, and atrial fibrillation at the same time. The occurrence of atrial tachycardia and subsequent bradycardia, until a secondary center kicks in with an escape rhythm is reflected in the term "tachycardia–bradycardia syndrome."

Sinus node dysfunction is often associated with AV conduction disturbances. This is termed a binodal lesion.

Epidemiology

In childhood, sinus node dysfunction develops primarily after atrial surgery, especially after an atrial baffle procedure, Fontan procedure, correction of an anomalous pulmonary venous connection, or rarely even after the closure of an atrial septal defect (especially in superior sinus venosus defects). In a structurally unremarkable heart, sinus node dysfunction is very rare.

Etiology

- Operations and procedures in the atrium (atrial baffle procedure, Fontan operation, ASD closure, correction of an anomalous pulmonary venous connection or superior sinus venosus defect)
- Inflammatory heart disease (myocarditis)
- Myocardial ischemia (coronary anomalies, Kawasaki disease)
- Cardiomyopathies
- Drugs (digoxin, beta blockers, calcium channel blockers, amiodarone)
- Hypothyroidism, hypothermia (temporary sinus node dysfunction)
- In adults, especially in coronary or hypertensive heart disease

Pathogenesis

Sinus node dysfunction usually develops as a result of direct or indirect injury or scarring of the sinus node, atrial wall, intranodal or intra-atrial conduction pathways, or the supplying coronary arteries.

18.5.2 Diagnostic Measures

Symptoms

Bradycardia may cause dizziness, syncopes, and symptoms of heart failure. Tachycardia may sometimes cause palpitations, dyspnea, and chest pain. Atrial fibrillation increases the risk of arterial embolism.

ECG

Various atrial arrhythmias are found concomitantly or alternately in the ECG. Typical findings are:

- Sinus bradycardia
- Pronounced sinus arrhythmia
- Sinus arrest
- SA block
- Slow escape rhythm (ectopic atrial rhythm, junctional escape rhythm, ventricular escape rhythm)
- Atrial flutter/fibrillation
- Bradycardia–tachycardia syndrome (bradycardia alternating with atrial tachycardia, usually in the form of atrial fibrillation or flutter)

In the ECG, special attention should be given to the occurrence of AV blocks (binodal lesion).

► **Holter ECG.** The 24-hour Holter ECG is used to document the different arrhythmias that occur concomitantly or alternately and to clarify whether the arrhythmias correlate with symptoms. In this way, the Holter ECG is useful for making a decision whether a pacemaker is required.

► **Exercise ECG.** In sinus node dysfunction, there is *chronotropic incompetence*, that is, the increase in the heart rate in the stress ECG is not adequate. The reaction of the sinus node to stimulation by the autonomic nervous system remains insufficient.

Electrophysiology Study

In some cases, an electrophysiology study may be useful, for example, when clinical symptoms suggest significant bradycardia that was not documented in the (24-hour Holter) ECG.

A typical finding of sinus node dysfunction is a prolonged sinus node recovery time, namely the time until the sinus rhythm is resumed after previous high-frequency atrial stimulation is prolonged. The SA conduction time can also be determined in the examination.

Laboratory

Useful laboratory tests are serum electrolytes including K, Mg, Ca, and CK/CK-MB, troponin I, drug levels (e.g., digoxin, amiodarone), and TSH on a case-by-case basis.

Echocardiography

Echocardiography is used to rule out or detect congenital heart defects and to assess cardiac function. After surgery such as an atrial baffle procedure or Fontan procedure, echocardiography is performed for postoperative followup.

18.5.3 Treatment

Asymptomatic patients usually do not require treatment.

In patients whose main symptom is bradycardia, medication that reinforces sinus bradycardia (e.g., beta blockers) should be discontinued if tenable.

Patients with severe bradycardia and corresponding symptoms are treated with a permanent pacemaker. The choice of a pacemaker system depends on whether additional chronotropic incompetence or AV conduction disturbances are present and how often tachycardia episodes occur. Often, a DDD mode is selected, because an AV block often develops in patients with sinus node dysfunction and after Fontan or atrial baffle procedures. A frequency-adaptive system that allows for an increase in the heart rate during exercise ("rate-response" function) should also be selected for patients with chronotropic incompetence. Patients with frequent atrial tachycardias can be fitted with a special system with an atrial antitachycardia function that recognizes and attempts to terminate atrial tachycardia by atrial overstimulation.

Patients with tachycardia may require additional antiarrhythmic treatment. Class III antiarrhythmic drugs (sotalol, amiodarone) are usually used; a combination of amiodarone with a beta blocker may be required. Pharmacological lowering of the basic heart rate may require the implantation of a pacemaker for antibradycardia therapy.

See Chapter 18.16 and Chapter 18.17 for the pharmacological treatment of atrial flutter or fibrillation.

The acute treatment of severe bradycardia is intravenous atropine, orciprenaline, isoprenaline, or epinephrine or implantation of a temporary external or transvenous pacemaker.

18.5.4 Prognosis

The prognosis is good for symptomatic patients who have been treated with an appropriate pacemaker system and have good ventricular function. But the prognosis is worse for patients with impaired ventricular function. This applies to quite a few patients after an atrial baffle or Fontan procedure.

18.6 AV Junctional Escape Rhythm

18.6.1 Basics

Synonyms: AV escape rhythm, atrioventricular nodal rhythm

Definition

If the sinus node fails to function as a pacemaker or there is a higher-grade conduction disturbance between the sinus node and atrium, the AV nodal region can assume the pacemaker function. The heart rate of the AV junctional escape rhythm is usually about two-thirds to three-quarters of the normal age-appropriate heart rate. If there is only one single heart action, it is called AV escape systole.

Epidemiology

In sinus bradycardia (e.g., during sleep or in physically fit individuals), a junctional escape rhythm occurs physiologically, even in persons with a healthy heart.

Etiology

In the following situations, the AV region can assume the pacemaker function:

- Sinus bradycardia of various causes (good physical condition, high vagal tone, but also increased intracranial pressure, hypothermia)
- Sinus node dysfunction (e.g., postoperatively, especially after operations in the atrium)
- SA block
- Myocarditis
- Drug intoxication (e.g., digoxin)

18.6.2 Diagnostic Measures

Symptoms

The patients are usually asymptomatic; symptoms of bradycardia such as dizziness or palpitations are rare.

ECG

Since the origin of the AV junctional escape rhythm is in the region of the AV node or the bundle of His, atrium excitation is retrograde. The P waves are therefore negative in leads II, III, and aVF. The P wave may precede or follow the QRS complex. Often, the P waves are also "hidden" in the QRS complex and are not visible in the surface ECG. The former classification of upper, middle and lower AV escape rhythm depending on the position of the P wave before, in, or after the QRS complex is incorrect from an electrophysiological standpoint.

Since the excitation of the ventricles originates from a center above the bifurcation of the bundle of His, the *QRS complexes are narrow.* Unlike supraventricular extrasystoles, which come earlier than the expected sinus beat, the AV escape beats follow the *QRS complex later* than expected.

An additional typical finding of AV junctional escape rhythm is *AV dissociation*—that is, atria and ventricles beat independently. The atrial rate and the frequency of the AV escape rhythm are approximately equal, so that the P waves of the sinus rhythm oscillate around the QRS complexes of the AV escape rhythm (▶ Fig. 18.6).

An *echo beat* (*re-entrant systole*) may also develop: An AV junctional escape beat is transmitted to the ventricles simultaneously with retrograde excitation of the atrium. The ECG has a negative P wave following the QRS complex. In the atrium, the excitation changes direction and runs through the AV node toward the ventricle. If the ventricle is no longer refractory, a second ventricular systole develops. There is thus a negative P wave in the ECG surrounded by two QRS complexes.

▶ **Holter ECG.** A 24-hour Holter ECG is indicated to document the bradycardia episodes and correlate them with symptoms.

▶ **Exercise ECG.** In physiological bradycardia, there is an adequate increase of the heart rate under physical exertion. In these cases, the sinus node again takes over the pacemaker function. In some pathological causes (e.g., sinus node dysfunction), the heart rate does not increase.

Laboratory

Laboratory tests are indicated only occasionally, such as in cases of suspected electrolyte disorders, hypothyroidism, or drug intoxication.

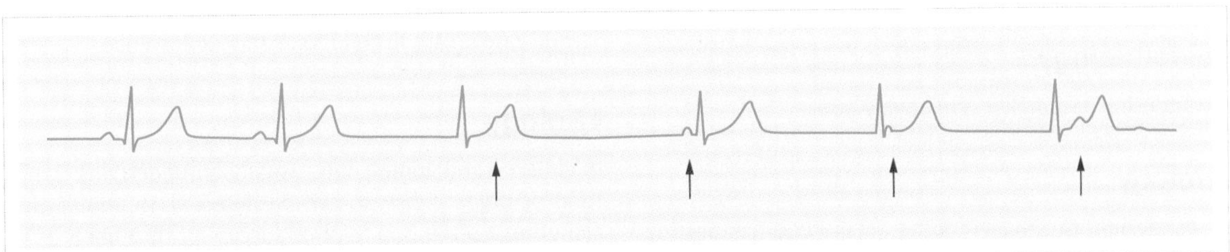

Fig. 18.6 AV junctional escape rhythm. In the ECG, after a long pause following the sinus rhythm, the AV junctional escape rhythm kicks in with narrow QRS complexes, after which AV dissociation develops. The P waves (arrows) oscillate around the QRS complexes because the atrial rate and the rate of the AV escape rhythm are similar.

Echocardiography

Echocardiography is sometimes useful for assessing cardiac function or investigating the causes of bradycardia.

Differential Diagnosis

In AV escape beats, supraventricular extrasystoles should be distinguished in the differential diagnosis. Unlike AV escape beats, the supraventricular extrasystoles come earlier than expected after the preceding sinus beat.

18.6.3 Treatment

The same principles apply to treatment as for sinus bradycardia. Asymptomatic patients do not require treatment. In secondary sinus bradycardia, the underlying cause is treated first.

For the acute treatment of sinus bradycardia, intravenous atropine, orciprenaline, isoprenaline, or epinephrine is administered in symptomatic patients. A temporary pacemaker may also be necessary.

After ruling out a treatable cause, symptomatic patients are treated with a permanent pacemaker (e.g., AAI or AAI-R system).

18.6.4 Prognosis

The prognosis depends on the underlying disease. If an underlying disease is ruled out, an AV junctional escape rhythm is not pathological in asymptomatic patients.

18.7 Wandering Pacemaker

18.7.1 Basics

Definition

A wandering pacemaker is said to exist when a secondary center in the atrium takes over the pacemaker function if there is a slow sinus node rate. In addition to the shape of the P wave, the PQ interval also changes between beats. These changes are explained by the fact that the pacemaker center "wanders" in the atrium.

Epidemiology

A wandering pacemaker is relatively rare.

Etiology

A wandering pacemaker occurs mainly in connection with sinus bradycardia and is observed with high vagal tone. A wandering pacemaker very rarely develops with sinus node dysfunction.

18.7.2 Diagnostic Measures

Symptoms

Patients are usually asymptomatic. Symptoms of bradycardia such as dizziness and palpitations are rare.

ECG

Different morphologies of the P waves can be noted in the ECG. For example, there is an increasing flattening of the P waves. In addition, the PQ interval changes (usually shortened). The rate remains approximately the same.

► **Holter ECG.** A 24-hour Holter ECG is occasionally indicated to document the bradycardia episodes and correlate them with the symptoms.

18.7.3 Treatment

Treatment is usually not indicated. Symptomatic bradycardia or sinus node dysfunction should be treated.

18.7.4 Prognosis

A wandering pacemaker is usually a benign rhythm disorder with no pathological significance in adolescents with increased vagal tone.

18.8 Accelerated Idioventricular Rhythm

18.8.1 Basics

Definition

In accelerated idioventricular rhythm, an ectopic automaticity center in the ventricular myocardium takes over the pacemaker function instead of the sinus rhythm. The heart rate is only slightly higher than the rate of the sinus rhythm.

Epidemiology

The disease is rare in childhood and adolescence.

Etiology

In children and adolescents, usually no underlying structural or organic disease can be detected. In adults, this arrhythmia often occurs after successful thrombolysis in the reperfusion phase after myocardial infarction. Rare causes include myocarditis or drug intoxication (e.g., digoxin).

Pathogenesis

The pathogenesis is not fully understood. It is assumed that it is caused by an abnormal automaticity in the ventricular myocardium.

18.8.2 Diagnostic Measures

Symptoms

Those affected are usually asymptomatic; they rarely have palpitations.

ECG

The ECG typically has bundle branch block–like widened ventricular complexes that have approximately the rate of the sinus rhythm. The ECG pattern shows the typical findings of a ventricular tachycardia, but the rate is much lower. There is AV dissociation or retrograde conduction from the ventricles into the atria (negative P waves after the QRS complexes).

Due to the similar rate, the sinus rhythm and accelerated idioventricular rhythm compete with each other, so that there is frequently a switch between the two rhythms. Fusion beats sometimes occur during the transition between the rhythms.

► **Holter ECG.** A 24-hour Holter ECG can detect which segments are marked by an accelerated idioventricular rhythm and which by a sinus rhythm. Ventricular extrasystoles can often be detected that have the same morphology as the beats of the idioventricular rhythm. Physical or emotional stress and an increase in heart rate can suppress the idioventricular rhythm.

► **Exercise ECG.** The idioventricular rhythm is typically replaced by a sinus rhythm under exertion.

Laboratory

Laboratory tests are usually not necessary. Sometimes they are indicated to rule out drug intoxication (e.g., digoxin.)

Echocardiography

Echocardiography may possibly be indicated to rule out (rare) structural or functional heart disease.

Differential Diagnoses

The following differential diagnoses must be ruled out:

- Ventricular tachycardia: In ventricular tachycardia, the rate is much higher than in accelerated idioventricular rhythm, which usually has nearly the same rate as the sinus rhythm.
- Third degree AV block with a ventricular escape rhythm: The rate in these cases is much slower than the sinus rhythm. The P waves in 3rd degree AV block have no regular relationship to the QRS complex.
- Ventricular escape rhythm with sinus arrest: In these cases, the rate is significantly slower than the sinus rhythm.

18.8.3 Therapy

No treatment is usually necessary. In rare cases where there is an organic or structural disease, this cause should be treated.

18.8.4 Prognosis

In most children and adolescents, the idioventricular rhythm subsides over time (but sometimes after years).

18.9 Supraventricular Extrasystoles

18.9.1 Basics

Definition

Supraventricular extrasystole(s) (SVES) is defined as an extrasystole with an origin above the bundle of His.

Epidemiology

SVES are very common and occur mostly in individuals with healthy hearts.

Etiology

In most cases, SVES are idiopathic in individuals with healthy hearts and have no pathological significance. SVES can also occur in the following disorders:

- Acquired heart disease (e.g., myocarditis, coronary artery disease)
- Congenital heart defects with atrial overload
- After atrial surgery (e.g., after Mustard or Senning atrial baffle procedures, Fontan procedure)
- Electrolyte imbalances (especially hypokalemia, hypomagnesemia, hypercalcemia)
- Drugs (e.g., antiarrhythmic drugs [proarrhythmogenic effect], digoxin, sympathomimetics)
- Stimulants/drugs: cocaine, caffeine, nicotine, alcohol
- Hyperthyroidism
- Acidosis, hypoxia

Pathogenesis

The automaticity center is located above the bundle of His.

Classification

SVES are classified according to their origin.

► **Sinus extrasystoles.** The excitation originates from the sinus node itself. The early P wave is identical in shape to the P waves of normal sinus beats and has the same vector as the sinus beats. After the extrasystole, the next sinus beat occurs at an interval equivalent to two normal sinus beats.

► **Atrial extrasystoles.** The premature P wave has a different shape than the P waves of sinus beats. It is often deformed or biphasic. Depending on the location of the excitation center in the atrium, the P vector is changed. The PQ interval varies in length depending on the distance to the AV node. The origin of the extrasystole is frequently in the lower segments of the atrium (negative P wave in leads II, III, aVF).

► **AV junctional extrasystoles.** The origin of the premature beats is located in the vicinity of the AV node. There is retrograde excitation of the atrium (negative P waves in leads II, III, aVF). The P wave comes before, in, or after the QRS complex. Formerly, a distinction was made between upper, middle, and lower AV nodal extrasystole. However, as the location of the origin of the extrasystole within the AV node area cannot be definitely determined based on the location of the P wave, this classification has been abandoned.

Excursus: Atrial bigeminy in fetuses and neonates

Atrial bigeminy is a special form of supraventricular extrasystole that occurs almost exclusively in fetuses and neonates. In atrial bigeminy, every second beat is an atrial extrasystole that meets refractory ventricle tissue and therefore does not result in ventricular excitation. That means that the ventricular rate is reduced to about half of the sinus rhythm. In the ECG, it can be seen that after the QRS complex of the sinus beat, there is a premature P wave that is not followed by a QRS complex. This is also called “blocked” atrial extrasystoles. Such “blocked” extrasystoles are important in the differential diagnosis of fetal or neonatal bradycardia. They usually disappear spontaneously over time and have a good prognosis.

18.9.2 Diagnostic Measures

Symptoms

The patients are usually asymptomatic; they rarely complain of palpitations. If there is a relevant disposition (accessory pathways, dual AV nodal physiology), SVES may trigger supraventricular tachycardias.

ECG

The typical features of SVES in the ECG are:

- Premature P waves that are often deformed and have a different P vector than the sinus beats.
- Usually no full compensatory pause: The interval between the sinus beat before and after the extrasystole is less than two normal R-R intervals. Explanation: The premature supraventricular extrasystole also depolarizes the sinus node. The next sinus beat then follows at the same interval of two normal sinus beats (► Fig. 18.7).
- Unremarkable narrow QRS complex: The QRS complex is usually narrow and not deformed. An exception is aberrantly conducted supraventricular extrasystoles. If a supraventricular extrasystole comes very early after a sinus beat, the ventricle may still be partially refractory and the QRS appears widened and has a bundle branch block pattern.

► **Holter ECG.** The 24-hour Holter ECG is used to assess the frequency of SVES and the effect of exercise on the SVES. Moreover, bursts and supraventricular tachycardia can be documented or ruled out. It is also used to assess the success of antiarrhythmic treatment.

► **Exercise ECG.** SVES that increase under exertion or in the recovery phase are classified as more significant than those that disappear under stress.

Differential Diagnosis

It is not always easy to differentiate between aberrantly conducted SVES and ventricular extrasystole(s) (VES). However, using the criteria listed below, the two can be reliably distinguished (► Fig. 18.8):

Typical features of aberrantly conducted SVES:

- Usually a deformed QRS complex as in a right bundle branch block. The refractory period of the left bundle branch is shorter than that of the right bundle branch, so that an SVES over the left bundle branch can often be normally transmitted, while it is still blocked in the right bundle branch.
- There is often triphasic QRS complex in V_1 (rsr′, rSR′, RSR′).
- The P wave can often be predicted in the preceding T wave.
- There is no full compensatory pause.
- The initial deflection of the extrasystole (initial vector, 10-ms vector) is identical to that of the sinus beat.

Typical features of VES:

- QRS complex in V_1 usually monophasic or biphasic
- No premature P wave
- Usually full compensatory pause
- The initial vector of the extrasystole has a different vector than that of the sinus beat.

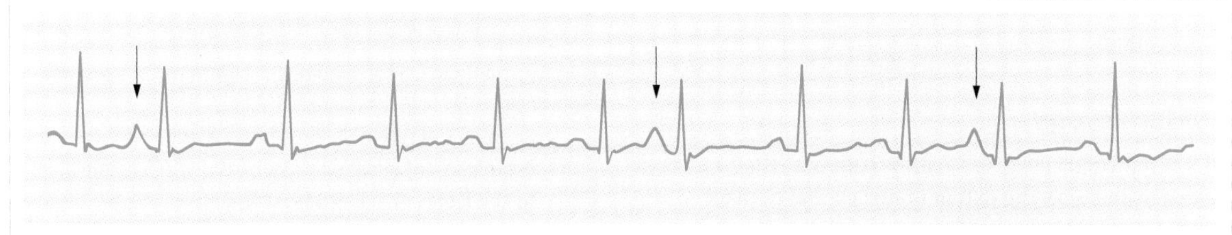

Fig. 18.7 Supraventricular extrasystole. In the ECG there is a premature P wave (arrows), followed by a narrow QRS complex with the same morphology as the QRS complexes of the sinus rhythm. The interval between the sinus beat before and after the extrasystoles is less than two normal R-R intervals (no full compensatory pause).

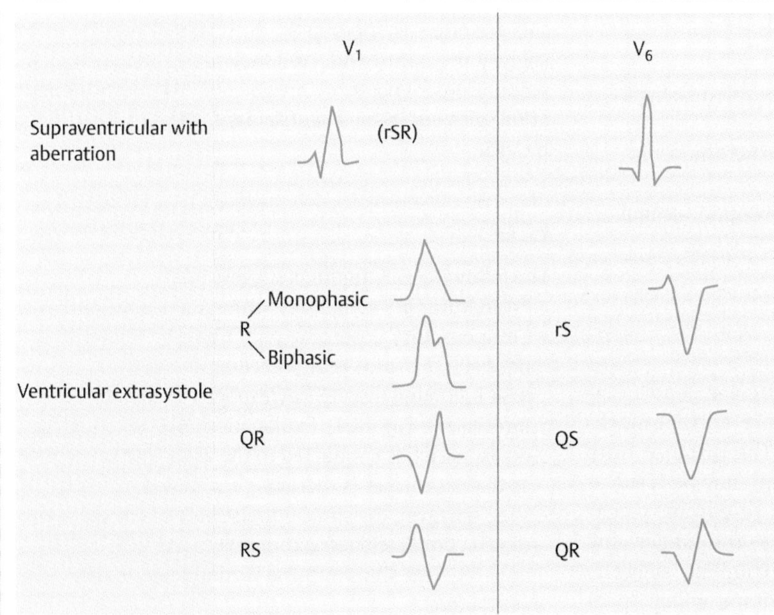

Fig. 18.8 Distinguishing between aberrantly conducted supraventricular (SVES) and ventricular (VES) extrasystoles. In aberrantly conducted SVES, the QRS complex in lead V_1 is usually triphasic, whereas in VES it tends to be monophasic or biphasic.[39]

Laboratory

If SVES are unusually frequent or if the diagnosis is suspected, the following laboratory tests may be useful: serum electrolytes including K, Mg, Ca, possibly CK/CK-MB, troponin I, TSH, drug screening and drug levels (e.g., theophylline, digoxin).

Echocardiography

Echocardiography can be used to rule out an underlying cardiac disease (e.g., heart defect, myocarditis), but it is not usually necessary.

18.9.3 Treatment

SVES in children with no structural heart defects that cause no symptoms or hemodynamic consequences do not need treatment.

In symptomatic patients, the underlying disease is first treated. Beta blockers are usually used as antiarrhythmic treatment. If this is unsuccessful or if beta blockers are contraindicated, class Ic antiarrhythmic drugs (e.g., propafenone), or class III (sotalol, amiodarone) can be used.

18.9.4 Prognosis

In asymptomatic children with no structural heart defects, SVES are usually not significant.

For blocked supraventricular extrasystoles (occurring primarily in fetuses and neonates as atrial bigeminy), a reduction of the ventricular rate may be hemodynamically significant.

18.10 Ventricular Extrasystoles

18.10.1 Basics

Definition

A ventricular extrasystole (VES) is defined as an extrasystole that has its origin in or below the bundle of His. In most cases, the origin is in the region of the ventricular myocardium.

Epidemiology

VES often occur even in healthy patients. They increase with age and with the extent of myocardial damage.

Etiology

VES are usually idiopathic in healthy patients, but they also occur in the following conditions:

- Heart disease such as cardiomyopathy, myocarditis, cardiac defects (particularly ventricular overload), and coronary heart disease
- Following cardiac surgery
- Electrolyte imbalance (especially hypokalemia, hypomagnesemia, hypercalcemia)
- Drugs such as antiarrhythmics (proarrhythmogenic effect!), digoxin, sympathomimetics
- Stimulants/drugs: cocaine, caffeine, nicotine, alcohol
- Hyperthyroidism
- Acidosis, hypoxia

Pathogenesis

VES is the result of premature ventricular depolarization due to increased automaticity, a re-entrant mechanism, or a triggered automaticity. The distance from the preceding QRS complex (coupling) may be fixed or variable. A fixed coupling suggests a re-entrant mechanism or triggered automaticity as the underlying pathogenic mechanism. A variable coupling suggests a more ectopic focus in the myocardium, which "produces" extrasystoles at its own rate (parasystolic automaticity).

Classification

VES are classified based on their morphology and frequency in relation to the sinus beats:

- Monomorphic (monotopic) VES: All QRS complexes of the VES have the same morphology.
- Polymorphic (polytopic) VES: QRS complexes of the VES have different morphologies.
- Bigeminy: Every sinus beat is followed by a VES.
- Trigeminy: A sinus beat is followed by two VES.
- 2:1 extrasystoles: Two sinus beats are followed by one VES.
- 3:1 extrasystoles: Three sinus beats are followed by one VES.
- Couplet: two consecutive VES.
- Triplet: three consecutive VES.
- Bursts: more than three consecutive VES.

Note

In German and US terminology, "trigeminy" is used differently:

- German definition: 1 sinus beat, 2 VES
- American definition: 2 sinus beats, 1 VES (equivalent to the German 2:1 extrasystoles).

18.10.2 Diagnostic Measures

Symptoms

VES are often asymptomatic, especially if the VES are only slightly premature. Affected individuals may complain of palpitations. Syncope or presyncope may occur in association with bursts or if ventricular tachycardia is triggered by VES.

ECG

The following ECG findings suggest VES:

- Premature QRS complexes without a preceding P wave.
- Compensatory postextrasystolic pause: The interval between the sinus beat preceding the VES and the sinus beat following the VES corresponds exactly to 2 R-R intervals (▶ Fig. 18.9). Explanation: In VES, no retrograde excitation is conducted to the atria. The sinus node as the pacemaker is therefore not at all affected by the VES; however, the sinus impulse spreads to a ventricle that is completely refractory due to the VES, so that only the next sinus impulse is conducted to the ventricle.
- Usually widened, bundle branch block pattern of the QRS complex: The more distal the origin of a VES, the more pronounced deformation and widening of the QRS complex are. In a right bundle branch block pattern of the QRS complex, the origin of the VES is likely in the left ventricle and vice versa.
- Discordant T wave: In VES, the T wave deflection is opposite to the deflection of the QRS complex.
- Combination systole / fusion beat: The QRS complex is formed as a mixture of the QRS complex of a sinus beat and a VES. The ventricles are thus partly depolarized by sinus beat and partly by the VES.
- Bundle of His extrasystole: Premature narrow QRS complex, full compensatory pause.

Interposed VES occur infrequently, usually in the context of sinus bradycardia: A VES is inserted between two sinus beats without affecting the sinus rhythm. In sinus bradycardia, after a VES, the ventricle can be excitable again for the next sinus impulse, so that no sinus beat is missed.

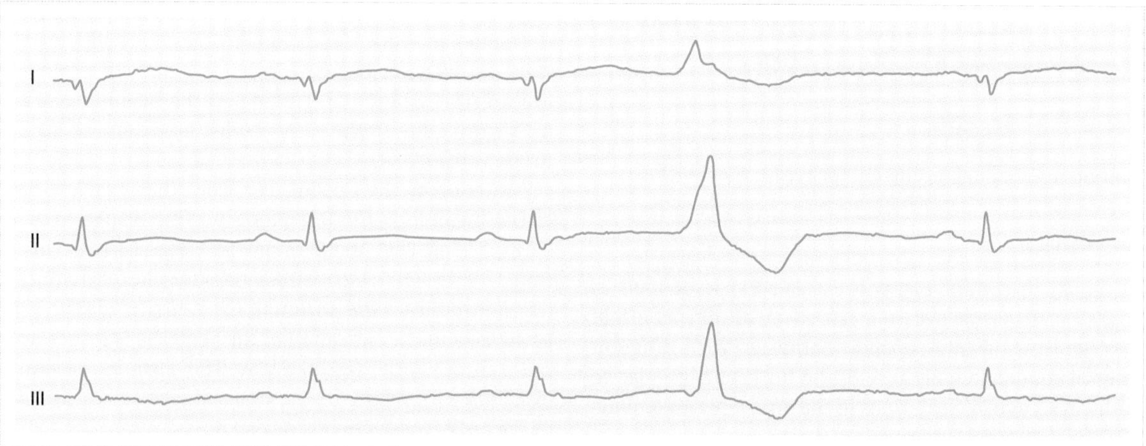

Fig. 18.9 Ventricular extrasystoles (VES). In the ECG there is a premature VES with a bundle branch block pattern of a widened QRS complex and a discordant T wave. The distance between the two sinus beats surrounding the VES corresponds exactly to 2 R-R intervals (full postextrasystolic compensatory pause).

▸ **Holter ECG.** A 24-hour Holter ECG may be conducted to investigate the following: assess the frequency of VES, assess the effect of physical exertion on the VES, rule out or detect bursts and ventricular tachycardia. It can also be used to monitor the success of antiarrhythmic treatment.

▸ **Exercise ECG.** VES that increase under stress or in the recovery phase are considered to be more severe than VES that disappear under stress (benign VES).

Differential Diagnosis

The distinction between an aberrantly conducted SVES and a VES is discussed in Chapter 18.9.

Laboratory

The following laboratory tests may be useful for frequent VES or associated tentative diagnosis: serum electrolytes including K, Mg, Ca, possibly TSH, CK/CK-MB, troponin I, drug screening, and drug levels (theophylline, digoxin).

Echocardiography

The echocardiography can rule out an underlying cardiac disease (e.g., cardiac defect, myocarditis, cardiac tumor).

MRI

An MRI may be indicated for VES and ventricular tachycardia to rule out arrhythmogenic right ventricular dysplasia (Chapter 17.4).

18.10.3 Treatment

In children with no structural heart defects, VES that do not cause symptoms or hemodynamic consequences require no therapy.

Children with symptomatic VES should be treated. The choice of medication depends on the underlying diseases:

- Patients with structurally and functionally healthy hearts: Class Ic antiarrhythmic agents (e.g., propafenone) or beta blockers often achieve success.
- Cardiomyopathy/arrhythmogenic right ventricular dysplasia: Beta blockers are the most promising.
- Complex heart defects (pre-/postoperative): Class III antiarrhythmic drugs (sotalol, amiodarone) are often required.

18.10.4 Prognosis

In asymptomatic children with no structural heart disease, VES are usually not significant. Single monomorphic VES that subside during exercise are generally harmless.

There is a higher risk if the following conditions are present:

- Structural heart disease
- History of syncopes or sudden cardiac death in the family
- VES triggered or increased in frequency by exercise
- Paroxysmal ventricular tachycardia

The *R-on-T phenomenon* appears to have no prognostic significance in children except in patients with a prolonged QT interval. The still frequently used Lown classification is of no prognostic value in children.

18.11 Atrioventricular Nodal Re-entrant Tachycardia

18.11.1 Basics

Synonym: AV nodal re-entrant tachycardia (AVNRT)

Definition

AV nodal re-entrant tachycardia (AVNRT) is defined as supraventricular tachycardia caused by an AV node that has two functionally separate pathways with different rates of conduction. Because of the functionally separate pathways, circular excitations in the atrioventricular node (AV nodal re-entry) may cause tachycardia.

Epidemiology

AV nodal re-entrant tachycardia is the second most common form of supraventricular tachycardia in children and adolescents and the most common form of supraventricular tachycardia in adults. AVNRT usually does not manifest until *adolescence*, rarely in schoolage children. AVNRT practically never occurs in neonates. The prevalence is about 2.25 per 1,000 people. Girls and women are more frequently affected.

Pathogenesis

In affected persons, the AV node has two functionally separate pathways: a fast and a slow conduction pathway. During normal sinus rhythm, excitation is conducted from the atrium to the ventricles only on the fast pathway. A supraventricular extrasystole can lead to a blockage of the fast pathway, so that the next excitation is conducted from the atrium to the ventricles via the slow pathway. In the ECG, there is a sudden prolongation of the PQ interval ("jump") at the beginning of the tachycardia due to the slow conduction from the atrium to the ventricle.

Excitation is then conducted from the ventricle back to the atrium via the fast pathway. This results in a re-entrant loop (AV nodal re-entry; ▶ Fig. 18.10). This is called "slow-fast" tachycardia because the excitation is transmitted from the atrium to the ventricle via the slow pathway and the excitation of the ventricle is returned to the atrium via the fast pathway. This form is present in over 90% of AVNRTs. In the unusual form of "fast-slow" tachycardia, conduction is reversed.

Classification

- "Slow-fast" tachycardia (more than 90% of cases): Conduction from the atrium to the ventricle is via the slow pathway, from the ventricle back to the atrium via the fast pathway.
- "Fast-slow"tachycardia (less than 10% of cases): Conduction from the atrium to the ventricle is via the fast pathway, from the ventricle back to the atrium via the slow pathway.

18.11.2 Diagnostic Measures

Symptoms

The symptoms depend on the heart rate during tachycardia and the duration of the tachycardia episodes. Typical symptoms during tachycardia are pallor, weakness,

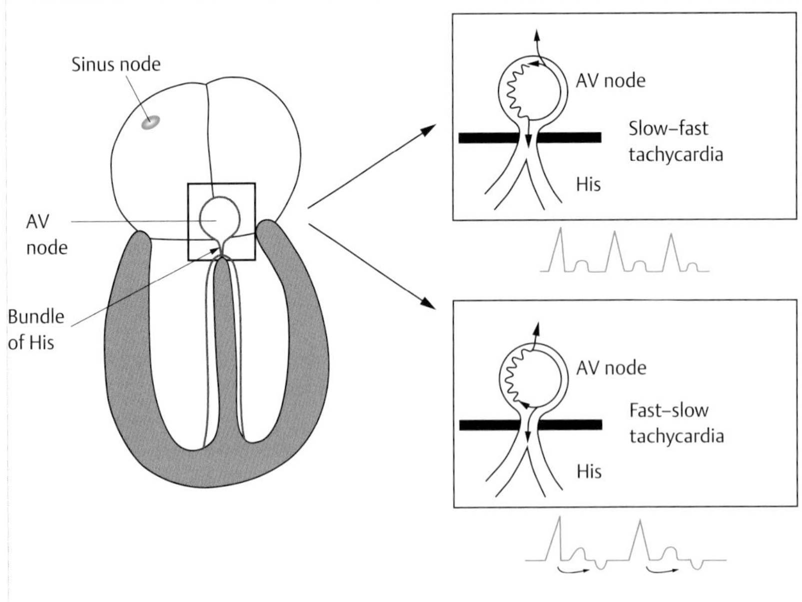

Fig. 18.10 Circular excitation in atrioventricular nodal re-entrant tachycardia (AVNRT). In "slow–fast" tachycardia (common form), excitation runs from the atrium to the ventricle via the fast pathway (wavy line) and excitation from the ventricle to the atrium via the slow pathway. Since there is rapid retrograde excitation of the atria, P waves are usually "hidden" in the QRS complex and are usually not visible in a surface ECG. In the rare "fast–slow" tachycardia, excitation is conducted from the atrium to the ventricle via the fast pathway, while excitation from the ventricle to the atrium is conducted via the slow pathway. Retrograde excitation of the atrium is thus slower, so the P waves follow the QRS complexes at some distance and are often visible in the surface ECG.

dyspnea, dizziness, discomfort, possibly angina if tachycardia is sustained, and rarely syncope.

A sudden onset and abrupt end of the tachycardia are typical.

ECG

During sinus rhythm, the ECG is normal. The PQ interval may be relatively short. In contrast to AV re-entrant tachycardia, there is no pre-excitation.

During the tachycardia, the following findings are typical, depending on the form of AVNRT:

► **"Slow-fast" tachycardia (common form).** The QRS complexes are narrow. Negative P waves may be found in leads II, III, and aVF very shortly following the QRS complex. In most cases, the P waves follow the QRS complex so fast that they are "hidden" in the QRS complex and cannot be detected in the surface ECG. The QP interval is usually shorter than 0.07 s. The heart rate is typically between 150 and 250 bpm.

► **"Fast-slow""tachycardia (unusual form).** The QRS complexes are also narrow. The P waves in leads II, III, and aVF are negative. Because of the slow spread of excitation from the ventricle to the atrium, the P waves follow the QRS complex late (RP interval > PR interval). The P waves are clearly visible between the QRS complexes and are located just before the next QRS complex. The heart rate is also 150 to 250 bpm. In the differential diagnosis, a permanent junctional re-entrant tachycardia (PJRT, Chapter 18.12) must be considered. In a PJRT, however, the heart rate during tachycardia is usually lower, but the tachycardia usually persists over long periods during the day in PJRT.

18.11.3 Treatment

Acute Treatment

In a hemodynamically unstable patient (rare), electrical cardioversion (synchronized with the QRS complex) with 0.5 J/kg is carried out under short anesthesia or deep conscious sedation. If this fails, the energy can be increased to 2 J/kg.

► **Vagal maneuvers.** However, most patients are generally hemodynamically stable and vagal maneuvers can first be attempted. The success rate for these measures is around 30 to 60%.

- Place a bag filled with ice water or a cool pack on the face for 15 to 30 s (always wrap ice bags or cool packs in a cloth).
- Induce a gag reflex
- In older children, Valsalva maneuver or abdominal pressure for 15 to 20 s
- Have patient drink ice water.

Table 18.6 Acute treatment of AV nodal re-entrant tachycardia (AVNRT) if vagal maneuvers and adenosine fail (from Paul et al. 2000)[93]

	Intravenous bolus	Continuous infusion
Flecainide	0.5–1 mg/kg	3–6 mg/kg/d
Amiodarone	5 mg/kg for 30–60 min	10–20 mg/kg/d
Propafenone	1–2 mg/kg	5–20 mg/kg/d
Verapamil (contraindicated in neonates and infants)	0.1 mg/kg	1–7 µg/kg/min
Transesophageal hyperstimulation		

- Unilateral carotid sinus massage
- Handstand

► **Adenosine.** If the vagal maneuvers fail, intravenous adenosine is used. Due to the extremely short half-life of adenosine, it must be injected quickly through a venous catheter placed as close to the heart as possible and flushed immediately afterward with NaCl 0.9%. Otherwise, adenosine is metabolized before it can affect the heart.

Initially 0.1 mg/kg is administered intravenously, if this fails, increase every 2 min up to a maximum 0.4 mg/kg as a single dose or 18 mg total dose (success rate 75–95%, but early recurrence of tachycardia occurs in about one-third of cases).

The side effects include flushing, nausea, vomiting, chest pain, dyspnea, bronchospasm, rarely arrhythmias, extremely rarely asystole or ventricular fibrillation (keep emergency equipment ready).

If adenosine fails, the drugs listed in ► Table 18.6 may be used.

Note

Caution: Verapamil is contraindicated as a bolus injection in newborns and infants (risk of electromechanical decoupling), but is safe and effective in school-age children and adolescents.

Digoxin can also be used for acute treatment, but it has the disadvantage that in most cases, high intravenous doses are required, which later leads to a very slow basic rhythm.

Adenosine is the drug of choice.

Long-term Pharmacological Treatment

There is an indication for long-term drug therapy in the following situations:

Table 18.7 Pharmacological prophylaxis of a recurrence of AV modal re-entrant tachycardia (AVNRT) (from Paul et al. 2000)[93]

Drug	Dosage	Remarks
Propafenone	5–20 mg/kg/d in 3–4 single doses	
Flecainide	1–8 mg/kg/d in 2–3 single doses	Note: proarrhythmogenic effect
Propranolol	2–6 mg/kg/d in 4 single doses	
Sotalol	2–8 mg/kg/d in 2–3 single doses	
Amiodarone	"Loading dose" 10 mg/kg/d in 1 single dose *for* 8–10 d, then 3–5 mg/kg/d in 1 single dose 5 days a week	Note: extracardiac side effects
Methyl digoxin	Maintenance: 10 µg/kg/d in 2 single doses	
Verapamil	2–7 mg/kg/d in 3 single doses	Not to be used as i.v. bolus in neonates and infants

- Recurrent persistent symptomatic AVNRT
- More than four supraventricular tachycardia episodes per year
- Recurrent, nonsustained AVNRT and the presence of a heart defect

The drugs that can be used to prevent the recurrence of AVNRT are listed in ▶ Table 18.7. In contrast to AVRT with an accessory conduction pathway, digoxin has proved to be successful in AVNRT. Beta blockers can also be used as an alternative. In case of failure, class Ic antiarrhythmics (e.g. propafenone, flecainide) or class III antiarrhythmics (sotalol, amiodarone) should be considered.

If treatment is not successful, the combination of a beta blocker with a class Ic antiarrhythmic drug or amiodarone may be useful.

Note

Unlike in AVRT with pre-excitation, digoxin and verapamil are not contraindicated in AVNRT.

Radiofrequency Ablation

In this method, the slow conductive pathway of the AV node is "ablated" in interventional catheterization by the local application of radiofrequency energy. Electrophysiologists call this "modulation" of the AV node.

The slow conductive pathway is modulated because the risk of inducing an AV block is clearly lower when this pathway is ablated.

Alternatively, cryoablation is sometimes used today. This is a new process, in which the arrhythmogenic substrate is iced (–75°C). The advantage of this method is that an initial reversible test icing is possible.

Radiofrequency ablation or cryoablation is indicated for recurrent symptomatic AVNRTs that do not respond to pharmacological treatment, or if pharmacological treatment is not tolerated.

These methods can usually be applied safely in patients weighing over 15 kg. The complication rate, however, is significantly higher in children weighing less than 15 kg. Meanwhile, catheter ablation has been established as a safe procedure, so today there is a broad indication for catheter ablation, especially in older children and adolescents.

18.11.4 Prognosis

There is practically no risk of sudden cardiac death in AVNRT in contrast to AVRT with an accessory pathway.

The success rate of the radiofrequency ablation is over 90%. The recurrence rate after electrophysiology intervention is about 3 to 5%. The risk of inducing an AV block as a result of the radiofrequency ablation is less than 1% for modulation of the slow pathway.

18.12 AV Re-entrant Tachycardia with an Accessory Pathway

18.12.1 Basics

Definition

AV re-entrant tachycardia with an accessory pathway (AVRT) is a supraventricular tachycardia that is partly caused by accessory pathways and is based on circular excitations (re-entry). An antegrade accessory conduction pathway (detectable delta wave on ECG) and the presence of supraventricular tachycardia is called Wolff-Parkinson–White syndrome (WPW syndrome).

Epidemiology

Accessory atrioventricular conduction pathways are the most common cause of supraventricular tachycardia in children. They usually occur without additional cardiac anomalies. They are sometimes are associated with heart

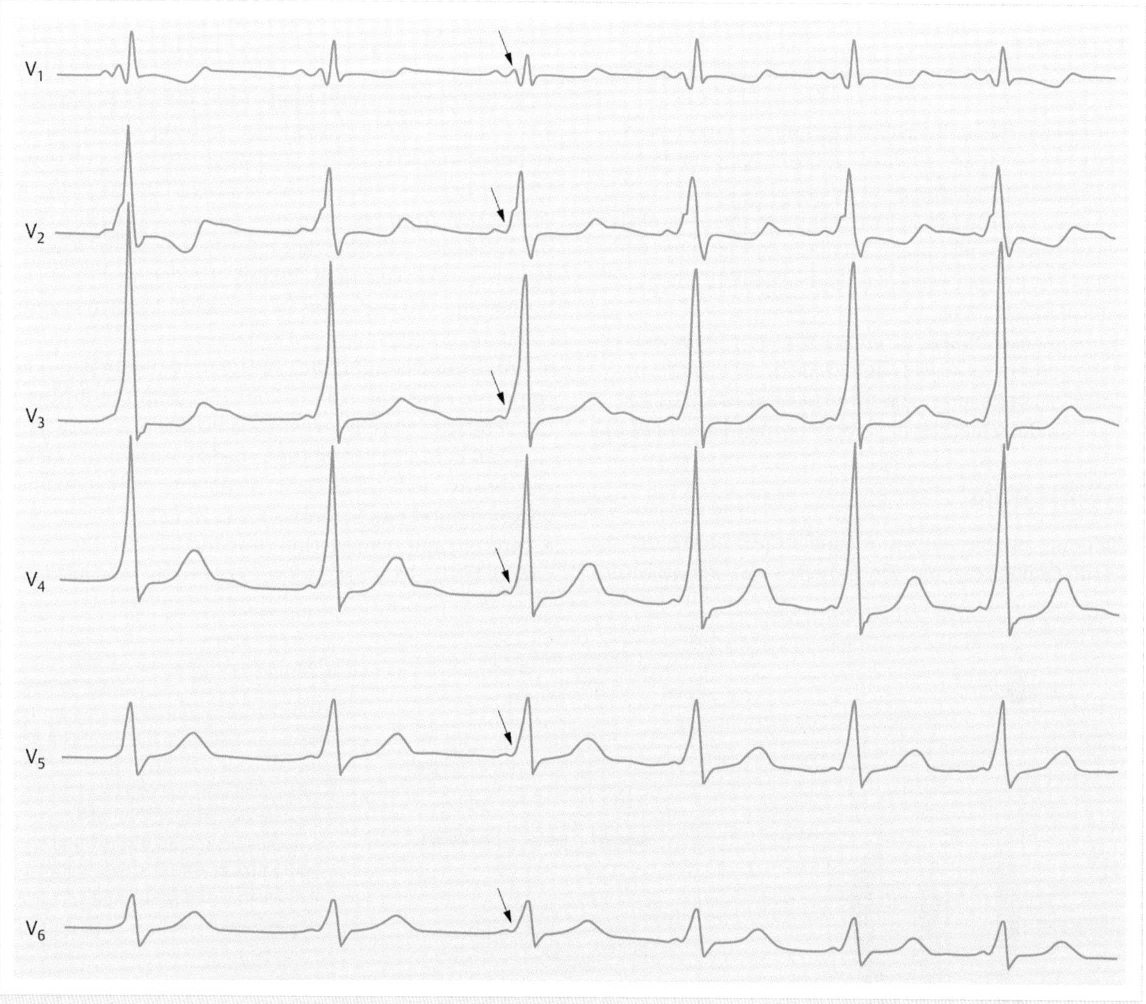

Fig. 18.11 Pre-excitation in the ECG. In this ECG of a patient with an Ebstein anomaly, there is clearly a delta wave at the beginning of the QRS complex (arrows) as well as a short PQ interval.

defects, mainly affecting the AV valve (Ebstein anomaly, tricuspid atresia, l-TGA). Boys are affected about twice as often as girls.

AVRT often manifests as early as the neonatal period. Other manifestation peaks occur in toddlerhood/adolescence and in young adulthood.

Pathogenesis

In an accessory conductive pathway, atrial excitation is conducted to the ventricular myocardium via two conduction pathways with different speeds. Conduction initially occurs via the rapid conduction accessory pathway. This is reflected in the surface ECG as a delta wave (pre-excitation) (▸ Fig. 18.11). In addition, atrial excitation is conducted to the ventricle normally through the slow conducting AV node. The result is a fusion beat. The PQ interval is shortened. The degree of the pre-excitation may vary in the same patient (accordion effect). The earlier the excitation is spread via the accessory pathway to the ventricular myocardium, the more pronounced are the repolarization disturbances in the ECG.

Whether the conduction proceeds from the atrium to the ventricle during the sinus rhythm mainly via the AV node or via accessory conduction pathway also depends on the autonomic tone. If the vagal tone is high (e.g., example during sleep), the conductivity of the AV node is reduced. The conduction then proceeds mainly via the accessory pathway (pronounced pre-excitation). When the sympathetic tone is high (e.g., during exercise), it is vice versa.

Due to an accessory conduction pathway, tachycardia may occur because of circular excitations (re-entry). The term "circular excitation" means that an electrical impulse circles around between the atrial and the ventricular myocardium by being conducted from the atrium to the ventricles via one pathway (AV node or accessory pathway) and from the ventricle back to the atrium via the other pathway. Since atrial excitation is retrograde in this circular excitation pattern, the P wave *comes after* the QRS complex.

The accessory pathways display the following individual properties:

- Location of the pathway: In principle, accessory pathways can be found anywhere at the AV valvular level. The exact location can be more precisely determined by the delta wave in the surface ECG or on the basis of the polarity of the QRS complex and the cardiac axis (see below). Some pathways (e.g., Mahaim fibers) show typical localizations.
- Direction of conduction: Some pathways can be bidirectional, others exclusively antegrade or retrograde.
- Speed of conduction: The speed of conduction can be fast (not decremental) or slow, delaying (decremental).

Classification

Depending on the nature of conduction during the re-entrant tachycardia and the properties of the accessory conduction pathway, the following types can be distinguished:

▸ **Orthodromic conduction.** This the most common form (about 80%). Conduction during tachycardia is orthodromic, that is, the excitation from the atrium to the ventricle takes the pathway through the AV node, and conduction from the ventricle back to the atrium is via the accessory pathway. Because the excitation from the atrium to the ventricle follows the "normal" pathway through the AV node, the QRS complex is narrow during tachycardia in this type (▸ Fig. 18.12).

▸ **Antidromic conduction.** Antidromic conduction is less common. Here, the conduction runs from the atrium to the ventricles during tachycardia via the accessory pathway and excitation from the ventricle back to the atrium via the AV node. The QRS complex is correspondingly widened during tachycardia (▸ Fig. 18.13).

▸ **Intermittent conduction.** Conduction via the accessory pathway (pre-excitation) occurs only intermittently.

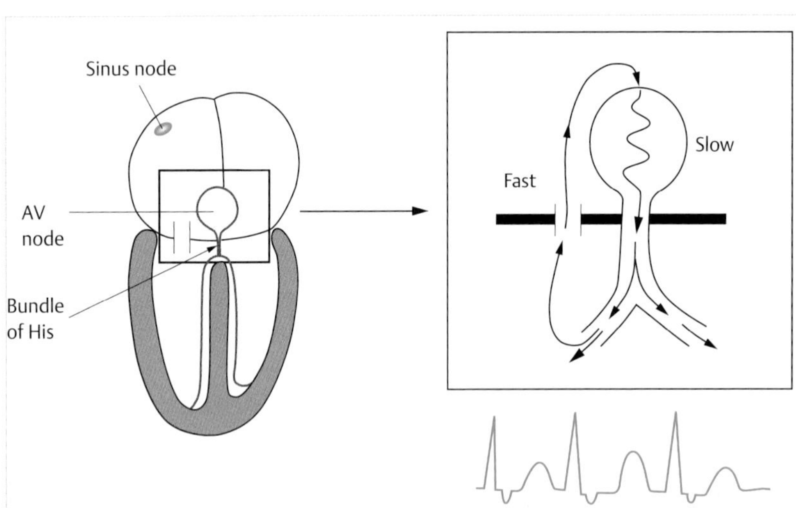

Fig. 18.12 Orthodromic conduction in AV re-entrant tachycardia (AVRT). In AVRT, orthodromic conduction is from the atrium to the ventricles via the AV node. During tachycardia, the QRS complexes are narrow. The retrograde excitation of the atrium proceeds via the accessory conduction pathway. The P waves follow shortly after the QRS complexes and are negative in leads II, III, and aVF.

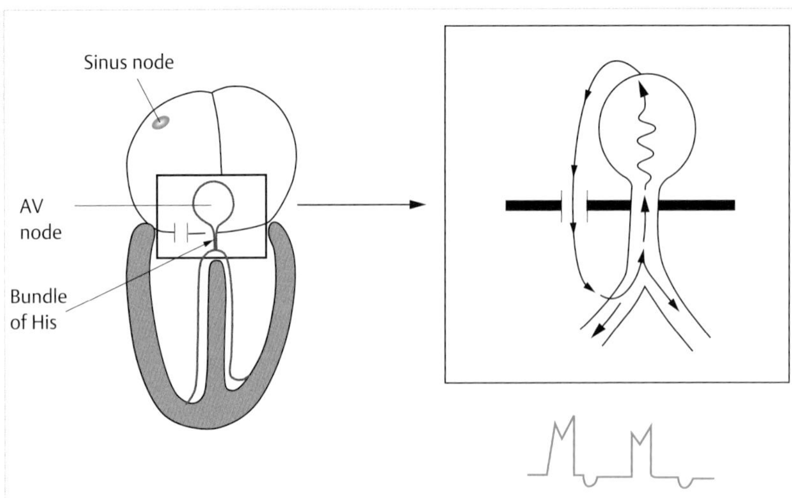

Fig. 18.13 Antidromic conduction in AV re-entrant tachycardia (AVRT). In AVRT, conduction is from the atrium to the ventricle via the accessory pathway. As one ventricle is excited considerably earlier than the other, the QRS complexes are widened as in a bundle branch block. Retrograde excitation of the atria occurs via the AV node. The P waves follow shortly after the QRS complex and are negative in leads II, III, and aVF.

A delta wave can therefore not always be detected in the ECG.

► **Concealed pathway.** If the accessory conduction pathway allows only retrograde conduction (i.e., from the ventricle to the atrium), it is a concealed accessory pathway. It is called a concealed accessory pathway because a delta wave in the surface ECG can never be detected. The ventricular complexes are narrow both during the sinus rhythm and during tachycardia. The incidence in children is assumed to be 50% of all accessory pathways. By contrast the "open" pathway is associated with pre-excitation in the surface ECG.

► **Conduction via Mahaim fibers.** The Mahaim fibers are an accessory pathway with only antegrade conduction and slowing and delaying conductive properties. Due to the slowing properties, pre-excitation is usually not very pronounced during the sinus rhythm. Because of the exclusive antegrade conduction via the accessory pathway, the QRS complexes are widened during tachycardia as in a bundle branch block.

► **Permanent junctional re-entrant tachycardia (PJRT).** This is a special form of re-entrant tachycardia. The accessory pathway allows only retrograde conduction and has slowing and strongly delaying properties. Often there is an orthodromic form of an AVRT that lasts over 12 hours per day ("permanent"). The QRS complexes are narrow. Due to the strong slowing conduction properties of the accessory pathway, the P waves do not follow the QRS complex until very late (RP/PR ratio > 1) and they are negative in leads II, III, and aVF (► Fig. 18.14). The heart rate during this form of tachycardia is usually much slower (usually between 120–180 bpm) in comparison with the other forms of AVRT. There is usually a long accessory pathway from the tricuspid valve annulus to the myocardium or to the fascicles of the right ventricle.

Note

A PJRT often remains undetected for a long time because of the relatively slow heart rate for tachycardia.

18.12.2 Diagnostic Measures

Symptoms

The symptoms depend on the heart rate during tachycardia and the duration of the tachycardia episodes.

The following symptoms may occur during tachycardia: pallor, weakness, dyspnea, dizziness, discomfort, possibly angina if there is a longer period of tachycardia, rarely syncopes.

A PJRT is often discovered only as an incidental finding in the ECG because of the relatively slow heart rates.

18.12.3 Complications

A much-feared complication is the induction of ventricular fibrillation. This risk exists in patients with (intermittent) atrial fibrillation and a very short refractory period of the accessory pathway (below 220 ms). In these cases, the high atrial frequencies of atrial fibrillation can be transmitted "unchecked" to the ventricles via the accessory pathway and induce ventricular fibrillation.

Also, a tachycardia-induced cardiomyopathy can develop in a long-standing tachycardia. This complication is not uncommon in patients with a PJRT that often remains undetected for a long time.

Note

If ventricular function is impaired, sustained tachycardia must always be ruled out as the cause. This condition is called tachycardia-induced cardiomyopathy.

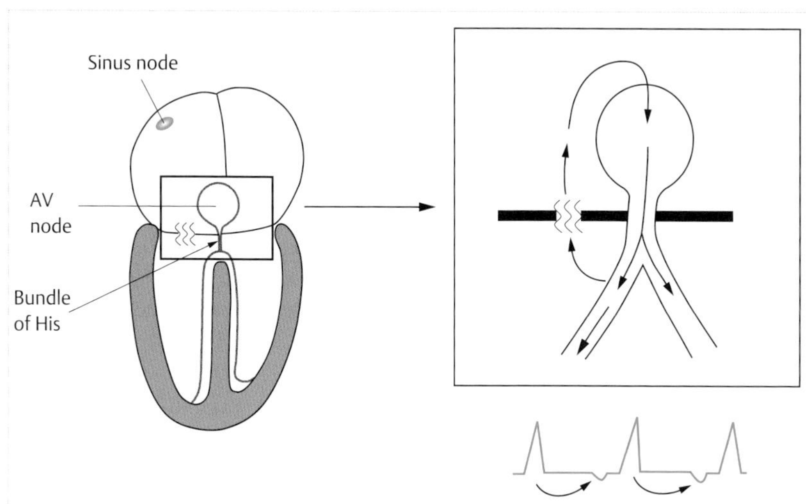

Fig. 18.14 Permanent junctional re-entrant tachycardia (PJRT). In PJRT, the accessory conduction pathway has strong delaying properties. In addition, the accessory pathway allows only retrograde conduction. The excitation from the atria to the ventricles runs via the AV node. The QRS complexes are narrow. The retrograde excitation of the atria occurs slowly via the accessory pathway. Correspondingly, the P waves follow the QRS complexes late, and they are negative in leads II, III, and aVF.

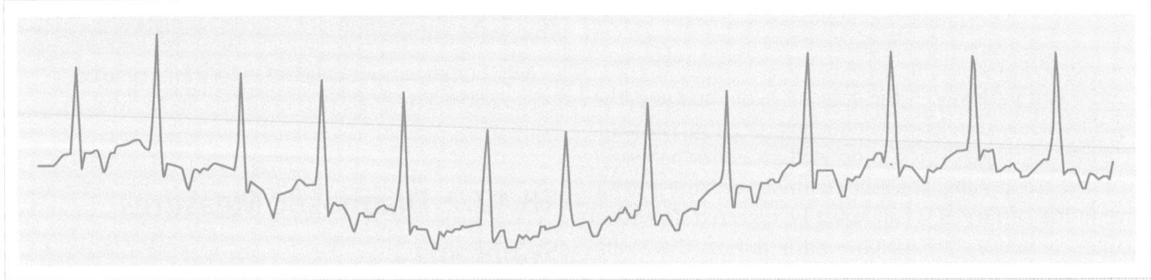

Fig. 18.15 AV re-entrant tachycardia (AVRT) with orthodromic conduction via an accessory pathway. The tachycardia is characterized by a narrow QRS complex. P waves follow shortly after the QRS complexes and are negative.

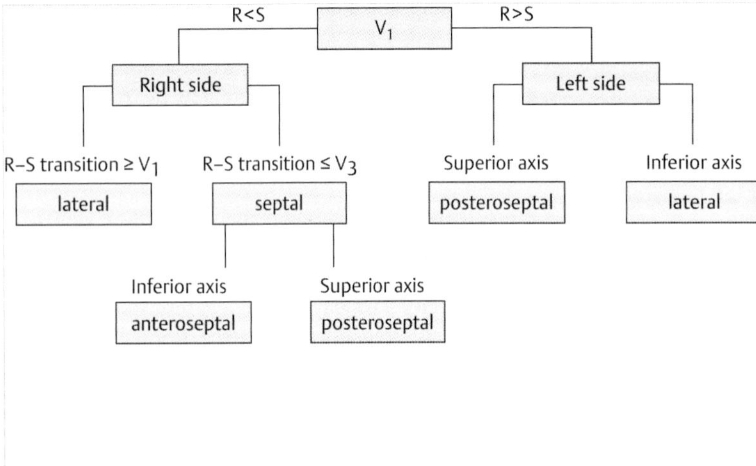

Fig. 18.16 Algorithm for locating an accessory pathway on the basis of the surface ECG.[26] There are numerous algorithms for locating accessory pathways on the basis of the surface ECG. The simplified algorithm uses the polarity of the QRS complex (R < S or R > S) in lead V_1, the R-S transition point in the chest leads, and the cardiac axis of the QRS complex. In the rare cases where the R-S transition is between V_3 and V_4, the right accessory pathway may be in a lateral or septal location.
Rule of thumb: If there is a predominantly positive QRS complex in V_1, the accessory pathway is located on the left side; in a predominantly negative QRS complex in V_1, the pathway is on the right side.

ECG

The typical ECG findings for the different conduction pathways are listed below:

- Orthodromic conduction:
  - *Sinus rhythm:* short PQ interval, widened QRS complex with a delta wave
  - *Tachycardia:* normal width of the QRS complex (▶ Fig. 18.15), no delta wave present, P wave follows shortly after QRS complex (negative in leads II, III, aVF), typical heart rate 180–250 bpm
- Antidromic conduction:
  - *Sinus rhythm*: short PQ interval, widened QRS complex with a delta wave
  - *Tachycardia*: widened QRS complex, P wave follows shortly after the QRS complex (but not usually detectable), typical heart rate 180–250 bpm
- Concealed conduction pathway:
  - *Sinus rhythm:* normal PQ interval, normal QRS complex with no delta wave
  - *Tachycardia:* normal width of the QRS complex, P wave follows shortly after the QRS complex (negative in II, III, aVF), typical heart rate 180–250 bpm
- Mahaim fiber:
  - *Sinus rhythm:* normal PQ interval, widened QRS complex with a delta wave
  - *Tachycardia:* widened QRS complex (left bundle branch block pattern), P wave before the QRS complex, typical heart rate 180–250 bpm
- Permanent junctional re-entrant tachycardia (PJRT):
  - *Sinus rhythm* (usually only a few hours per day): normal PQ interval, normal QRS complex without delta wave
  - *Tachycardia* (during most of the day): normal width of the QRS complex, P wave follows very late after the QRS complex (ratio RP/PR > 1), negative P wave in leads II, III, aVF. Typical heart rate relatively low (120–180 bpm)

▶ **Location of the accessory pathway.** The location of the accessory pathway can be narrowed down for orientation purposes according to the polarity of the delta wave and the QRS complexes in the surface ECG (▶ Fig. 18.16).

▶ **Exercise ECG.** Pre-excitation that disappears under exertion suggests a low risk to the patient. In these patients, the effective refractory period of the accessory pathway is likely to be relatively long.

Electrophysiology Study

One use of the electrophysiology study is to determine the precise location of the accessory pathway. The effective refractory period, which provides information on the risk of suffering ventricular fibrillation or sudden cardiac death, can also be determined. Radiofrequency ablation of the accessory pathway may be performed in the same session.

18.12.4 Treatment

Acute Treatment

The acute treatment of AVRT with an accessory pathway is the same as for AVNRT (Chapter 18.11).

Long-term Pharmacological Treatment

The indications for long-term pharmacological treatment vary with age.

In *neonates and infants*, relapse prevention treatment is carried out after the first tachycardia episode. Without long-term medication, the risk of recurrence in this age group is above 90%. Because of the high spontaneous cure rate within the first year of life, a treatment-free interval can be attempted if the patient has had no recurrence for one year.

In *older children*, long-term therapy is required after two tachycardia episodes requiring pharmacological treatment within 6 months or if the children are greatly endangered by tachycardia, syncope, or presyncope. In chronic or permanent tachycardia, long-term treatment is necessary to prevent tachycardia-induced cardiomyopathy.

► **Choice of drug.** Long-term treatment is initiated with monotherapy of a class Ic antiarrhythmic agent, a beta blocker, or a class III antiarrhythmic agent. If this treatment is not sufficiently successful, the combination of a beta blocker with a class Ic antiarrhythmic agent or amiodarone can be useful. In patients without pre-excitation, treatment is often limited to monotherapy with digoxin or a combination of digoxin with another antiarrhythmic agent.

Note

Caution: Digoxin and verapamil are contraindicated in classic pre-excitation due to a possible shortening of the effective refractory period of the antegrade accessory pathway.

Radiofrequency Ablation

In radiofrequency ablation, the accessory pathway is "ablated" by radiofrequency energy in interventional catheterization. Radiofrequency ablation is a safe procedure in children weighing over 15 kg. For smaller children, the complication rate is higher.

The following are considered indications for radiofrequency ablation:

- WPW syndrome after successful resuscitation
- WPW syndrome with a high risk of sudden cardiac death. A high risk is assumed after syncope and rapid conduction via the accessory pathway (effective refractory period < 220 ms or QRS interval < 220 ms in patients with atrial fibrillation)
- Poor left ventricular function as a result of tachycardia-induced cardiomyopathy

Other indications include children and adolescents over 15 kg with frequent symptomatic tachycardias refractory to antiarrhythmic therapy. Many centers also offer elective radiofrequency ablation as an alternative to long-term antiarrhythmic treatment.

The value of radiofrequency ablation in patients with pre-excitation in the ECG without tachycardia is not yet fully known.

Radiofrequency and cryoablation have been established as safe procedures, so that especially in older children weighing more than 15 kg and adolescents, there is a tendency toward a broad indication for ablation of the accessory pathway.

18.12.5 Prognosis

In infants under 1 year, the spontaneous cure rate through fibrotic changes of the accessory pathway is 85%; in children aged 5 years it is only 20%. The success rate of interventional catheter radiofrequency ablation of the accessory pathway is over 95% in children and adolescents. Pharmacological treatment of a WPW syndrome with propafenone has a success rate of about 80%. In a PJRT, long-term pharmacological treatment is usually much more difficult. Treatment is often limited to lowering the heart rate with medication.

The risk of sudden cardiac death in patients with an accessory pathway depends mainly on the effective refractory period of the accessory pathway. The shorter the effective refractory period, the more vulnerable the patient is. The critical level for children is 220 ms.

- The following suggest a *low risk*:
  - Intermittent pre-excitation in the surface ECG. There is a long effective refractory period of the accessory pathway.
  - Disappearance of the pre-excitation during exercise
  - In atrial fibrillation, the distances between the QRS complexes are greater than 220 ms. This means that the effective refractory period of the accessory pathway is longer than 220 ms.
- The following suggest a *high risk*:
  - History of presyncope, syncope, or resuscitation
  - Permanent pre-excitation in the surface ECG

- Persistence of the pre-excitation during exercise
- In atrial fibrillation, the intervals between the QRS complexes are shorter than 220 ms. This means that the effective refractory period is shorter than 220 ms. Due to the rapid conduction of the atrial impulses, high ventricular frequencies may occur in atrial fibrillation that may develop into ventricular fibrillation.

18.13 Ectopic Atrial Tachycardia

18.13.1 Basics

Synonym: focal atrial tachycardia (FAT)

Definition

Ectopic atrial tachycardia (EAT) is triggered by a focus with increased automaticity located in the atria outside the sinus node (▶ Fig. 18.17). The focus is affected by impulses from the autonomic nervous system, so there is diurnal and stress-related variation of the heart rate during tachycardia.

Epidemiology

EAT represents less than 10% of all supraventricular tachycardias.

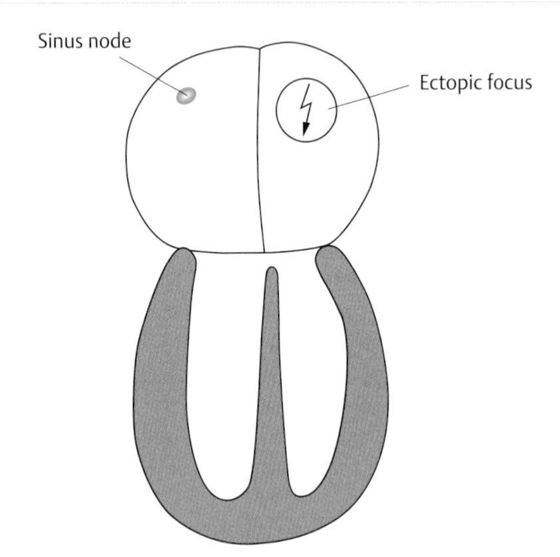

Fig. 18.17 Ectopic atrial tachycardia (EAT). In EAT, the focus of the tachycardia is located in the atrium outside the sinus node.

Etiology

Often no structural cardiac anomaly is detected. Sometimes EAT occurs after operations in the atrial area (Fontan procedure, atrial baffle procedure, ASD closure, correction of anomalous pulmonary venous connection). It is rarely caused by myocarditis or cardiac tumors.

Pathogenesis

EAT is caused by increased automaticity of the atrial cells. These cells are often located in the vicinity of the sinus node or in the left atrium in the vicinity of the ostium of the pulmonary vein, but theoretically, they can be present anywhere in the atria.

18.13.2 Diagnostic Measures

Symptoms

Depending on the frequency of the tachycardia, EAT may remain asymptomatic or only rarely cause symptoms such as palpitations and dizziness. Similar to a permanent junctional tachycardia (Chapter 18.12), a long-lasting EAT impairs cardiac function and leads to the clinical picture of a tachycardia-induced cardiomyopathy.

Note

When investigating heart failure or cardiomyopathy, an EAT should not be overlooked or confused with a sinus tachycardia. Cardiac function can recover after successful treatment of an EAT.

ECG

The morphology of the P waves in an EAT differs from that of a sinus rhythm. Depending on the location of the ectopic focus, there may be only slight changes. The atrial rate is usually between 150 and 200 bpm and is therefore often only slightly above the age-appropriate norm. However, the heart rate at rest is usually inadequately high and continues to increase under stress. A slow gradual increase in the heart rate at the beginning of the tachycardia ("warming up") and a similar slow decline in the heart rate at the end ("cooling down") are typical. Often there is a 1st or 2nd degree AV block during tachycardia.

Especially during sleep, the rate often switches to a sinus rhythm. Particular attention should be given to possible differences in P wave morphology during sleep and during the tachycardia episodes.

▶ **Holter ECG.** The 24-hr Holter ECG can be used to document the tachycardia episodes and compare the P wave morphology between tachycardia and the sinus rhythm.

▶ **Exercise ECG.** EAT typically results in an increase in the heart rate under exertion.

Electrophysiology Study

An ectopic focus can be located ("mapping") in the electrophysiological study. In older children and persistent cases, catheter ablation of the focus may be performed.

Laboratory

Laboratory tests are performed to rule out differential diagnoses as the cause of sinus tachycardia. Factors that must be ruled out include anemia, electrolyte imbalances, myocarditis, hyperthyroidism, and drug intoxication.

Echocardiography

Echocardiography is performed to assess cardiac function and to rule out structural anomalies (heart tumor).

Differential Diagnosis

It is often difficult to distinguish EAT from sinus tachycardia and may require, for example, a detailed analysis of the P wave morphology. Other supraventricular tachycardias, in particular a PJRT, are possible differential diagnoses.

18.13.3 Treatment

EAT usually cannot be terminated for a longer period with adenosine, cardioversion, or atrial overstimulation. However, adenosine can be used to make the differential diagnosis: After administering adenosine, an AV block can be detected, but the ectopic atrial focus remains unaffected. However, adenosine leads to a brief sinus bradycardia at the sinus node level.

The aim of drug therapy is to slow down the heart rate by influencing the ectopic focus directly or by slowing down AV conduction. Beta blockers or class III antiarrhythmics (amiodarone, sotalol) are usually used.

In otherwise refractory cases, catheter ablation of the focus may be considered in older children.

18.13.4 Prognosis

Particularly in neonates, infants, and toddlers, the spontaneous cure rate is quite high, so these patients can be given medication and a wait-and-see approach applied. On the other hand, pharmacological treatment is often difficult, so that in older children, catheter ablation of the focus should be considered. After effective treatment of tachycardia, any previously impaired cardiac function almost always recovers.

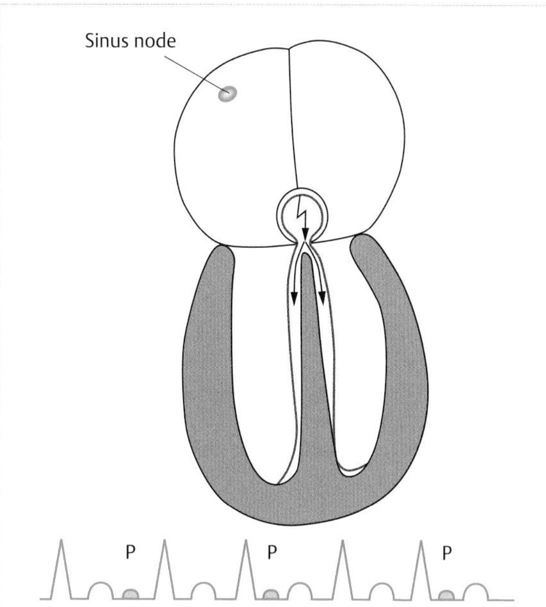

Fig. 18.18 Junctional ectopic tachycardia (JET). In JET, there is a fast ectopic impulse in the region of the AV node or proximal bundle of His. The excitation is usually not conducted from the AV nodal region to the atria. The atria and the ventricles each beat independently of the other (AV dissociation). A JET is a typical problem in the early postoperative period after cardiac surgery.

18.14 Junctional Ectopic Tachycardia

18.14.1 Basics

Definition

In junctional ectopic tachycardia (JET), there is an ectopic impulse center in the region of the AV node or the proximal bundle of His (▶ Fig. 18.18). Ventricular excitation follows this from this ectopic center. Usually there is no retrograde conduction to the atria; excitation of the atria originates from the sinus node independently of the ventricles. AV dissociation occurs and atria and ventricles each beat independently of the other. A JET occurs mainly in the early phase after cardiac surgery.

Epidemiology

JET is very rare in individuals with a healthy heart; it occurs especially in neonates and has a high familial incidence. After heart surgery, JET is a greatly feared complication and usually occurs postoperatively in the warming-up period after cardiopulmonary bypass or within the first 24 hours after surgery.

Etiology

- Cardiopulmonary bypass surgery (e.g., after correction of tetralogy of Fallot)
- Idiopathic, particularly in neonates and young infants, familial clustering described
- Very rarely myocarditis or drug intoxication (e.g., digoxin)

Pathogenesis

The cause is an ectopic automaticity center in the AV node or proximal bundle of His. In the postoperative form, a direct trauma of the AV node, an inadequate reaction to reperfusion after cardiopulmonary bypass, or the effect of anesthetics are some of the factors that have been discussed as possible triggers.

18.14.2 Diagnostic Measures

Symptoms

Patients often have severe hemodynamic impairment from the JET. Especially in the postoperative period, patients may rapidly develop cardiac decompensation as a result of uncoordinated atrial and ventricular activity, tachycardia, and increased oxygen consumption.

ECG

In a healthy neonate, the ventricular rate in JET is usually between 170 and 250 bpm. In the postoperative form, ventricular rates may be as high as 300 bpm. Since the ventricles are stimulated by an automaticity center above the bifurcation of the bundle of His, the QRS complexes are narrow. They are widened only if there is a pre-existing bundle branch block. Irrespective of the QRS complexes, P waves arising from the sinus node with the slower sinus rhythm rate can be detected. There is thus AV dissociation, where the ventricles beat faster than the atrium. In the post-op setting the external pacing wires can be used for diagnostic purposes to obtain an atrial ECG. Only rarely is retrograde excitation conducted from the ventricles to the atria. Then a P wave, which is negative in leads II, III, and aVF, can be detected after the QRS complex. Occasionally there are "capture beats," which are ventricular systoles that are "captured" by the atrial activity.

▸ **Holter ECG.** Permanent tachycardia can usually be detected. The 24-hr Holter ECG is also used for monitoring antiarrhythmic treatment.

Electrophysiology Study

In some treatment-refractory individuals, ablation of the ectopic automaticity center may be considered, but this method is not an option for the postoperative form.

Laboratory

Laboratory tests may possibly rule out myocarditis and drug intoxication (digoxin).

Echocardiography

Echocardiography is useful for assessing myocardial function.

Differential Diagnosis

The following tachycardias are possible differential diagnoses:

- Sinus tachycardia: In a sinus tachycardia, there is no AV dissociation.
- AVNRT, AVRT: In AVNRT or AVRT, the P waves are hidden in the QRS complex or follow shortly after the complex. The P waves are negative in leads II, III, and aVF.
- EAT, MAT: In EAT or MAT, there are different P wave morphologies. No AV dissociation is present.

18.14.3 Therapy

In both the congenital and the postoperative form, the most common antiarrhythmic drugs are not effective. Frequently, only the ventricular rate can be reduced in order to stabilize the condition. In the congenital form, amiodarone is the most effective drug. Catheter ablation of the ectopic focus may be considered in refractory cases.

In the postoperative form, the following procedure has proven effective:

- Amiodarone: Amiodarone has been found to be the most effective pharmacological treatment of postoperative JET. It is often only possible to lower the JET rate, but this can then make effective AV sequential pacemaker stimulation possible.
- Initially, an intravenous bolus or short infusion of 5 mg/kg is administered over 30 to 60 min, followed by a continuous infusion of 10 to 20 mg/kg/d. The bolus can be repeated two or three times if needed.
- Catecholamines should be reduced or discontinued if hemodynamically possible (proarrhythmogenic effect of catecholamines).
- Atrial pacing: The temporary epicardial pacemaker wires that are routinely implanted intraoperatively

make AV sequential pacing possible. An atrial rate is selected higher than the JET rate so the atrial and ventricular contractions are coordinated again. The disadvantage is that a very high, abnormal atrial pacing rate is usually required.

Cooling the patient was formerly often recommended for reducing the rate. Because of improved treatment options, this measure is now rarely necessary.

18.14.4 Prognosis

In healthy newborns with congenital JET, spontaneous remission of the tachycardia usually occurs within the first year of life, but drug therapy is difficult until then. In most cases, medication does not lead to a conversion to sinus rhythm; it can only reduce the ventricular rate.

Postoperative JET is a dreaded complication after cardiopulmonary bypass surgery and, if left untreated, has a high mortality rate in the early postoperative period. After 24 to 72 hours, there is usually spontaneous remission. Until then, the patient must be stabilized with the measures described above.

After a JET, there is possibly an increased risk of developing an AV block at a later stage, so a 24-hour Holter ECG follow-up is recommended.

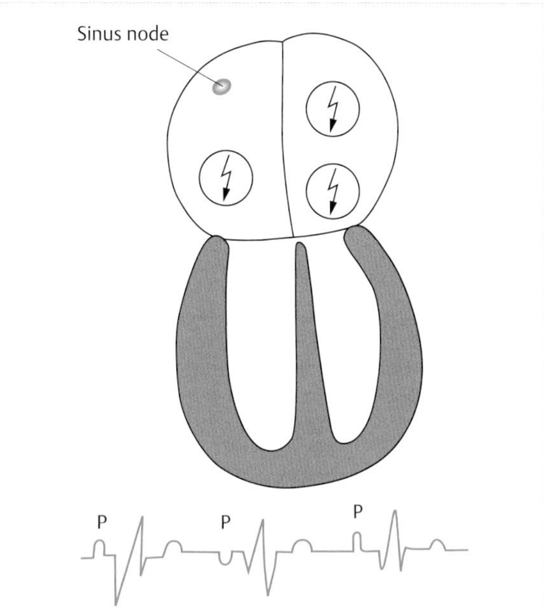

Fig. 18.19 Multifocal atrial tachycardia (MAT). In MAT, there are at least three other ectopic impulse centers apart from the sinus node. The morphology of the P waves in the ECG is correspondingly varied. The P-R interval varies in length depending on the location of ectopic centers.

18.15 Multifocal Atrial Tachycardia

18.15.1 Basics

Synonym: chaotic atrial tachycardia (CAT)

Definition

In multifocal atrial tachycardia (MAT), there are at least three different ectopic impulse centers in the atrium apart from the sinus node (▶ Fig. 18.19). Accordingly, at least three different P wave morphologies can be detected in the ECG in addition to the sinus rhythm P wave.

Epidemiology

MAT is very rare. It can be found in all age groups, but is most common in newborns.

Etiology

Usually no structural heart disease is detected. In elderly patients, it is often associated with pulmonary diseases that lead to right atrial overload (pulmonary hypertension, bronchopulmonary dysplasia, pulmonary embolism, pneumonia). Other causes of MAT are:

- Cardiac surgery
- Cardiac tumors
- Myocarditis
- Drugs (e.g., theophylline, digoxin)
- Hypoxia, acidosis, electrolyte imbalances
- Virus infection with accompanying myocarditis

Pathogenesis

There are probably multiple atrial centers with increased automaticity present in MAT. Atrial myocarditis has also been discussed.

18.15.2 Diagnostic Measures

Symptoms

Tachycardia is usually well tolerated. Depending on the frequency of tachycardia, symptoms such as palpitations or dizziness sometimes occur. In long-standing tachycardia, the ventricular function may deteriorate and in these cases, a tachycardia-induced cardiomyopathy may develop.

ECG

Different P waves (usually best seen in leads II, III, and V_1), variable PQ intervals and P-P segments, and variable AV transitions are typical. Depending on the heart rate, conduction can be sometimes aberrant, so that the QRS complexes that follow may have a bundle branch block pattern. The atrial rate is highly variable and is usually between 100 and 300 bpm. These findings lead to great variation in the ECG. Accordingly, the MAT is also called chaotic atrial tachycardia (CAT).

▸ **Holter ECG.** The 24-hour Holter ECG is used to document the tachycardia phases and to assess the different P wave morphologies.

Electrophysiology Study

Catheter ablation is usually not an option because of the multiple centers.

Laboratory

Laboratory tests are used to rule out electrolyte imbalances, myocarditis, and drug intoxication e.g., (theophylline, digoxin).

Echocardiography

Echocardiography is useful for assessing cardiac function and ruling out structural anomalies (heart tumor).

Differential Diagnosis

The following supraventricular rhythm disorders must be considered as a differential diagnosis:

- Atrial flutter or intra-atrial re-entrant tachycardia: Typical flutter waves in leads II, III, and aVF. In contrast to MAT, no isoelectric line can be detected between the flutter waves.
- EAT: In EAT, there is only one other P wave morphology in addition to the sinus rhythm P wave.

18.15.3 Treatment

Similar to EAT, the MAT usually cannot be terminated by adenosine, cardioversion or atrial overstimulation for a long period. Treatment is based on principles similar to those of EAT therapy. The goal is to slow down the heart rate by directly influencing the ectopic centers or a slowing AV conduction. Beta blockers or class III antiarrhythmic drugs (amiodarone, sotalol) are usually used.

Suppressing the ectopic centers often requires a combination treatment with amiodarone and propafenone or flecainide.

If there is an underlying disease, it must be treated first.

18.15.4 Prognosis

Overall, a spontaneous remission rate of 50 to 80% has been described. It is highest in the first year of life.

18.16 Atrial Flutter and Intra-atrial Re-entrant Tachycardia

18.16.1 Basics

Definition

Atrial flutter and intra-atrial re-entrant tachycardia (IART) are caused by circular excitations based on a macro-re-entrant mechanism in the atrium area. Conduction from the atrium to the ventricles can be irregular or regular. In atrial flutter, the excitations circle around the tricuspid valve. In IART, re-entrant circuits occur in the area of scars or prosthetic material after atrial procedures.

Epidemiology

Atrial flutter and IART are very rare in children with no cardiac disease. There is usually an underlying structural heart disease affecting primarily the right atrium. In the absence of a structural heart disease, atrial flutter occurs mainly in fetuses and neonates and is the second most common intrauterine tachycardia.

Etiology

IART occurs after atrial surgery such as a Mustard or Senning atrial baffle procedure or Fontan operation, less often after the closure of an atrial septal defect or correction of an anomalous pulmonary venous connection or tetralogy or Fallot.

Frequent causes of atrial flutter are cardiomyopathy, atrial septal aneurysm, AV septal defects, and muscular diseases (e.g., muscular dystrophy).

Pathogenesis

▸ **Atrial flutter.** Atrial flutter or IART is caused by circular electrical excitation in the atrium. In typical atrial flutter, electrical excitation runs *counter clockwise* in the right atrium along the tricuspid valve annulus and through the "posterior isthmus"—the area between the ostium of the inferior vena cava in the right atrium, the ostium of the coronary sinus, and the tricuspid valve annulus (▸ Fig. 18.20).

Because of the "protective" function of the AV block, not all atrial impulses are conducted to the ventricles. In patients with an accessory pathway (WPW syndrome), there may be 1:1 conduction of the atrial impulses to the ventricles with a correspondingly rapid ventricular rate.

In an atypical atrial flutter, the excitation runs *clockwise* along the anatomical structures described above.

▸ **Intra-atrial re-entrant tachycardia.** After surgery in the atrial area, macro-re-entry can also develop around the scar tissue or the prosthetic material, which is called intra-atrial re-entrant tachycardia (IART).

18.16.2 Diagnostic Measures

Symptoms

Atrial flutter with an almost normal ventricular rate (e.g., 3:1 conduction) can be asymptomatic. Typical clinical symptoms are usually palpitations, tachycardia, arrhythmic pulse, or a pulse deficit.

Signs of heart failure develop especially in patients with impaired ventricular function or very fast or slow conduction to the ventricles. Syncopes are rare, but may develop especially in patients with a WPW syndrome and "unprotected" conduction of atrial flutter to the ventricles. Thromboembolism is less common than in atrial fibrillation.

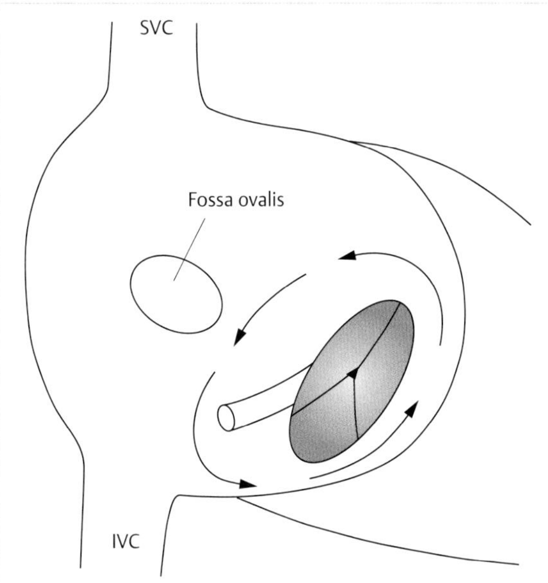

Fig. 18.20 Macro-re-entrant mechanism in typical atrial flutter. In typical atrial flutter, the electrical excitation runs counterclockwise around the tricuspid valve. This macro-re-entrant circuit includes the "posterior isthmus" between the inferior vena cava, tricuspid valve, and the ostium of the coronary sinus. SVC, superior vena cava; IVC, inferior vena cava.

ECG

A typical atrial flutter has saw-tooth waves without isoelectric lines between the P waves. The P waves are negative in the inferior leads II, III, and aVF, as well as in lead V_1 in typical atrial flutter.

In atypical atrial flutter and in IART, the P waves are positive or isoelectric in leads II, III, and aVF. In contrast, in IART there is a return to the isoelectric zero line between the P waves.

The atrial rate is between 250 and 400 bpm. Due to the "protective" function of a 2nd degree AV block, the ventricular rate is usually much lower (▶ Fig. 18.21). Usually there is 2:1 or 3:1 conduction to the ventricles. Conduction may be regular or irregular. If a bundle branch block is not already present, the QRS complexes are narrow.

Differential Diagnosis

- Atrial fibrillation: In atrial fibrillation, P waves cannot usually be identified. There is also absolute arrhythmia.
- Multifocal atrial tachycardia: In MAT, there are different P wave morphologies. The atrial rate is usually lower than in ventricular flutter.

Note

If the flutter waves cannot be identified in the surface ECG with certainty, adenosine can be administered intravenously for diagnostic purposes. The flutter waves are unmasked by the adenosine-induced transient AV block.

Echocardiography

Echocardiography is used to rule out an underlying cardiac disease (heart defect with atrial overload or after atrial surgery). The different atrial and ventricular rates are also visible in echocardiography.

A transesophageal echocardiography should always be performed prior to cardioversion for long-standing atrial flutter to rule out atrial thrombi.

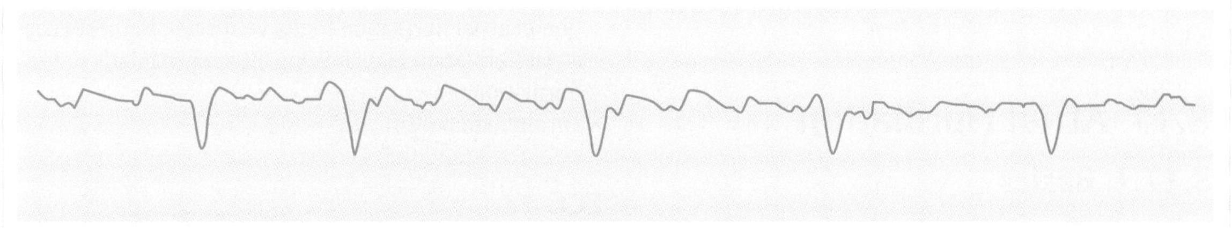

Fig. 18.21 Atrial flutter. The atrial flutter waves are clearly visible in the ECG. Due to the 2nd degree AV block, not every atrial excitation is conducted to the ventricle.

18.16.3 Treatment

In acute atrial flutter or acute IART, transesophageal overdrive stimulation or ECG-triggered cardioversion is performed (starting with 0.5–2 J/kg).

In atrial flutter or in IART *lasting more than 48 hours* or of unknown duration, a transesophageal echocardiography should be performed to rule out atrial thrombi, which could lead to emboli. If atrial thrombi are found, oral anticoagulation with phenprocoumon or warfarin should be started at least 4 weeks prior to the restoration of normal rhythm.

If electric cardioversion or overdrive stimulation is not possible, beta blockers may be used to reduce the ventricular rate.

After a successful conversion to sinus rhythm, *relapse prophylaxis* is required in some cases. In postoperative patients, class III antiarrhythmic drugs (amiodarone, sotalol) or beta blockers are the drugs of choice. Class Ic antiarrhythmic drugs should not be used alone because the reduction of the flutter rate may lead to 1:1 conduction to the ventricles. Class Ic antiarrhythmic drugs are therefore suitable for inhibiting 1:1 conduction only when combined with a beta blocker or a calcium antagonist.

Catheter ablation is indicated in refractory cases or in cases of intolerable side effects of the antiarrhythmic therapy. In some cases, rhythm surgery may be required.

Oral *anticoagulation* is required for recurrent atrial flutter or recurrent IART.

> **Note**
>
> If atrial flutter or IART is combined with sinus node dysfunction (sick sinus syndrome), significant bradycardia may develop after successful cardioversion, so that a temporary pacemaker must be available during the cardioversion.

18.16.4 Prognosis

The prognosis depends on the underlying disease. In neonates with structurally inconspicuous hearts, the prognosis of atrial flutter is usually very good.

Patients who develop IART soon after complex operations in the atrial area are at an increased risk for IART in the later postoperative course as well. IART in cardiac surgery patients clearly increases morbidity and mortality rates.

18.17 Atrial Fibrillation

18.17.1 Basics

Definition

In atrial fibrillation, intra-atrial conduction is disordered. Due to the irregular spread of excitation to the ventricles, there is absolute arrhythmia. Functionally, there is atrial standstill, so that there is a high risk for the formation of atrial thrombi.

Epidemiology

In adulthood, atrial fibrillation is the most common cardiac rhythm disorder. The incidence increases with age. In childhood, atrial fibrillation is rare and develops mainly after cardiac surgery in children and adolescents or in heart defects associated with enlargement of the left atrium (e.g., mitral valve defects).

Etiology

In childhood, atrial fibrillation is usually caused by a structural heart disease that is either associated with atrial overload (especially mitral or aortic valve defects) or required surgical intervention in the atrial area (e.g., atrial baffle procedure, Fontan procedure, rarely after ASD closure). Other causes include myocarditis, cardiomyopathy, hyperthyroidism, electrolyte imbalance, or drug intoxication (e.g., digoxin). Idiopathic atrial fibrillation is extremely rare. Familial forms have also been described. In some families, gene mutations that code for potassium channels can be detected.

Pathogenesis

Atrial fibrillation occurs due to multiple polytopic reentrant circuits that are located in the atria and are conducted chaotically in different directions. Atrial fibrillation is hemodynamically relevant due to the absence of atrial contraction and the irregular conduction of electrical excitation to the ventricles (▸ Fig. 18.22).

18.17.2 Diagnostic Measures

Symptoms

Typical symptoms of atrial fibrillation are:

- Palpitations, tachycardia, arrhythmic pulse, pulse deficit
- Signs of heart failure in patients with impaired ventricular function or with very fast or slow conduction to the ventricles
- Syncope is rare, but may develop, especially in patients with WPW syndrome and with "unchecked" conduction of atrial fibrillation to the ventricles. In these cases, atrial fibrillation may develop into ventricular fibrillation.
- Thromboembolism

ECG

In the ECG, the *fibrillation waves* are an expression of disordered atrial depolarization. The fibrillation waves undulate around the zero line at a low amplitude and

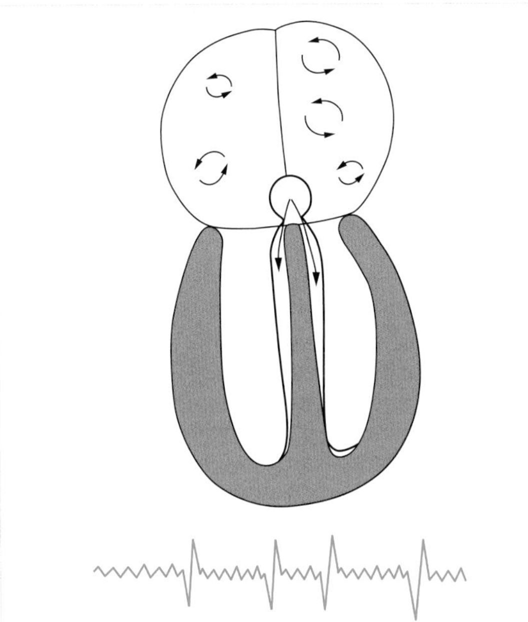

Fig. 18.22 Pathogenesis of atrial fibrillation. In atrial fibrillation there are numerous re-entrant circuits in the atria. Functionally, atrial standstill occurs. The excitations are randomly conducted to the ventricles. The result is absolute arrhythmia. The ECG has atrial fibrillation waves that undulate around the zero line at a low amplitude.

have very different characteristics and morphology. The atrial rate is between 400 and 700 bpm.

Due to the completely irregular AV conduction, *absolute arrhythmia* develops with irregular R-R intervals. If a bundle branch block was not already present, the QRS complexes are usually narrow, but QRS complexes with bundle branch block patterns may occur intermittently as the result of aberrant conduction of the atrial activity. Such aberrant conduction develops especially after a change of the R-R intervals from a long to a short R-R interval (Ashman phenomenon).

Differential Diagnosis

The following arrhythmias must be differentiated for the differential diagnosis:

- Atrial flutter or intra-atrial re-entrant tachycardia (IART): In atrial flutter or in IART, there are saw-tooth P waves with a frequency of 250–400 bpm.
- Multifocal atrial tachycardia (MAT): In MAT there are different P wave morphologies. Atrial stimuli are usually conducted to the ventricles 1:1. No absolute arrhythmia is present.
- Junctional escape rhythm: If the fibrillation waves are so flat that they are virtually undetectable, the narrow QRS complexes "without" preceding P waves may resemble a junctional escape rhythm. However, there is no absolute arrhythmia in a junctional escape rhythm.

Laboratory

The following laboratory tests are useful if the situation is unclear: serum electrolytes including K, Mg and Ca. Other tests include CK/CK-MB, troponin I, drug levels (such as digoxin, theophylline), and TSH.

Echocardiography

Echocardiography is used to rule out an underlying cardiac disease (e.g., myocarditis, mitral valve defects or other cardiac defects with atrial overload or after atrial surgery).

If atrial fibrillation lasts more than 48 hours, a transesophageal echocardiography should be performed before cardioversion to rule out atrial thrombi.

18.17.3 Treatment

Two basic treatment strategies need to be distinguished:

- Frequency regulation: normalization of the ventricular rate if there is absolute tachyarrhythmia due to a rapid AV conduction or absolute bradyarrhythmia due to a very slow AV conduction
- Rhythm regulation: converting the atrial fibrillation to a sinus rhythm with drugs or by external electrical cardioversion

Conservative Treatment

If atrial fibrillation has lasted *less than 48 hours*, the risk of atrial thrombi and associated thromboembolism is low. Therefore, in such cases ECG-triggered cardioversion under sedation can be performed (starting with 0.5–2 J/kg) to normalize the rhythm. Alternatively, in hemodynamically stable patients, class Ic (propafenone, flecainide) or class III (sotalol, amiodarone) antiarrhythmic agents may be used to restore rhythm.

In atrial fibrillation lasting *longer than 48 hours* or with unclear time of onset, a transesophageal echocardiogram should be performed. If there are no thrombi, the process to restore rhythm can start.

However, if atrial thrombi are detected, anticoagulation treatment with phenprocoumon or warfarin should should be commenced and the restoration of the sinus rhythm should not be attempted until at least 4 weeks later. Otherwise there is a high risk that after conversion to sinus rhythm and resumption of atrial contractions, an atrial thrombus may break free and may lead to thromboembolism.

If it is necessary to reduce the ventricular rate in absolute tachyarrhythmia until conversion, drugs that block AV conduction may be used (e.g., beta blockers, digoxin, or verapamil; caution: digitalis and verapamil should not be used in a WPW syndrome). If ventricular function is impaired, amiodarone is used to control the rate; ajmaline, flecainide or amiodarone are used in a WPW syndrome.

After successful cardioversion, *anticoagulation* treatment should be continued with phenprocoumon or warfarin for at least 4 weeks with a target INR between 2 and 3. If atrial fibrillation is recurrent, anticoagulation treatment may also be permanent.

After successful cardioversion, *long-term pharmacological prophylaxis* with a beta blocker or a class III antiarrhythmic has proven effective.

Interventional Treatment

Interventional catheter ablation of atrial fibrillation is an option nowadays available in most centers. The success rate for permanent relief of AF is about 60%.

Surgical Treatment

The Maze procedure and its numerous modifications are among the surgical options. These are complex and costly surgical procedures in which electrically isolated areas are created through incisions in the atrium region, thus eliminating atrial fibrillation. The electrical isolation of the pulmonary veins by circular incisions in the posterior wall of the left atrium is especially significant in this technique.

18.17.4 Prognosis

The prognosis depends on the underlying disease. Chronic atrial fibrillation can often no longer be converted to an atrial rhythm. In most of these cases, only drugs are given for controlling the atrial rate and for anticoagulation to prevent thromboembolism.

18.18 Ventricular Tachycardia

18.18.1 Basics

Definition

In ventricular tachycardia (VT), the origin of the tachycardia is located distally to the bundle of His bifurcation. The QRS complexes are accordingly widened in a bundle branch block pattern. By definition, VT occurs if there is a series of more than three such beats. There is usually dissociation between the atria and the ventricles (AV dissociation). In about half of cases, however, there is retrograde conduction of ventricular excitation to the atria.

Classification

VT is classified according to duration and morphology:

- Duration:
  - Nonsustained: duration < 30 s
  - Sustained: duration > 30 s
- Morphology:
  - Monomorphic: identical morphology of the QRS complexes
  - Polymorphic: different morphology of the QRS complexes (e.g., torsades de pointes)

Epidemiology

VT is rare in childhood and is almost always caused by a cardiac disease.

Etiology

VT may occur in connection with cardiac diseases such as cardiomyopathy, congenital heart disease, myocardial ischemia, or cardiac tumors. There are also a number of congenital syndromes that pose a risk for the development of VT such as long QT syndrome, short QT syndrome, or Brugada syndrome.

Other causes include metabolic disorders such as hypoxia, acidosis, electrolyte imbalances (hypomagnesemia, hyper-/hypokalemia), hypothermia, and drug intoxication (e.g., catecholamines, digoxin, psychostimulants, antidepressants, antiarrhythmic drugs, narcotics).

Idiopathic VT is rare in childhood.

Pathogenesis

There is either a ventricular focus with increased automaticity, triggered activity, or a re-entrant mechanism. A re-entrant mechanism may be caused by scar tissue or prosthetic material.

18.18.2 Diagnostic Measures

Symptoms

The symptoms depend largely on ventricular rate and ventricular function. Typical symptoms include palpitations, dizziness, chest pain, dyspnea, and syncope up to functional circulatory arrest. In chronic tachycardia, tachycardia-induced cardiomyopathy may develop.

ECG

Tachycardia with widened QRS complexes with a bundle branch block pattern is typical. The R-R intervals are regular in monomorphic VT and irregular in polymorphic VT. The ventricular rate is usually between 150 and 300 bpm. The QRS complexes usually present an atypical configuration, that is, not corresponding with the typical image of a right bundle branch block or a left bundle branch block. The QRS vector in the precordial leads is typically concordant, being consistently positive or consistently negative.

An indicative finding for VT is AV dissociation, which can be detected in approximately half of cases. In such

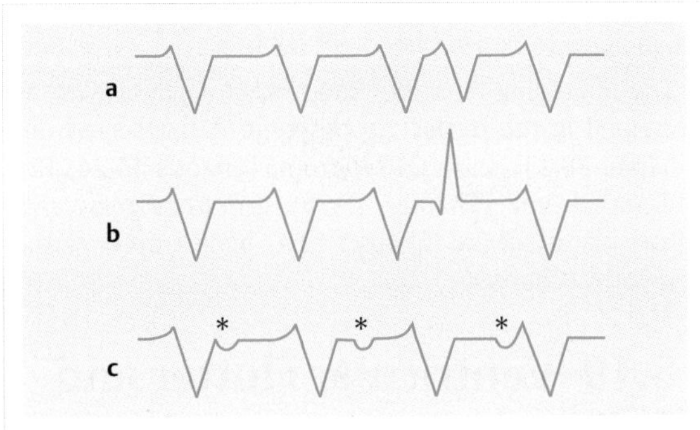

Fig. 18.23 Typical ECG phenomena in ventricular tachycardia.[16] **a** Fusion beat. **b** Capture beat. **c** AV dissociation. * = p-waves

cases, P waves can be identified with no relation to the QRS complexes (▸ Fig. 18.23 **c**).

Other typical findings are:

- Fusion beats: These are early single beats with a different QRS morphology caused by the fusion of a sinus beat with an impulse from a ventricular ectopic center (mixed image between sinus beats and the QRS complex of the VT; ▸ Fig. 18.23 a).
- Capture beats: On rare occasions, a P wave is conducted via the AV node to nonrefractory ventricular tissue that is excited by it. The morphology of the QRS complex then corresponds to that of the sinus beat (▸ Fig. 18.23 b).

▸ **Holter ECG.** The 24-hour Holter ECG is used to document the VT and to assess frequency, triggers, rate, and correlation with symptoms.

Electrophysiology Study

In certain circumstances, an electrophysiology study is indicated to accurately locate the origin of the VT. Catheter ablation of the arrhythmogenic focus may also be an option. In addition, it can be tested whether VT can be triggered by ventricular stimulation.

Laboratory

In many cases it is useful to determine the following laboratory parameters: electrolytes including Ca and Mg, also CK, CK-MB and troponin I, and possibly drug levels to rule out drug intoxication. In cases of suspected genetic disorders (e.g., long QT syndrome), corresponding molecular genetic testing may be arranged.

Echocardiography

Echocardiography is necessary to rule out or detect heart defects, other cardiac anomalies (e.g., tumor), or myocarditis, and to assess cardiac function.

Differential Diagnosis

The following tachycardias may resemble VT and must be considered in the differential diagnosis:

- Supraventricular tachycardia (SVT) with pre-existing bundle branch block or aberrant AV conduction: It can be difficult to distinguish between VT and SVT with bundle branch block or aberrant AV conduction, in which the QRS complexes are also widened. AV dissociation, fusion beats, or capture beats suggest a VT. Furthermore, the QRS complexes in a VT—although widened—do not correspond morphologically with the typical image of a right or left bundle branch block.
- SVT in a pre-excitation syndrome with antidromic conduction (rare): Here there is a bizarre widening of the QRS complex with maximum pre-excitation.
- Accelerated idioventricular rhythm: In this usually benign arrhythmia, the ventricular rate is only slightly higher than the sinus rhythm rate.

18.18.3 Treatment

Acute Treatment

In *hemodynamically unstable* patients, ECG-triggered cardioversion is performed under short anesthesia. The initial energy dose is 1 to 2 J/kg. A continuous infusion of amiodarone to prevent recurrence is necessary afterward.

In *hemodynamically stable* patients, intravenous amiodarone is the drug of choice. A bolus of 5 mg/kg BW is slowly injected intravenously; the setting for an acute electrical cardioversion should be prepared. Alternatively, intravenous lidocaine or an intravenous beta blocker may be used.

If the onset of VT is observed (e.g., in the ICU or in the cardiac catheterization laboratory), one immediate precordial thump is often effective.

Long-Term Treatment

In asymptomatic patients with structurally unremarkable hearts, no long-term drug treatment is usually required. However, it is relative rare for children with VT to have a structurally normal heart.

In a structurally conspicuous heart or after corrective surgery of congenital heart defects, long-term treatment with an oral beta blocker or amiodarone is usually indicated. Catheter ablation of the focus may be an option for monomorphic VT.

An ICD implantation is indicated in polymorphic and hemodynamically relevant VT.

For the treatment of individual special forms, see the section "Specific Ventricular Tachycardia" below.

18.18.4 Prognosis

The prognosis depends mainly on the specific type of the arrhythmia, the underlying heart defect, or genetic factors. After cardiac surgery, VT—which may occur even years after surgery—contributes greatly to mortality. A particularly high risk for sudden cardiac death is posed by torsades de pointes tachycardia and other polymorphic VTs, which often develop into ventricular fibrillation.

Monomorphic VT in structurally normal hearts has a relatively good prognosis in asymptomatic patients.

18.18.5 Specific Ventricular Tachycardias

► **Catecholamine-induced VT.** This is a rare form of VT. The name refers to the fact that the tachycardia occurs during exercise or stress. The cause is an underlying genetic disorder that leads to disruption of calcium regulation of the sarcoplasmic reticulum. The treatment of choice is high-dose beta blockers. In cases that do not respond to beta blockers, an AICD very likely prevents sudden cardiac death. In bidirectional tachycardia, catheter ablation may lead to success.

► **"Incessant" VT.** In this form, the VT is permanent. It characteristically occurs more than 10% of the time. It is usually caused by hamartomas or Purkinje cell tumors. It occurs mainly within the first 3 years of life. No pathognomonic ECG findings are present. Often this VT is relatively well tolerated, but may lead to the development of tachycardia-induced cardiomyopathy. Acute treatment is not effective and the usual antiarrhythmic drugs often do not lead to success either. Where possible, treatment consists of the removal of the pathological substrate by catheter ablation or surgical resection.

► **Right ventricular outflow tract tachycardia.** This is a focal monomorphic tachycardia that originates in the right ventricular outflow tract and occurs mainly in young adults. It is the most common idiopathic VT in children. The ECG during tachycardia shows the image of a left bundle branch block and a QRS vector of approximately + 90° (normal cardiac axis). Because of the slow rate, this VT is often well tolerated, but over time may lead to tachycardia-induced cardiomyopathy. Symptomatic patients with good cardiac function can be treated with beta blockers. Otherwise, catheter ablation of the focus is promising.

► **Left ventricular fascicular VT.** Synonyms: Verapamil-sensitive VT, Belhassen tachycardia. The cause of this VT is a re-entrant mechanism involving the left ventricular septum and the posterior fascicle of the left bundle branch. This VT can be easily confused with an SVT as it has several similar features: abrupt beginning, relatively narrow QRS complex, and good response to verapamil (the only VT that can be terminated with a calcium antagonist). There is a right bundle branch block pattern and left axis deviation in the ECG depending on the location of the re-entrant circuit. Long-term treatment with verapamil is most effective, but catheter ablation also has a high success rate.

The following specific ventricular tachycardias are described in the respective chapters: long QT syndrome (Chapter 18.23), short QT syndrome (Chapter 15.24), Brugada syndrome (Chapter 15.25), arrhythmogenic right ventricular dysplasia (Chapter 17.4), hypertrophic cardiomyopathy (Chapter 17.2).

18.19 Ventricular Flutter and Fibrillation

18.19.1 Basics

Definition

Ventricular flutter consists of ventricular impulses with a frequency between 200 and 300 bpm that have a typical hairpin curve in the ECG. The transitions to ventricular tachycardia and ventricular fibrillation are fluid. In *ventricular fibrillation*, there is very rapid ventricle excitation that leads to functional circulatory arrest. The ECG has irregular flutter waves; the individual QRS complexes cannot be distinguished.

Epidemiology

In childhood, both ventricular flutter and fibrillation are very rare and almost always occur in the context of an underlying cardiac disease. The most common cause in childhood is long QT syndrome.

Etiology

The causes generally correspond with those of ventricular tachycardia (Chapter 18.18). Ventricular flutter or fibrillation usually develops in children with long QT syndrome. Other common causes include congenital heart defects, especially those associated with myocardial hypertrophy or cyanosis. Hypoxia, electrical accidents, hypothermia, or drugs can trigger ventricular flutter or fibrillation even in an otherwise healthy heart.

There is a high risk of transition to ventricular flutter or fibrillation for polymorphic ventricular tachycardias.

Pathogenesis

Ventricular micro-re-entrant circuits, often associated with a previously damaged myocardium, constitute the underlying cause. Ventricular flutter usually develops from ventricular tachycardia.

18.19.2 Diagnostic Measures

Symptoms

Ventricular flutter and fibrillation result in functional circulatory arrest.

ECG

In the ECG there are the following pathognomonic findings (▶ Fig. 18.25):

- Ventricular flutter: Ventricular tachycardia with a rate between 200 and 300 bpm. ST segments can no longer be identified; no isoelectric line can be detected (hairpin curve).
- Ventricle fibrillation: Typical fibrillation waves of different morphology and low amplitude in the vicinity of the baseline. No individual QRS complexes can be identified.

18.19.3 Treatment

Ventricular fibrillation and flutter are life-threatening situations.

Acute Treatment

A precordial thump may be effective when cardiovascular arrest is observed immediately after the onset of a ventricular flutter/fibrillation (e.g., in the ICU or in the cardiac catheterization laboratory).

If the patient has no pulse, according to the APLS or EPLS guidelines cardiopulmonary resuscitation (CPR) must start immediately. The patient is ventilated with 100% oxygen. While continuing CPR, defibrillation is prepared. If several defibrillations are required, resuscitation must be continued between the defibrillations.

Treatment algorithm for ventricular flutter and fibrillation:

- **Defibrillation with 4 J/kg** (for the first and all subsequent defibrillations)
- Continue resuscitation immediately, rhythm analysis after 2 min
- If a shockable rhythm persists, second defibrillation with 4 J/kg
- Continue resuscitation immediately, rhythm analysis after 2 min
- If a shockable rhythm persists:
  - **Intravenous or intraosseous adrenaline 0.01 mg/kg** (equivalent to 0.1 mL/kg of the 1:10000 diluted solution)
  - Immediately thereafter, third defibrillation with 4 J/kg
- Continue resuscitation immediately, rhythm analysis after 2 min
- If a shockable rhythm persists:
  - **Amiodarone 5 mg/kg,** intravenous or intraosseous
  - Immediately thereafter, fourth defibrillation with 4 J/kg
- If a shockable rhythm persists:
  - Continue defibrillation, alternating with 2 min resuscitation
- During resuscitation, intravenous or intraosseous adrenaline 0.01 mg/kg every 3 to 5 min

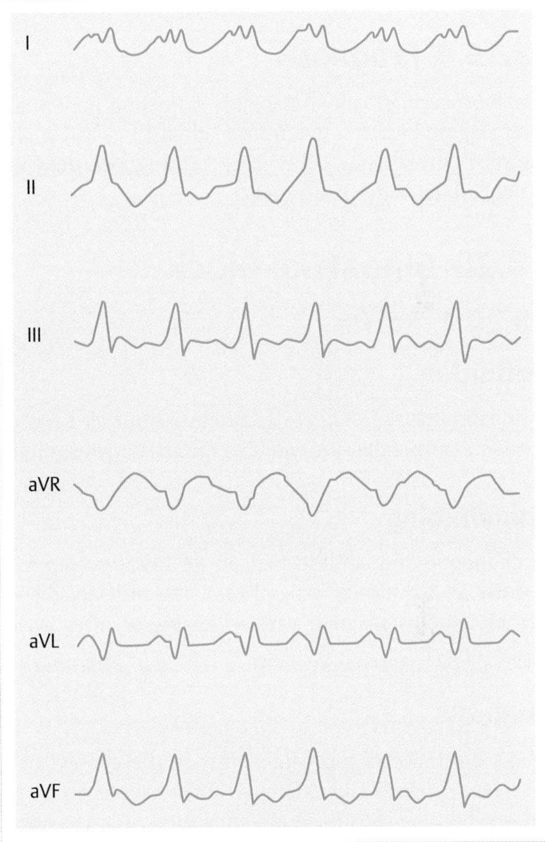

Fig. 18.24 ECG findings in ventricular tachycardia.

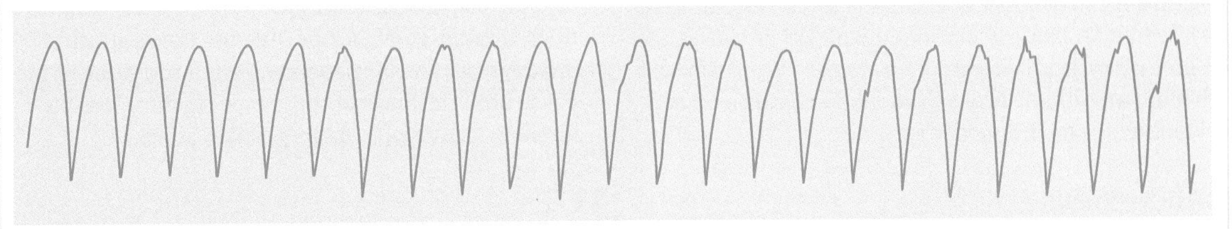

Fig. 18.25 Ventricular flutter. Typical findings in ventricular flutter are the hairpin-shaped QRS complexes. No isoelectric line or ST segments can be distinguished.

- Elimination of causative factors: hypoxia, hypovolemia, electrolyte imbalance, hypothermia, cardiac tamponade, thromboembolism, intoxication, tension pneumothorax
- In torsades de pointes or hypomagnesemia, intravenous or intraosseous magnesium 0.3 to 0.5 mmol/kg

After successful conversion to sinus rhythm, prophylaxis with a continuous infusion of amiodarone is recommended.

If it must be assumed that ventricular fibrillation has developed from a different arrhythmia, an electrophysiology study should always be performed to assess the continued risk. In most cases, the implantation of an AICD is indicated for secondary prevention.

18.19.4 Prognosis

The short-term prognosis depends mainly on how much time elapsed between the onset of circulatory arrest and the start of treatment. Otherwise, the prognosis depends mainly on the underlying disease.

18.20 Sinoatrial Block

18.20.1 Basics

Definition

A sinoatrial block (SA block) is an obstruction or delay of conduction from the sinus node to the atrial myocardium.

Epidemiology

In childhood and adolescence, an SA block occurs frequently as a clinically insignificant, intermittent disorder in patients in good cardiac health or after atrial procedures.

Etiology

An SA block occurs most frequently in the context of a sick sinus syndrome. In childhood and adolescence, a sick sinus syndrome usually occurs after surgery in the atrial area close to the sinus node (Mustard/Senning atrial baffle procedure, Fontan procedure, correction of an anomalous pulmonary venous connection, ASD closure). But even in children and adolescents in good cardiac health or with a high vagal tone (e.g., in athletes) an intermittent 2nd degree SA block is not infrequent. Other causes are inflammatory heart disease or overdose of digoxin and other antiarrhythmic drugs (beta blockers, calcium channel blockers, sotalol, amiodarone).

Pathogenesis

Conduction from the sinus node to the atria is delayed or completely blocked. The sinus node excitation and conduction from the sinus node to the atrial myocardium are not reflected in the surface ECG. Depolarization of the atria is the first to appear as a P wave. In a surface ECG, it is thus not possible to diagnose a 1st degree SA block or distinguish a 3rd degree SA block from sinus node arrest.

Classification

Similar to an AV block, the SA block is divided into three degrees:

- 1st degree SA block: There is a *delay in the conduction* of the excitation from the sinus node to the atrial myocardium without loss of atrial and ventricular excitation. Since conduction from the sinus node to the atria is not shown in the surface ECG, a 1st degree SA block cannot be detected in the surface ECG.
- 2nd degree SA block: *intermittent interruption* of conduction from the sinus node to the atria.
  - Type I (Wenckebach): With a constant PQ interval, the P-P intervals become increasingly *shorter* until eventually an atrial action (P wave) is completely absent. The following pause is then shorter than twice the previous P-P interval. Explanation for the increasingly shorter P-P intervals: The delay in the conduction from the sinus node to the atria is most pronounced at the beginning and then decreases with each sinus beat until conduction is completely absent. Accordingly, the P waves come closer to each other until one is finally absent.
  - Type II (Mobitz): *intermittent complete interruption* of conduction from the sinus node to the atria. The resulting pause in the ECG is twice as long as or a multiple of the normal P-P interval.
- 3rd degree SA block: *complete interruption* of conduction from the sinus node to the atria over a varying period. After a pause of varying length, an escape rhythm (usually AV escape rhythm) develops. In the surface ECG, a 3rd degree SA block is indistinguishable from sinus node arrest.

18.20.2 Diagnostic Measures

Symptoms

The symptoms depend mainly on the length of the resulting pauses:

- 1st degree SA block: always asymptomatic
- 2nd degree SA block: depending on the length of the ensuing pauses and ventricular rate, possibly palpitations, dizziness, or syncope (Adams–Stokes attack)
- 3rd degree SA block: depending on the duration of the pause until the onset of the escape rhythm, possibly dizziness or syncope (Adams–Stokes attack).

ECG

First degree SA block cannot be detected in the surface ECG. A 3rd degree SA block is indistinguishable from sinus node arrest in the surface ECG.

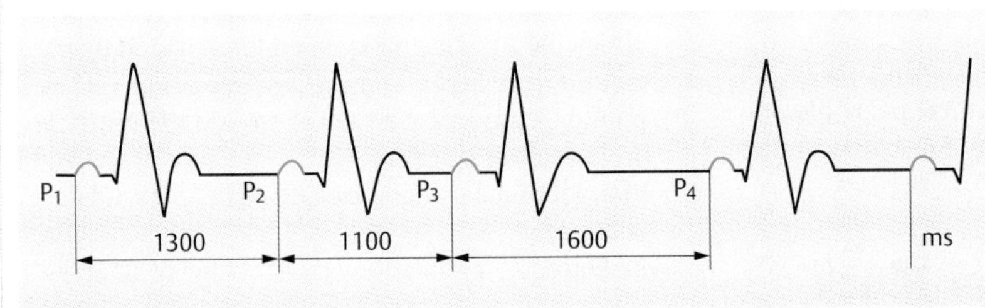

Fig. 18.26 ECG findings of a 2nd degree SA block, type I (Wenckebach). The P-P intervals become increasingly shorter until a P wave and the QRS complex disappear completely.[38]

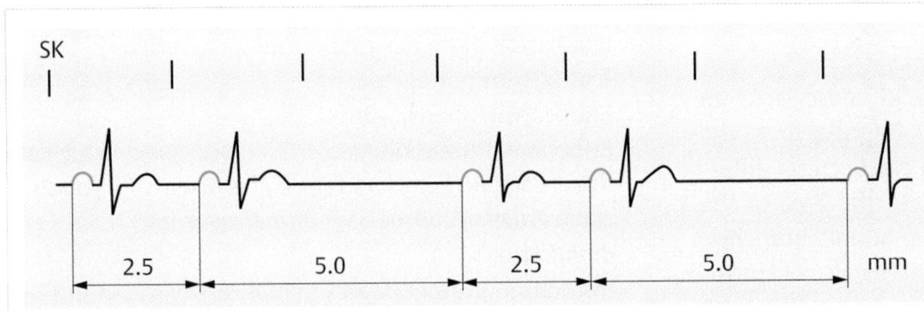

Fig. 18.27 ECG findings of a 2nd degree SA block, type II (Mobitz). The P-P intervals are constant. There is a sudden disappearance of a P wave and the QRS complex. The pause is equivalent to twice the previous P-P intervals.[38]

Characteristic findings in 2nd and 3rd degree SA block are:

- 2nd degree SA block, type I (Wenckebach): increasingly shorter P-P intervals with constant PQ intervals until a P wave and the QRS complex are completely absent. The resulting pause is shorter than twice the previous P-P interval (▸ Fig. 18.26).

- 2nd degree SA block, type II (Mobitz): absence of one P wave and QRS complex with constant P-P intervals. The pause is twice as long or a multiple of the previous P-P interval (▸ Fig. 18.27).

- 3rd degree SA block: complete absence of the P waves and QRS complexes (= asystole) until the onset of the escape rhythm. The ventricular rate depends on the rate of the escape rhythm.

Differential Diagnoses

The following differential diagnoses are possible depending on the type of SA block:

- 1st degree SA block: sinus bradycardia.
- 2nd degree SA block: sinus arrhythmia, sinus bradycardia. Longer lasting regular 2:1 or multiple blockage of type II (Mobitz) leads to bradycardia.
- 3rd degree SA block: sinus node arrest.
- Sick sinus syndrome: In sinus node dysfunction, there are different atrial arrhythmias simultaneously: sinus bradycardia, SA block, sinus arrest, atrial tachycardia, atrial flutter/fibrillation.

Laboratory

Laboratory tests may rule out electrolyte disorders, myocarditis, or drug intoxication.

▸ **Holter ECG.** The 24-hour Holter ECG is used to assess bradycardia (frequency, duration, heart rate), pauses (frequency, duration), and escape rhythms (frequency, duration, rate). If other arrhythmias such as atrial tachycardia, atrial flutter/fibrillation are detected, this suggests a sick sinus syndrome.

▸ **Exercise ECG.** A 2nd degree SA block in children and adolescents has usually clinically little significance if there is an adequate increase in the heart rate during exercise.

Echocardiography

Echocardiography allows an underlying cardiac disease (e. g., myocarditis, heart defects with atrial overload after an operation in the atrium area) to be ruled out or assessed.

18.20.3 Treatment

An intermittent SA block needs no treatment in asymptomatic persons. Otherwise, the focus is on causal treatment if possible for hemodynamically stable patients: compensation of electrolyte imbalances, possibly pausing high-dose medication, and discontinuation of drugs that can induce bradycardia.

In symptomatic bradycardia or cardiac arrest, emergency treatment consists of the following drugs:

- Atropine 0.01 to 0.03 mg/kg intravenously
- If this fails, isoprenaline or orciprenaline (Alupent) 0.01 mg/kg slow intravenously or adrenaline (epinephrine) 0.01 mg/kg intravenously (equivalent to 0.1 mL of 1:10,000 diluted solution)

The long-term treatment of symptomatic patients (syncope/presyncope) is a pacemaker with an atrial pacing system (e.g., AAIR).

18.20.4 Prognosis

The prognosis depends on the underlying cause. In asymptomatic patients without structural heart disease, an intermittent 1st or 2nd degree SA block is not pathological.

18.21 Atrioventricular Block

18.21.1 Basics

Definition

An atrioventricular block (AV block) describes an impaired conduction of the electrical impulse from the atria to the ventricles. The impairment can occur at different points of the conduction system: in the area of the AV node, in the bundle of His, or in the bundle branches. They are termed supra-Hisian, intra-Hisian, or infra-Hisian blocks, respectively. If there is a complete blockage of the electrical impulse, an escape rhythm kicks in to take over electrical excitation of the ventricles.

Epidemiology

The exact incidence is unclear. First degree or 2nd degree AV block type I (Wenckebach) is found in many individuals with no clinical significance—for example, during sleep. Men are affected slightly more often than women, and the prevalence increases with age. An AV block can also occur in a fetus or neonate as a congenital AV block.

Etiology

If vagal tone is increased (e.g., during sleep or in athletes), a 1st or 2nd degree AV block may be physiological. Otherwise AV block occurs in childhood particularly if there is structural heart disease (especially ccTGA, Ebstein anomaly, and AV canal) or as a complication after cardiac surgery. AV block is less often caused by inflammatory heart disease.

The many different causes of an AV block are listed below:

- Physiological:
  - Increased vagal tone (1st/2nd degree AV block, e.g., in sleep or in physically fit athletes).
- Iatrogenic:
  - Postoperatively after cardiac surgery: Postoperative AV block can be temporary or permanent. Cardiac surgery is the most common cause of acquired AV block. An injury or irritation of the conduction system may occur especially after operations on the AV junction, such as closure or enlargement of a VSD, ASD-I closure, AV canal correction, Fallot correction, Mustard/Senning atrial baffle procedure, or mitral or aortic valve replacement.
  - Cardiac catheterization: Patients with a ccTGA in which the AV node is displaced forward and upward and the bundle of His at the anterior margin of the pulmonary artery is displaced toward the ventricle are particularly at risk.
  - Interventional catheter closure of an ASD with an occluder.
  - Radiofrequency ablation / cryoablation of an accessory pathway or an atrioventricular nodal re-entry.
  - Drugs: beta blockers, digoxin, calcium antagonists, tricyclic antidepressants, clonidine
  - Irradiation of mediastinal or thoracic tumors.
- Infectious/immunogenic:
  - Endocarditis/myocarditis
  - Infectious/immunological: rheumatic fever, Lyme carditis (*Borrelia burgdorferi*), Chagas disease (*Trypanosoma cruzii*), diphtheria (*Corynebacterium diphtheriae*)
  - Immunological: neonates of mothers with autoimmune antibodies (anti-SSA/Ro and anti-SSB/La): Maternal autoimmune antibodies are the most common cause of congenital 3rd degree AV block. The mothers are often asymptomatic. AV block should be ruled out in all children of mothers with positive autoimmune antibodies.
- Structural heart disease:
  - Congenital heart defects (especially ccTGA, Ebstein anomaly, AV canal, ASD I)
  - Cardiac tumors
- Neuromuscular diseases/mitochondropathy:
  - Kearns–Sayre syndrome (typical features: retinopathy, external ophthalmoplegia, ataxia, increased protein concentration in the cerebrospinal fluid, AV block, mitochondrial inheritance pattern). Patients with Kearns–Sayre syndrome are at high risk for sudden cardiac death, so prophylactic pacemaker implantation is indicated in 1st to 3rd degree AV block.
  - Duchenne muscular dystrophy, myotonic dystrophy
- Others:
  - Congenital or acquired long QT syndrome: The significantly prolonged repolarization phase in QT prolongation may cause the atrial impulse to meet a still refractory ventricle and thus not be transmitted. The result is a functional AV block.
  - Familial atrioventricular block: An autosomal dominant inheritance pattern has been described in some cases. One affected gene is SCN5A, for example, which codes for a potassium channel.
  - Idiopathic progressive fibrosis or sclerosis of the conduction system (Lenègre disease) or the connective tissue of the heart (Lev disease). In elderly patients, Lev disease is often associated with calcification of the aortic and mitral valves.
  - Sickle cell crisis: There is probably an ischemic disorder of the AV node in these cases.

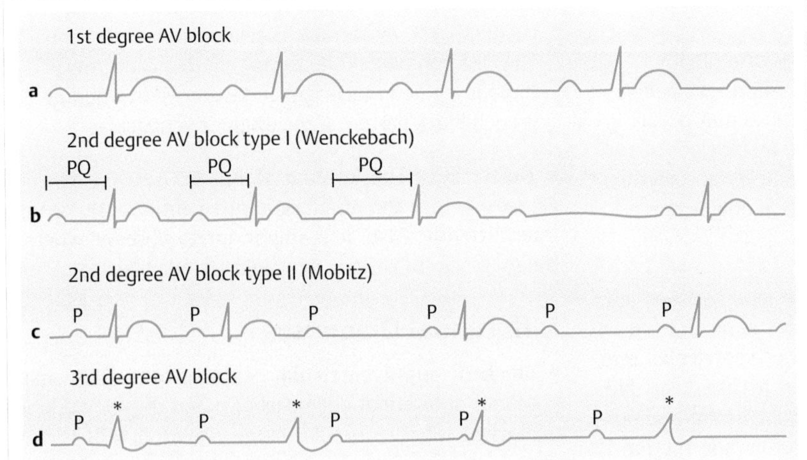

Fig. 18.28 ECG diagram of the various forms of AV block.[16] **a** 1st degree AV block: prolongation of the PQ interval. **b** 2nd degree AV block Mobitz type I (Wenckebach): increasing prolongation of the PQ interval until ventricular action stops completely. **c** 2nd degree AV block Mobitz type II: PQ interval remains constant with intermittent failure of ventricular action. **d** 3rd degree AV block: complete blockage of AV conduction. Atrial (P wave) and ventricular actions (QRS complexes) are each independent of the other.

- ◦ After a heart transplant, an AV block may be the result of a rejection crisis, coronary angiopathy, or complications related to surgery or cardiac catheterization.
- ◦ Myocardial infarction

Note

The most common cause of a congenital AV block is damage to the fetal cardiac conduction system by maternal antibodies associated with maternal autoimmune disease (especially lupus erythematosus, Sjögren syndrome). The mothers can possibly be asymptomatic, so the maternal autoimmune disease is often first diagnosed by the child's AV block. Heart failure with hydrops fetalis may already develop in utero.

Classification

AV blocks are classified as 1st to 3rd degree:

- 1st degree AV block: prolongation of the PQ interval with regular conduction of atrial activity to the ventricles (▶ Fig. 18.28 a).
- 2nd degree AV block: periodic blocking of the AV conduction:
  - Mobitz type I (Wenckebach periodicity): increasing prolongation of the PQ interval until AV conduction fails completely. In these cases, blockage is usually in the AV node itself (▶ Fig. 18.28 b).
  - Mobitz type II: atrial excitation is suddenly no longer conducted, with no prior prolongation of the PQ interval. The blockage is usually in or distal to the bundle of His (▶ Fig. 18.28 c). There is an increased risk for transition to a 3rd degree AV block.
    If there is no regular periodicity (e.g., 2:1, 3:1, or 4:1) of AV conduction, it is termed *advanced 2nd degree AV block.*

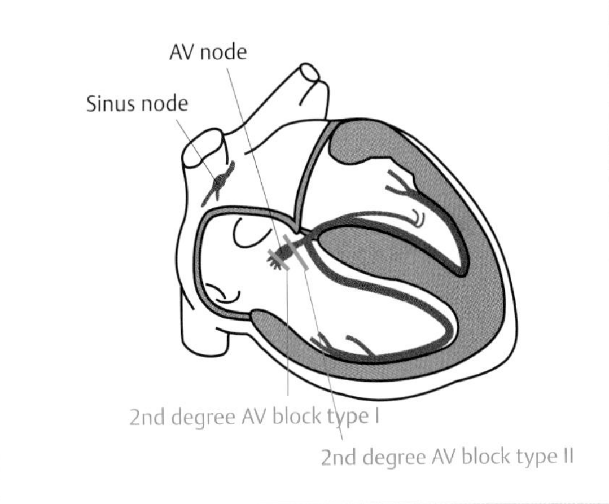

Fig. 18.29 Different locations of the various forms of AV block. In 2nd degree AV block type I (Wenckebach periodicity), the conduction defect is generally in the area of the AV node; in 2nd degree AV block type II it is usually in or distal to the bundle of His.[16]

- 3rd degree AV block: AV conduction is completely blocked. Atria and ventricles beat independently (complete dissociation of atria and ventricles). The ventricles are depolarized by a ventricular escape rhythm (▶ Fig. 18.28 d). The further distal the blockage, the slower the escape rhythm usually is (▶ Fig. 18.29).

18.21.2 Diagnostic Measures

Symptoms

The symptoms depend mainly on the type of the AV block and the resulting ventricular rate. The following symptoms may occur depending on the type of the AV block:

- 1st degree AV block: asymptomatic
- 2nd degree AV block:

- Mobitz type I (Wenckebach periodicity): almost always asymptomatic
- Mobitz type II: Most patients are asymptomatic. Depending on the ventricular rate, dizziness, pallor, reduced physical capacity, or syncopes may occur; possible transition to a 3rd degree AV block.

• 3rd degree AV block: Depending on the escape rhythm, dizziness, pallor, physical deterioration or syncope (Adams–Stokes attacks) may occur.

In a congenital AV block, intrauterine fetal hydrops may develop. The hydrops in these cases is the result of heart failure that can develop due to a low ventricular rate. Postnatally, depending on the escape rhythm, heart failure may develop, but asymptomatic courses are also possible. The heart rate of the ventricular escape rhythm is usually 60 to 80 bpm. Affected neonates may have discoid skin lesions as a result of maternal antibodies.

ECG

- 1st degree AV block: Regular P waves followed by QRS complexes, prolonged PQ interval.
- 2nd degree AV block:
  - Mobitz type I (Wenckebach periodicity): Regular P waves, increased prolongation of the PQ interval followed by QRS complexes until conduction stops completely and no QRS complex follows the P wave.
  - Mobitz type II: Regular P waves, although not every P wave is conducted and followed by a QRS complex. Conduction and blocking of the P wave often occur at a fixed ratio, for example, 2:1 or 3:1. The ventricular rate depends on the ratio between conduction and blocking. If the disruption of conduction is in the bundle His, the subsequent QRS complexes are relatively narrow and not very deformed. If the disruption is more distal, the transmitted QRS complexes are widened and have a bundle branch block pattern.
- 3rd degree AV block: Regular P waves that are not conducted to the ventricles. The ventricular rate depends on the escape rhythm. P waves and QRS complexes thus occur independently of each other (AV dissociation; ▶ Fig. 18.30). The P-P intervals that include a QRS complex are often shorter than the P-P intervals without ventricular complexes. This phenomenon is called "ventriculophasia" or "ventriculophasic sinus arrhythmia." The QRS complex of the escape rhythm is narrow if there is a junctional origin and widened in a bundle branch block pattern if the origin is ventricular.

▶ **Holter ECG.** The 24-hour Holter ECG can be used to assess whether the AV block occurs continuously or only intermittently. Also, it is important to observe whether the AV block transitions to a higher-grade blockage.

Differential Diagnoses

▶ **Blocked supraventricular extrasystoles.** The main potential differential diagnosis of a 2nd degree AV block is blocked supraventricular extrasystoles, in which the P wave is premature and is often hidden in the preceding T wave. This occurs mainly in fetuses and neonates.

▶ **Idioventricular rhythm.** A 3rd degree AV block must also be distinguished from an idioventricular rhythm, whose rate is just below that of the sinus rhythm, so the idioventricular rhythm is usually faster than the ventricular escape rhythm. In addition, no P waves can be detected in an idioventricular rhythm.

Laboratory

Useful laboratory tests depend mainly on the suspected causes of the AV block:

- Serum electrolytes including K, Mg, Ca
- CK/CK-MB, troponin I
- Serology: Borrelia burgdorferi, Streptococcus, etc., if infection is suspected
- CK, AST, ALT if muscular dystrophy is suspected
- Blood gas analysis, including lactate if mitochondriopathy is suspected
- Possibly drug levels (e.g., digoxin)
- In fetuses and neonates with congenital AV block: anti-SSA/Ro and anti-SSB/La titers in maternal (and child's) serum

Electrophysiological Study

An electrophysiological study may be necessary, decided on a case-by-case basis. It is used to determine the exact

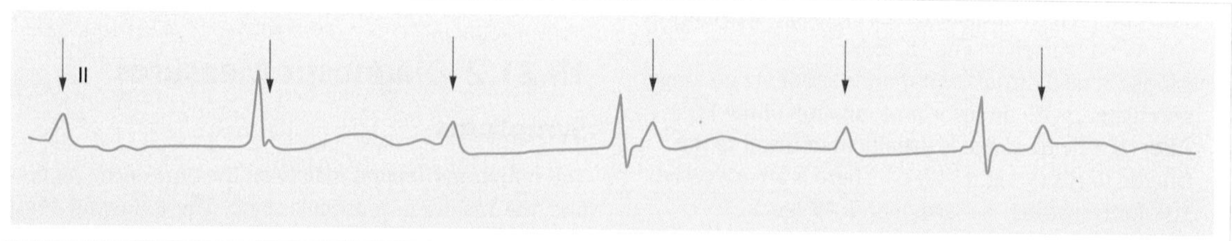

Fig. 18.30 ECG of a 3rd degree AV block. The atrial (P waves, arrows) and ventricular actions (QRS complexes) are completely independent of each other.

location of the AV block (above, in, or below the bundle of His). In an infra-Hisian block, the escape rhythm is usually much slower. There is an increased risk of asystole. It can also be tested when an escape rhythm occurs. If myocarditis is suspected, a myocardial biopsy may also be considered.

Echocardiography

Echocardiography is used primarily to rule out an underlying cardiac disease (e.g., myocarditis, ccTGA, Ebstein anomaly, atrioventricular canal, ASD I).

18.21.3 Treatment

Emergency Treatment

For symptomatic bradycardia or cardiac arrest, the following drugs and measures are used:

- Atropine 0.01 to 0.03 mg/kg IV (minimum dose 0.1 mg), if unsuccessful orciprenaline (Alupent) 0.01 mg/kg in a slow IV or adrenaline (epinephrine) 0.01 mg/kg IV (equivalent to 0.1 mL/kg of the 1:10,000 diluted solution)
- If the effect is insufficient, temporary (transcutaneous, transesophageal, or transvenous) pacemaker stimulation

During these measures, if circulatory arrest occurs, according to the APLS/EPLS guidelines cardiopulmonary resuscitation following to the ABC principle must be performed.

Causal Treatment

Any underlying cause of the AV block must be treated. Possible measures are:

- Discontinuation of drugs that prolong the PQ interval (e.g., digoxin, beta blockers, calcium channel antagonists)
- Treatment of myocarditis, Lyme carditis, etc.

Symptomatic Treatment

Symptomatic treatment consists mainly of implantation of a pacemaker. The need for a pacemaker depends on the degree and cause of the AV block. A pacemaker is practically always indicated for symptomatic patients. The main indications are:

- 1st degree AV block: no treatment needed.
- 2nd degree AV block:
  - Mobitz type I (Wenckebach periodicity): Usually asymptomatic, so no treatment is necessary. Exceptions are patients with an infra-Hisian block (rare in Mobitz type I). These patients, who generally have wide QRS complexes, have a greater risk of developing higher-degree AV block. In all patients with a 2nd degree AV block Mobitz type I and wide QRS complexes, an electrophysiological study is recommended to determine the location of the AV block. Symptomatic patients are treated with a pacemaker.
  - Mobitz type II: All symptomatic patients are fitted with a pacemaker. In addition, implantation of a pacemaker is indicated in infranodal blockage.
- 3rd degree AV block:
  - All symptomatic patients are fitted with a pacemaker.
  - Prophylactic pacemaker therapy is also recommended for wide QRS complexes of an escape rhythm because these patients have a greater risk of sudden cardiac death.
  - Prophylactic pacemaker treatment is recommended if the heart rate is below 50 bpm (children) or below 45 bpm (adolescents) to prevent heart failure.
- Kearns–Sayre syndrome: Prophylactic permanent pacemaker treatment is indicated in 1st to 3rd degree AV block.
- Postoperative advanced 2nd or 3rd degree AV block: If a postoperative advanced 2nd or 3rd degree AV block persists more than 7 to 14 days, a pacemaker is usually implanted because recovery of the AV conduction is no longer expected. As an interim measure, temporary stimulation is applied via the epicardial pacemaker electrodes that are routinely placed intraoperatively.
- Congenital 3rd degree AV block:
  - If a 3rd degree AV block has already been diagnosed prenatally, treatment of the mother with steroids or plasmapheresis may be considered and pharmacological treatment of the mother with chronotropic and/or inotropic agents should be considered for hydrops fetalis, but the success of such measures has not been sufficiently proven.
  - Pacemaker therapy of the neonate is generally recommended in the following situations:
    - Average heart rate < 50 bpm or < 45 bpm during sleep without structural heart disease
    - Average heart rate of 70 bpm with hemodynamically significant structural heart disease
    - Pauses longer than 3 s as a result of AV block
    - Additional indications for pacemaker treatment: cardiomegaly, ventricular dysfunction, high atrial rate, escape rhythm with wide ventricular complexes, complex ventricular ectopy, inadequate reaction of the escape rhythm under stress, and QT prolongation.

A two-chamber system (DDD or DDDR mode) that allows AV sequential pacing is usually indicated for an AV block. In young children, the implantation of a transvenous system is often not possible or not useful because of the risk of mechanical or thromboembolic vascular occlusion. In these cases, myocardial or epicardial electrodes are necessary, which, however, require a thoracotomy. In young children, subpectoral pacemaker implantation is not yet possible, and the generator unit is placed under the abdominal skin or in the intrapleural area, for example. In newborns, it is usually not possible to implant the relatively large DDD generator units, so a VVI unit is first implanted as a temporary solution.

18.21.4 Prognosis

The prognosis depends on the type and cause of the AV block:

- 1st degree AV block: harmless, not pathological
- 2nd degree AV block:
  - Mobitz type I (Wenckebach periodicity): This form has a good prognosis. It rarely transitions to a higher-grade block.
  - Mobitz type II: A 2nd degree AV block Mobitz type II often transitions to 3rd degree AV block.
- 3rd degree AV block: Most patients with 3rd degree AV block require a pacemaker.
- Postoperative AV block: Most postoperative AV blocks are a temporary problem. The AV block is often the result of edema or hemorrhage in the area of the conduction system. In general, AV conduction recovers within 7 to 10 days. An advanced 2nd or 3rd degree AV block is an indication for implantation of a permanent pacemaker.
- Congenital AV block: The fetal mortality rate in an AV block is as high as 30 to 50%. Patients who were diagnosed and treated in the neonatal period have a survival rate of 94%. Risk factors include a confirmed AV block in utero, hydrops fetalis, preterm birth, fibroelastosis, and impaired ventricular function.

18.22 Bundle Branch Block

18.22.1 Basics

Definition

A bundle branch block is an intraventricular conduction disorder caused by a complete interruption or delay of conduction in certain segments of the bundle branches. Depending on the location of the disruption, excitation of the corresponding regions of the ventricles is delayed.

Classification

The classification depends on the location of the interruption of the conduction pathway (▶ Fig. 18.31):

- Right bundle branch block (RBBB): blockage in the right bundle branch
- Left bundle branch block (LBBB): blockage in the two fascicles of the left bundle branch
- Left anterior hemiblock (LAH): blockage in the anterior fascicle of the left bundle branch

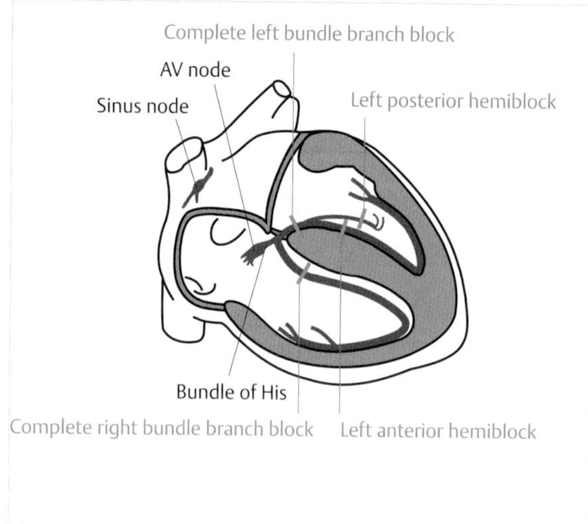

Fig. 18.31 Location of the various bundle blocks in the conduction system.[16]

- Left posterior hemiblock (LPH): blockage in the posterior fascicle of the left bundle branch

Depending on the number of affected pathways, the following are also distinguished:

- Unifascicular block: blockage of one of the two bundle branches
- Bifascicular block: In a bifascicular block, there is a right bundle branch block and in addition a left anterior *or* left posterior hemiblock. A bifascicular block occurs mainly after cardiac surgery. A right bundle branch block with left anterior hemiblock is not uncommon, for example, after tetralogy of Fallot correction. A trifascicular block may also develop, making regular follow-up necessary.
- Trifascicular block: In a trifascicular block, there is a right bundle branch block with a left posterior hemiblock *and* left anterior hemiblock. The result is a complete AV block with the corresponding consequences.

Depending on the extent of conduction disturbances, a distinction is made between a complete and incomplete bundle branch block:

- Complete bundle branch block: right or left bundle branch block with complete interruption of conduction in one of the bundle branches. The QRS duration is prolonged.
- Incomplete bundle branch block: right or left bundle branch block with slight disturbance of conduction in one of the bundle branches. The QRS duration is normal.

18.22.2 Complete Right Bundle Branch Block

Epidemiology

This is the most common form of a complete bundle branch block.

Etiology

In children and adolescents, a right bundle branch block (RBBB) occurs especially after cardiac surgery with VSD closure. After correction of a tetralogy of Fallot, a RBBB is almost always present, after a VSD closure in 20 to 50% of individuals. RBBB can also be the result of right ventricular volume overload, inflammatory heart disease, coronary heart disease, cardiomyopathy, or hypertension. Especially in older adults, RBBB can occur even without organic heart disease.

Pathogenesis

There is an interruption of conduction in the right bundle branch. In a VSD closure, for example, the patch is sutured from the right ventricle so a lesion of the right bundle branch is more likely to occur than a lesion of the left bundle branch.

In RBBB, the excitation initially spreads in the ventricles via the left bundle branch. The right ventricle is not excited until later from the left bundle through the septal wall. The ECG therefore has a widened QRS complex and altered repolarization.

ECG

Typical ECG findings in RBBB are (▶ Fig. 18.32):

- Widened QRS complex
- The right precordial leads (V_1, V_2) have high, wide, M-shaped, fragmented QRS complexes (RsR′, rsR′, rSR′); delayed upper transition point
- The left precordial leads have wide S waves
- Repolarization disturbances in the form of ST segment depression, possibly negative T waves in lead III, and in the right precordial leads. Accordingly, there is a slight ST segment elevation in the left precordial leads.

18.22.3 Incomplete Right Bundle Branch Block

Synonyms: incomplete RBBB, right delay

Epidemiology

Relatively common finding in healthy children and adolescents. An incomplete RBBB may also suggest volume overload of the right heart (e.g., in an ASD II).

Etiology

There is usually no organic cause. The affected individuals are healthy. The most common pathological causes of an incomplete RBBB are:

- Right volume overload (e.g., ASD II)
- Hypothyroidism
- Funnel chest
- Consequence of myocarditis

Pathogenesis

In children and adolescents with healthy hearts, it is presumed that a relatively small number of the Purkinje fibers at the base of the right ventricle slow the spread of the excitation in this area.

ECG

Typical ECG findings are (▶ Fig. 18.33):

- Normal QRS interval (!)
- QRS complexes in the right precordial leads are fragmented similar to a complete RBBB.
- Repolarization disturbances are either absent or less pronounced than in a complete RBBB.

> **Note**
>
> An incomplete right bundle branch block with an Rsr′ configuration usually has no clinical significance in children and adolescents. However an rsR′ configuration (second R wave greater than the first) may be a sign of volume overload of the right heart and often occurs in an ASD II (▶ Fig. 18.33).

18.22.4 Complete Left Bundle Branch Block

Epidemiology

In children and adolescents, a left bundle branch block (LBBB) is rare. It occurs practically only in the context of organic heart disease or postoperatively after cardiac surgery.

Etiology

The most common causes of a complete LBBB are:

- Cardiomyopathy
- After procedures in the left ventricular outflow tract (e.g., correction of aortic or subaortic stenosis)
- Heart defects with left heart hypertrophy (e.g., aortic stenosis, hypertrophic obstructive cardiomyopathy)

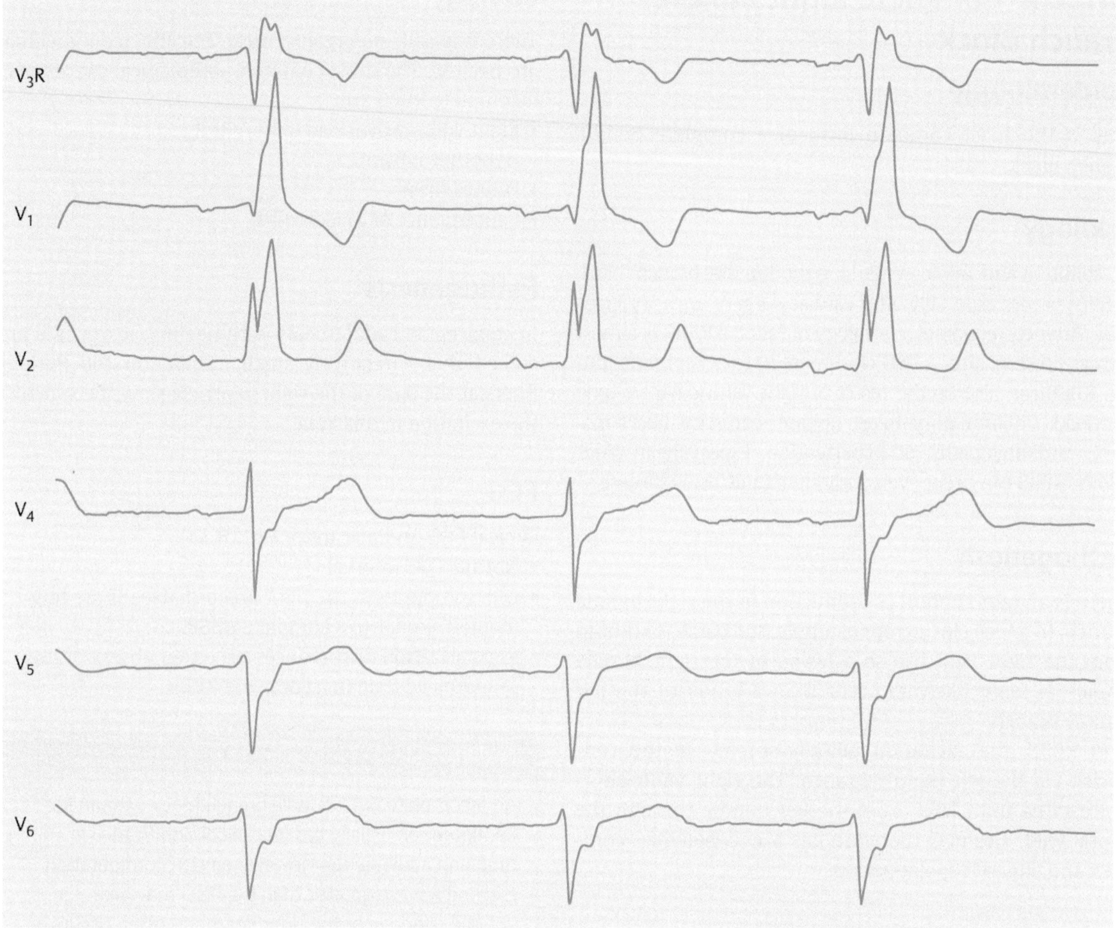

V_3R

V_1

V_2

V_4

V_5

V_6

Fig. 18.32 ECG of a complete right bundle branch block. The QRS complex is widened with M-shaped fragmentation in the right precordial leads. There are also the typical repolarization disturbances.

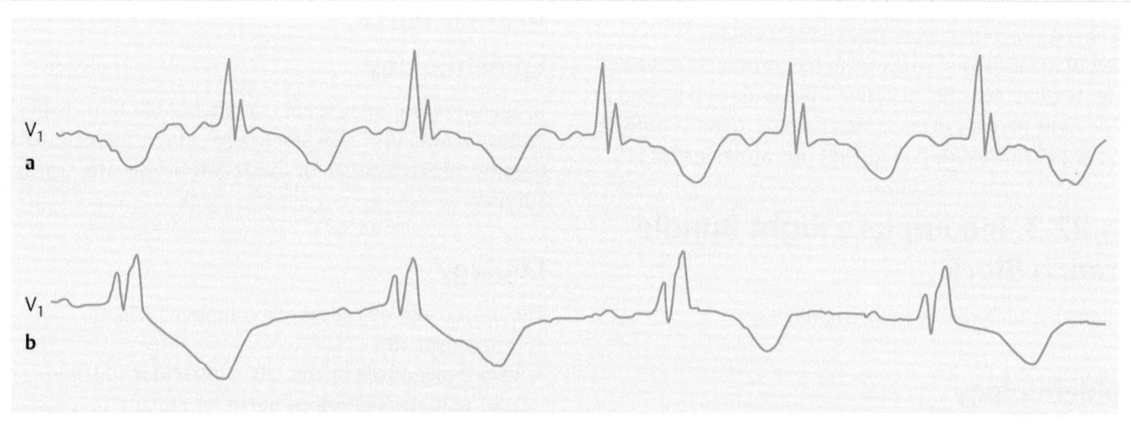

Fig. 18.33 ECG findings in an incomplete right bundle branch block of the physiological type and the volume overload type. In incomplete right bundle branch block of the physiological type (**a**), the first R wave is higher than the second (Rsr′ configuration). In the volume overload type (**b**), the configuration is reversed: the first R wave is smaller than the second (rsR′ configuration). The most common cause is an ASD II.

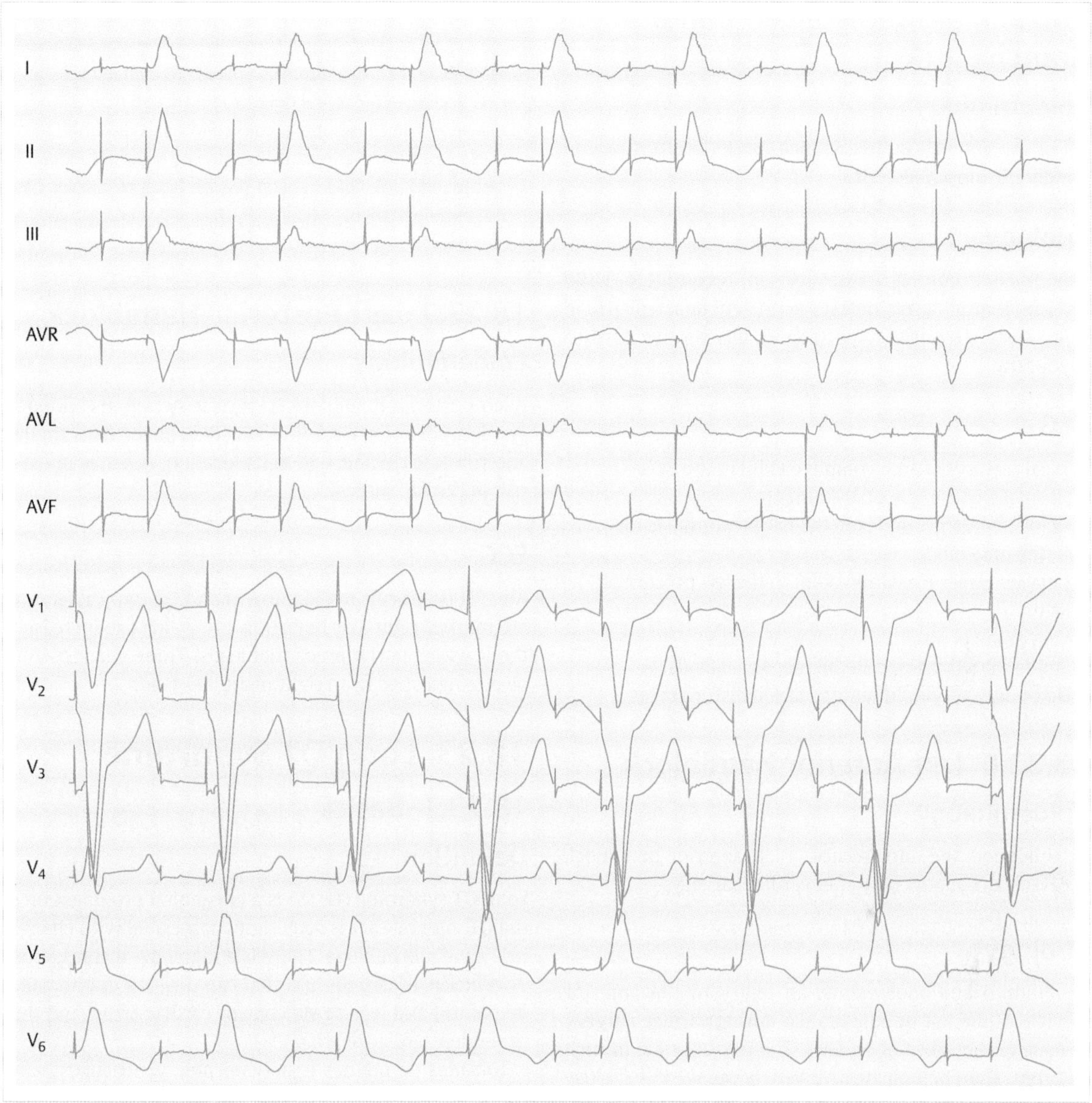

Fig. 18.34 ECG in a complete left bundle branch block. The fragmentation of the widened QRS complex in the left precordial leads and the typical repolarization disturbances in a complete left bundle branch block can be seen. In the right precordial leads, the S wave is distinctively deep.
Note: This case is a pacemaker ECG (DDD mode). Since the ventricular pacemaker electrode is located in the right ventricle, the right ventricle is stimulated before the left ventricle. This results in an ECG image of a complete left bundle branch block.

- Myocardial ischemia
- Hypertension
- Myocarditis

ECG

Characteristic findings in a complete LBBB are (▶ Fig. 18.34):

- Widened QRS complex with distinct notching or M-shaped fragmentation in the left precordial leads (V_4–V_6)
- Delayed upper transition point
- Deep S waves in the right precordial leads
- Repolarization disturbances (ST segment depression or elevation, negative T waves) in the left precordial leads

18.22.5 Incomplete Left Bundle Branch Block

Epidemiology

An incomplete left bundle branch block (LBBB) is rare in childhood and adolescence.

Etiology

The most common causes of an incomplete LBBB are congenital heart defects with left heart overload (e.g., aortic stenosis, hypertrophic obstructive cardiomyopathy).

ECG

Typical features of an incomplete LBBB in the ECG:

- Normal QRS complex duration (!)
- Deformed QRS complex in the left precordial leads (often only mild)
- Delayed upper transition point in the left precordial leads
- Very small or absent R waves in V_1 and V_2
- Sudden R-S transition in the precordial leads
- No or only very mild repolarization disturbances

18.22.6 Left Anterior Hemiblock

Epidemiology

In childhood and adolescence, a left anterior hemiblock (LAH) occurs almost only after cardiac surgery.

Etiology

In children and adolescents, an injury to the anterior fascicle of the left bundle branch during cardiac surgery is usually the cause of an LAH. The right bundle branch is often simultaneously involved because of its close proximity. This then results in a bifascicular block (RBBB + LAH).

LAH can also be caused by myocardial ischemia, cardiomyopathy, or inflammatory heart disease. Since the left anterior fascicle of the left bundle branch is supplied along with the right bundle branch by the left coronary artery, the development of a bifascicular block (RBBB + LAH) is relatively common in myocardial ischemia due to the left coronary artery.

ECG

The leading finding in the ECG is marked left axis deviation. Typically there are also deep S waves in the left precordial leads. The QRS complex is of normal width and is not deformed.

> **Note**
>
> Marked left axis deviation also occurs as a characteristic ECG finding in AV septal defects and tricuspid atresia. However, the cause of the marked left axis deviation in these cases is the abnormal location of the conduction system and not a blockage in the left anterior fascicle of the bundle branch.

18.22.7 Left Posterior Hemiblock

Epidemiology

A left posterior hemiblock (LPH) is very rare in childhood. The left posterior fascicle is much stronger than the left anterior fascicle and, due to its location, is not as much at risk in cardiac surgery.

ECG

An LPH is difficult to diagnose in an ECG. Typical features are marked right axis deviation and a sluggish increase in the R waves in the precordial leads. These changes must be distinguished from right heart overload.

18.23 Long QT Syndrome

18.23.1 Basics

Definition

Long QT syndrome (LQTS) is a congenital prolongation of the QT interval that is sometimes associated with changes in T wave morphology. There is a markedly increased risk of ventricular arrhythmias that can develop into torsades de pointes and lead to syncope or cardiac arrest and thus to sudden cardiac death.

Torsades de pointes is polymorphic ventricular tachycardia whose amplitude twists around the zero line and can develop into ventricular fibrillation. Torsades de pointes typically occurs in the context of long QT syndrome. Torsades de pointes is very rare in a normal QT interval.

In addition to a congenital prolongation of the QT interval, there is also acquired prolongation of the QT interval (e.g., due to drugs, electrolyte imbalance, or myocarditis).

▸ **QT interval.** The QT interval (▸ Table 18.8) is defined as the time from the beginning of the QRS complex to the end of the T wave. The QT interval thus represents the duration of activation and recovery of the ventricle myocardium. Since the duration of the QT interval depends on heart rate, it is corrected to a heart rate of 60 bpm (QTc interval) using the Bazett formula. The QT interval in lead II is usually the longest and is best measured there.

$$\text{QT}_C \text{ time} = \frac{\text{QT time}}{\sqrt{\text{RR interval}}}$$

Example: In a patient, the measured QT interval is 0.4 s. The distance between the two previous R waves is 0.5 s. The QTc interval in this example is 0.56 s.

Epidemiology

The prevalence of LQTS is approximately 1 per 10,000 people. But it is probably underestimated, since 10 to 15% of patients with LQTS have a normal QT interval in the ECG. The most common LQT syndromes are types 1 to 3.

LQTS causes an estimated 4,000 deaths in the United States each year. Teenagers and young adults are particularly affected. Up to 10 years of age, the risk of sudden cardiac death is higher for young boys than girls; after age 10 the risk is equal for both sexes.

Table 18.8 Normal QTc values

Patient group	Normal value	Borderline prolonged QTc interval	Prolonged QTc interval
Children and adolescents under 15 years	< 0.44 s	0.44–0.46 s	> 0.46 s
Men	< 0.43 s	0.43–0.45 s	> 0.45 s
Women	< 0.45 s	0.45–0.46 s	> 0.46 s

Pathogenesis

The QT interval represents the duration of activation and recovery of the ventricular myocardium. Delayed recovery of electrical excitation increases the occurrence of transmural re-entries in the ventricular myocardium and may lead to ventricular arrhythmias including torsades de pointes and ventricular fibrillation.

LQTS usually occurs in familial clusters. It is caused by mutations of genes for cardiac ion channels (K, Na, and Ca channels). Several genes have now been identified that cause LQTS and at least 10 forms of LQTS can currently be distinguished.

Classification

LQT syndromes 1 to 6 are grouped as the *Romano-Ward syndrome* and have an autosomal dominant inheritance pattern.

JLN 1 and 2 are referred to as *Jervell–Lange–Nielsen syndrome* and affect the same genes as LQT syndromes 1 and 5, but are also associated with congenital inner ear hearing loss. Inheritance is autosomal recessive.

LQTS 7 is referred to by many authors as *Anderson syndrome*. In addition to cardiac ion channels, muscular channels are also affected. Additional features include skeletal abnormalities (e.g., scoliosis, short stature and neuromuscular problems such as periodic paralysis).

LQTS 8 is also known as *Timothy syndrome* and is associated with congenital heart defects, behavioral problems, musculoskeletal diseases, and disorders of the immune system. ▶ Table 18.9

Table 18.9 Classification of long QT syndromes

LQTS type	Chromosomal locus	Affected gene	Affected ion channel	Associated anomalies	Prevalence
LQT 1	11p15.5	KVLQT1, KCNQ1	Potassium (IKs)		45%
LQT 2	7q35–36	HERG, KCNH2	Potassium (IKr)		45%
LQT 3	3p21–24	SCN5A	Sodium (INa)		7%
LQT 4	4q25–27	ANK2, ANKB	Sodium, potassium, calcium		Rare
LQT 5	21q22.1–22.2	KCNE1	Potassium (IKs)		Rare
LQT 6	21q22.1–22.2	MiRP1, KNCE2	Potassium (IKr)		Rare
LQT 7 (Andersen syndrome)	17q23	KCNJ2	Potassium (IK1)	Skeletal abnormalities, periodic paralysis	Rare
LQT 8 (Timothy syndrome)	12q13.3	CACNA1C	Calcium (ICa-Lalpha)	Congenital heart defect, behavioral abnormalities, cognitive disorders, musculoskeletal diseases, immune system disorders	Rare
JLN 1	11p15.5	KVLQT1, KCNQ1	Potassium (IKs)	Inner ear hearing loss	Rare
JLN 2	21q22.1–22.2	KCNE1	Potassium (IKs)	Inner ear hearing loss	Rare

Etiology

There are multiple possible causes of LQTS and they include numerous drugs. The following list contains only a portion of the drugs that cause a prolongation of the QT interval. A complete list is available on the Internet at www.longqt.org or www.torsades.org.

Causes of acquired prolongation of the QT interval include:

- Antibiotics: erythromycin, trimethoprim, ampicillin, levofloxacin, chloroquine
- Antifungals: fluconazole, itraconazole, ketoconazole
- Antidepressants: imipramine, amitriptyline, desipramine, doxepin
- Antipsychotics: haloperidol, risperidone, chlorpromazine
- Antiarrhythmics: Class Ia: quinidine, procainamide, disopyramide, Class Ic: flecainide, Class III: amiodarone, sotalol
- Antihistamines: astemizole, terfenadine, diphenhydramine
- Immunosuppressive drugs: tacrolimus
- Prokinetics: droperidol, cisapride
- Other medications: methadone
- Electrolyte imbalances: hypokalemia, hypocalcemia, hypomagnesemia
- Bradycardia: complete AV block, severe bradycardia, sick sinus syndrome, hypothermia
- Myocardial dysfunction: cardiomyopathy, congestive heart failure, myocarditis, cardiac tumors
- Endocrine diseases: hypothyroidism, hyperparathyroidism, pheochromocytoma
- Neurological diseases: encephalitis, brain trauma, cerebral hemorrhage, stroke
- Eating disorders: alcoholism, anorexia, starvation

The drugs listed above can lead to a prolongation of the QT interval. In patients with LQTS, there may therefore be additive effects that considerably increase the risk of torsades de pointes tachycardias.

There may also be a risk of excessive QT prolongation when the metabolism of a QT interval-prolonging substance competes with another drug. Therefore, the inhibitors and substrates of the respective cytochrome P-450 isoenzymes must be considered.

In addition, there are drugs that have a proarrhythmogenic effect (e.g., sympathomimetics such as adrenaline, beta-2 mimetics, amphetamines, methylphenidate) or may lead to electrolyte disorders (e.g., diuretics), which should be avoided or at least used with extreme caution in affected individuals.

18.23.2 Diagnostic Measures

Medical History

LQTS is usually diagnosed following a cardiac event (syncope, cardiac arrest) or as an incidental finding in the ECG or in family studies.

The following questions must be included in the medical history in patients with long QT intervals in the ECG:

- History of syncopes/presyncopes
- Triggers of syncopes/symptoms
- Palpitations
- Family history: sudden deaths, events requiring resuscitation of relatives (especially at a young age), death of relatives at an early age
- Hearing loss in the patients themselves or in family members (Jervell–Lange–Nielsen syndrome)
- Muscular problems, skeletal abnormalities in the patients themselves or in family members (Andersen syndrome)
- Behavioral disorders, cognitive disorders in the patients themselves or in family members (Timothy syndrome)
- Drug history: use of medications that prolong the QT interval, reduce potassium or magnesium levels, or have a proarrhythmogenic effect

Note

Some types of LQTS have typical triggers that can cause syncope:

- LQTS 1: physical exertion, swimming
- LQTS 2: emotional stress, sudden acoustic signals (alarm clock, telephone ringing, and doorbell)
- LQTS 3: night sleep

Laboratory

Electrolytes including K, Mg, and Ca should be determined routinely. A thyroid disorder must be ruled out. Increased myocardial enzymes could suggest myocarditis.

Molecular genetic testing for LQTS mutation is generally sought in suspected cases. However, genetic testing is time consuming and expensive due to pronounced heterogeneity. A known mutation can be found in only around half of the patients. The other half probably have unknown mutations. Thus, molecular genetic evidence has a high specificity, but low sensitivity.

ECG

The typical ECG findings of LQTS are (▶ Table 18.10):

- Prolonged QTc interval (normal values, see ▶ Table 18.8)
- Abnormal T wave morphology:
  - Wide-based T waves (common in LQTS 1)
  - Notched T waves (common in LQTS 2)
  - T wave alternans (T waves with varying morphology)
- Long isoelectric ST segments (common in LQTS 3; ▶ Fig. 18.35)
- Bradycardia (20%)
- QT dispersion: Variability of the QT intervals among the different ECG leads. QT dispersion of about 100 ms is considered to be pathological and suggests heterogeneous repolarization. It promotes the occurrence of arrhythmias.

In addition, the following findings can occur in the context of LQTS:

- 2nd degree AV block: Due to the long repolarization period, an atrial impulse may still encounter refractory ventricular myocardium and not be conducted. This causes a functional 2nd degree AV block.
- Polymorphic ventricular extrasystoles, ventricular tachycardias.

► **Exercise ECG.** An exercise ECG is indicated for a borderline long QTc interval in the resting ECG. QTc prolongation can sometimes be detected only under stress. Maximum prolongation of the QTc interval typically occurs in the recovery phase after about 2 minutes. Caution: Ventricular arrhythmias develop in one-third of patients during or after the exercise test.

► **Holter ECG.** In the assessment of a 24-hour Holter ECG, the following points should be particularly noted:

- Changes in the QTc interval depending on stress and events during the day
- T wave morphology, T wave alternans
- Bradycardia, AV block
- Tachycardia or ventricular arrhythmias including torsades de pointes

Table 18.10 Clinical features of the most common forms of LQTS

LQTS type	Trigger	Characteristic ECG findings
LQTS 1	Physical exertion, swimming	Broad-based T wave
LQTS 2	Acoustic signals, emotional stress	Notched T wave
LQTS 3	Rest and sleep (higher risk due to low heart rates)	Long isoelectric segment with high peaked T wave

Echocardiography

In congenital long QT syndromes, the echocardiography findings are usually normal. However, there are acquired forms of prolonged QT interval that may be caused by cardiac abnormalities such as cardiomyopathy or cardiac tumors.

Confirmation of the Diagnosis

The clinical diagnosis of LQTS is made on the basis of findings published by Schwartz in 1993 (► Table 18.11). Diagnostic criteria are the ECG findings, clinical findings, and family history. Care should be taken that ECG findings are not falsified by drugs that affect the ECG criteria. The basis for calculating the QTc interval is the Bazett formula. In the family history, a family member with confirmed LQTS who died suddenly before the age of 30 years is not counted in both categories. Based on the diagnosis criteria, a maximum possible score is 9. LQTS is confirmed with a score over 3.

Differential Diagnoses

In the differential diagnosis, LQTS must be distinguished mainly from acquired prolongation of the QT interval and other diseases that may lead to syncope, life-threatening arrhythmias, or cardiac arrest:

- Drug-induced QT prolongation
- Endocrine or neurological QT prolongation
- Myocardial function disorders
- Bradycardia (bradycardia may cause a prolonged QT interval, on the other hand bradycardia is also an important criterion for the diagnosis of LQTS, see ► Table 18.11)

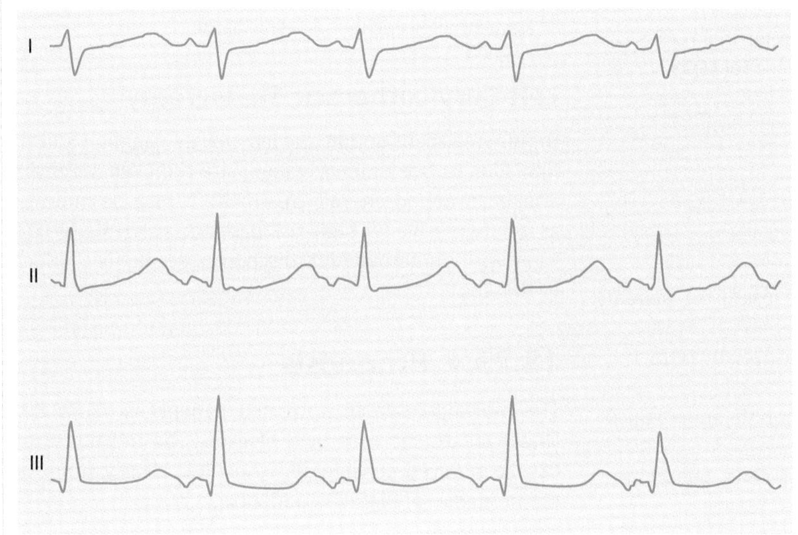

Fig. 18.35 ECG in long QT syndrome type 3.

Table 18.11 Schwartz diagnostic criteria for LQTS (Circulation 1993; 88: 782–784)

Criterion		Points
ECG finding		
QTc interval	> 480 ms	3
	460–470 ms	2
	450 ms in males	1
Torsades de pointes		2
T wave alternans		1
Notched T wave in at least 3 leads		1
Heart rate too low for age (heart rate at rest below the 2nd percentile		0.5
Clinical findings		
Syncope	Under stress	2
	Without stress	1
Congenital hearing loss		0.5
Family history		
Family member with confirmed LQTS		1
Unclear sudden death of a close relative under age 30 years		0.5

- Vasovagal syncopes
- Seizures
- Other causes of syncope or sudden cardiac death at a young age:
  - Hypertrophic obstructive cardiomyopathy
  - Arrhythmogenic right ventricular dysplasia
  - Brugada syndrome

Note

If there is evidence or reasonable suspicion of an LQTS, family members should also be examined for LQTS.

18.23.3 Treatment

General Measures

The following general measures are useful in patients with LQTS:

- Competitive sports are prohibited (especially LQTS 1 and 2).
- Avoid swimming and water sports or only under supervision (especially LQTS 1).
- Minimize acoustic alarms (e.g., alarm clock, telephone ringing, especially LQTS 2).
- Instruct family members and teachers in cardiopulmonary resuscitation.
- Avoid drugs that prolong the QT interval, lead to loss of potassium and magnesium, or are arrhythmogenic.

Pharmacological Treatment

Prophylactic beta-blocker treatment is indicated for all patients with LQTS. Propranolol is most often used. Other beta blockers, however, are probably similarly effective. The propranolol dosage is normally around 3 mg/kg/d in three to four single doses, but lower doses may also be effective.

For LQTS 3, mexiletine (sodium channel blocker) is used in combination with a beta blocker. Potassium and magnesium are substituted in case of deficiency.

AICD

The implantation of an AICD is the most effective therapy for the prevention of sudden cardiac death in high-risk patients. Indications are:

- High-risk patients (previous cardiac arrest, recurrent cardiac events such as syncope or torsades de pointes, despite conventional therapy)
- Possibly patients with a family history of sudden cardiac death

Pacemaker Treatment

Bradycardia, sinus pauses, and AV blocks occur more frequently in patients with LQTS and predispose them to torsades de pointes. Pacemaker implantation should prevent arrhythmogenic bradycardia. Bradycardia-induced torsades de pointes is common especially in LQTS 3, so pacemaker treatment should be considered especially for these patients.

Most AICDs now also have a pacemaker function. Therefore, it is usually better to use such an AICD instead of a pacemaker without a defibrillator.

Left Cervicothoracic Stellectomy

In this treatment option, the left stellate ganglion and the first four to five thoracic ganglia are removed surgically. This is an antiadrenergic treatment. It may be indicated as an alternative for high-risk patients (particularly LQTS 1) or with numerous AICD discharges despite beta-blocker therapy.

18.23.4 Prognosis

The mortality rate in untreated patients is 75 to 80%. Under treatment with beta blockers, the mortality rate can be reduced considerably. An AICD clearly improves the prognosis of high-risk patients.

Pregnancy is not associated with an increased risk for cardiac events, but affected women are particularly vulnerable in the postpartum period.

Risk factors for syncope or sudden cardiac death are:

- Pronounced prolongation of the QTc interval
- Young age at the first episode
- History of syncope
- Documented torsades de pointes or ventricular fibrillation
- Congenital hearing loss

18.24 Short QT Syndrome

18.24.1 Basics

Definition

Short QT syndrome is an ion channel disease associated with shortening of the QT interval in the ECG and a tendency for syncope, atrial fibrillation, and life-threatening arrhythmias. There is an increased risk of sudden cardiac death.

Epidemiology

Short QT syndrome is very rare. It affects mainly young, otherwise healthy individuals without an underlying structural heart disease. Both familial clustering and isolated cases have been described.

Etiology

Short QT syndrome is a genetic ion channel disease. To date, three mutations in genes that code for potassium channels have been described as a cause of short QT syndrome. The affected genes are KCNH2, KCNQ1, and KCNJ2.

18.24.2 Diagnostics

Symptoms

The clinical symptoms range from asymptomatic forms to atrial fibrillation and syncope and to sudden cardiac death. Short QT syndrome can sometimes manifest very early. Sudden deaths can often be found in the family history.

ECG

The following ECG findings are typical for short QT syndrome:

- Short QT interval: A QT interval of 330 ms is very suggestive of short QT syndrome
- High T wave
- Well-defined U wave

Another typical feature of the short QT syndrome is atrial fibrillation. After atrial fibrillation is converted to a sinus rhythm, the above findings can be observed.

Differential Diagnoses

Other conditions that cause a shortening of the QT interval must be ruled out in the differential diagnosis. The main ones are:

- Hypercalcemia
- Tachycardia
- Medication: catecholamines, acetylcholine

18.24.3 Treatment

The only established treatment is implantation of an AICD. The significance of pharmacological treatment with antiarrhythmic agents that prolong the QT interval (e.g., sotalol or quinidine) has not yet been definitely established.

18.24.4 Prognosis

Since the short QT syndrome has only recently been described as an entity, it is still difficult to make any concrete statements on prognosis. It is striking, however, that short QT syndrome sometimes manifests even in very young children in the form of malignant cardiac arrhythmias or even sudden cardiac death.

18.25 Brugada Syndrome

18.25.1 Basics

Definition

Brugada syndrome is a genetic disorder that is associated with typical changes in the surface ECG (atypical right bundle branch block and ST segment elevation in leads V_1–V_3) in otherwise healthy people and involves an increased risk for syncope, ventricular tachycardia, and sudden death.

Epidemiology

The incidence of this syndrome, which was defined only in 1991, is unknown. Figures for the prevalence of typical ECG abnormalities range between 0.4% and 1%, depending on the study and ethnic group investigated. Brugada syndrome affects mainly young, otherwise healthy men. Men are affected about eight times more frequently than women. Brugada syndrome is rarely diagnosed in children; it typically manifests in the 4th decade of life.

In Asia, Brugada syndrome is supposedly the most common cause of natural death in young men under 50 years old. The diseases known as "bangungut" in the

Table 18.12 Classification of the Brugada syndrome based on ECG features in leads V_1 to V_3

Feature	Type 1	Type 2	Type 3
Amplitude of the J wave	≥ 2 mm	≥ 2 mm	≥ 2 mm
T wave	Negative	Positive or biphasic	Positive
ST segment	Coved type	Saddle type	Saddle type
Terminal ST segment	Gradually descendent	Elevated ≥ 1 mm	Elevated < 1 mm

Philippines, "pokkuri" in Japan, and "lai tai" in Thailand probably correspond with Brugada syndrome.

Etiology

Brugada syndrome is a genetic disorder that is inherited in an autosomal dominant pattern. The fact that mainly men are affected suggests gender-specific penetrance. The SCN5A gene located on chromosome 3 that codes for a cardiac sodium channel is affected. There are already more than 60 known mutations of the SCN5A gene. However, mutations of this gene can be detected in only 20 to 30% of patients with Brugada syndrome.

Long QT syndrome type 3 also involves a mutation of the SCN5A gene.

18.25.2 Diagnostic Measures

Symptoms

The Brugada syndrome typically manifests with no prior symptoms as sudden episodes of ventricular tachycardia or ventricular fibrillation. Depending on the duration of the arrhythmia, the following may occur:

- Asymptomatic development
- Palpitations
- Dizziness
- Syncopes
- Sudden cardiac death

It is important to ask about a family history of sudden deaths or survived resuscitations.

> **Note**
>
> Because of the familial clustering, family members of affected patients should also be examined for a Brugada syndrome.

Laboratory

In a Brugada syndrome, there are no specific changes in blood chemistry apart from the molecular genetic detection of mutations in the SCN5A gene. It is important to determine certain laboratory parameters to eliminate differential diagnoses:

- Serum electrolytes, especially calcium and potassium: Hypercalcemia or hyperkalemia can cause similar ECG changes as a Brugada syndrome (ST segment elevation).
- CK-MB, troponin I: to rule out myocardial ischemia, which leads to ST segment elevation
- Molecular genetic analysis: If there is clinical suspicion of a Brugada syndrome, the SCN5A gene should be tested for mutations, although mutations can be detected in only 20 to 30% of the cases.

ECG

The diagnosis of Brugada syndrome is established in the 12-lead surface ECG (visual diagnosis). The typical criteria are an atypical right bundle branch block and saddle-shaped or curved ("coved type") ST-segment elevation. These changes may occur permanently, only intermittently, or only after specific provocation tests (see Provocation Tests, concealed Brugada syndrome).

It is significant that there is a risk of fatal ventricular tachycardia irrespective of whether the ECG changes are permanent, intermittent, or only on provocation.

On the basis of the ECG changes, three types of Brugada syndrome can be differentiated (▶ Table 18.12, ▶ Fig. 18.36).

Provocation Tests

It is especially important to identify patients with a concealed Brugada syndrome, in which the ECG changes are only temporary or not visible at all in the normal ECG. After administration of class I antiarrhythmic drugs, hidden forms can be "unmasked" or the previously only mild ST elevation can be amplified. The test is considered positive if the amplitude of the J wave increases to 2 mm or more.

The provocation tests should always be carried out under ECG monitoring and resuscitation conditions. The following drugs may be used for the provocation test:

- Ajmaline 1 mg/kg IV over 5 min

  or
- Flecainide 2 mg/kg (max. 150 mg) IV over 10 min

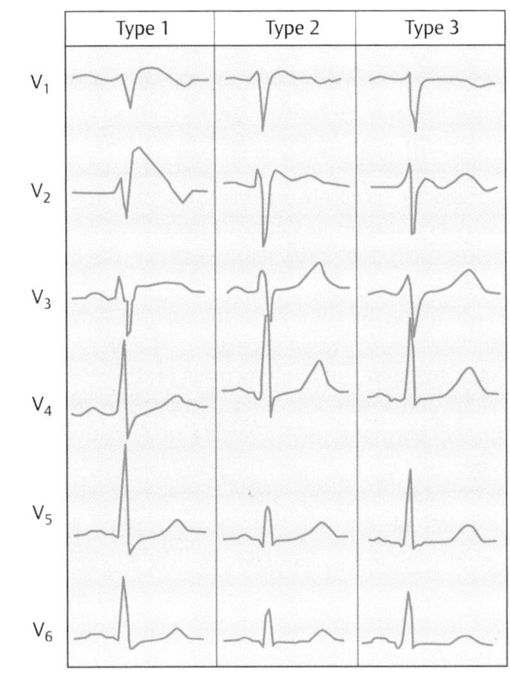

Fig. 18.36 Typical changes of the ST segment in various Brugada syndromes (see also ▶ Table 18.12). (Wilde et al. 2002)[112]

Discontinuation criteria are:

- positive result,
- ventricular arrhythmias,
- widening of the QRS complex by more than 30%.

Isoproterenol should be available as an antidote. The adrenergic stimulation by isoproterenol leads to a reduction of the provoked ECG changes.

Note

In patients with unexplained syncopes or ventricular tachycardia, a concealed Brugada syndrome should be considered and a drug provocation test should be performed if necessary.

Imaging Procedures

Echocardiography and/or MRI are used to rule out possible differential diagnoses such as arrhythmogenic right ventricular dysplasia, hypertrophic cardiomyopathy, myocarditis, or coronary anomalies.

Electrophysiological Study

An electrophysiological study is used to check whether ventricular tachycardia can be induced. However, the predictive value is not clear. In about half of patients, prolongation of the HV interval is also found (slowed conduction in the AV bundle of His system).

Differential Diagnoses

The differential diagnosis includes mainly right precordial ST-segment elevation of other causes and other causes of syncopes or sudden cardiac death.

- Right precordial ST-segment elevation of other causes:
  - Myocardial ischemia, myocardial infarction
  - Myocarditis, pericarditis
  - Arrhythmogenic right ventricular dysplasia (epsilon wave), cardiomyopathies
  - Atypical right bundle branch block
  - Left ventricular hypertrophy
  - Changes in the autonomic nervous system (e.g., high vagal tone)
  - Hypercalcemia, hyperkalemia
- Other causes of syncopes or sudden cardiac death
  - Hypertrophic cardiomyopathy
  - Long QT syndrome

18.25.3 Treatment

The only effective treatment is the implantation of an AICD. Antiarrhythmic drugs cannot definitely prevent sudden death. In Brugada syndrome, the implantation of an AICD is definitely indicated in patients who had syncopes and ventricular tachycardia in the past or survived cardiac arrest. However, it is controversial whether completely asymptomatic patients should also be fitted with an AICD without a family history of sudden death. Furthermore, there are drugs that are associated with arrhythmias in Brugada syndrome patients. These drugs should be avoided. The drug list can be found on www.brugadadrugs.org.

18.25.4 Prognosis

Without appropriate therapy (AICD), patients with Brugada syndrome have a poor prognosis. The risk of sudden death is high even in concealed Brugada syndrome. Life-threatening arrhythmias reoccur within 2 to 3 years in about one-third of patients who have already suffered syncopes or ventricular tachycardias.

19 Heart Failure

19.1.1 Basics

Definition

Heart failure is defined as the inability of the heart to pump sufficient cardiac output to meet the metabolic needs of the body and supply it with enough oxygen. Depending on the section of the heart affected, a distinction is made between left heart, right heart, and global failure. Heart failure is also divided into acute and chronic heart failure according to the course of the disease.

Epidemiology

No precise epidemiological data are available on heart failure in children and adolescents. Congenital heart defects in neonates occur with a frequency of 8 to 11 per 1,000 live births—that is, about 1% of all live births. Only a fraction of these individuals develop symptoms of heart failure, estimated to be 0.1–0.2% of all live births.

Etiology

Heart failure is a result of congenital or acquired heart disease that leads to a volume or pressure overload of the heart or to myocardial insufficiency (▶ Table 19.1). Furthermore, arrhythmias can lead to insufficient cardiac output.

In childhood, congenital heart defects that lead to volume or pressure overload of the heart are the most common causes of heart failure. Examples of volume overload are a large ventral septal defect (VSD), patent ductus arteriosus (PDA), or atrioventricular septal defect (AVSD). Pressure overload develops in aortic stenosis, coarctation of the aorta, or mitral stenosis, for example.

The clinical symptoms of heart failure in the various congenital heart defects typically manifest at certain times (▶ Table 19.2). Congenital heart defects with a large left-to-right shunt, for example, usually lead to heart failure when pulmonary resistance drops at the age of 6 to 8 weeks. An atrial septal defect (ASD) usually does not lead to heart failure until adulthood. In most cases, children with tetralogy of Fallot do not develop heart failure, as they are protected from a large shunt volume and corresponding volume overload due to pulmonary stenosis.

Pathophysiology

The body reacts to the decreased pumping capacity of the heart with various compensatory mechanisms that initially improve the blood supply to the body, but over time contribute considerably to deterioration of cardiac condition.

▶ **Neuroendocrine activation.** The increase in the sympathetic tonus, and thus the increased release of catecholamines initially leads to an increase in the heart rate and contractility. However, over time, downregulation of the beta-adrenergic receptors occurs so that the effectiveness of the catecholamines in the heart decreases. Because of an increase in systemic vascular resistance, the afterload increases.

The activation of the renin–angiotensin–aldosterone system (RAAS) leads to an increase in the afterload due to vasoconstriction and to an increase in the preload due to sodium and water retention. Increased secretion of antidiuretic hormone (ADH) results in excessive water retention.

The increased pressure and volume load also leads to activation of the NO and the natriuretic peptides ANP (atrial natriuretic peptide), BNP (brain natriuretic

Table 19.1 Causes of acute and chronic heart failure

Pathological preload
• Shunt defects
• Valve regurgitations
Pathological afterload
• Valve stenosis
• Outflow tract obstructions
• Arterial hypertension
• Pulmonary hypertension, pulmonary embolism, bronchial obstruction
Diminished myocardial contractility or restricted ventricular filling
• Cardiomyopathies
• Myocarditis
• Pericarditis
• Myocardial ischemia
• Kawasaki disease
• Endocarditis
• Sepsis
• Acidosis
• Severe hypoxia, peripheral asphyxia
• Metabolic disorder
• Toxic myocardial damage (e.g., anthracycline)
Pathological heart rate
• Tachycardia and bradycardia

Table 19.2 Typical manifestation times of congenital heart defects

Heart disease	Remark
Manifestation in the fetal period	
• Fetal tachyarrhythmia • Complete AV block • Severe valve regurgitation (e.g., severe form of Ebstein anomaly) • Large AV anomalies • Severe anemia	Clinical manifestation: hydrops fetalis
Manifestation at birth	
• HLHS with restrictive foramen ovale • Severe valve regurgitation (e.g., Ebstein anomaly) • Severe AV anomalies	Clinical manifestation: cardiogenic shock
Manifestation in the 1st week of life	
• TGA • Total anomalous pulmonary venous connection with pulmonary venous obstruction • Critical aortic or pulmonary stenosis • HLHS	Clinical manifestation: cyanosis and cardiogenic shock
• PDA in premature infants	Premature infants do not compensate volume overload as well as mature neonates
Manifestation in the 1st month of life	
• High grade coarctation of the aorta	
• VSD in premature neonates	Premature infants do not compensate volume overload as well as mature neonates
Manifestation in the 2nd–4th month of life	
• AVSD • Large VSD • Large PDA • Truncus arteriosus	Heart defects with a large left-to-right shunt usually manifest at the age of 6–8 weeks when the pulmonary vascular resistance drops
• Bland–White–Garland syndrome, ALCAPA	A steal phenomenon develops when the pulmonary vascular resistance drops

peptide), and CNP (C-type natriuretic peptide). They cause vasodilatation and an inhibition of the RAAS as well as natriuresis, in effect a counter-regulatory mechanism.

NT-pro-BNP (N-terminal pro brain natriuretic peptide), a precursor of BNP, is also used as a laboratory chemical marker of heart failure. The serum levels of the natriuretic peptides rise with increasing heart failure.

The recombinant form of BNP, nesiritide, is currently used in clinical trials for the treatment of acute heart failure due to its vasodilator properties.

▸ **Frank–Starling mechanism.** An increase in the preload (e.g., through activation of RAAS and increased secretion of ADH) initially causes an improvement in contractility and an increase in stroke volume, but over time, the increases in end-diastolic pressure and afterload (also consequences of the neuroendocrine compensatory mechanisms) lead to a decrease in cardiac pump function.

▸ **Myocardial hypertrophy.** Chronic volume overload leads to dilatation and thus to eccentric hypertrophy. By contrast, pressure overload leads to concentric hypertrophy with an increase of heart wall thickness. These remodeling processes initially improve the pumping function of the heart, but with increasing hypertrophy, the oxygen demand of the myocardium increases disproportionately.

19.1.2 Diagnostics

Symptoms

Most affected children have global heart failure; it is rarely possible to distinguish between right heart failure and left heart failure.

Infants and younger children have a history of poor feeding, failure to thrive, tachypnea (especially under exertion, such as drinking), and increased sweating (especially on the forehead). In older children, the main symptoms are dyspnea or shortness of breath under stress, rapid fatigability, and eyelid or foot edema.

On clinical examination, the following findings are indicative of heart failure:

- Tachycardia: due to increased sympathetic tone.
- Gallop rhythm: A third or fourth heart sound is probably a sign of rapid filling of a relatively stiff ventricle.
- Cool limbs, pallor, prolonged capillary refill time: signs of peripheral vasoconstriction and reduced peripheral perfusion in sympathetic activation.
- Tachypnea, dyspnea, subcostal and intercostal retractions, orthopnea: Tachypnea is the clinical manifestation of the excessive pulmonary blood flow and pulmonary edema. With advancing heart failure, ventilation function is increasingly impaired. Dyspnea with subcostal and intercostal retractions develops. Manifest pulmonary edema causes fine bubbly crackles. Frequent pulmonary infections are also a result of excessive pulmonary blood flow. A dry cough can also be a sign of excessive pulmonary blood flow or pulmonary congestion.
- Pulsus tardus: Arterial pulses weak on palpation.
- Pulsus paradoxus
- Cyanosis: Sign of increasing oxygen utilization in the periphery or deterioration of gas exchange as a result of pulmonary edema. Cyanosis may also be indicative of an increasing right-to-left shunt.
- Hepatomegaly: Sign of systemic venous congestion in the context of right heart failure or global failure.
- Jugular vein distention: Occurs mainly in older children and adults as a sign of a systemic venous congestion. It is rarely observed in younger children.
- Edema: Mainly eyelid edema in children. Peripheral edema is less common than in adults.

Similar to adults, the clinical severity of heart failure is divided in four NYHA classes. The criteria have been modified for children (▶ Table 19.3).

ECG

The ECG is not particularly indicative for assessing heart failure. A typical finding is sinus tachycardia. Cardiac arrhythmias must also be ruled out as a cause of heart failure. In addition, the ECG provides evidence of a heart defect or underlying cardiac disease (e.g., myocarditis).

Chest X-ray

The main finding in heart failure is cardiomegaly. In addition, there are often signs of excessive pulmonary blood flow. In *interstitial* pulmonary edema, there are increased streaky hilar markings; in *alveolar* edema there is diffuse opacification ("ground glass").

Echocardiography

Underlying congenital or acquired heart defects can be diagnosed by echocardiography. Pericardial or pleural effusion can be reliably detected or ruled out. In addition, size and wall thickness of both ventricles as well as systolic and diastolic function should be assessed. The left ventricular systolic function is easily described by fractional shortening and ejection fraction; left ventricular diastolic function can be described using the inflow profile across the mitral valve, for example.

Laboratory

The following characteristic laboratory changes occur as a result of the deterioration of the organ and tissue perfusion or as a sign of compensatory mechanisms that occur during heart failure:

- Hyponatremia: consequence of water retention or increased natriuresis
- Increased lactate: sign of tissue hypoxia. In shunt defects, tissue hypoxia suggests an imbalance between pulmonary and systemic circulation (increased lung perfusion, decreased systemic perfusion).
- Respiratory acidosis: As a result of excessive pulmonary blood flow or pulmonary edema, carbon dioxide accumulates and oxygen partial pressure is reduced.

Table 19.3 New York Heart Association (NYHA) classification of heart failure in children

NYHA class	Symptoms
I	No limitation of physical activity • Ordinary physical activity does not induce symptoms (undue fatigue, sweating, shortness of breath)
II	Slight limitation of physical activity • No discomfort at rest • Greater physical activity (depending on age: drinking, crawling, walking, climbing stairs) causes symptoms (fatigue, sweating, shortness of breath)
III	Marked limitation of physical activity • Still no discomfort at rest • Slight physical activity leads to symptoms (fatigue, sweating, dyspnea)
IV	Discomfort during all physical activity and at rest • Symptoms such as sweating, dyspnea, or cyanosis from all physical activity and at rest • Bedridden, cardiac dystrophy or cachexia

- Increased transaminases: Due to liver congestion, liver enzyme levels may increase.
- Increased renal function parameters: Increased levels of creatinine and urea suggest renal failure as a result of heart failure.
- Increased specific gravity of urine: result of increased excretion of protein and sodium
- Increased plasma catecholamine level: Due to neurohumoral compensatory mechanisms, the plasma levels of noradrenaline and adrenaline are increased in heart failure patients. In adults, increased noradrenaline levels are associated with a poor prognosis.
- NT-pro-BNP: This precursor of the brain natriuretic peptide is now being used as a laboratory heart failure marker in clinical routine.

19.1.3 Treatment

In the treatment of chronic heart failure, the priority is treatment of the cause. In addition, conditions that exacerbate heart failure must be eliminated (e.g., arrhythmia, infection, anemia). Different drugs are used in the various stages to improve the clinical symptoms and the long-term course. Sometimes pharmacological treatment is used as an interim measure until definitive treatment (e. g., corrective surgery for congenital heart defects).

Causal Treatment

Causal treatment can be given for the following diseases:

- *Congenital or acquired heart defects*: Most heart defects can now be corrected by surgery or catheter intervention or at least treated palliatively. Anticongestive drug treatment may be required later for residual defects.
- *Arrhythmias*: Arrhythmias that cause heart failure or have an adverse effect on it are treated with antiarrhythmic agents, cardioversion, or with a pacemaker to restore rhythm.
- *Arterial hypertension*: Arterial hypertension is treated with antihypertensive agents.
- *Metabolic and storage diseases*: Some metabolic or storage disorders can be treated causally. Myocardial failure due to iron storage disease (e.g., thalassemia) is treated with desferal to reduce the iron overload. For a thyroid function disorder, appropriate hormone replacement therapy is a priority.

General procedures

- Bed rest and elevation of the upper body ("cardiac chair")
- Oxygen administration if there are respiratory symptoms. Caution: In heart defects with left-to-right shunt and in hypoplastic left heart syndrome (HLHS), caution is required when oxygen is administered. When oxygen is administered, the pulmonary resistance decreases and the left-to-right shunt increases. The result is excessive pulmonary blood flow to the detriment of systemic perfusion. There is an increase in lactate levels in the laboratory tests and the clinical signs of heart failure increase.
- In acute decompensation, fluid restriction to 75% of the usual age-appropriate requirements. Hospitalized patients are balanced and weighed daily.
- Weight normalization
- Moderate exercise (sports ban if there is decompensation)
- Low-salt diet: It is enough to avoid very salty foods such as chips and to dispense with the adding of salt to food.
- In acute decompensation, sedation may be indicated to avoid unnecessary consumption of oxygen through agitation and restlessness. Caution: Most sedatives cause a drop in blood pressure and can lead to acute cardiac decompensation. In critical situations, therefore, ketamine is used, which leads to an increase in blood pressure. Emergency medication must be ready in case of sedation.
- Mechanical ventilation if necessary: By eliminating the breathing work, oxygen demand decreases.
- Compensation of metabolic acidosis: The catecholamine effect is reduced if acidosis is present.
- Compensation for anemia: Severe anemia means that cardiac output must be additionally increased to supply the body with enough oxygen. Depending on the underlying disease, the target hematocrit level is between 30% and 45%.

Rising lactate levels, increasing metabolic acidosis, an increasing need for catecholamines to achieve sufficient blood pressure for diuresis, and low central venous oxygen saturation (more than 40% lower than arterial oxygen saturation as a sign of increased peripheral oxygen extraction) suggest a deteriorating situation.

Pharmacological Treatment of Chronic Heart Failure

The pharmacological treatment of chronic heart failure is a staged therapy (▸ Table 19.4). The primary aim of modern therapy is to break through the neurohumoral compensatory mechanisms that ultimately lead to a deterioration of the prognosis. Accordingly, ACE inhibitors and beta blockers are used. Diuretics and cardiac glycosides are used mainly for symptomatic treatment.

▸ **ACE inhibitors.** ACE inhibitors are the basis of the pharmacological treatment of chronic heart failure and are indicated for NYHA class I and above (▸ Table 19.5). They improve the hemodynamic situation and ventricular function and their inhibitory effect on the RAAS reduces neurohumoral activity. However, ACE inhibitors should be administered carefully and gradually increased because they may lead to a drop in blood pressure and cause renal

Table 19.4 Staged pharmacological therapy of chronic heart failure

Drug	NYHA I	NYHA II	NYHA III	NYHA IV
ACE inhibitor	+	+	+	+
Beta blocker	Only for hypertension	+	+	+
Loop diuretic	–	Only for fluid retention	+	+
Thiazide	Only for hypertension	Only for fluid retention	To enhance the effect of loop diuretics	To enhance the effect of loop diuretics
Aldosterone antagonist	–	Only for hypokalemia	+	+
Cardiac glycoside	–	–	+	+

Table 19.5 Dosage recommendations for the treatment of chronic heart failure (DGPK German Society of Pediatric Cardiology guidelines of 2007)

Drug	Initial dose (mg/kg/d)	Target dose (mg/kg/d)
ACE inhibitors		
Captopril	3 × 0.1	1–3
Enalapril	2 × 0.03	0.15–0.3
Beta blockers		
Metoprolol	2 × 0.1–0.2	1–2.5
Carvedilol	2 × 0.05–0.1	0.5–0.8
Bisoprolol	1 × 0.02	0.15
Diuretics		
Furosemide		2 (–10)
Hydrochlorothiazide		2–4
Spironolactone		2–4
Cardiac glycosides		
Digoxin	Target plasma levels: 0.5–0.9 ng/mL	

failure. They may also cause an increase in potassium, which may be relevant, especially if combined with spironolactone. If ACE inhibitors are not tolerated due to a dry, irritating cough (typical adverse effect, but very rare in children), they can be switched to angiotensin antagonists.

► **Beta blockers.** Beta blockers are also an integral part of long-term anticongestive treatment (► Table 19.5). They protect the heart from chronic beta-adrenergic stimulation and decrease the oxygen demand of the heart. Beta blockers without intrinsic sympathomimetic activity are used to treat heart failure—in childhood mainly metoprolol, propranolol, bisoprolol, or carvedilol.

Beta blockers are indicated for NYHA class II and above (for class I if hypertension is present). However, they should be administered only to stable patients and must be increased gradually and under close monitoring. The dosage is increased so the target dose is not reached until 2 to 3 months (!). If heart failure deteriorates or there is a relevant drop in blood pressure during beta-blocker therapy, the dosage increase must be slowed and anticongestive therapy must be optimized. Bronchial obstructions and pronounced AV blocks are considered contraindications.

► **Aldosterone antagonists.** Aldosterone antagonists are indicated as additional therapy for NYHA class III and above. In adults, favorable effects of aldosterone antagonists on the prognosis have been described that go beyond the diuretic effect. However, there is a tendency to develop hyperkalemia, which may be particularly relevant in combination with ACE inhibitors. An aldosterone antagonist may also be useful for NYHA class II patients with hypokalemia.

► **Diuretics.** Diuretics are indicated if there is fluid retention and in general for NYHA class III and above (► Table 19.5). However, diuretics lead to an unfavorable stimulation of neurohumoral compensatory mechanisms, so they should always be combined with ACE inhibitors, beta blockers, and possibly aldosterone antagonists. Loop diuretics are usually used, which can be combined with thiazide diuretics if the effect is insufficient. Patients should be monitored for potassium and magnesium loss. Hypochloremic metabolic alkalosis may develop as a result of chloride loss that may lead to increased absorption of bicarbonate. In addition, loop diuretics may be ototoxic and can also cause nephrocalcinosis.

► **Cardiac glycosides.** The importance of cardiac glycosides in the treatment of heart failure has declined in recent years. Cardiac glycosides are currently considered

Table 19.6 Dosage of essential drugs for the treatment of acute heart failure (modified according to DGPK guidelines of 2007)

Drug	Dosage
Catecholamines	
• Dobutamine	5–10 (–15) µg/kg/min
• Adrenaline	0.01–0.5–2 µg/kg/min
• Noradrenaline	0.01–0.1–1 µg/kg/min
Phosophodiesterase inhibitors	
• Milrinone	50 µg/kg as a loading dose over at least 15 min, then 0.25–1 µg/kg/min
Vasodilators	
• Sodium nitroprusside	0.5–5 µg/kg/min (for prolonged use and high doses, add 10-fold dose of sodium thiosulfate)
• Nitroglycerin	0.5–3 µg/kg/min (reduce preload) 3–20 µg/kg/min (reduce afterload)
• NO	2–5–40 ppm (administer with breathing gas)
• Prostacyclin (epoprostenol)	5–20 ng/kg/min
• Iloprost IV	0.5–4 ng/kg/min
Diuretics	
• Furosemide	0.5–1–2 mg/kg/dose IV, 10 (–20) mg/kg/d as continuous infusion

to be indicated for NYHA class III and above (▸ Table 19.5). Low normal serum levels are targeted. Cardiac glycosides have a potential positive effect on rate reduction and neurohumoral compensation. Patients should be monitored for increased digitalis toxicity in hypokalemia that may occur under diuretic therapy.

▸ **Phosphodiesterase inhibitors and calcium sensitizers.** Phosphodiesterase inhibitors (e.g., milrinone) and calcium sensitizers (levosimendan) may be used as intravenous therapy in otherwise treatment-refractory heart failure. They can often be used to bridge the time until other measures such as implantation of a mechanical assist device or heart transplantation are possible.

▸ **Intracardiac defibrillators.** An intracardiac defibrillator (ICD) is indicated in patients with heart failure for secondary prevention after a syncope or resuscitation due to ventricular tachycardia.

Table 19.7 Hemodynamic effects of different catecholamines

Catecholamine	CO	Contractility	Heart rate	SVR	PVR
Dobutamine	↑↑↑	↑	↑	↓	↓
Noradrenaline	↑	↑	↔	↑↑	↔
Adrenaline	↑↑	↑	↑	↑	
• 0.5–3 µg/kg/min	↑	↑	↑	↓	↓
• 3–8 µg/kg/min	↑↑	↑	↑	↓	↓
• >8 µg/kg/min	↑↑	↑	↑	↑↑	↔(↑)

CO, cardiac output; SVR, systemic vascular resistance; PVR, pulmonary vascular resistance.

▸ **Cardiac resynchronization therapy.** Biventricular pacemaker stimulation may optimize myocardial contraction processes. It may be indicated in patients with severe heart failure and asynchronous ventricular contraction as a result of a left bundle branch block.

▸ **Heart transplantation.** Heart transplantation is the last treatment option for otherwise treatment-refractory patients with a high mortality rate.

Pharmacological Treatment of Acute Heart Failure

The priority in the pharmacological treatment of acute heart failure is to increase myocardial contractility, maintain adequate blood pressure, and reduce afterload (▸ Table 19.6). In refractory cases, mechanical circulatory assist devices (VAD or ECMO; Chapter 27) may be required as interim measures.

▸ **Catecholamines.** Catecholamines act on the heart by stimulating beta-1 and beta-2 receptors. They lead to an increase in contractility and heart rate and to an acceleration of the spread of excitation and impulse formation. Alpha receptors mediate vasoconstriction and beta-2 receptors mediate vasodilatation. It should be noted that catecholamines increase myocardial oxygen demand.

The various catecholamines stimulate the individual receptors in different ways. The mode of action of catecholamines varies accordingly (▸ Table 19.7).

▸ **Dopamine.** Dopamine has a positive inotropic effect via beta-1 stimulation and causes vasoconstriction by alpha stimulation. The stimulation of specific dopamine receptors causes vasodilation of mesenteric and renal vessels. However, the effect of dopamine is dose dependent. At a low dose, the main effect is to increase renal perfusion, an intermediate dose increases inotropy, and at high doses, dopamine primarily causes vasoconstriction.

Dopamine was formerly often used at a low dose ("renal dose") to stimulate diuresis, but dopamine is now viewed much more critically and it should no longer be used routinely. The renal protective effect has been disproven. Dopamine also leads to deterioration of microcirculation of the intestinal villi, inhibits the formation of neurohypophysial hormones, and causes changes in cellular and humoral immunity. Therefore, dopamine no longer plays a role in the treatment of heart failure.

► **Dobutamine.** Dobutamine improves myocardial contractility and reduces systemic resistance by stimulating beta-1 and beta-2 receptors. Dobutamine is the catecholamine of choice for increasing inotropy. Due to the increase in the heart rate and stroke volume, cardiac output is increased. However, because of the vasodilator effect, blood pressure may drop if there is an insufficient increase in cardiac output. Dobutamine is often combined with milrinone. In combination with noradrenaline it is useful for increasing blood pressure.

► **Adrenaline.** Adrenaline stimulates alpha and beta receptors very effectively. At a low dosage, it leads to an increase of myocardial contractility and heart rate; at high doses, vasoconstriction is the main effect. Adrenaline is indicated as interim therapy for severe acute heart failure, but it increases myocardial oxygen consumption. It is also the catecholamine of choice in resuscitation and is often combined with milrinone or sodium nitroprusside.

► **Noradrenaline.** Compared with adrenaline, the increase in contractility is less pronounced than the increase in resistance. Noradrenaline is therefore especially indicated when systemic resistance must be increased, for example, in critical hypotension associated with sepsis or anaphylaxis.

► **Phosphodiesterase inhibitors.** Phosphodiesterase inhibitors inhibit the breakdown of cAMP and thus lead to an increase in cellular cAMP levels. This results in an increase in contractility and vasodilation (reduction of systemic resistance). For this reason, phosphodiesterase inhibitors are known as "inodilators." Because of the longer half-life compared to catecholamines, phosphodiesterase inhibitors are more difficult to control.

The most common phosphodiesterase inhibitors used are milrinone and enoximone. Phosphodiesterase inhibitors are indicated for the treatment of severe acute heart failure and are often combined with catecholamines.

► **Vasodilators.** Sodium nitroprusside and nitroglycerin are the main vasodilators used in pediatric cardiology intensive therapy to reduce systemic afterload. Nitric oxide and prostanoids (prostacyclin, iloprost) are used to reduce pulmonary vascular resistance.

► **Sodium nitroprusside.** Sodium nitroprusside is a potent NO donor and has a strong vasodilator effect on the smooth vascular muscles. Its half-life is only a few minutes. It must be infused continuously and protected from light. However, sodium nitroprusside contains cyanide and for prolonged infusion at higher doses, a 10-fold quantity of thiosulfate should be added to the infusion to aid cyanide detoxification. Sodium nitroprusside is indicated in the acute treatment of (left) heart failure.

► **Nitroglycerin.** Nitroglycerin is also an NO donor, but is less potent than sodium nitroprusside. At low doses, it acts as a vasodilator mainly on the veins, at higher doses also on the arteries as well.

► **Nitric oxide (NO).** NO acts as a direct vasodilator on the smooth vascular muscles. When NO is added to breathing gas, it acts highly selectively on pulmonary vascular resistance. It is used especially when pulmonary vascular resistance must be selectively reduced, for example, in pulmonary hypertension. However, the reaction of NO with hemoglobin causes methemoglobin. The methemoglobin concentration must be monitored regularly and may not exceed 3%. In addition, the NO_2 concentration in breathing gas must be monitored continuously, as NO_2 levels over 3 ppm may cause toxic pulmonary edema.

► **Prostacyclin.** Prostacyclin belongs to the prostanoids group and it is a short-acting vasodilator that must be infused continuously. Synthesized prostacyclin is called epoprostenol. It affects both the pulmonary and the systemic arterial vascular system and it is used primarily to reduce pulmonary vascular resistance, for example, in the treatment of critical pulmonary resistance crises, but also as an interim measure in pulmonary hypertension and cor pulmonale. Major side effects include a drop in systemic pressure and inhibition of platelet aggregation.

► **Iloprost.** Iloprost also belongs to the group of prostanoids, but has a longer half-life of 20 to 30 minutes compared with epoprostenol. It can also be administered as an inhalation solution using a special nebulizer system.

► **Diuretics.** Diuretics are generally administered intravenously for the treatment of acute heart failure. Furosemide is often used, sometimes in combination with ethacrynic acid, another loop diuretic. Diuretics inhibit preload.

▸ **Mechanical circulatory support.** Mechanical circulatory support may become necessary for treatment-refractory heart failure. In childhood, options include the implantation of a "ventricular assist device" (VAD) or an ECMO (Chapter 27). However, these are only interim measures until cardiac function recovers or definitive therapy with a heart transplant is possible.

▸ **Heart transplantation.** A heart transplant is the last treatment option, but this option is limited by the severe shortage of donor organs.

19.1.4 Prognosis

The prognosis of heart failure depends largely on the underlying cause. Congenital heart defects, the most common cause of heart failure in children, can usually be corrected or at least palliated by surgery or interventional catheterization. For the prognosis of cardiomyopathies and heart transplants, please refer to the corresponding chapters.

20 Arterial Hypertension

20.1.1 Basics

Definition

Arterial hypertension is defined as an increase in systolic and/or diastolic blood pressure over the gender-specific 95th percentile for the age or size of the patient (▶ Table 20.1). At least three independent measurements are needed.

The following formulas can be used as a rule of thumb for the upper blood pressure limits:

- Children age 1 to 10 years:
  - Systolic blood pressure (mmHg): 100 + (age in years × 2)
  - Diastolic blood pressure (mmHg): 60 + (age in years × 2)
- Children and adolescents age 11 to 17 years:
  - Systolic blood pressure (mmHg): 100 + (age in years × 2)
  - Diastolic blood pressure (mmHg): 70 + (age in years)

Epidemiology

The incidence of arterial hypertension in children and adolescents in Germany is at present 1 to 3% but increasing.

Classification and Etiology

Arterial hypertension is classified as primary (essential) hypertension or secondary hypertension. Secondary hypertension is due to a treatable cause.

Primary (Essential) Hypertension

The cause of essential hypertension is unknown. It is assumed that there are multiple factors, among them genetic predisposition, environmental factors, lifestyle, and ethnic origin. Studies in the United States show that essential hypertension is on the increase, even in children and adolescents. Many of these patients are obese and have a positive family history of hypertension. This form of hypertension is often associated with lipid metabolism

Table 20.1 Normal values for 24-hour long-term blood pressure measurement in children and adolescents in relation to gender and height (Soergel et al. 1997)[101]

Mean values for boys (mmHg)						
	Daytime		Nighttime		24 hours	
Height (cm)	50th percentile	95th percentile	50th percentile	95th percentile	50th percentile	95th percentile
120	112/73	123/85	95/55	104/63	105/65	113/72
130	113/73	125/85	96/55	107/65	105/65	117/75
140	114/73	127/85	97/55	110/67	107/65	121/77
150	115/73	129/85	99/56	113/67	109/66	124/78
160	118/73	132/85	102/56	116/67	112/66	126/78
170	121/73	135/85	104/56	119/67	115/67	128/77
180	124/73	137/85	107/56	122/67	120/67	130/77
Mean values for girls (mmHg)						
	Daytime		Nighttime		24 hours	
Height (cm)	50th percentile	95th percentile	50th percentile	95th percentile	50th percentile	95th percentile
120	111/72	120/84	96/55	107/66	103/65	113/73
130	112/72	124/84	97/55	109/66	105/66	117/75
140	114/72	127/84	98/55	111/66	108/66	120/76
150	115/73	129/84	99/55	112/66	110/66	122/76
160	116/73	131/84	100/55	113/66	111/66	124/76
170	118/74	131/84	101/55	113/66	112/66	124/76
180	120/74	131/84	103/55	114/66	113/66	124/76

disorders and impaired glucose tolerance (metabolic syndrome), especially in overweight patients.

Secondary Hypertension

- Renal disease: Kidney diseases constitute around 90% of secondary hypertension:
  - Renovascular diseases: Renovascular disease is found in about half of neonates with hypertension. Examples:
    - Congenital renal artery stenosis
    - Complex anomaly of the entire aorta (mid-aortic syndrome)
    - Renal artery stenosis due to a fibromuscular dysplasia (association with neurofibromatosis type I)
    - Renal vascular thrombosis (especially after umbilical vessel catheters)
    - After kidney transplantation
  - Renal parenchymal diseases: Renal parenchymal diseases are the most common causes of secondary hypertension in infants and school-age children. Examples:
    - Focal segmental glomerulosclerosis
    - Mesangial proliferative glomerulonephritis
    - Membranoproliferative glomerulonephritis
    - Rapid progressive glomerulonephritis
    - IgA nephritis
    - Diabetic nephropathy
    - HIV nephropathy
    - Renal parenchymal scarring and reflux nephropathy
    - Vasculitis (systemic lupus erythematosus, Wegener granulomatosis, polyangiitis)
    - Hemolytic uremic syndrome
    - Polycystic kidney disease (in autosomal recessive forms, severe hypertension is often already present at birth)
    - Alport syndrome
    - Renal hypoplasia/dysplasia
    - Metabolic diseases (cystinosis, oxalosis)
- Cardiovascular diseases:
  - Coarctation of the aorta—leading symptom: increased blood pressure in the upper limbs, decreased blood pressure in the lower limbs. (Even after surgery or interventional catheterization, hypertension often persists in the upper limbs.)
  - Rarely:
    - Hypoplastic aortic arch
    - Mid-aortic syndrome
    - Takayasu arteritis
    - Aortic aneurysm
    - Stenosis of the carotid artery
    - After Kawasaki disease
- Endocrine diseases:
  - Cushing syndrome, steroid treatment
  - Adrenogenital syndrome
  - Pheochromocytoma (rare in childhood, usually associated with neurofibromatosis type I)
  - Neuroblastoma (however, usually no hypertension present)
  - Hyperthyroid crisis
  - Hyperaldosteronism, Liddle syndrome (hypokalemia, alkalosis)
- Neurogenic diseases:
  - Intracranial pressure (brain tumors, trauma)
  - CNS inflammation (Guillain–Barré syndrome, encephalitis)
- Drugs and toxic causes:
  - Drugs: steroids, cyclosporine A, sympathomimetics, caffeine
  - Excessive consumption of liquorice
  - Mercury poisoning
- Other causes:
  - Bronchopulmonary dysplasia
  - Hypercalcemia
  - Porphyria
  - Turner Syndrome
  - Marfan syndrome
  - Sickle cell anemia
  - Sleep apnoe

Note

Essential hypertension is a diagnosis of exclusion. The younger the patient and the higher the blood pressure, the more likely secondary hypertension is. In children, more than 75% of cases are secondary hypertension. About half of cases among adolescents involve secondary hypertension.

The most common cause of secondary hypertension is kidney disease. The most common cardiovascular cause is coarctation of the aorta.

20.1.2 Diagnostic Measures

Symptoms

Arterial hypertension does not initially lead to symptoms and is discovered as an incidental finding when blood pressure is measured.

Typical symptoms include headache, dizziness, vomiting, nosebleeds, pallor, blurred vision, and in secondary hypertension, symptoms of the underlying disease. In a hypertensive crisis, the main signs are neurological symptoms such as headaches, blurred vision, and loss of consciousness up to seizures. Severe dyspnea may also develop in the context of pulmonary edema.

Medical History

Important points to be clarified:

- Neonatal period: umbilical vessel catheters, prematurity, bronchopulmonary dysplasia

Table 20.2 Indicative findings of the physical examination for the investigation of hypertension

Finding	Suspected diagnosis
Blood pressure gradient between upper and lower limbs, attenuated inguinal pulses	Coarctation of the aorta, mid-aortic syndrome
Abdominal vascular sound	Renal artery stenosis, mid-aortic syndrome
Striae, obesity, delayed growth	Cushing syndrome
Photosensitivity, arthralgia	Systemic lupus erythematosus
Café-au-lait spots	Neurofibromatosis type I
Hypopigmentations (white spots)	Tuberous sclerosis
Short stature and anemia	Chronic renal failure
Tachycardia, goiter	Hyperthyroidism
Syndromic stigmata	Turner syndrome, Marfan syndrome

- Drug history: use of steroids, sympathomimetics, hormones (contraceptives), cyclosporine A
- Family history: arterial hypertension, myocardial infarction, stroke, metabolic disorders (diabetes mellitus, lipid metabolism disorders)

Physical Examination

Indicative findings of the physical examination are summarized in ▸ Table 20.2:

▸ **Blood pressure.** Regularly measuring blood pressure as screening or before surgery is useful, especially for patients with the following risk factors: kidney disease, heart disease, diabetes mellitus, neurofibromatosis type I, Turner syndrome, Marfan syndrome, obesity, premature birth, family history, and patients under steroid, cyclosporine A, sympathomimetic, or hormone therapy.

Blood pressure is measured in a sitting position. The cuff width should be about two-thirds the length of upper arm. A cuff that is too narrow results in a high blood pressure value, a cuff that is too wide yields a low value.

Note

In all patients with high blood pressure on the arm, the pressure must also be measured on the other arm and the legs.

In *long-term blood pressure measurement*, the blood pressure cuff is attached to the nondominant arm, in a coarctation of the aorta, pressure is always measured on the right arm. Blood pressure is measured during the day, usually at 15-minute intervals and at night at half-hour intervals. The patient should record a log of his/her activity.

It is important that in addition to the systolic, diastolic, and mean pressure values, a sufficient drop in the blood pressure must be assessed during the night. Normally, the blood pressure falls at night by 10 to 20%. A lack of nocturnal drop in blood pressure may suggest secondary hypertension.

Echocardiography

Echocardiography is used to rule out coarctation of the aorta, a hypoplastic aortic arch, or a mid-aortic syndrome. Moreover, left ventricular hypertrophy can be ruled out and the diastolic and systolic posterior wall thickness should be determined.

Sonography of the Abdomen and Retroperitoneum

In ultrasound examination, renal size and renal parenchyma are assessed and renal anomalies (cysts, reflux) and parenchymal scars are ruled out. The Doppler ultrasound scan of the renal arteries is used as screening to rule out renal artery stenosis. Furthermore, the adrenal glands are assessed and abdominal tumors are ruled out.

Renal Scintigraphy

Following the administration of an ACE inhibitor, there is a visible decrease in the renal blood flow behind a renal artery stenosis. If this examination is positive, a renal angiography should follow.

Angiography of the Renal Vessels

Angiography of the renal vessels is the gold standard for diagnosing a renal artery stenosis. Stenosis of the renal vessels may possibly be treated in the same session with catheter interventional balloon dilation or stent. In addition, a selective determination of renin activity in the left and right renal artery can be made.

Note

Angiography of the renal vessels is the gold standard for diagnosing stenosis of the renal artery.

Spiral CT/Magnetic Resonance Tomography

In general, a good assessment of the renal vessels in older patients can be made.

Fundoscopy

A fundoscopy is performed to rule out or to follow up on hypertensive retinopathy.

Laboratory

The standard diagnostics include:

- Complete blood count, Na, K, Cl, Ca, pH, creatinine, urea, blood sugar, cholesterol, total protein, albumin, plasma renin, TSH
- Urine: urinalysis, catecholamine excretion (vanillylmandelic acid)

Other diagnostic tests to consider are 24-hour cortisol, aldosterone, ACTH, C3/C4 complement, ANA, blood gas analysis, and HIV serology.

20.1.3 Treatment

The treatment goals aside from treating the causes are to relieve symptoms, prevent end-organ damage, and reduce complications such as increased cardiovascular morbidity.

General Measures

The following general measures may have a positive effect on arterial hypertension:

- Low-salt diet (less than 100 mmol or 2.5 g/d)
- Potassium and calcium-rich diet (except in renal failure)
- Reduction of overweight
- Increased physical activity (but isometric stress such as strength training or competitive cycling are contraindicated in uncontrolled hypertension)
- Avoidance of alcohol and tobacco consumption
- Treatment of accompanying diseases such as hypercholesterolemia or diabetes mellitus

Causal Treatment

In secondary hypertension, the priority is causal treatment. Typical examples are listed below:

- Coarctation of the aorta: surgical correction or interventional catheterization with balloon dilation or stent implantation
- Renal artery stenosis: surgical correction or interventional catheterization with balloon dilation or stent implantation
- Hormone producing tumors: surgical removal
- Hyperthyroidism: antithyroid drugs
- Drug-induced hypertension: switch medication

Pharmacological Treatment

Pharmacological treatment is indicated in severe hypertension for the symptoms of or already existing end-organ damage. If there are additional risk factors such as diabetes mellitus or chronic renal failure, drug treatment of mild hypertension should be started at an early stage (definition: in mild hypertension, the blood pressure is > 95th percentile; in moderate/severe hypertension, the blood pressure is 10 mmHg > 95th percentile). The appropriate drug classes are summarized in ▶ Table 20.3; the dosages are found in ▶ Table 20.4.

Principles of Antihypertensive Therapy

The choice of an antihypertensive agent depends on the underlying disease (▶ Table 20.5). The medication should be administered slowly under regular monitoring of the blood pressure. Drugs with a longer half-life improve compliance.

Treatment is usually started with one agent. If the effect is inadequate, a combination therapy follows, where drugs with a complementary mechanism of action have an advantage. Examples of favorable combinations are diuretics and ACE inhibitors or diuretics and beta blockers.

Treatment of a Hypertensive Crisis

In a hypertensive crisis, the blood pressure is more than one-third dover the corresponding 95th percentile. The main clinical signs may be neurological symptoms of a hypertensive encephalopathy such as headache, altered consciousness, visual disturbances, or seizures. In addition, acute pulmonary edema may develop.

In a hypertensive crisis, it is sufficient to reduce blood pressure by about 25% within 1 hour. A complete normalization of blood pressure should be sought only within 12 hours to avoid the complications of a too rapid lowering of the blood pressure. Suitable drugs are listed in ▶ Table 20.6.

20.1.4 Prognosis

Arterial hypertension is a major risk factor for the development of diseases such as atherosclerosis, coronary heart disease, cerebrovascular diseases, and chronic renal failure and is a crucial cause of morbidity and mortality.

Table 20.3 Antihypertensive drugs

Drug class	Mechanism of action	Side effects	Contraindications	Remarks
ACE inhibitors	Inhibit the conversion of angiotensin I into angiotensin II, thereby vasorelaxation, aldosterone ↓	Hyperkalemia, dry cough	Pregnancy, coarctation of the aorta, bilateral renal artery stenosis, acute and chronic renal failure, hyperkalemia	
Angiotensin II antagonists	Block the angiotensin II receptor at the vessels	Hyperkalemia	Pregnancy, coarctation of the aorta, bilateral renal artery stenosis, acute and chronic renal failure, hyperkalemia	Dry cough is not a side effect, otherwise similar to ACE inhibitors, relatively little experience in children
Calcium antagonists	Reduction of Ca influx into the smooth muscle cells	Tachycardia, headache, flushing, edema, lower glucose tolerance, gingival hyperplasia	Heart failure Verapamil/diltiazem: AV block, atrial flutter, fibrillation, neonates	Nifedipine is used especially in hypertensive crises because of the short half-life; amlodipine has a long half-life and is used in long-term treatment
Beta blockers	Block activity of the sympathetic nervous system	Negative inotropic, bradycardia, bronchoconstriction, lipid metabolism disorders, hypoglycemia, fetopathy	Bronchial asthma, pregnancy, AV block Caution in diabetes mellitus and heart failure!	
Diuretics	Increased renal excretion of water and sodium, reducing intravascular volume	Loop diuretics: hypokalemia, hypercalciuria, nephrocalcinosis, ototoxicity Thiazides: hyperglycemia, hyperlipidemia	Hypovolemia Thiazides: hyperbilirubinemia Loop diuretics: hypercalciuria, nephrocalcinosis Potassium-sparing diuretics: hyperkalemia, diabetic nephropathy	
Vasodilators	Direct effect on vascular smooth muscles	Sodium and water retention, headache, tachycardia	Minoxidil: pheochromocytoma, congestive heart failure. Sodium nitroprusside: increased intracranial pressure, coarctation of the aorta	Sodium nitroprusside: for treatment of a hypertensive crisis in the ICU (note risk of cyanide poisoning)
Peripheral alpha blockers	Vasodilatation by inhibiting the postsynaptic alpha adrenoreceptors	Orthostatic hypotension, sodium and water retention		Rarely used in children
Central alpha 2 agonists	Central inhibition of the sympathetic nerve	Sedation, dry mouth, rebound phenomenon after discontinuation		Very potent antihypertensive drugs, only second choice because of relevant side effects

Table 20.4 Dosages of relevant antihypertensive drugs (modified from Bald 2007)

Drug	Dosage	Highest dosage
ACE inhibitors		
Captopril	0.3–6 mg/kg/d in 2–3 single doses orally	450 mg/d
Enalapril	0.08–0.6 mg/kg/d in 1–2 single doses orally	40 mg/d
Ramipril	0.05–0.2 mg/kg/d in 1–2 single doses orally	10 mg/d
Angiotensin II antagonists		
Losartan	0.7–1.4 mg/kg/d in 1 single dose orally	100 mg/d (little experience in children)
Calcium antagonists		
Nifidipine retard	0.5–2 mg/kg/d in 3 single doses orally	80 mg/d
Amlodipine	0.1–0.6 mg/kg/d in 1–2 single doses	10 mg/d
Beta blockers		
Metoprolol retard	1–6 mg/kg/d in 2 single doses orally	200 mg/d
Atenolol	0.5–2 mg/kg/d in 1–2 single doses orally	100 mg/d
Propranolol	1–5 mg/kg/d in 3–4 single doses orally	640 mg/d
Diuretics		
Furosemide	0.5–6 mg/kg/d in 2–4 single doses orally	600 mg/d
Hydrochlorothiazide	1–3 mg/kg/d in 2 single doses orally	50 mg/d
Spironolactone	1.5–4 mg/kg/d in 1–2 single doses orally	100 mg/d
Direct vasodilators		
Hydralazine	0.75–7.5 mg/kg/d in 4 single doses orally	200 mg/d
Minoxidil	0.2–0.5 mg/kg/d in 1–2 single doses orally	50–100 mg/d
Central alpha-2 agonists		
Clonidine	2.5–25 μg/kg/d in 3 single doses orally	2.4 mg/d
Peripheral alpha blockers		
Prazosin	0.05–0.5 mg/kg/d in 2–3 single doses orally	20 mg/d

Table 20.5 Antihypertensive drugs depending on the underlying disease or accompanying disease

Form of hypertension / concomitant disease	Preferred antihypertensive drug	Remark
Essential hypertension	ACE inhibitors	Especially in obese patients in whom beta blockers have an unfavorable effect on fat metabolism and obesity
	Beta blockers	Caution in diabetes mellitus
Diabetes mellitus	ACE inhibitors	No beta blockers if possible
Renal artery stenosis/untreated coarctation of the aorta and residual hypertension after correction	Beta blockers	Treatment of choice: operation or interventional catheterization
Renal parenchymal diseases	ACE inhibitors	Additionally antiproteinuric; possibly beneficial effect on the progression of renal parenchymal diseases; dosage must be increased gradually; monitor creatinine and potassium
Hypercortisolism	Diuretics	
Pheochromocytoma		Beta blockers are contraindicated without simultaneous alpha blockade
Dialysis patients, kidney transplant patients	Calcium antagonist (possibly in combination with a beta blocker)	ACE inhibitors usually not suitable because of hyperkalemia and increased creatinine
Cyclosporine A treatment	Calcium antagonist	

Table 20.6 Drugs for the treatment of hypertensive crisis

Drug	Dosage	Remark
Nifedipine drops	0.1–0.5 mg/kg orally or sublingually (up to 10 mg per single dose)	Repeat after 15–30 min if necessary
Urapidil	1–3 mg/kg in a slow infusion, then 0.5–1 mg/kg/h as a continuous infusion	
Sodium nitroprusside	0.5–5 (–10) µg/kg/min as a continuous infusion	Potent antihypertensive drug. Titrate according to effect. Risk of cyanide poisoning at high doses and prolonged therapy. Therefore, add 10 times the amount of sodium thiosulfate. Infuse protected from light.
Furosemide	0.2–1 mg/kg IV	For imminent pulmonary edema

21 Pulmonary Hypertension

21.1.1 Basics

Definition

Pulmonary hypertension is present when the mean pulmonary artery pressure is greater than 25 mmHg at rest or greater than 30 mmHg during exercise.

Elevated pulmonary vascular resistance is defined as an increase in the pulmonary vascular resistance to 3 Wood units × m^2. It is a sign of pulmonary artery vasculopathy, which is initially reversible but is later irreversible (fixed).

Epidemiology

Idiopathic or familial pulmonary hypertension is extremely rare in childhood. It is assumed that their incidence is 2 patients per 1 million inhabitants.

Pathogenesis

The pulmonary artery pressure (PAP) is determined by three factors:

- LAP = left atrial pressure
- Q_P = pulmonary blood flow
- R_P = pulmonary vascular resistance

$$PAP = LAP + Q_P \times R_P$$

Normally, the pulmonary artery pressure, which is increased at birth, drops rapidly within the first few weeks of life. After 6 to 8 weeks, it usually reaches the normal adult value of 1 to 3 Wood units × m^2. Later, the muscles of the pulmonary vessels become thin, the arteries increase in size, and new arteries and arterioles develop.

An increase in pulmonary artery pressure leads to changes in the pulmonary vascular bed with *vasoconstriction, thrombosis* in the small vessels, and remodeling including *proliferation of smooth muscle and endothelial cells*. These processes increase pulmonary hypertension, leading to *pulmonary arterial vasculopathy* and are sustained by an imbalance between protective and aggressive factors. Vasodilators (e.g., prostacyclin, NO) have a protective effect and vasoconstrictors (e.g., thromboxane, endothelin) have an aggressive effect. Prostacyclin and NO also have a very beneficial effect by inhibiting platelet aggregation and the proliferation of smooth muscle and endothelial cells. Hypoxia adversely affects pulmonary hypertension.

If pulmonary hypertension is due to an increased blood flow caused by a heart defect with a left-to-right shunt, the continuous overload on the pulmonary vessels leads to pulmonary arterial vasculopathy with an increase in pulmonary vascular resistance. If pulmonary vascular resistance exceeds the systemic resistance, shunt reversal develops with cyanosis (Eisenmenger reaction, Chapter 22). The time at which the Eisenmenger reaction occurs varies and depends not only on the shunt volume, but also on structural heart defects and other factors not yet fully understood. Patients with AV septal defects, TGA with a VSD, and with truncus arteriosus are at particularly high risk. For them, irreversible pulmonary hypertension may already occur in the first year of life if the heart defect is not corrected in time. In an ASD, however, pulmonary hypertension often does not develop for several decades. In children with trisomy 21 and a shunt defect, an Eisenmenger reaction often occurs earlier than in other children. The reason for this may be an obstruction of the upper airways that causes hypoxia and high endothelin levels.

Another cause of pulmonary artery hypertension is pulmonary venous congestion, for example, if there is increased pressure in the left atrium in left heart diseases (mitral stenosis, mitral regurgitation, cor triatrium, left ventricular dysfunction) or stenosis of the pulmonary veins.

The high pressure overload in pulmonary hypertension causes hypertrophy of the right ventricle. If the right ventricle becomes insufficient and cannot overcome the pulmonary resistance, there is insufficient filling of the left heart, and hypotension and cardiovascular shock occur. If there is a connection between the right and left heart (e.g., an ASD or VSD), this connection may function as an overflow valve and leads to sufficient filling of the left heart for maintaining adequate cardiac output. Because of the right-to-left shunt, however, cyanosis occurs. Since such an overflow valve in an Eisenmenger reaction is vital for maintaining adequate cardiac output, corrective surgery to close the shunt is contraindicated in such cases.

Etiology

Pulmonary hypertension in childhood occurs most often with the following disorders:

- Congenital or acquired heart defects
- Persistent pulmonary hypertension of the newborn
- Idiopathic or familial pulmonary hypertension
- Chronic lung diseases such as bronchopulmonary dysplasia, cystic fibrosis

Classification

Classification of pulmonary hypertension (from Simonneau et al. 2004)[100]:

- I. Pulmonary arterial hypertension:
  - Idiopathic
  - Familial

 - Associated with
   - Collagen diseases
   - Congenital shunt defects (ASD, VSD, PDA, AVSD, aortopulmonary window, truncus arteriosus communis, single ventricle with nonobstructive pulmonary blood flow)
   - Portal hypertension, HIV infection, pertussis
   - Drugs and toxins: e.g., amphetamines, cocaine, appetite suppressants, L-tryptophan, canola oil
   - Other diseases: e.g., thyroid disorders, storage diseases (glycogen storage diseases, Gaucher disease), congenital hemorrhagic telangiectasia, myeloproliferative disorders, splenectomy
- II. Pulmonary arterial hypertension with relevant venous and capillary involvement:
  - Pulmonary veno-occlusive disease
  - Pulmonary capillary hemangiomatosis
- III. Persistent pulmonary hypertension of the newborn (PPHN)
- IV. Pulmonary hypertension in left heart diseases:
  - Left heart disease, pulmonary vein stenosis, cor triatrium
- V. Pulmonary arterial hypertension in lung diseases and/or hypoxia
  - Chronic obstructive lung disease, interstitial lung disease
  - Bronchopulmonary dysplasia, congenital diaphragmatic hernia, hypoplastic lungs
  - Sleep apnea syndrome, chronic tonsillar hypertrophy, craniofacial anomalies, thoracic deformities, disorders of the respiratory muscles
  - Developmental disorders
  - Exposure to high altitudes
- VI. Pulmonary arterial hypertension in chronic thrombotic or embolic disease:
  - Thrombotic occlusion of the proximal pulmonary arteries
  - Thrombotic occlusion of the distal pulmonary arteries
  - Sickle cell anemia
  - Nonthrombotic lung embolism (tumor, parasites, foreign body)
- VII. Other diseases:
  - Sarcoidosis, histiocytosis X, lymphangiomatosis, scleroderma, compression of the pulmonary vessels (e.g., tumors)

Idiopathic hypertension and familial pulmonary hypertension were formerly known as primary pulmonary hypertensions, all others as secondary forms.

21.1.2 Diagnostic Measures

Symptoms

- Rapid fatigue, deteriorating physical capacity
- Exertional dyspnea, syncope: caused by the inability to adequately increase cardiac output during exercise
- Headache
- Angina pectoris symptoms: result of right ventricular ischemia (unfavorable ratio between right ventricular muscle mass, increased right ventricular pressure, and coronary supply)
- Signs of right heart failure (edema, hepatomegaly, venous congestion, ascites)
- Cyanosis at rest (blue lips disease): sign of mixed venous saturation and reduced cardiac output, another underlying disease (e.g., parenchymal lung disease), or a right-to-left shunt.
- Bronchial obstruction: often associated with pulmonary hypertension
- Hemoptysis: late symptom

The clinical severity of pulmonary hypertension is classified into four classes similar to those of heart failure (▶ Table 21.1).

Auscultation

In pulmonary hypertension, a loud ("popping") second heart sound is typical. If the right ventricle is dilated, there is possibly a low-frequency systolic murmur as a result of a tricuspid regurgitation. A diastolic decrescendo murmur may suggest pulmonary valve regurgitation.

ECG

In the ECG there are signs of right heart hypertrophy (moderate right axis deviation, P pulmonale), possibly repolarization disturbances in the right precordial leads, an (incomplete) right bundle branch block, tachycardia, or arrhythmia.

Table 21.1 Clinical classification (New York Heart Association) of the severity of pulmonary hypertension

NYHA class	Symptoms
I	No limitation of physical activity: • Normal activity induces no symptoms (dyspnea, fatigue, chest pain, syncope)
II	Slight limitation of physical capacity: • No symptoms at rest • Normal physical activity does not induce excessive symptoms
III	Clear limitation of physical capacity: • Still no symptoms at rest • Normal physical activity induces excessive symptoms
IV	Incapacity with respect to any stress: • Signs of right heart failure • Dyspnea and/or fatigue even at rest • Increase of the symptoms with any activity

Chest X-ray

Depending on the stage and the extent of the disease, the following changes are found in the chest X-ray:

- Prominent pulmonary artery segment, widened hilar vessels, and breakup of the vessels in the lung periphery (hilar amputation, pruning phenomenon)
- Right heart enlargement, in the lateral image, the enlarged right ventricle fills the retrosternal space
- Pulmonary edema if there is acute exacerbation

Echocardiography

Echocardiography is the standard method for noninvasive determination of pulmonary pressure. In addition, it serves the following purposes or may show the following typical findings:

- Ruling out or detection of shunt defects or left heart diseases as a cause of pulmonary hypertension
- Assessment of the right ventricle (hypertrophy, dilation) and atrium (dilation)
- Dilatation of the inferior vena cava and hepatic veins
- Flattened or paradoxical septal movement
- Estimation of the right ventricular and pulmonary arterial pressure via the flow velocity of a tricuspid or pulmonary regurgitation. In a VSD, the right ventricular pressure can also be estimated using the flow velocity across the defect. In a PDA, the pulmonary arterial pressure can be approximately estimated via the maximum flow velocity in the ductus arteriosus.
- Typical pulmonary artery flow curve in Doppler: steep rise in the flow velocity across the right ventricular outflow tract with a shortened acceleration time (normal ≥ 120 ms)
- Possible exclusion of intracardiac thrombi (with transesophageal echocardiography if needed)

Cardiac Catheterization

Cardiac catheterization is the gold standard for diagnosing pulmonary hypertension. In addition to the hemodynamic measurements—including pressures in the right atrium, right ventricle, and pulmonary arteries—the pulmonary vessels can be visualized in the angiography. In shunt defects, the degree of the shunt can also be determined.

An essential part of the examination is testing *pulmonary vascular reactivity*. For this purpose, standardized vasodilators (NO, iloprost, oxygen) may be administered intravenously or by inhalation. Vasoreactivity is assumed to be preserved if the ratio of the mean PAP to the systemic pressure, or the ratio of pulmonary vascular resistance to systemic resistance, is reduced by 20% or more. These "responders" benefit from a high-dose treatment with calcium antagonists.

Scintigraphy

Ventilation-perfusion scintigraphy can be used to rule out chronic embolism and a ventilation–perfusion mismatch.

MRI/High-resolution CT

Tomographic techniques are used to rule out parenchymal lung disease or a heart defect. In spiral CT, chronic pulmonary embolism can be ruled out or visualized after contrast medium is administered.

Abdominal Sonography

To rule out liver cirrhosis and portal hypertension.

Lung Function Test

The lung function test often shows a slight restriction and peripheral airway obstruction, but it can also be completely normal. Nonspecific provocation tests are often positive and thus lead to a misdiagnosis of bronchial asthma. The CO diffusion capacity is usually reduced. A significant reduction may indicate lung disease or collagen disease.

Lung Biopsy, Bronchoalveolar Lavage

These tests are indicated only for unclear lung parenchymal disorders.

Six-minute Walk Test, Cardiopulmonary Exercise Test

Both tests are used to assess physical capacity and monitor the course of the disease.

Nocturnal Oximetry/Polysomnography

These tests can rule out sleep apnea syndrome.

Laboratory

The following laboratory tests are recommended for the assessment of pulmonary hypertension (from Schranz 2006):

- Complete blood count, ESR, CRP, electrolytes, uric acid, LDH, liver function tests, iron, ferritin, BNP
- Thrombophilia screening including PTT, D-dimers, APC (activated protein C) resistance, protein C, protein S, factors II, V, VII, and VIII, von Willebrand antigen, von Willebrand ristocetin cofactor, antithrombin III, phospholipid antibodies
- Hb electrophoresis, quantitative immunoglobulins, fractionated plasma catecholamines, thyroid parameters, lipid profile including Lp(a), HIV test, exclusion of collagen storage diseases (lupus anticoagulant, ANA,

anti-DNA antibodies, CH-50 complement and complement components, anti-centromeres, rheumatoid factor, HLA typing, serum ACE levels)
- Genetic tests: Mutations in the bone morphogenetic protein receptor type II (BMPR2) can be detected in approximately half of patients with familial pulmonary hypertension.

21.1.3 Treatment

General Measures

Physical stress that leads to symptoms such as dyspnea, chest pain, dizziness, or syncope must be avoided. A stay in the mountains is not a problem up to an altitude of 1,200 m. However, supplemental oxygen should be available for air travel.

As patients are particularly susceptible to pulmonary infections, in addition to the usual vaccinations they should be vaccinated against influenza and pneumococcus. Bacterial infections must be treated systematically with antibiotics.

▸ **Oxygen.** Nocturnal oxygen is indicated for patients who hypoventilate during sleep. In addition, it may be useful to improve the respiratory mechanics in some patients, for example, to perform a tonsillectomy or adenoidectomy. Generally, oxygen is indicated in hypoxemia with an oxygen partial pressure of less than 60 mmHg, and oxygen saturation under 90 to 93%.

▸ **Phlebotomy.** Patients with high hematocrit levels with symptoms of hyperviscosity syndrome (headache, blurred vision, transient ischemic attack) benefit from a phlebotomy. Phlebotomy is recommended only at a hematocrit of about 65 to 70% and hemoglobin greater than 20.5 g/dL. As a hyperviscosity syndrome is often associated with a decreased iron level, appropriate substitution should be considered.

▸ **Anticoagulation.** If there is no increased risk of bleeding, anticoagulation is indicated. Anticoagulation is used to prevent secondary thrombosis in the pulmonary vascular bed as a result of decreased pulmonary blood flow. The target INR for warfarin or phenprocoumon treatment is 1.5 to 2.5. Note, however, that especially patients with Eisenmenger syndrome often have a high risk of bleeding, so that in these cases the decision to administer anticoagulation drugs must be taken on a case-by-case basis.

▸ **Digoxin.** The benefit of digoxin in pulmonary hypertension is not conclusively defined. Digoxin can be considered for chronic heart failure or in combination with a high-dose calcium antagonist to compensate its negative inotropic effect.

▸ **Diuretics.** Diuretics are indicated for right heart failure (edema). But marked intravascular volume depletion must be avoided. Otherwise, the right ventricular preload may drop substantially and an acute drop in the cardiac output can occur. Furthermore, the risk of thrombosis is increased by a fluid deficit.

Specific Pharmacological Treatment

The objective of specific pharmacological treatment is to achieve vasodilation of the pulmonary vessels and to slow down the remodeling processes in the lungs (▸ Table 21.2).

Patients with a positive finding in the pulmonary vascular reactivity test probably benefit from different drugs more than those with a negative vascular reactivity test.

▸ **Calcium antagonists.** Calcium antagonists are indicated for patients with confirmed vascular reactivity. Compared with the treatment for arterial hypertension, high doses are required for pulmonary hypertension, which must be determined on a case-by-case base by slowly increasing the dose (risk of severe hypotension). Children often respond better than adults to treatment with calcium antagonists.

▸ **Prostacyclin/prostanoids.** Prostanoids are used regardless of the result of the vascular reactivity test. Prostanoids have vasodilatory properties, inhibit platelet aggregation, and improve the quality of life, physical capacity, and survival rate in patients with pulmonary hypertension. Various formulations are available:
- Epoprostenol must be administered continuously intravenously (e.g., Broviac catheter). If there is an abrupt interruption of administration, life-threatening crises can occur.
- Treprostinil can be injected continuously subcutaneously. However, there are often local side effects at the injection site, so use is very limited, especially in young children with thin subcutaneous tissue.
- Iloprost may be administered by inhalation, but special nebulizers are required. Moreover, iloprost is also available as an intravenous form for continuous infusion.
- Berapost is administered orally. Its effectiveness is judged to be controversial.

▸ **Phosphodiesterase inhibitors.** Phosphodiestarese V inhibitors block the breakdown of cGMP and in this way increase the NO activity. Sildenafil is now also established for children and infants. Additive effects result through the combination—for example, with inhaled iloprost or bosentan, which is often used in the treatment of pulmonary hypertension as a result of bronchopulmonary dysplasia.

▸ **Endothelin antagonists.** Bosentan improves the clinical symptoms in long-term oral administration. The administration is limited mainly due hepatotoxicity and

Table 21.2 Specific medication for pulmonary hypertension

Drug	Dosage	Main side effects
Calcium antagonists		
Amlodipine	Gradual increase of the dosage over months until a maximum dose of 0.2–0.6 mg/kg/d in 1–2 single doses orally	Hypotension, regular blood pressure monitoring required
Phosphodiesterase inhibitors		
Sildenafil	1–2 (max. 3) mg/kg/d in 3–4 single doses orally	Headaches, flushing, swelling of the mucosa
Endothelin antagonists		
Bosentan	< 10 kg: 1 × 15.6 mg for 4 weeks, then 2 × 15.6 mg orally. (Alternatively 2 × 1–2 mg/kg for 4 weeks, then 2 × 2–4 mg/kg orally) 10–20 kg: 1 × 31.25 mg for 4 weeks, then 2 × 31.25 mg orally 20–40 kg: 2 × 31.25 mg for 4 weeks, then 2 × 62.5 mg orally > 40 kg: 2 × 62.5 mg for 4 weeks, then 2 × 125 mg orally	Hepatotoxic, teratogenic, anemia, flushing, syncope, enzyme induction (vitamin K antagonists, contraceptives)
Prostacyclin/prostanoids		
Iloprost inhalation	6–8 × 0.25–0.5 µg/kg as inhalation (dosage for children not uniform)	Headache, diarrhea, nausea, flushing, syncope
Iloprost IV	0.5–2 ng/kg/min, possibly increase over time	
Epoprostenol IV	Initially 2–4 ng/kg/min, then increase every 2–4 weeks by 1–2 ng/kg/min depending on the symptoms and tolerance. Do not discontinue abruptly, taper off gradually.	
Beraprost oral	Not recommended for children due to insufficient long-term effect	
Treprostinil continuous subcutaneous infusion	Not recommended for children (local irritation)	
Nitric oxide		
NO inhalation	5–20 ppm, do not discontinue abruptly	Rebound effect after discontinuation, methemoglobinemia

teratogenicity. Furthermore, anemia often develops under bosentan treatment. It should also be noted that bosentan may lead to enzyme induction and thus to an increased metabolism of vitamin K antagonists and contraceptives.

▶ **Inhaled NO.** Inhaled NO is a pulmonary vasodilator with a very short half-life. It also inhibits platelet aggregation. It is used primarily in mechanically ventilated patients, such as in persistent pulmonary hypertension of the newborn or postoperatively for the treatment of pulmonary hypertension after correction of congenital heart defects. In some cases, successful outpatient treatment has been reported. An abrupt discontinuation of treatment may lead to a rebound effect, so treatment should be tapered off gradually. In addition, methemoglobin and NO_2 may form, so corresponding monitoring is required.

▶ **Combination therapy.** If there is insufficient improvement under a monotherapy, a combination therapy may be considered, such as prostanoids (IV or inhalation) in combination with sildenafil or bosentan.

Interventional and Surgical Treatment

▶ **Atrial septostomy.** If conservative treatment is unsuccessful, and especially if syncopes occur, an atrial septostomy may be useful. This is the case especially if right heart failure or decreased filling of the left ventricle occur as a result of pulmonary hypertension. The right ventricle is relieved by the artificially created atrial opening that serves as an overflow valve. In addition, the left atrium and the left ventricle are again sufficiently filled by the shunt, which leads to increased cardiac output. However, due to the right-to-left shunt, cyanosis develops. The risk of this procedure is not insignificant. Under certain circumstances, an atrial septostomy may also be performed to bridge the time until transplantation. Another possibility is the establishment of a Pott's anastomosis (i.e. a shunt between the left pulmonary artery and the descending aorta, surgically or interventionally). This has the benefit of providing adequate pressure relief for the right heart and directing the blood flow of the deoxygenated blood to the lower part of the body, thus avoiding cyanosis for the heart and brain.

▸ **Lung transplantation.** A (heart and) lung transplantation is the last treatment option for severe treatment-refractory cases. The results so far are still unsatisfactory. An additional significant problem is the lack of donor organs. The prognosis after lung transplantation for pulmonary hypertension is worse than after lung transplantation for other pulmonary diseases. Slightly more than half of the patients survive the first year. After 5 years, only about 40% are still alive.

21.1.4 Prognosis

Pulmonary hypertension is a serious disease with a poor prognosis. Idiopathic or familial pulmonary hypertension cannot be cured, but progression can be significantly slowed down and the symptoms can be improved. Before effective drugs were available for treatment, most patients with idiopathic pulmonary hypertension died within a year of diagnosis. In patients with Eisenmenger reaction, the 5-year survival rate is 80%. In congenital shunt defects, the most significant measure is the timely surgical or interventional catheter correction before irreversible pulmonary hypertension has developed.

22 Eisenmenger Syndrome

22.1.1 Basics

Synonym: Eisenmenger reaction

Definition

The Eisenmenger syndrome is a secondary form of pulmonary hypertension, in which, due to a heart defect with an originally left-to-right shunt, increased pulmonary resistance leading to a shunt reversal has occurred.

As a result of the left-to-right shunt with increased pulmonary blood flow, the pulmonary arterial resistance increases more and more until it becomes irreversible due to pulmonary vascular remodeling (fixed increased pulmonary vascular resistance). When the pulmonary arterial resistance exceeds the systemic resistance, shunt reversal occurs with right-to-left shunt and cyanosis. An Eisenmenger syndrome is not a congenital heart defect, but rather the long-term result of an uncorrected shunt defect.

Epidemiology

Patients with Eisenmenger syndrome are now rare in industrialized nations, since nearly all congenital heart defects are surgically corrected before an Eisenmenger reaction has occurred. Most patients with Eisenmenger are now adults, for example, patients with trisomy 21 and an AVSD channel whose defects were not previously corrected surgically, or patients with complex congenital heart defects who were treated with a palliative aortopulmonary shunt.

Pathogenesis

As a result of a congenital heart defect with left-to-right shunt, there is increased pulmonary blood flow. In addition, in a large VSD, for example, the pressure of systemic circulation is transferred unprotected to the pulmonary circulation. Over time, the increased pulmonary blood flow, in particular in combination with pressure overload, leads to remodeling of the pulmonary vascular circulation. Histologically, hypertrophy of the media, proliferation of the intima, and fibrosis of the pulmonary vessels develop. The result is a gradual increase in pulmonary vascular resistance. If the pulmonary resistance exceeds systemic resistance, the blood flow in the lungs is impeded, leading to a reversal of the original left-to-right shunt; a right-to-left shunt with cyanosis develops. Moreover, cardiac output cannot be adequately increased during exercise due to limited pulmonary arterial blood flow.

Note

A cardiac defect must be corrected surgically before fixed increased pulmonary resistance develops.

Etiology

In theory, an Eisenmenger reaction can occur with any heart defect with a relevant left-to-right shunt, but it is most often found with the following diseases:

- Complete AVSD channel
- Truncus arteriosus
- d-TGA with VSD
- VSD
- PDA
- Aortopulmonary window
- After surgical creation of an aortopulmonary shunt for palliative treatment of a complex congenital heart defect

22.1.2 Diagnostic Measures

Symptoms

The morphological changes of the pulmonary vessels associated with Eisenmenger syndrome usually begin in childhood. However, the affected children often have few symptoms. With increasing pulmonary resistance, the symptoms of heart failure in shunt defects initially even decrease. Severe symptoms usually do not occur in Eisenmenger patients until adolescence or adulthood. The main symptoms are severe cyanosis and increasing deterioration of physical capacity. Later, severe heart failure develops.

▸ **Later complications.** The complications are mainly the result of chronic hypoxemia or the inability to adequately increase pulmonary blood flow under stress.

- Cardiac complications:
  - Increasing heart failure as a result of hypoxemia
  - Arrhythmias (especially atrial flutter/fibrillation)
  - Angina pectoris
  - Syncopes, sudden cardiac death (e.g., as a result of arrhythmias or the inability to increase the cardiac output under stress due to limited pulmonary blood flow)
  - Paradoxical embolism (result of right-to-left shunt, high risk for embolism due to increased blood viscosity)
  - Endocarditis
  - Enlargement of the central pulmonary vessels

- Hematological complications:
  - Increased erythropoiesis as a result of chronic hypoxemia
  - Hyperviscosity syndrome (as a result of high hematocrit and iron deficiency that adversely affects the deformability of the erythrocytes)
  - Iron deficiency (often as a result of bleeding or bloodletting)
  - Neutropenia and thrombocytopenia
  - Tendency to bleed (decreased synthesis of clotting factors, platelet dysfunction, thrombocytopenia)
- Pulmonary complications:
  - Hemoptysis, intrapulmonary bleeding
  - Lung abscesses
- Neurological complications:
  - Stroke, transient ischemic attacks (due to bleeding or thromboembolic events, promoted by atrial fibrillation)
  - Brain abscess
  - Tinnitus, vision disorders, paraesthesia, myalgia, headache (as a result of hyperviscosity, "hyperviscosity syndrome")
- Renal complications:
  - Proteinuria, hematuria
  - Progressive renal failure
- Metabolic complications:
  - Hyperuricemia
  - Hyperbilirubinemia and gallstones
  - Nephrolithiasis
- Orthopedic complications:
  - Joint pain (hypertrophic osteoarthropathy, localized cell proliferation with periostitis)

Clinical Examination

A major finding in the clinical examination is central cyanosis, usually with oxygen saturation at rest around 80% measured by pulse oximetry. Under stress, the oxygen saturation decreases further.

Watch-glass nails and finger clubbing develop as characteristic trophic disorders due to chronic hypoxemia.

Auscultation

As a result of pulmonary hypertension there is typically a loud ("popping") second heart sound, depending on the heart defect. If there is dilation of the right ventricle, there may be a low-frequency systolic murmur (tricuspid regurgitation). A diastolic decrescendo murmur suggests pulmonary regurgitation. Due to the approximately equal pressures in both ventricles, the typical murmur of a VSD can no longer be heard in patients with Eisenmenger syndrome.

Laboratory

Typical laboratory findings in Eisenmenger patients are:

- High hematocrit (up to 70–90%)
- Thrombocytopenia (50–150/nL)
- Leukocytopenia
- Microcytic and hypochromic erythrocytes, iron deficiency
- Elevated uric acid and bilirubin
- Low Quick, elevated INR, prolonged PTT and bleeding time
- Urine: proteinuria, hematuria

ECG

Depending on the heart defect, the ECG typically has signs of right heart hypertrophy (right axis deviation, P pulmonale), possibly repolarization disturbances in the right precordial leads, an (incomplete) right bundle branch block, tachycardia or arrhythmia, particularly atrial flutter or fibrillation.

Chest X-ray

Depending on the stage and the extent of the disease, the following changes are found in the chest X-ray:

- Prominent pulmonary artery segment, widened hilar vessels, and breakup of vessels in the lung periphery ("hilar amputation," pruning phenomenon)
- Possibly right heart enlargement: in the lateral image the enlarged right ventricle fills the retrosternal space.

Echocardiography

Echocardiography is the standard noninvasive method for diagnosing the underlying shunt defect. In Eisenmenger patients, the following conditions may also be assessed by echocardiography:

- Visualization of the right-to-left shunt
- Assessment of ventricular function
- Assessment of the right ventricle (hypertrophy, dilation) and atrium (dilation)
- Estimate of the right ventricular and pulmonary arterial pressure via the flow velocity of the tricuspid regurgitation or pulmonary regurgitation. In a VSD, the right ventricular pressure can be also estimated based on the flow velocity across the defect. It is possible to estimate the pulmonary artery pressure in a PDA using the maximum flow velocity across the ductus arteriosus; likewise in an aortopulmonary shunt using the flow velocity in the shunt.
- The typical finding of pulmonary hypertension in a Doppler examination is a steep increase of the flow velocity across the right ventricular outflow tract with a shortened acceleration time (normal: ≥ 120 ms).

Cardiac Catheterization

In addition to the hemodynamic measurements including pressures in the right atrium, right ventricle, and pulmonary arteries as well as the resistance in the pulmonary circulation, the pulmonary vessels can be visualized by angiography. The extent of the right-to-left shunt can also be determined.

An essential part of cardiac catheterization is testing the pulmonary vascular reactivity. For this purpose, standardized pulmonary vasodilators (NO, iloprost, oxygen) may be administered intravenously or by inhalation.

MRI

The right-to-left shunt can be quantified in an MRI. In addition, the cardiac structures can be visualized in detail.

Six-minute Walk Test, Cardiopulmonary Exercise Test

Both tests are used to assess physical capacity and to monitor the course of the disease (in particular under medication), but special caution is required.

22.1.3 Treatment

Causal treatment is not usually available. Treatment is symptomatic and aims at improving the symptoms of heart failure and pulmonary hypertension as well managing and preventing complications of chronic hypoxemia.

General Measures

Fluid depletion should be avoided. High temperatures and high humidity should be avoided since these may cause peripheral vasodilatation and thus increase the right-to-left shunt. Vasodilators should be avoided for the same reason. Air travel is usually not a problem, but additional oxygen should be available.

Some patients benefit clinically from nocturnal oxygen administration.

Pharmacological Treatment of Heart Failure

► **Digoxin.** The benefit of digoxin for patients with right heart failure in Eisenmenger syndrome is not fully understood.

► **Diuretics.** Diuretics are indicated in right heart failure with edema. Marked intravascular volume depletion must be avoided. Otherwise, right ventricular preload may be excessively reduced and cause an acute drop in cardiac output. In addition, the rheological properties of blood deteriorate if there is fluid depletion.

Pharmacological Treatment of Pulmonary Hypertension

The pharmacological treatment of pulmonary hypertension with pulmonary vasodilators (prostacyclin, endothelin antagonists, sildenafil) is described in Chapter 21. For Eisenmenger patients, similar principles apply as for patients with idiopathic pulmonary hypertension. Very little evidence-based data for Eisenmenger patients is currently available.

► **Anticoagulation.** Since patients with Eisenmenger sydrome present an increased risk of bleeding, routine anticoagulation—unlike in the treatment of idiopathic pulmonary hypertension—is not recommended.

Platelet aggregation inhibitors should also be avoided due to platelet dysfunction in these patients.

► **Phlebotomy.** A phlebotomy is not routinely recommended, but only if the hematocrit is over 65%, provided that there are hyperviscosity-related symptoms. As a rule, in such cases, 500 to 1500 mL of blood is removed and replaced with an equal amount of crystalloid and colloid fluid. Fluid depletion as the cause of the elevated hematocrit should of course be ruled out beforehand.

► **Iron substitution.** Iron deficiency should be substituted immediately in Eisenmenger patients. Iron deficiency, which is often the result of bloodletting, leads to reduced red blood cell deformability and thus has an unfavorable effect on the hyperviscosity of the blood.

► **Contraception.** Women with Eisenmenger syndrome must avoid pregnancy. The best method of contraception is tubal ligation for these patients. Contraception with estrogens increases the risk of thrombosis.

► **Endocarditis prophylaxis.** There is a high risk of endocarditis, so that in addition to good dental hygiene for interventions that may be associated with bacteremia, antibiotic endocarditis prophylaxis is necessary. Systematic antibiotic therapy is required for manifest bacterial infections.

Surgical Treatment

Heart–lung transplantation is possible as surgical treatment in certain cases, but this treatment option is severely limited by a lack of donor organs as well as poor short- and long-term prognosis (5-year survival rate below 30%). In addition, there are individual case reports of a combination of surgical correction of the heart defect and lung transplantation. The optimal time for the transplant is yet not clear.

22.1.4 Prognosis

► **Long-term prognosis.** The Eisenmenger reaction is a serious disease with a poor prognosis, but the average life expectancy after diagnosis is higher than that for patients with idiopathic pulmonary hypertension. Studies that include pediatric patients have shown that patients with

Eisenmenger syndrome have an average life expectancy of 25 to 35 years. Risk factors are syncope, elevated right atrial pressure, and severe cyanosis at rest with pulse oximetry saturation below 80%. Among the most common causes of death are sudden cardiac death, heart failure, and hemoptysis, less often they are consequences of pregnancy or brain abscess.

► **Outpatient checkups.** Eisenmenger patients require continuous cardiac care. Due to the complex problems, it is useful to have close links to a specialist for adolescents and adults with congenital heart defects.

► **Lifestyle and physical capacity.** Adolescents and adults with Eisenmenger syndrome have severely limited physical capacity. Competitive sports are prohibited because of the considerable risk of sudden cardiac death. Light exercise can be individually permitted if the oxygen saturation is above 80%, ventricular function is good, and there are no symptomatic arrhythmias.

Pregnancy must be prevented in Eisenmenger patients because of the significant risk to the mother and the unborn child. The fetal mortality rate is 25% and the maternal mortality rate is as high as 50%.

Note

Women with Eisenmenger syndrome should be informed that pregnancy must be absolutely avoided.

Operations pose a significant risk to patients with Eisenmenger syndrome (anesthesia-induced drop of systemic resistance, bleeding, intravascular volume depletion, thrombosis, paradoxical embolism).

23 Syndromic Diseases with Cardiac Involvement

23.1 Overview of Syndromic Diseases with Cardiac Involvement

An overview of the most common syndromic diseases associated with congenital heart defects is presented in ▶ Table 23.1. Marfan and Marfanlike syndromes are discussed separately in Chapter 23.2.

23.2 Marfan Syndrome

23.2.1 Basics

Definition

Marfan syndrome is an autosomal dominant disorder of the connective tissue. Typically, several organ systems are involved (e.g., skeleton, eyes, heart and circulatory system). Typical symptoms include tall stature, arachnodactyly, ectopia lentis, mitral valve prolapse, and dilation of the aortic root, which may lead to aortic dissection. The involvement of the cardiovascular system is decisive for the prognosis.

Epidemiology

The incidence is approximately 1:10,000, possibly higher.

▶ **Genetics.** Usually there is a genetic mutation of the fibrillin-1 gene (FBN1). Inheritance is autosomal dominant. Up to one-third of the cases involve a new mutation. Fibrillin is a glycoprotein of the microfibrils and the main component of the extracellular matrix.

In some patients with a Marfan phenotype, however, no mutation of the FBN1 gene is found. Some of these patients have mutations in the genes (TGFBR1 or TGFBR2) that code for the receptors of transforming growth factor β (TGFβ). The TGFβ is a transcription factor that plays a significant role in the development of various organ systems.

23.2.2 Diagnostic Measures

Marfan syndrome is diagnosed on the basis of family history, mutation analysis, and clinical symptoms.

Symptoms

▶ **Ghent nosology.** The diagnostic criteria are summarized in the Ghent nosology (▶ Table 23.2) and include the clinical symptoms in several organ systems. The diagnostic process requires clinical and imaging techniques as well as the family history and genetic testing. Adult patients with Marfan syndrome often meet the criteria of the Ghent nosology. Children often have only some symptoms, which makes the clinical diagnosis difficult.

Marfan syndrome can be diagnosed if the following criteria are met:

- Evidence of one major criterion in two organ systems and the involvement of a third system

or

- Evidence of a pathological mutation, one major criterion, and organ involvement

or

- A relative with Marfan syndrome and evidence of a major criterion and organ involvement

▶ **Cardiac symptoms.** The cardiac symptoms in patients with Marfan syndrome are summarized in the following list:

- Dilatation of the ascending aorta with risk of aortic dissection
- Dilatation of the descending aorta or abdominal aorta
- Aortic regurgitation
- Dilatation of the proximal pulmonary trunk
- Thickening or prolapse of one or both AV valves (in particular mitral valve prolapse) with or without valve regurgitation
- Calcification of the mitral valve annulus
- Vascular aneurysm aside from the aorta
- Cystic media necrosis of the proximal coronary artery (coronary heart disease)
- ECG changes: AV block, repolarization disturbances (QT prolongation, U wave), ventricular arrhythmias (in particular in patients with impaired diastolic left ventricular function)
- Dilative cardiomyopathy
- Sudden cardiac death

Note

The leading symptom of acute aortic dissection is a sudden, tearing pain that may be located in the chest, interscapular, or even epigastric or thoracoabdominal region. Other symptoms may include: syncope, shock, pulse deficit (depending on the location of the dissection).

Predilection sites for aortic dissection are the ascending aorta 2–3 cm distal to the aortic valve and the transition between the aortic arch and the descending aorta.

Auscultation

A systolic click caused by the penetration of the prolapsed leaflet into the left atrium suggests a mitral valve prolapse. The click is often clearer after isometric stress

Table 23.1 Overview of the most common syndromic diseases associated with congenital heart defects

Syndrome	Characteristics	Associated heart defects	Remark
Trisomy 21 (Down syndrome)	Short stature, generalized muscle hypotonia, simian crease, sandal gap (large distance between the 1st and 2nd toes), clinodactyly of the 5th finger, brachycephalus with mongoloid eye slant, epicanthus, macroglossia, Brushfield spots, psychomotor retardation, average IQ of 50 (considerable variation), pancreas annulare, Hirschsprung disease	**AVSD**, VSD, Fallot tetralogy, PDA, rarely coarctation of the aorta, aortic stenosis	Most common chromosomal abnormality with an incidence of 1:650 of all live births; the incidence increases with maternal age. Approximately 40–50% of children have a heart defect, approximately half of these have AVSD
Trisomy 18 (Edwards syndrome)	Intrauterine growth retardation, short trunk, small nipples, microcephaly, craniofacial anomalies (prominent occiput, low-set ears, small mouth, micrognathia), renal anomalies. Typical hand position: flexion of the fingers where the index finger and little finger are bent over the middle and ring fingers	**VSD** (almost always present, often as malalignment VSD), cardiac valvulopathy (**"polyvalvular disease,"** such as thickened leaflets, long chordae, hypoplastic or absent papillary muscles), DORV, Fallot tetralogy	Second most common chromosomal abnormality with an incidence of 1:3,500 of all live births. The prognosis is poor. Most children die within the first weeks of life, only 10% survive the first year. Survival into adulthood has been described in some cases, but severe mental retardation is always present
Trisomy 13 (Patau syndrome)	Microcephaly, scalp defects, microphthalmia, coloboma, cleft lip and palate, flexion contractures of the fingers, rocker bottom feet, polydactyly, renal anomalies, mental retardation	PDA, VSD, ASD, valvular anomalies, coarctation of the aorta	Incidence 1:4000–10,000 of all live births. Cardiac defects occur in 80%, the majority of those affected have complex cardiac defects. The prognosis is as poor as that of trisomy 18, the mortality rate in the first year of life is 80–90%
Trisomy/tetrasomy 22p ("cat-eye" syndrome)	Mild mental retardation, hypertelorism, iris coloboma, ear tags, kidney dysplasia (large variability of the phenotype)	Anomalous pulmonary venous connections, Fallot tetralogy, VSD, left persistent superior vena cava, interrupted inferior vena cava, tricuspid atresia	Cardiac defects occur in 40% of patients
Turner syndrome (45, X0)	Congenital lymphedema (almost pathognomonic), short stature, pterygium colli, short fingers, widely spaced nipples, ovarian dysgenesis, renal anomalies	**Coarctation of the aorta**, bicuspid aortic valve, aortic stenosis, hypoplastic left heart syndrome, aortic dilation, aortic dissection	Incidence 1:2,500 of all female newborns. Cardiac defects occur in 20–40% of patients, usually obstruction or hypoplasia of the left heart. The spectrum ranges from asymptomatic bicuspid aortic valve up to hypoplastic left heart syndrome. The most common is coarctation of the aorta
Noonan syndrome	Short stature, pterygium colli, chest deformities, congenital lymphedema, cryptorchismus, mental retardation (usually mild)	Myxomatous valvular pulmonary stenosis, hypertrophic cardiomyopathy, ASD, VSD	Affected genes: mostly PTPN11 mutation, rarely KRAS, SOS1, autosomal dominant inheritance. The phenotype is similar to Turner syndrome

Syndrome	Characteristics	Associated heart defects	Remark
Microdeletion 22q11 (DiGeorge syndrome, velo-cardio-facial syndrome, Shprintzen syndrome, "conotruncal anomaly face" CATCH 22)	Cardiac anomalies, abnormal facies, thymus hypoplasia, cleft palate, hypocalcemia, mental retardation of varying degrees. Pronounced genotype-phenotype variability	Interrupted aortic arch, truncus arteriosus communis, Fallot tetralogy, pulmonary atresia with VSD, VSD, aortic arch anomalies	Incidence 1:5,000 of all live births. Malformation of the 3rd/4th pharyngeal pouch. The great variability of expression is reflected in the different names of the syndrome, all of which are now summarized as microdeletion 22q11. Cardiac defects occur in approximately 80% of patients. Typical defects are conotruncal anomalies, i.e., heart defects affecting mainly the great vessels. Patients with 22q11 microdeletion should always be examined for immune defects
Holt–Oram syndrome	Malformations of the upper extremities	**ASD**, VSD, anomalous pulmonary venous connection, conduction disturbances	Affected gene: TBX5, autosomal dominant inheritance, cardiac anomalies occur in about 75% of patients, an ASD is typical
Alagille syndrome	Intrahepatic cholestasis (biliary atresia), typical face (prominent forehead and chin, deep-set eyes, and anomalies of the anterior chamber [posterior embryotoxon]), butterfly vertebrae	**Peripheral pulmonary stenosis**, Fallot tetralogy, valvular pulmonary stenosis, ASD, VSD	Affected genes: JAG1, NOTCH2, autosomal dominant inheritance, cardiac defects occur in approximately 90% of patients, peripheral pulmonary stenosis is typical
Ellis–van Creveld syndrome (chondroectodermal dysplasia)	Short stature, short limbs, ectodermal dysplasia (hypoplastic nails, dental abnormalities), polydactyly, narrow thorax, usually normal intelligence	Common atrium, ASD I, AVSD	Affected gene: EVC, autosomal recessive inheritance. Cardiac defects occur in approximately 50% of cases, anomalies that affect the embryonic AV channel are typical
Williams–Beuren syndrome ("elfin face" syndrome)	Short stature, mental retardation, elflike facies with midface hypoplasia, hypodontia, very good verbal skills, friendly behavior, sometimes social disinhibition, hoarse voice, hypercalcemia, hypogenitalism, early tendency to arterial hypertension	**Supravalvular aortic stenosis**, (peripheral) pulmonary stenosis, coarctation of the aorta, coronary artery stenosis, renal artery stenosis	Incidence 1:10,000–20,000 of all live births. Affected gene: elastin gene (ELN1), microdeletion 7q11.2. Cardiac defects occur in approximately 75% of cases. Supravalvular aortic stenosis is typical, less often peripheral pulmonary stenosis, coarctation of the aorta, and stenosis of the peripheral arteries
VATER association (VACTERL association)	Combination of vertebral, anorectal, cardiac, tracheo-esophageal (tracheal fistulas), esophageal (esophageal atresia), renal, and limb anomalies, intrauterine growth retardation	Broad range of cardiac anomalies, most common are VSD, single umbilical artery	Incidence 1:6,000 of all live births, mostly sporadic occurrence, cardiac defects are present in approximately 50% of the cases
CHARGE association	Coloboma, cardiac anomalies, choanal atresia, retarded development, genital hypoplasia, ear anomalies	**Conotruncal anomalies** (Fallot tetralogy, DORV, truncus arteriosus communis), **aortic arch anomalies** (vascular rings, arteria lusoria, interrupted aortic arch)	Affected genes: CHD7, SEMA3E. Cardiac defects are present in approximately 70% of cases, conotruncal and aortic arch anomalies are typical
LEOPARD Syndrome	Lentiginosis (pigmentation of the skin), ECG changes, ocular anomalies, pulmonary stenosis, genital anomalies, retardation, deafness	**Valvular pulmonary stenosis**, hypertrophic cardiomyopathy, conduction disorders	Affected gene: PTPN11. Cardiac defects are present in more than 70% of cases, valvular pulmonary stenosis is typical
Smith–Lemli–Opitz syndrome	Syndactyly of the 2nd and 3rd toes, short stature, microcephaly, genital anomalies	ASD, VSD, AVSD, anomalous pulmonary venous connection	Incidence 1:20,000 of all live births, affected gene DHCR7, autosomal recessive inheritance

Table 23.2 Clinical symptoms of Marfan syndrome according to the Ghent nosology

Organ system	Major criterion	Minor criterion	Criterion for organ system involvement
Skeleton	4 of the following components = 1 major criterion: • Pigeon chest • Funnel chest with surgical indication • Reduced ratio upper/lower half of the body or arm span/height > 1.05 • Positive thumb or wrist sign ▶ Fig. 23.1 • Scoliosis > 20° or spondylolisthesis • Pes planus due to medial displacement of the medial malleolus • Protrusio acetabuli • Elbow extension deficit (< 170°)	• Mild funnel chest • Loose flexible joints • High (Gothic) palate with dental deformity due to lack of space • Dolichocephaly, endophthalmus, retrognathia, cheek bone hypoplasia • Downward slanted eyes	2 major criteria or 1 major criterion and 2 minor criteria
Eyes	• Ectopia lentis	• Abnormally flat cornea • Elongated bulbus • Hypoplastic iris / ciliary muscle hypoplasia	1 major criterion or 2 minor criteria
Cardiovascular	• Dilatation of the ascending aorta including the aortic sinus of Valsalva with or without aortic valve regurgitation • Aortic dissection	• Mitral valve prolapse • Dilatation of the pulmonary artery before age 40 (pulmonary stenosis ruled out) • Mitral valve annulus calcification before age 40 • Dilatation or dissection of the thoracic/abdominal aorta before age 50	1 major criterion or 1 minor criterion
Lungs		• Spontaneous pneumothorax • Apical emphysema	1 minor criterion
Skin		• Striae atrophicae (not caused by weight loss, pregnancy) • Recurrent hernias or scar hernias	1 minor criterion
Dura	• Lumbosacral dural ectasia		1 major criterion
Family history / genetic findings	• 1st degree relative with Marfan syndrome • FBN1 mutation, with a known causative relationship to Marfan syndrome • Evidence of a haplotype in the FBN1 gene inherited from a relative with a clinically manifest Marfan syndrome		1 major criterion

(e.g., squats). An accompanying mitral regurgitation causes a systolic, usually rough murmur that can be heard over the entire precordium and radiates to the axilla.

Aortic regurgitation causes a usually relatively soft, early diastolic murmur with decrescendo character. Typically, it has a high frequency and is often described as "pouring."

ECG

Possible ECG findings in Marfan patients: AV block, repolarization disturbances (QT prolongation, U wave), and ventricular arrhythmias (especially in patients with impaired diastolic left ventricular function).

Echocardiography

Echocardiography is often made difficult due to thorax deformities. The following possible cardiac manifestations in Marfan syndrome should be noted:

- Dilatation of the ascending aorta. The upper normal limit of the aortic root diameter is 1.9 cm/m^2 body surface and is independent of age and gender
- Dilatation of the remaining aorta or the main pulmonary artery
- Mitral valve prolapse with or without mitral regurgitation
- Aortic regurgitation

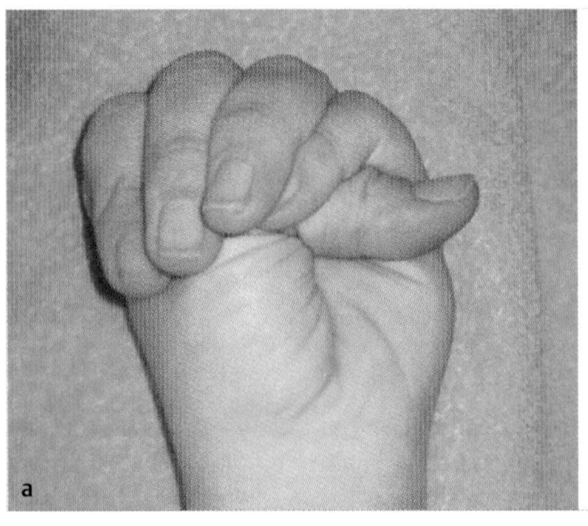

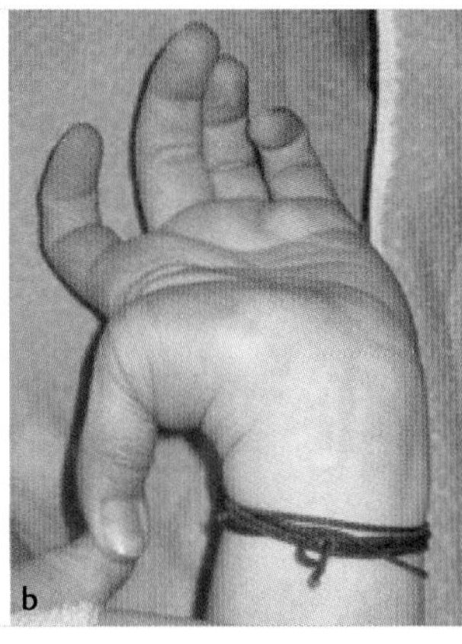

Fig. 23.1 Positive thumb sign (**a**) and hyperextension of the metacarpophalangeal joint (**b**) in a patient with Marfan syndrome.

Table 23.3 Differential diagnosis of Marfan syndrome[45]

Syndrome	Symptoms	Mutation	Remark
MASS syndrome	Mitral valve prolapse, aortic dilation, skeletal and skin involvement	FBN1 or unknown	
Marfan syndrome type II	Similar to classic Marfan syndrome but no ectopia lentis	TGFBR1 or 2	Probably more aggressive vascular complications
Weil–Marchesani syndrome	Patients tend to have short stature, short fingers, stiff joints, ectopia lentis	FBN1 (autosomal dominant) ADAMTS10 (autosomal recessive)	
Congenital contractural arachnodactyly	Similar to Marfan syndrome, typically: joint contractures, ear deformities	FBN2	
Loeys–Dietz syndrome type I	Similar to the classic Marfan syndrome, additionally cleft palate, bifid uvula, hypertelorism	TGFBR1 or 2	Vascular complications in relatively young patients
Loeys–Dietz syndrome type II	Similar to the Loeys–Dietz syndrome type I and the vascular type of Ehlers-Danlos syndrome	TGFBR1 or 2	
Shprintzen–Goldberg syndrome	Similar to Marfan and Loeys–Dietz syndromes, typically: craniosynostosis	FBN1	
Familial thoracic aortic aneurysm	Familial aortic aneurysm	TGFBR1 or 2 MYH11 ACTA2	

- Aneurysms of the descending aorta and abdominal aorta or other vessels
- Aortic dissection

In doubtful cases, transesophageal echocardiography may be required to visualize the aortic dissection.

MRI/CT

MRI is the diagnostic procedure of choice for visualizing aortic dissection in all segments of the aorta. This procedure should be performed at least in all patients in whom the measured diameter of the aortic root is more than 1.5 times the upper normal limit. In acute aortic dissection and a hemodynamically unstable patient, there may not be enough time to perform this investigation.

Differential Diagnoses

Syndromes with features similar to Marfan syndrome that do not fully meet the criteria of the Ghent nosology or where a FBN1 mutation is not present are called fan-like syndromes. As in a classic Marfan syndrome, there is a greatly increased risk of a dissecting aortic aneurysm. The differential diagnoses of Marfan syndrome are listed in ▶ Table 23.3.

23.2.3 Treatment

The care of Marfan patients is an interdisciplinary task that requires the cooperation of (pediatric) cardiologists, ophthalmologists, and orthopedic surgeons. The cardiology aspects are discussed below.

Cardiac treatment involves beta blockers and the prohibition of competitive sports. A regular review of the aortic root diameter is necessary in order not to miss the right time for an elective surgical aortic root replacement.

▸ **Beta-blocker therapy.** Beta blockers are considered standard treatment for all Marfan patients, regardless of the diameter of the aortic root. In children, the evidence regarding the optimal timing of the start of the beta-blocker therapy is inconclusive. Beta blockers reduce hemodynamic stress on the aorta and thus counteract the development of aortic dissection. Propranolol or atenolol are usually used. The dose should be adjusted so that the heart rate does not exceed 110 bpm after submaximal exercise. For adults, it is also recommended that the heart rate should not exceed 60 bpm at rest. If beta blockers are not tolerated, calcium antagonists may be considered.

▸ **Angiotensin II antagonists.** There is growing evidence that Losartan not only has positive effects on blood pressure management but also remodelling effects in patients with Marfan disease based on the intracellular reversal of cystic media necrosis. This effect leads to a reduction of the diameter of the ascending aorta, an improvement of mitral competence and a reduction of the left ventricular enddiastolic diameter.

▸ **Limitation of physical activity.** Sports with mainly isometric stress such as weightlifting or strength training are contraindicated in Marfan patients because of the rise in blood pressure and the high hemodynamic stress on the proximal aorta. Most dynamic sports are allowed; however, a maximum heart rate of 110 bpm should not be exceeded in children. Competitive sports are thus not allowed. Marfan patients should also avoid contact sports.

▸ **Prophylactic replacement of the aortic root.** In children, surgical replacement of the aortic root should be performed only after growth is completed. The indication for this is very rare in children under age 12 years.

The risk of aortic dissection increases with aortic root diameter. In adults, the following criteria are the indications for prophylactic replacement of the aortic root:

- Aortic root diameter greater than 45 mm
- Aortic root diameter greater than 40 mm and other risk factors (e.g., aortic dissection or rupture in a relative, rapid increase in the aortic root diameter)

In children: The assessment of the aortic root diameter is based on the adult criteria. Should there be a sudden increase in the aortic root diameter that has always run parallel above the normal range for years, there is also an indication for surgery.

▸ **Mitral valve surgery.** A mitral valve prolapse occurs in 50 to 80% of Marfan patients. The extent of the accompanying mitral regurgitation varies. In echocardiography, the chordae tendineae of the mitral valve appear elongated, the mitral valve annulus is widened, sometimes also calcified. The indication for mitral valve surgery is not significantly different from the general recommendations for mitral valve surgery (Chapter 15.29).

▸ **Pregnancy.** Pregnancy is associated with an increased risk of aortic dissection and rupture in female patients with Marfan syndrome. There is a particularly high risk if the aortic root diameter is over 40 mm. Therefore, women with such an aortic root diameter should undergo elective prophylactic aortic root replacement prior to pregnancy. Women in whom no cardiovascular involvement was detected before pregnancy may also develop an aortic dissection during pregnancy.

Vaginal delivery is usually possible in women with an aortic root diameter of less than 40 mm if cardiac failure has not developed due to valve incompetence or cardiomyopathy. Regular echocardiography checkups (e.g., at 3-month intervals) are required during pregnancy and for at least 3 months postpartum.

Note, however, that the probability of inheritance of Marfan syndrome is 50%.

23.2.4 Prognosis

The involvement of the cardiovascular system is decisive for the prognosis. The mean life expectancy of untreated patients with Marfan syndrome was previously about 32 years; today it is 70 years. Prophylactic beta-blocker therapy and elective aortic root replacement have contributed significantly to improving the life expectancy.

Outpatient echocardiography follow-up is required at least annually. If the aortic root diameter approaches 40 mm or the patient is pregnant, checkups should be made at shorter intervals.

Part IV

Treatment

24 Interventional Catheterization

24.1 Basics

Today, an increasing number of cardiac catheterization procedures are no longer used for diagnostic purposes only. This means that more and more catheter-based treatment is now performed with interventional catheterization. In many centers today, more interventional catheterizations are performed than cardiac surgeries and catheter interventions constitute 60 to 80% of all cardiac catheterizations. The number of diagnostic catheterization procedures is steadily decreasing as echocardiography and magnetic resonance imaging of the heart gradually replace diagnostic cardiac catheterization. Many simple cardiac defects such as coarctation of the aorta, ASD, PDA, and some VSDs, can now be treated very well by interventional measures. The same is true for almost all valvular stenoses that were previously the domain of surgery. In addition, the development of materials and devices used is continually advancing, so that new areas are becoming accessible for the interventional cardiologist (e.g., percutaneous valve implantation, AV valve reconstruction, pulmonary artery banding, Fontan completion, treatment of subaortic or subpulmonary stenosis).

In the following sections some standard routines will be presented as examples of how patients can be treated using interventional procedures.

24.1.1 Preparation

Careful preparation is essential before a planned intervention, just as it is before surgery. This process usually includes the following preparations and examinations:

- Organization of the existing documents, especially outpatient records, old medical reports, operation reports, cardiac catheterization reports, previous imaging (MRI, CT), and other details prior to the investigation
- Discussion and clarification of the indication
- General admission examination, especially
  - Neurological status
  - Ruling out infection
  - Ruling out clotting disease (petechiae, bruising, medical history)
  - Pulse or vascular status
- Pulse oximetry
- Blood pressure in all four limbs
- Recent ECG—that is, obtained within the last 2 (to 3) months
- Recent echocardiography
- Insertion of a peripheral intravenous access port (routine blood sampling is usually not necessary)

► **Patient information.** The patient should always be informed by an experienced colleague from the cardiac catheterization team who knows the nature of the intended catheter investigation and intervention and can explain it accordingly. Ideally, the procedure should be discussed with the patient and his or her parents before the cardiac catheterization. The general and specific risks associated with the planned cardiac catheterization and intervention should always be explained. The risks should also be documented in the patient information sheet. Examples of general risks are:

- Sedation → Overreactions → Intubation → Intensive care monitoring
- Puncture → Bleeding → Transfusion
- Puncture → Thrombosis → Perfusion disturbance → Lysis treatment
- Puncture → Thrombosis → Embolism
- Puncture → Vascular lesion, vascular occlusion → Operation
- Infection → Antibiotic treatment
- Rhythm disorder → Pharmacological treatment, pacemaker treatment
- Air embolism, systemic thromboembolism
- Contrast medium intolerance → Shock→ Intensive care
- Perforation → Pericardial effusion → Tamponade → Puncture/surgery
- Radiation exposure

The specific complications of the individual cardiac defects and interventions and alternative treatment options are discussed in the respective chapters of this book.

In addition, the cardiac defect and the planned intervention should be illustrated in a diagram in the information sheet, and the questions of the parents and the patient should be discussed in detail. It should be emphasized that the overall risk for a simple diagnostic cardiac catheterization is 5% and the risk is somewhat higher for an interventional procedure. For complex interventions, the risk is sometimes comparable to that of surgery.

Sometimes a vascular puncture in the area of the neck and upper chest is necessary. For example, access to the jugular vein or to the subclavian vein is chosen following an upper cavopulmonary anastomosis or if there is known thrombosis of the leg/pelvic vessels. In these cases, the following additional complications have to be pointed out (risk < 5%):

- Accidental puncture of the carotid artery
- Puncture of the trachea/larynx
- Pneumothorax
- Hematothorax

► **Blood tests.** For most interventional procedures, no "routine" blood tests are necessary before the planned operation. Should a patient have clinical signs of infection, for example, cardiac catheterization may be allowed or not based on the clinical examination. Likewise for electrolytes, Hb tests, kidney or liver enzymes: during cardiac catheterization, blood tests can be performed at any time, so electrolytes, Hb levels, and blood gases can be determined if necessary, using modern equipment in the catheterization laboratory. A clinical history of coagulation disorders is an important consideration that may trigger specific additional clotting tests.

When there is an increased risk for blood loss or myocardial perforation in certain examinations or interventions, additional laboratory tests can be ordered on a case-by-case basis (blood typing and cross-matching). An example of such an intervention is the catheter interventional opening of pulmonary atresia.

24.1.2 Sedation/Anesthesia/ Monitoring

In most centers, cardiac catheterization is almost always performed in deep conscious sedation. General anesthesia is not usually necessary. This also applies to studies in which transesophageal echocardiography is needed (e.g., ASD closure). However, the safety measures and standards which apply for continuous monitoring by specialized medical and nursing staff are the same as those for surgery and anesthesia.

▸ **Premedication.** A premed is given before the patient is moved to the cardiac catheterization laboratory (e.g., midazolam 0.1 mg/kg IV).

▸ **Monitoring.** During catheterization, the patient is monitored continuously with ECG, pulse oximetry, and frequent checks of blood pressure. If necessary, oxygen is administered.

▸ **Deep conscious sedation.** For deep conscious sedation with ketamine (and atropine) and propofol, the following regimen is recommended:

- Monitoring with pulse oximetry, ECG, blood pressure
- Oxygen mask / resuscitation bag at hand
- Initiate sedation with ketamine 2 mg/kg IV
- Atropine: at least 100 µg, max. 500 µg IV
- Propofol bolus of 1 mg/kg IV
- Propofol infusion of 5 mg/kg/h
- If necessary, further doses of ketamine and propofol as indicated

▸ **Monitoring after cardiac catheterization.** After completion of the procedure, patients are brought directly to the recovery area or ward for further monitoring. Monitoring in an intensive care setting or unit is not necessary in most cases. A physician accompanies the patient during transport to the aftercare station. The patient is given oxygen during transport and is continuously monitored with pulse oximetry and ECG.

▸ **Transfer to the ward.** The patient is then handed over to the physicians and the nursing staff on the aftercare ward. The clinical condition is documented jointly (oxygen saturation, breathing, circulation).

24.1.3 Postinterventional Measures

Every interventional catheterization should be followed by a standardized and well-defined treatment schedule consisting of pharmacological treatment, checkups, and monitoring according to the procedure performed.

Such an algorithm may be as follows:

- Heparinization
  - Not usually needed after a venous puncture. In cyanotic patients, 200 IU/kg/d until the next morning, continuous IV administration
  - After an arterial puncture, for 24 hours or until the next morning: 400 IU/kg/d, continuous IV administration
  - After interventions, for 36 to 48 hours or until the morning of the second day: 400 IU/kg/d, continuous IV administration
- Infusion treatment: until the patients are awake and able to drink
- Food/drink: As soon as the patients are awake, start with clear liquids; if well tolerated, give food and drink as desired.
- Monitoring: Carry out continuous monitoring of pulses, blood pressure, and oxygen saturation through a central monitoring system with documentation; include assessment of the leg perfusion and neurological status.
- Post-catheterization bleeding: If there is bleeding at the puncture site, renew (compression) dressing and extend monitoring for 12 hours.

24.2 Special Interventional Catheterization Procedures

24.2.1 Interventional Catheterization for Valvular, Vascular, and Outflow Tract Stenosis

Basics of Balloon Valvuloplasty

▸ **Definition.** In balloon valvuloplasty, the narrow site of a vessel or a stenotic valve is stretched when the balloon catheter is inflated so that, ideally, only little or no residual stenosis remains.

▸ **Material.** Balloon catheters of different lengths and diameters are available as well as balloons with different pressure capacities (low-pressure and high-pressure balloons). In addition, there are special balloons with special shapes (e.g., Inoue balloon for mitral valve valvuloplasty) or with special features (such as cutting balloons with small blades attached).

▸ **Procedure.** First the pressure gradient is determined and the anatomy of the stenosis as well as the upstream and downstream vessels is visualized. A combination of angiography and previous echocardiography or MRI findings is useful for this. Then a guidewire is advanced through the stenosis into the downstream vascular area (e.g., in pulmonary valve stenosis into the pulmonary artery) or, if retrograde probing is performed, into the upstream area (e.g., for aortic stenosis into the left ventricle). Then the deflated balloon catheter is placed in the stenotic area, oriented by cardiac catheter angiography.

When the balloon catheter has been placed correctly in the stenotic area, it is briefly inflated to the maximum pressure specified by the manufacturer. This process is documented (usually 6 frames/s). Then the balloon is deflated and the balloon catheter is withdrawn with the guidewire remaining. An angiography catheter is then placed at the site of the former stenosis, the pressure is measured and an angiography performed. If the stenosis is not sufficiently widened, the dilation procedure may be repeated with a larger or harder balloon or a cutting balloon, or a stent is implanted.

▸ **Complications.** Uncontrolled tearing of the vessel wall may develop during the dilation process. There is a risk of dissection or rupture, later thrombosis, embolism or even restenosis depending on the tissue repair process. In valvular stenosis, accidental laceration or avulsion of a leaflet may cause severe regurgitation.

▸ **Treatment.** The procedure is often followed by heparinization for 1 to 2 days and by giving low-dose aspirin (3–5 mg/kg orally) to avoid excessive thrombosis, embolism, or vascular occlusion.

▸ **Checkups.** Depending on the treated site (valve or vessel), echocardiography checkups are usually sufficient, but sometimes an MRI is also necessary.

Valvular Aortic Stenosis

▸ **Indication.** Overall, the indication criteria for balloon valvuloplasty of the aortic valve are still evolving as, on the one hand, the interventional results are promising while, on the other hand, the risk of the procedure is relatively low. Generally accepted indications are:

- Gradient related (Doppler gradient > 50 mmHg)
- Cardiac decompensation or decreasing left ventricular function
- Increasing cardiac overload (left ventricular hypertrophy, poor diastolic function)
- ST segment changes under stress
- A still-competent aortic valve is a precondition (aortic regurgitation ≤ 2°)

▸ **Preliminary examinations.** An ECG that is no more than 2 months old is recommended; if it is suspicious, a 24-hour Holter ECG or exercise ECG is also recommended. Moreover, a recent echocardiography may be useful including determination of the valve annulus diameter, anatomy of the valve (bicuspid, tricuspid), mean and maximum gradient, aortic regurgitation, left ventricular function, mitral regurgitation, isthmus, ductus, and exclusion of a Shone complex.

▸ **Risks/patient information.** The overall risk is below 10%, including the risk of rupture of the valve, acute and severe aortic regurgitation, emergency surgery with possible valve replacement, myocardial ischemia, arrhythmias, AV block, development of mitral regurgitation, infection/endocarditis, perfusion disorder, or vascular occlusion at the arterial puncture site.

▸ **Procedure.** In small children, an antegrade approach (across an ASD or a patent foramen ovale) may be attempted, otherwise a retrograde approach via an arterial puncture should be undertaken.

▸ **Cardiac catheterization/treatment.** First, pressure measurement and ascendogram, measurement of the valve annulus, probing and angiography of the left ventricle (▸ Fig. 24.1). Then switch the catheter to a long exchange wire, then place the balloon catheter. Balloon dilation (balloon diameter 80–110% of the valve annulus diameter). Check of pressure in the left ventricle, re-angiography of the left ventricle and again ascendogram (aortic regurgitation?). In older children, pacemaker stimulation of the right ventricle. For this, quick VVI stimulation (300–400/min) during balloon dilation can briefly reduce ejection from the left ventricle due to tachycardia so the balloon is not displaced too much by the pulsation of blood flow.

▸ **Heparinization.** Administration of 100 IU/kg intravenously during cardiac catheterization, then 400 IU/kg/d as a continuous infusion until the morning of the second day.

▸ **Echocardiography after cardiac catheterization.** Possible aortic regurgitation, the mean and maximum residual gradient, left ventricular function, and a possible new occurrence of mitral regurgitation should be noted.

▸ **Medication.** Aspirin 3 to 5 mg/kg for 3 months, endocarditis prophylaxis for 6 months if needed.

Critical Aortic Stenosis of the Neonate

▸ **Indication.** Owing to the typical hemodynamic situation (ductal-dependent systemic perfusion) and the fact that the left ventricular function is usually considerably impaired, there is an indication regardless of the gradient in a still-competent aortic valve (aortic regurgitation < 2°).

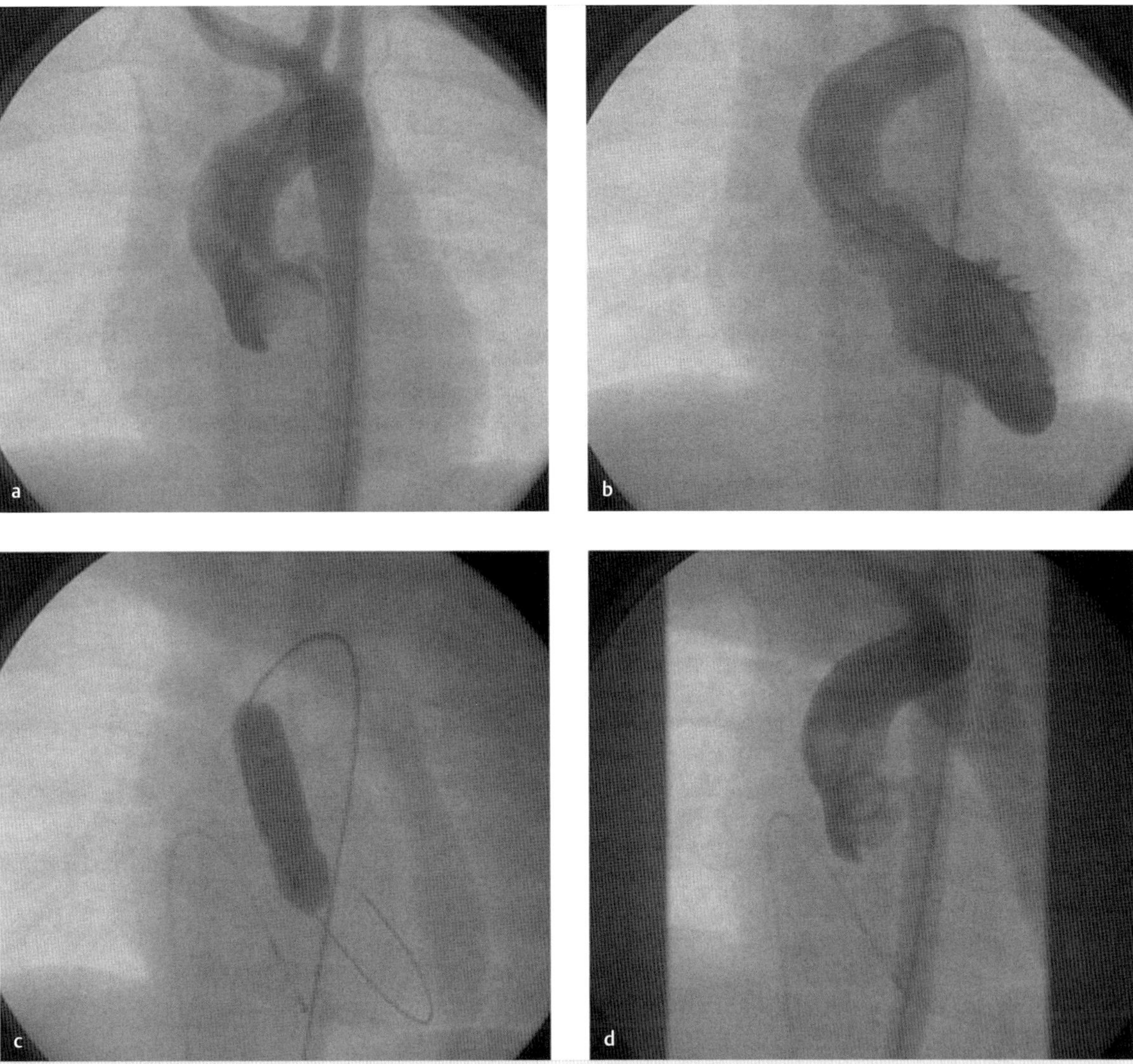

Fig. 24.1 Dilation of a valvular aortic stenosis. **a** First an ascendogram is made. **b** Then angiography of the left ventricle and visualization of the valvular stenosis, the thickened valve, and the jet across the stenotic valve. **c** Dilation of the valve under high-frequency stimulation around 350/min. **d** Finally angiography to document possible newly developed aortic regurgitation.

▸ **Preliminary examinations.** Patients are usually admitted under intensive care conditions; they are very often ventilated, critically ill newborns. ECG, detailed echocardiography, chest X-ray, and preparation for surgery with cardiopulmonary bypass is necessary.

▸ **Echocardiography.** Visualization of the valve annulus diameter, aortic regurgitation, valve anatomy (bicuspid, tricuspid), mean and maximum gradient, left ventricular function, mitral regurgitation, isthmus, ductus arteriosus, pulmonary artery diameter, exclusion of a Shone complex.

▸ **Preparation.** Preparation should be the same as for cardiopulmonary bypass surgery as dictated by hospital standards. If necessary, this may include first inserting an arterial catheter (umbilical) and a central venous catheter, catecholamine treatment, and in every case prostaglandin treatment. If still possible, give umbilical care (keep navel moist) so that antegrade cardiac catheterization via the umbilical vein remains possible.

▸ **Risks/patient information.** The risk is high because the patient is usually a critically ill neonate with impaired ventricular function. Risks include a valve rupture, acute and severe aortic regurgitation, emergency surgery, possibly with valve replacement (homograft implantation) or Ross procedure, myocardial ischemia, arrhythmias, AV block, mitral regurgitation, infection/endocarditis; for an arterial puncture, perfusion disturbance or vascular occlusion.

► **Procedure.** Whenever possible, an antegrade approach across an ASD or a patent foramen ovale should be attempted, possibly via the umbilical vein, otherwise a retrograde approach via an arterial puncture should be undertaken.

► **Cardiac catheterization/treatment.** Ascendogram, measurement of the valve annulus, probing and angiography of the left ventricle, switch to an exchange wire, then balloon dilation (balloon diameter max. 80–100% of the valve annulus diameter), check of left ventricular pressure, angiography of the left ventricle, ascendogram (aortic regurgitation?). In a critically ill child, the dilation is often performed based solely on echocardiography findings and without pressure measurements or angiographies.(► Fig. 24.2).

► **Monitoring.** Intensive care monitoring, catecholamines and prostaglandin reduced depending on the clinical status, regular echocardiography checkups.

► **Heparinization.** Administration of 100 IU/kg as an intravenous bolus during cardiac catheterization, then 400 IU/kg/d in a continuous infusion until the morning of the second day.

► **Echocardiography after cardiac catheterization.** Aortic regurgitation, mean and maximum residual gradient, left ventricular function, mitral regurgitation, mitral stenosis, PDA, isthmus, exclusion of a Shone complex.

Note

The balloon valvuloplasty of critical aortic stenosis in the neonate is carried out regardless of the gradient. The children often need an adaption phase of varying length until the left ventricle has recovered sufficiently. Long-term catecholamine support and possibly ventilation are often required.

Supravalvular Aortic Stenosis

► **Indication.** In a supravalvular aortic stenosis, an indication for intervention is relatively rare. The results for a "classic" supravalvular aortic stenosis in Williams–Beuren syndrome are poor. Postoperative supravalvular stenosis (e.g., after Damus–Kaye–Stansel anastomosis is practically the only indication):

- Gradient related (Doppler gradient over 50 mmHg)
- Cardiac decompensation or decreasing ventricular function
- Increased cardiac overload
- ST segment changes under stress

► **Preliminary examinations.** ECG no more than 2 months old; 24-hour Holter ECG and exercise ECG only if the most recent ECG was abnormal.

► **Echocardiography.** The following questions should be answered: valve annulus diameter, aortic regurgitation, anatomy of the stenosis, mean and maximum gradient,

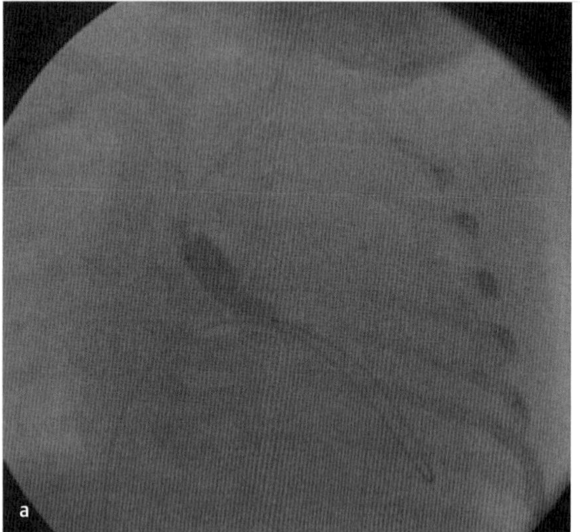

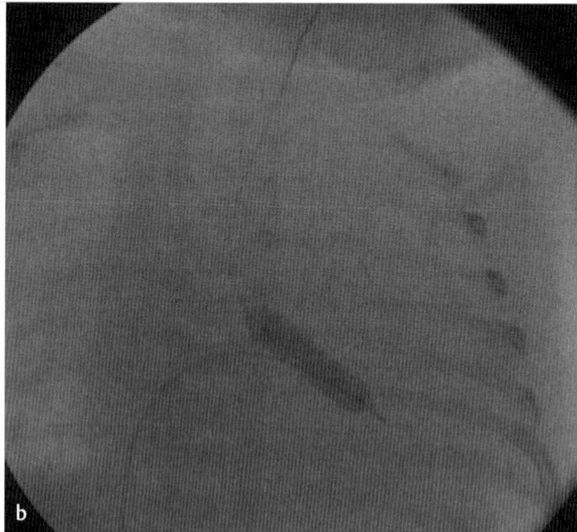

Fig. 24.2 Antegrade dilation of critical aortic valve stenosis. **a** First, antegrade probe of the stenotic aortic valve with a thin guidewire. For this a guide catheter is inserted through the inferior vena cava, the right atrium, and across the septal shunt into the left atrium and left ventricle. After passing the aortic valve, the guidewire finally crosses the aortic valve into the ascending aorta. The dilation balloon is positioned in the stenotic valve. When the dilation balloon is inflated, a distinct notch forms in the balloon, which is a sign of the valvular stenosis. **b** After repeated dilations, the notch in the dilation balloon is no longer visible. The stenotic valve is widened.

left ventricular function, isthmus, other stenosis of the head and neck vessels.

▶ **Risks/patient information.** The risk is less than 5%, dissection and coronary problems could lead to myocardial ischemia, arrhythmias, and AV block; perfusion disturbance or vascular occlusion for arterial punctures.

▶ **Procedure.** In univentricular hearts, an antegrade approach may be possible (across an ASD or the ventricle), otherwise a retrograde approach via an arterial access is used.

▶ **Cardiac catheterization/treatment.** Ascendogram, measurement of the valve annulus, probe of the left and right ventricle, angiography, switch to exchange wire, balloon dilation, check of ventricular pressure, ventricular angiography, ascendogram (aortic regurgitation?).

▶ **Monitoring.** Routine monitoring and a 12-lead ECG after the intervention, additional monitoring on an ECG monitor with ST-segment analysis, 24-hour Holter monitoring only if the ECG is abnormal.

▶ **Heparinization.** Administration of 100 IU/kg as an intravenous bolus during cardiac catheterization, then 400 IU/kg/d as a continuous infusion until the morning of the second day, and aspirin 3 to 5 mg/kg for 3 months.

▶ **Echocardiography after cardiac catheterization.** Aortic regurgitation, mean and maximum residual gradient, ventricular function, and wall dyskinesia should be documented.

▶ **Medication.** Aspirin 3 to 5 mg/kg for 3 months, endocarditis prophylaxis for 6 months.

Mitral Stenosis

▶ **Indication.** Overall, balloon valvuloplasty of the mitral valve is only rarely indicated in children in Europe. From a global perspective, it is a common procedure after rheumatic fever or—rarely—because of endocarditis. The results are satisfactory for stenosis of previously normal valves. In primarily anomalous valves (e.g., parachute or hammock valve), or especially after surgical reconstruction, the results are unsatisfactory. Indications are:

- Gradient dependency (Doppler gradient of 10 mmHg)
- Signs of "left decompensation" (pulmonary edema, pulmonary congestion)
- Atrial arrhythmias
- Ectatic left atrium with thrombi
- Intermittent pulmonary edema—congestive cough
- Significant pulmonary hypertension
- Progressive deterioration of physical capacity

▶ **Preliminary examinations.** ECG no more than 2 months old, 24-hour Holter ECG and exercise ECG only if the most recent ECG was abnormal, cardiopulmonary exercise test for larger patients.

▶ **Echocardiography.** Valve annulus diameter, anatomy, mean and maximum gradient, left ventricular function, mitral regurgitation, ASD or patent foramen ovale, and pulmonary hypertension should be investigated.

▶ **Risks/patient information.** Risk less than 5%, rupture of the valve, acute severe mitral regurgitation (often not well tolerated), emergency operation (low risk), valve replacement, dissection, tamponade, death, myocardial ischemia, arrhythmias, AV block, infection/endocarditis.

▶ **Procedure.** Antegrade approach through the femoral veins.

▶ **Cardiac catheterization/treatment.** Transseptal probing of the left atrium, if necessary by transseptal puncture; rarely, left atrial angiography and pressure measurement, probe of the left ventricle with wire, insertion of the balloon catheter (e.g., Inoue balloon) and dilation, check of left atrial and left ventricular pressure, angiography of the left ventricle (mitral regurgitation?).

▶ **Echocardiography after cardiac catheterization.** Mitral regurgitation, mean and maximum residual gradient, left ventricular function, pulmonary hypertension.

▶ **Medication.** Aspirin 3 to 5 mg/kg for 3 months, endocarditis prophylaxis for 6 months if necessary, possibly treatment/prophylaxis of rheumatic fever.

Note

Balloon valvuloplasty of the mitral valve has become very rare in Europe, but in other countries with more frequent rheumatic fever, it is one of the most commonly performed interventional procedures. Congenital mitral valve defects are not successfully treated by interventional catheterization.

Balloon Valvuloplasty of Coarctation of the Aorta

▶ **Indication.** Overall, the indication criteria for balloon valvuloplasty of coarctation of the aorta are evolving as, on one hand, the results are promising while, on the other hand, the risk of the procedure is relatively low. In neonates and children under 6 months, the recurrence rate is unsatisfactory (elastic ductal tissue), which is why this

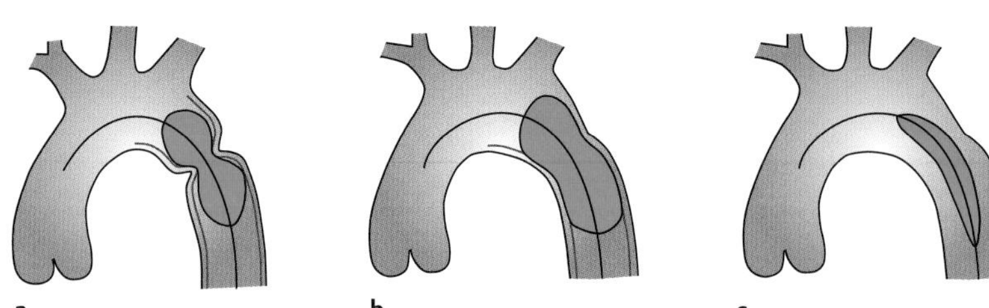

Fig. 24.3 Balloon dilation of coarctation of the aorta. **a** First the balloon is advanced up to the stenosis. **b** The stenosis is widened by inflating the balloon. **c** After dilation, the balloon is deflated and the catheter is retrieved.

group is usually treated surgically. Clinical as well as pharmacological exercise tests (e.g., orciprenaline stress test) are often helpful in determining the indication. Accepted indications are:

- Doppler gradient well above 20 mmHg
- Absent or severely attenuated inguinal pulses
- Blood pressure difference arm/leg well above 20 mmHg
- Hypertension (exercise test, long-term blood pressure measurement)
- Cardiac decompensation or decreasing left ventricular function
- Increasing cardiac overload (left ventricular wall thickness)
- ST segment changes on exertion
- Increasing aortic regurgitation

▶ **Preliminary examinations.** ECG not more than 2 months old, echocardiography; if possible, in older children, MRI with 3D reconstruction and dimensions of the aortic arch and isthmus.

▶ **Echocardiography.** Visualization of the diameter of the arch, the coarctation, the descending aorta at the diaphragm level, aortic valve, valve annulus diameter, aortic regurgitation, mean and maximum gradient, left ventricular function, mitral regurgitation, isthmus, ductus arteriosus, possibly gradient under stress, exclusion of a Shone complex.

▶ **Risks/patient information.** The risk is well below 5%. There are a few patients beyond the neonatal age who still require surgery owing to insufficient success of catheter intervention (elastic tissue). Possible complications are dissection due to massive overdilation, aneurysm formation, hematothorax, transfusion, chest tube, emergency stent implantation, emergency surgery, death, paraplegia (extremely rare). The restenosis rate is over 20% (same as for a surgical procedure), and perfusion problems or vascular occlusion may occur after the arterial puncture. There is typically mild chest pain after the intervention.

▶ **Procedure.** In young children, an antegrade approach (across ASD or patent foramen ovale) may be possible. In most patients, however, a retrograde approach via an arterial puncture is undertaken access is used. (▶ Fig. 24.3).

▶ **Cardiac catheterization/treatment.** Ascendogram, measurement of each arc segment and determining the anatomy, pull-back pressure, possibly orciprenaline stress test (Alupent), switch to an exchange wire, balloon dilation, control angiography, pull-back pressure, possibly another pharmacological stress test.

▶ **Monitoring after dilatation.** Additional monitoring and documentation of blood pressure at least every 30 minutes through the night and for 24 hours if any questions remain, blood pressure, apply generous analgesia and, systematic antihypertensive therapy (e.g., carvedilol, ACE inhibitors).

▶ **Heparinization.** Administration of 100 IU/kg as an intravenous bolus during cardiac catheterization, then 400 IU/kg/d in a continuous infusion until the morning of the second day.

▶ **Checkups after cardiac catheterization.** Echocardiography: documentation of mean and maximum residual gradient, left ventricular function, perfusion of the inguinal vessels.

MRI: Routinely after 6 months to document the result as well as to rule out aneurysms.

▶ **Medication.** See Aortic Stenosis.

Dilation of Coarctation of the Aorta of the Neonate

▶ **Indication.** There are currently very few generally accepted indications for the interventional treatment of the coarctation of the aorta of the neonate. Children are not usually treated by interventional catheterization before the age of 6 months because the risk of recurrence is very high (over 70%). The procedure is indicated for sick newborns with additional problems that impede rapid surgery (e.g., necrotic enterocolitis, unclear syndromes, brain hemorrhage) or in critically ill children with cardiac decompensation, as well as children with cardiomyopathy and mild coarctation of the aorta.

▸ **Preliminary examinations.** Cranial ultrasound (to rule out brain hemorrhage), other organ diagnostic workups under intensive care conditions (the neonate is usually ventilated and critically ill). ECG, echocardiography, chest X-ray, surgical preparation, prostaglandin treatment, possibly catecholamines.

▸ **Echocardiography.** The diameter of the aortic arch, coarctation of the aorta, descending aorta at diaphragm level, aortic valve, valve annulus diameter, aortic regurgitation, valvular anatomy, mean and maximum gradient, left ventricular function, mitral regurgitation, isthmus, ductus arteriosus should be documented; a Shone complex should be ruled out.

▸ **Preparation.** Same as for cardiopulmonary bypass surgery; if necessary, insertion of an arterial catheter (umbilical) as well as a central venous catheter, catecholamine treatment, prostaglandin treatment obligatory in all patients.

▸ **Risks/patient information.** The risk is high as the neonate is critically ill. There is a very high recurrence rate due to elastic ductal issue. Dissection in massive overdilation, hematothorax, transfusion, chest drainage, emergency stent implantation, emergency surgery, death, and perfusion disturbance or vessel occlusion and rupture after arterial puncture may occur. Surgery is usually required soon afterward as the intervention is only a palliative measure.

▸ **Procedure.** An antegrade approach may be possible (across an ASD or patent foramen ovale), but in most cases a retrograde approach via an arterial access is used.

▸ **Cardiac catheterization/treatment.** Ascendogram, measurement of each segment of the arch and assessment of the anatomy, change to wire, balloon dilation (▸ Fig. 24.4). Switch to an exchange wire, control angiography, leave arterial catheter in place. Dilation may also be performed also based only on the echocardiography.

▸ **Monitoring.** Use intensive care monitoring, taper catecholamines, discontinue prostaglandin, carry out regular echocardiography checkups. In addition, blood pressure is monitored every 30 minutes overnight, perfusion of the legs should be monitored with continuous pulse oximetry. Early enteral nutrition intake should be instigated on the same day, and possibly antihypertensive treatment (e.g., diuretics, ACE inhibitors, carvedilol).

▸ **Heparinization.** Administration of 100 IU/kg as an intravenous bolus during cardiac catheterization, otherwise proceed according to intensive care guidelines and patient need.

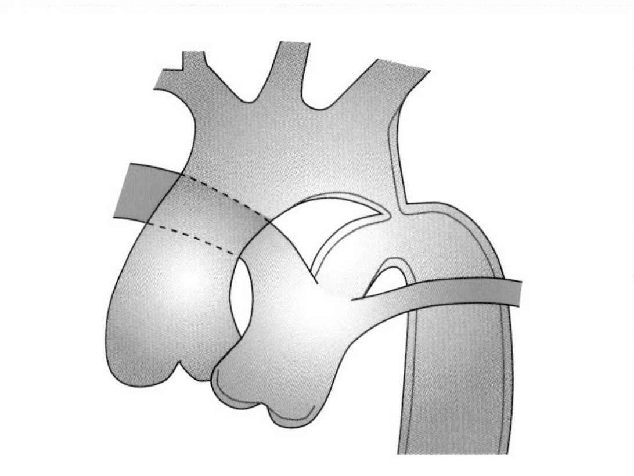

Fig. 24.4 Anatomy of coarctation of the aorta in the neonate with perfusion of the lower half of the body across the patent ductus arteriosus.

▸ **Echocardiography after cardiac catheterization.** Access aortic regurgitation, mean and maximum residual gradient, left ventricular function, mitral regurgitation, mitral stenosis, PDA, exclusion of a Shone complex.

Stent Implantation in Coarctation of the Aorta

▸ **Indication.** The indication criteria for stent implantation as treatment of coarctation of the aorta are still evolving because the results are promising and the risk of the procedure is low—also due to the development of new materials with small sheath sizes. The issue as to whether covered stents should be used or not, is still under discussion.

In small children, stents are used only as an emergency solution intraoperatively in hypoplastic vessels. Coronary stents or small vascular stents are used as bailout options in neonates or small children. Specifically designed stents for neonates that can be redilated to adult size are under clinical development. Exercise tests are useful for determining the indication in so called "mild coarctations". The acceptable indications for body weight of at least 20 kg are the same as for unstented coarctation of the aorta:

- Doppler gradient well above 20 mmHg
- Absent or severely attenuated inguinal pulses
- Blood pressure difference arm/leg well above 20 mmHg
- Hypertension (exercise test, long-term blood pressure measurement)
- Cardiac decompensation or decreasing left ventricular function
- Increasing cardiac overload (left ventricular wall thickness)
- ST segment changes under stress
- Increasing aortic regurgitation

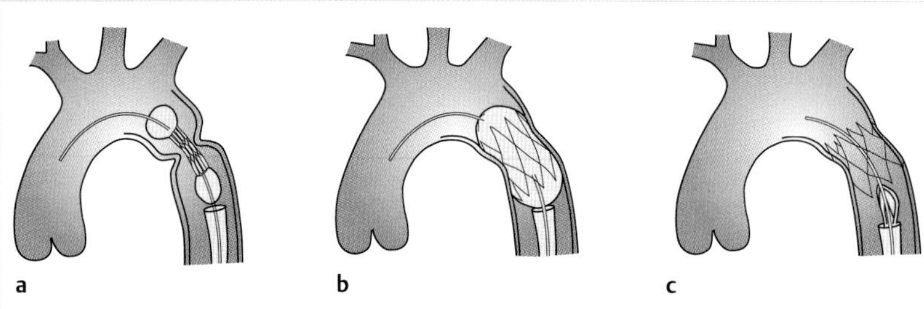

Fig. 24.5 Stent implantation for coarctation of the aorta. **a** First a balloon catheter with a stent is inserted up to the stenosis. **b** The balloon is inflated to widen the stenosis and expand the stent. **c** After dilation the balloon is deflated and the catheter is retrieved. The stent maintains the dilation.

▶ **Preliminary examinations.** ECG no more than 2 months old, current echocardiography with documentation of the diameter of the vessels, MRI with 3D reconstruction and dimensions; possibly, exercise tests, 24-hour blood pressure monitoring.

▶ **Echocardiography.** The diameter of the aortic arch and coarctation, the descending aorta at diaphragm level, aortic valve, valve annulus diameter, aortic regurgitation, valvular anatomy, mean and maximum gradient, left ventricular function, mitral regurgitation, isthmus, ductus arteriosus should be documented; a Shone complex should be ruled out.

▶ **Risks/patient information.** The risk is less than 5%, possible dissection due to massive overdilation, hematothorax, transfusion, chest drainage, aneurysm formation, emergency implantation of covered stents, emergency surgery, death, paraplegia (rare), low rate of restenosis (< 5%), possibly two-stage procedure with re-dilation in 6 to 12 months, perfusion disorders or vessel occlusion for an arterial puncture. Typically there is mild chest pain after the stent implantation.

▶ **Procedure.** Usually an antegrade approach via an arterial puncture is attempted.

▶ **Cardiac catheterization/treatment.** Ascendogram, measurement of each arch segment and determination of the anatomy, pull-back pressure, possibly orciprenaline (Alupent) stress test, switch to an exchange wire (balloon dilation, control angiography), insertion of the long transport sheath, control angiography using hand injections, stent implantation (▶ Fig. 24.5), pull-back pressure, possibly repeated pharmacological stress test. In larger children and arch stenosis, pacemaker stimulation (rare) may be instigated to ensure proper stent placement.

▶ **Monitoring.** Heparinization, medication, and monitoring are the same as for balloon dilation.

Balloon Valvuloplasty of Pulmonary Stenosis

▶ **Indication.** The indication for balloon valvuloplasty of the pulmonary valve is made generously today because the results are usually very satisfactory and the risk of the intervention is relatively low. Accepted indications are:

- Gradient related (Doppler gradient over 50 mmHg)
- Cardiac decompensation or decreasing right ventricular function
- Increasing cardiac overload, pressure in the right ventricle over 60 mmHg
- Increasing poststenotic ectasia of the pulmonary artery
- Intermittent peripheral edema as a sign of right heart failure
- Progressive decrease in physical exercise capacity
- Cyanosis with an ASD or patent foramen ovale

▶ **Preliminary examinations.** ECG no more than 2 months old, recent echocardiography, 24-hour Holter ECG and stress ECG if the most recent ECG was abnormal, cardiopulmonary exercise test in larger, cooperative patients.

▶ **Echocardiography.** The valve annulus diameter, pulmonary regurgitation, anatomy (bicuspid, tricuspid valve), mean and maximum gradient, pressure and function of the right ventricle, tricuspid regurgitation, ASD or patent foramen ovale, PDA, and subvalvular stenosis should be documented and additional stenoses ruled out.

▶ **Risks/patient information.** The risk is below 1%, rupture of the valve, acute and severe pulmonary regurgitation (usually well tolerated), emergency operation (minimal risk), dissection, tamponade, death, myocardial ischemia, arrhythmias, AV block, tricuspid regurgitation, infection/endocarditis, infundibulum stenosis (beta-blocker therapy). In myxomatous (i.e., massively thickened), deformed valves, the result is less satisfactory, possibly requiring a repeat of the intervention or surgery.

▶ **Procedure.** An antegrade approach via the femoral vessels, possibly via the jugular vein, is performed.

▶ **Cardiac catheterization/treatment.** Angiography of the right ventricle, measurement of the valve annulus, probing of the pulmonary artery, switch to exchange wire, balloon dilation (ratio of balloon/valve annulus 1.3–1.5: 1; ▶ Fig. 24.6), thereafter, check of pressure in the pulmonary artery and in the right ventricle, pulmonary artery angiography (pulmonary regurgitation), angiography of

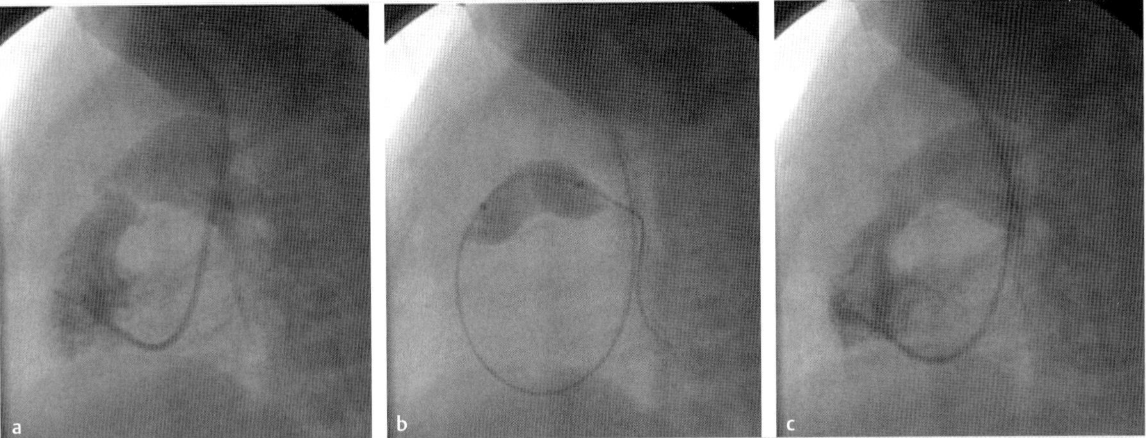

Fig. 24.6 Balloon dilation of a valvular pulmonary stenosis. **a** First angiography of the right ventricle and measurement of the valve annulus. **b** The stenosis is widened by inflating the balloon. **c** After dilation, angiography of the pulmonary artery documents possible development of pulmonary regurgitation.

the right ventricle. Possibly, give beta blocker treatment for new occurrence of a reactive subvalvular stenosis.

▶ **Monitoring.** Heparinization, ECG after the intervention, in addition to monitoring of saturation.

▶ **Echocardiography after cardiac catheterization.** Pulmonary regurgitation, mean and maximum residual gradient, pressure in the right ventricle, tricuspid regurgitation, documentation of the subvalvular anatomy (residual gradient, infundibulum stenosis?).

▶ **Medication.** See Aortic Stenosis.

Critical Pulmonary Stenosis in the Neonate

▶ **Indication.** Owing to the typical hemodynamics (PDA-dependent pulmonary perfusion), treatment is indicated regardless of the gradient. It is important to have a sufficiently large right ventricle with all three anatomical segments, that is, inlet segment (for sufficiently large right ventricle, tricuspid valve annulus > 7–10 mm), ventricular segment, and infundibulum. Oxygenation is ensured by prostaglandin administration. The children are cyanotic due to the right-to-left shunt at the atrial level.

▶ **Preliminary examinations.** The children are usually under intensive care and are sometimes ventilated (prostaglandin side effect); they are rarely critically ill newborns. ECG, echocardiography, and chest X-ray should be documented, otherwise the preparation is the same as for surgery.

▶ **Echocardiography.** Visualization of valve annulus diameter, size of the right ventricle, right ventricular anatomy, infundibulum, pulmonary regurgitation, right ventricular function, right ventricular systolic pressure, tricuspid regurgitation, pulmonary valve anatomy (bicuspid, tricuspid valve), mean and maximum gradient, size of the ASD or patent foramen ovale, isthmus, ductus arteriosus, diameter of the main pulmonary artery as well as the right and left pulmonary artery.

▶ **Preparation.** Same as for surgery with cardiopulmonary bypass; the insertion of an arterial access (umbilical) as well as a central venous catheter may be indicated. Possibly give catecholamines; prostaglandin treatment obligatory in all patients.

▶ **Blood tests.** Same as for surgery with cardiopulmonary bypass.

▶ **Risks/patient information.** The risk is increased for critically ill neonates. Theoretically, rupture of the valve, acute and severe pulmonary regurgitation with inadequate systemic perfusion caused by the run-off across a large PDA, emergency surgery—possibly with creation of a shunt or a transannular patch, myocardial ischemia, arrhythmias, AV block, development of tricuspid regurgitation, infection/endocarditis, perfusion disturbance or vascular occlusion if an arterial puncture is made. If treatment fails, surgery after an interval may be performed; possibly re-intervention after an interval of weeks and months.

▶ **Procedure.** An antegrade approach is undertaken, possibly via the umbilical vein, otherwise via the femoral vein or jugular vein; in addition arterial pressure measurement is made. If apnea is present (prostaglandin side effect), sometimes intubation is necessary.

▶ **Cardiac catheterization/treatment.** Contrast hand-injection into the right ventricle, measurement of the valve annulus (echocardiography), probing of the pulmonary artery, switch to an exchange wire, balloon dilation, check of pressure in the pulmonary artery and in the right ventricle, pulmonary artery (PA) angiography (pulmonary regurgitation), angiography of the right ventricle, possibly dilatation and checks without angiography based on echocardiography parameters, possibly switch the catheter to a central venous catheter.

► **Monitoring.** Intensive care monitoring, taper catecholamines (if previously necessary), discontinue or taper prostaglandin, carry out regular echocardiography checkups; a saturation of around 75-80% is acceptable in a closed PDA because the right ventricle is usually hypertrophic, and if there is a large ASD and a significant tricuspid regurgitation, there is initially still a large volume flow via the right-to-left shunt despite the free outflow in the pulmonary artery.

► **Heparinization.** Administration of 100 IU/kg as an intravenous bolus during the cardiac catheterization, then 400 IU/kg/d as a continuous infusion until the morning of the second day.

► **Echocardiography after cardiac catheterization.** Check for pulmonary regurgitation, mean and maximum residual gradient, pressure, volume and function of right ventricle, tricuspid regurgitation, tricuspid stenosis, PDA, isthmus, ASD or patent foramen ovale, shunt reversal.

Note

The indication for balloon dilation of critical pulmonary stenosis of the neonate is independent of the gradient. After successful treatment, some children require adaptation phases of varying lengths before the right ventricle can produce a sufficient antegrade blood flow into the pulmonary circulation. In significant pulmonary regurgitation and a large PDA, a critical drop in systemic cardiac output may develop.

Balloon Dilatation of the Pulmonary Valve in Untreated Tetralogy of Fallot

► **Indication.** These children are usually relatively sick and, in particular, severely cyanotic; occasionally they are neonates with a closed PDA or children with hypercyanotic spells. The indication for treatment may vary. Possible reasons for palliative intervention are:

- Hypoplastic pulmonary vessels (antegrade perfusion improves the size of the pulmonary artery)
- Ductal-dependent children (to delay the time of surgery)
- Severe cyanosis (saturation below 75% without PDA or oxygen supplementation)
- If necessary before interventional closure of MAPCAs
- In very small children (preterm) as a palliative measure
- To postpone surgery in children with hypercyanotic spells despite adequate pharmacological treatment

► **Preliminary examinations.** Often the patient will be in intensive care, occasionally ventilated, and may be a critically ill child. ECG, echocardiography, chest X-ray, preparation for surgery; arterial pressure measurement is optional.

► **Echocardiography.** Documentation of the valve annulus diameter, pulmonary regurgitation, valve anatomy (bicuspid, tricuspid valve), mean and maximum gradient, subvalvular anatomy, right ventricular pressure and function, tricuspid regurgitation, size of the ASD or the patent foramen ovale, isthmus, ductus arteriosus, pulmonary artery diameter left/right.

► **Preparation.** Same as for surgery with cardiopulmonary bypass. Based on the clinical condition it may be necessary to insert an arterial catheter, central venous catheter, administer catecholamines. Treatment with prostaglandines is always indicated in neonates. Possibly intubation anesthesia. Generous volume substitution is necessary before the Catheter investigation and intervention and an additional intravenous bolus of 20 mL/kg of colloidal volume after puncturing the inguinal vessels should be given to minimize the risk of hypercyanotic spells.

► **Risks/patient information.** The risk is higher because the children are often critically ill. Main risk: hypercyanotic spells, resuscitation and death, increasing infundibulum stenosis (beta-blocker treatment), emergency surgery possibly with creation of a shunt or transannular patch, myocardial ischemia, arrhythmia, AV block, development of tricuspid regurgitation, infection/endocarditis, reperfusion edema of the pulmonary vessels (ventilation needed); in case of failure of treatment, repeat cardiac catheterization or surgery after an interval.

► **Procedure.** In neonates, an antegrade approach via the umbilical vein may be possible. Usually an access via the femoral vein or jugular vein is performed. In addition, arterial pressure monitoring is helpful.

► **Cardiac catheterization/treatment.** (Manual) injection right ventricle, measurement of the valve annulus, probing of the pulmonary artery, rapid switch to an exchange wire, rapid balloon dilation (► Fig. 24.7), In stable patients check pressure in the pulmonary artery and right ventricle, optional PA angiography (pulmonary regurgitation), angiography of the right ventricle. In unstable patients, dilation without angiography according to echocardiography findings is possible. The aim is to achieve an

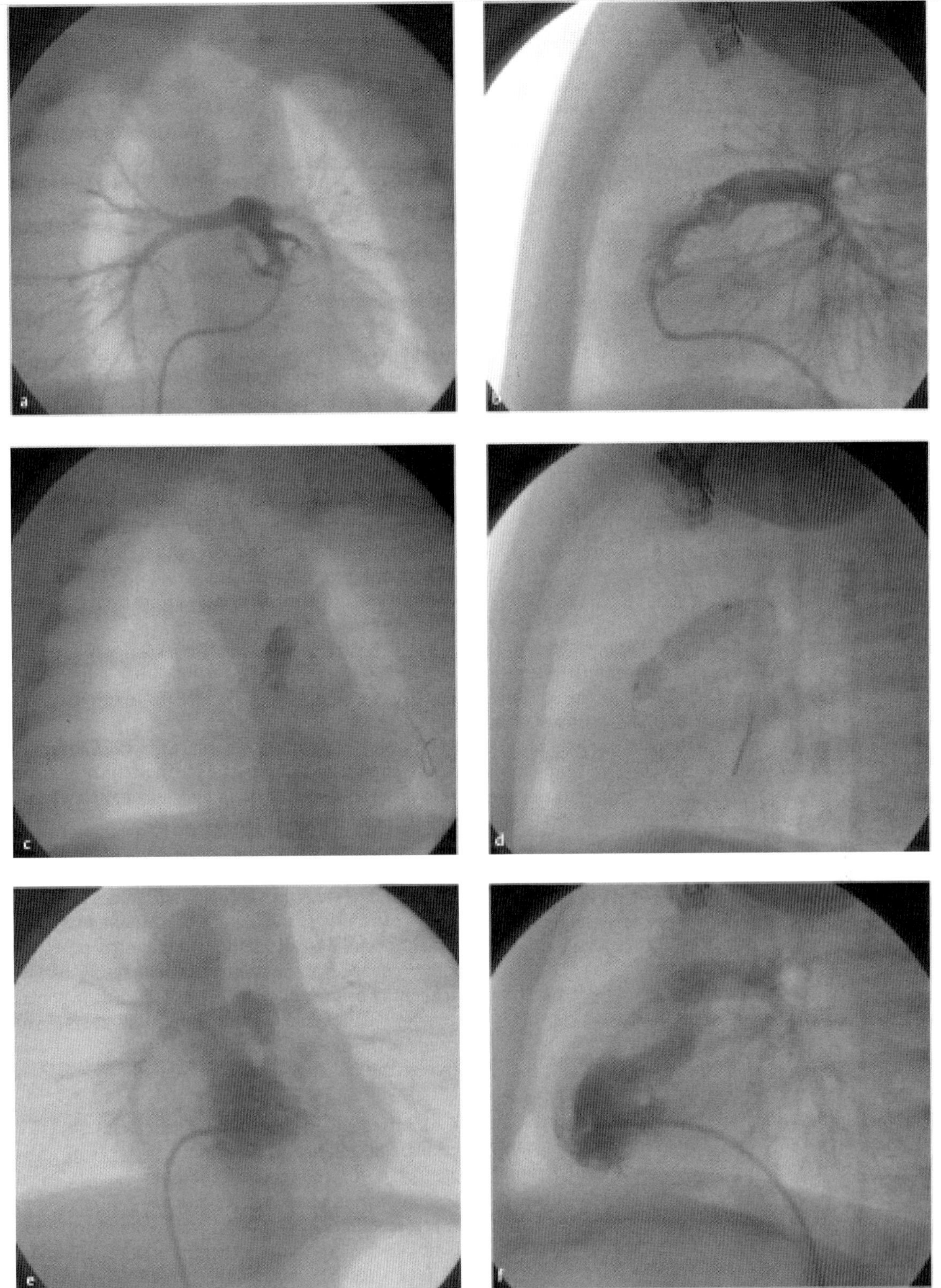

Fig. 24.7 Dilatation of the pulmonary valve and the right ventricular outflow tract in untreated tetralogy of Fallot. Initial saturation is around 70%, after the intervention it is 90%. First, angiography of the right ventricle and measurement of the valve annulus (**a**, **b**). The stenosis is widened by inflating the balloon (**c**, **d**). After the dilation, angiography of the pulmonary artery to document a possible development of pulmonary regurgitation and repeat angiography of the right ventricle (**e**, **f**).

increase in the saturation. Thereafter switch to a central venous catheter. The individual steps depend the stability of the patient. In addition, intravenous beta blockers should be kept at hand (e.g., propranolol, esmolol) and noradrenaline for the treatment of a hypercyanotic spell.

► **Heparinization.** Administration of 100 IU/kg as intravenous bolus during the procedure; then 400 IU/kg/d in continuous infusion until the morning of the second day.

► **Monitoring.** Standard intensive care monitoring; possibly taper off catecholamine treatment, discontinue prostaglandin, carry out regular echocardiography checkups; documentation of the saturation trend on the monitor, chest X-ray (pulmonary edema).

► **Echocardiography after cardiac catheterization.** Documentation of pulmonary regurgitation, anatomy and gradient across the infundibulum, tricuspid regurgitation, flow across the PDA if present.

Interventional Treatment of Pulmonary Atresia

► **Indication.** In neonates, the indication is based on the typical hemodynamic situation (PDA-dependent lung perfusion) just as in severe or critical pulmonary stenosis and sufficiently large right ventricle (tricuspid valve annulus > 7–10 mm). Other indications exist for older children after creation of an aortopulmonary shunt as a palliative measure to improve perfusion of the pulmonary artery and as a preparatory step toward corrective surgery. Anatomy can vary considerably if MAPCAs and multifocal lung perfusion are present. Indications are:

- Hypoplastic pulmonary artery (antegrade perfusion improves the size of the pulmonary artery)
- Ductal-dependent children (avoid or delay surgery)
- Severe cyanosis (saturation below 75% without a PDA or oxygen supplementation)
- Possibly before interventional closure of MAPCAs
- As a palliative measure in very young children (preterm)
- Preparation for surgery

► **Preliminary examinations.** Newborn patients are often in intensive care, sometimes ventilated, but rarely are critically ill neonates. ECG, echocardiography, chest X-ray, preparation for surgery, arterial pressure measurement is optional. In larger children an MRI with 3D reconstruction, if possible, may help in procedure planning.

► **Echocardiography.** Visualization of the valve annulus diameter, anatomy of the right ventricular outflow tract and the rudimentary pulmonary artery, right ventricular function, tricuspid regurgitation, size of the ASD or patent foramen ovale, isthmus, ductus arteriosus, pulmonary artery diameter left/right, MAPCAs.

► **Preparation.** In neonates, same as for cardiopulmonary bypass surgery, possibly insertion of an arterial catheter and a central venous catheter beforehand, rarely catecholamine treatment, prostaglandin treatment in all patients, Sometimes intubation may be requested. Routine preparation is appropriate for larger children.

► **Risks/patient information.** In neonates the risk is increased (around 10%), it includes perforation with pericardial tamponade, possibly emergency surgery, possibly shunt or transannular patch, myocardial ischemia, arrhythmia, AV block, tricuspid regurgitation, infection, reperfusion edema (possibly ventilation); if treatment fails, surgery or interventional catheterization may be performed later; if antegrade perfusion is inadequate, long term intensive care may be necessary and prostaglandin therapy needs to be tapered down.

In larger children, the risk assessment is relatively predictable (well below 5%) and includes the following risk factors: perforation, tamponade with subsequent pericardial drainage, emergency surgery, reperfusion edema (ventilation); if treatment fails, surgery or additional interventional catheterization later.

It may be necessary to implant a stent across the right ventricular outflow tract to stabilize the antegrade pulmonary perfusion.

► **Procedure.** An antegrade approach via the umbilical vein is undertaken if possible, otherwise via the femoral vein or jugular vein; in addition, angiographic visualization of the rudimentary pulmonary artery.

► **Cardiac catheterization/treatment.** Contrast medium injection into the right ventricle and probing of the right ventricular outflow tract, probe of the pulmonary artery, simultaneous visualization of both structures, then radiofrequency perforation, switch to exchange wire, sequential balloon dilation (► Fig. 24.8). For hypoplastic anatomy, subsequent stent implantation is usually needed. The objective is to increase saturation. Possibly change the catheter to a central venous catheter.

► **Monitoring.** Intensive care for neonates, taper off catecholamine treatment, discontinue or taper off prostaglandin, carry out regular echocardiography checkups. Documentation of saturation: around 75-80% saturation is accepted for a closed PDA because the right ventricle is usually hypertrophic; if there is a large ASD and significant tricuspid regurgitation, blood flow across the right-to-left shunt is still adequate initially despite the free outflow into the pulmonary artery.

► **Heparinization, echocardiography, aftercare.** Same as for a critical pulmonary stenosis of the neonate.

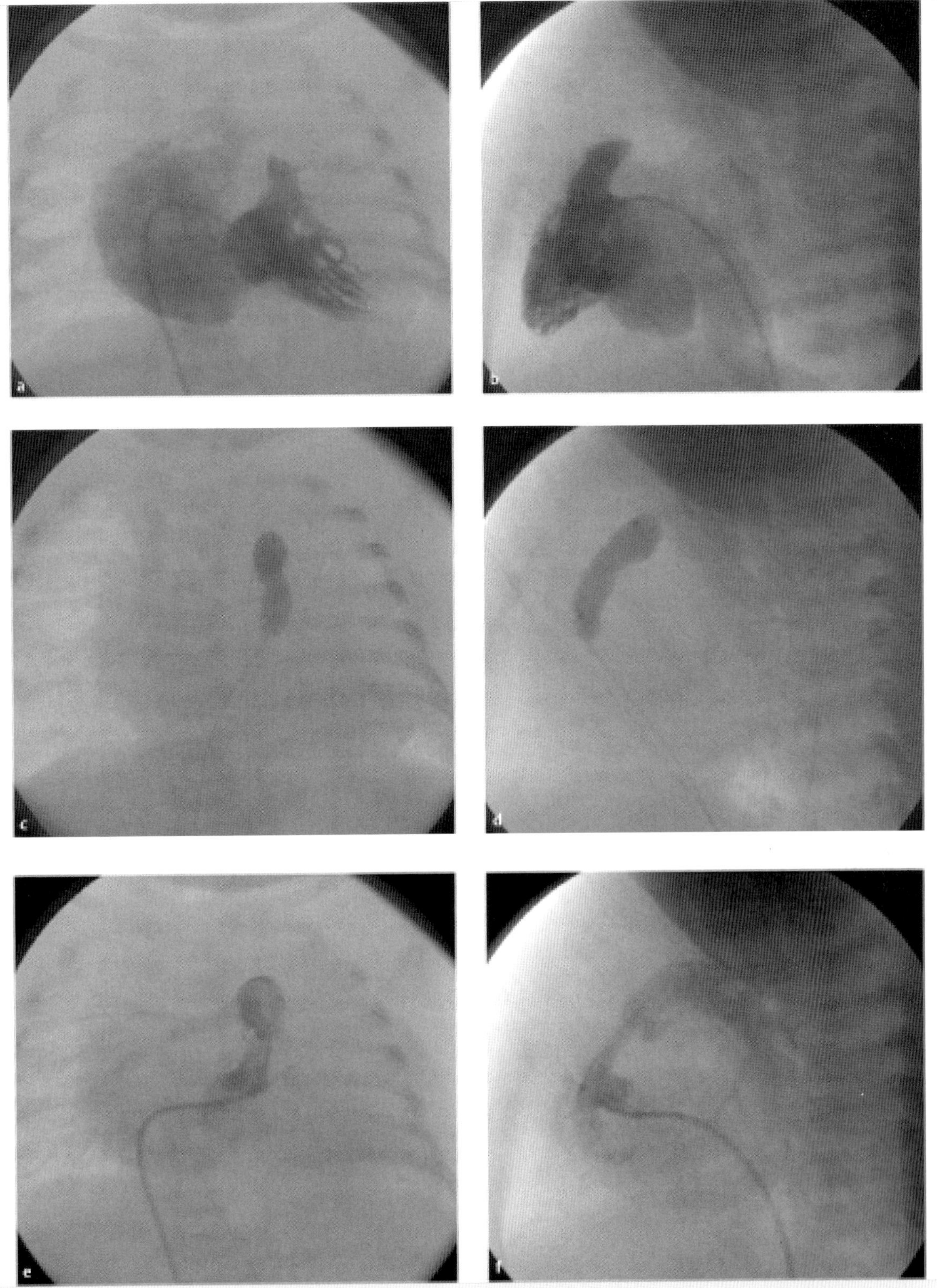

Fig. 24.8 Interventional opening of a pulmonary atresia. First, the right ventricle is visualized and the right ventricular outflow tract is probed (**a**, **b**). There is significant tricuspid regurgitation and no antegrade flow across the right ventricular outflow tract. Then radiofrequency perforation and sequential balloon dilatation (**c**, **d**). After dilation there is sufficient antegrade flow and the tricuspid regurgitation is much lower (**e**, **f**). Decrease of the right ventricular pressure from 150 to 50 to 60 mmHg.

Balloon Dilation of Supravalvular Pulmonary Stenosis

▶ **Indication.** In untreated supravalvular pulmonary stenosis (Williams–Beuren syndrome, Turner syndrome) the results are often less satisfactory, since elastic and muscular vessel wall segments cause the stenosis. In postoperative stenosis (after pulmonary artery banding, Fallot tetralogy surgery, homograft implantation) there is usually a significant improvement in the hemodynamic situation after the dilation. The risk of the intervention is relatively low. Accepted indications are:

- Gradient dependent (Doppler gradient over 50 mmHg)
- Cardiac decompensation or decreasing right ventricular function
- Increasing cardiac overload, pressure in the right ventricle over 50–60 mmHg
- Readily visualized circumscribed stenosis in echocardiography
- Poststenotic ectasia of the pulmonary artery
- Intermittent peripheral edema as a sign of right heart failure
- Progressive deterioration of physical exercise capacity

▶ **Preliminary examinations.** ECG no more than 2 months old, 24-hour Holter ECG and exercise ECG only if the ECG was abnormal, cardiopulmonary exercise test in larger and cooperative patients, optional MRI with 3D reconstruction.

▶ **Echocardiography.** Valve annulus diameter, pulmonary regurgitation, anatomy of the valve, mean and maximum gradient, diameter of the left and right pulmonary artery (LPA and RPA), right ventricular pressure and function, tricuspid regurgitation, ASD or patent foramen ovale, subvalvular stenosis, other stenoses.

▶ **Risks/patient information.** The risk is low (< 1%), rupture or dissection of the pulmonary artery wall, possibly acute and severe pulmonary regurgitation (usually well tolerated), emergency surgery (minimal risk), dissection, tamponade, death, myocardial ischemia, arrhythmia, AV block, development of tricuspid regurgitation, infection/endocarditis, infundibular stenosis (beta-blocker treatment), lung embolism, postembolic pneumonia, reperfusion edema.

▶ **Procedure.** An antegrade approach is undertaken via the femoral vessels, also feasible via the jugular vein.

▶ **Cardiac catheterization/treatment.** Angiography of the right ventricle and pulmonary artery, measurement of the valve annulus and the right ventricular outflow tract and the pulmonary artery, probing of the pulmonary artery, switch to exchange wire, balloon dilation of the stenosis and the right ventricular outflow tract and pulmonary artery branches (▶ Fig. 24.9, ▶ Fig. 24.10), check of the pressure in the pulmonary artery and right ventricle, PA angiography (pulmonary regurgitation, dissection?), angiography of the right ventricle. High pressure balloons are often necessary to achieve satisfactory results for homograft stenosis and calcification.

▶ **Heparinization/medication.** Same as for valvular pulmonary stenosis.

▶ **Echocardiography after cardiac catheterization.** Documentation of pulmonary regurgitation, mean and maximum residual gradient, right ventricular pressure and function, tricuspid regurgitation.

Dilatation of Peripheral Pulmonary Stenosis

▶ **Indication.** Sometimes postoperative patients (e.g., with scarred strictures or calcifications after multiple surgeries), but more often patients with congenital heart defects (e.g., tetralogy of Fallot, pulmonary atresia, truncus arteriosus communis, etc.) or with syndromic disorders (e.g., Williams–Beuren syndrome, Alagille syndrome) are affected by multiple peripheral pulmonary stenoses. The results are often promising. The indication is an additional improvement of the hemodynamic situation and right ventricular overload, sometimes for recruitment of additional vascular areas in a rarefied vascular bed. The risk of the intervention is relatively low. Accepted indications are:

- Gradient related (Doppler gradient over 50 mmHg)
- Cardiac decompensation or deteriorating right ventricular function
- Increasing cardiac load, right ventricular pressure over 60 mmHg
- Readily visualized circumscribed stenosis in echocardiography
- Apparent hypoperfusion of a lung area with inadequate distribution of the pulmonary perfusion (MRI)
- Cyanosis due to right ventricular overload
- Reduced physical capacity (in cardiopulmonary exercise test)

▶ **Preliminary examinations.** ECG no more than 2 months old, 24-hour Holter ECG and stress ECG if the ECG was abnormal, cardiopulmonary exercise test for larger and cooperative patients, optional MRI with 3D reconstruction and segmental perfusion, in selected but exceptional cases lung perfusion scintigraphy.

▶ **Echocardiography.** Valve annulus diameter, pulmonary regurgitation, mean and maximum gradient, right ventricular pressure and function, tricuspid regurgitation, ASD or patent foramen ovale, other stenoses.

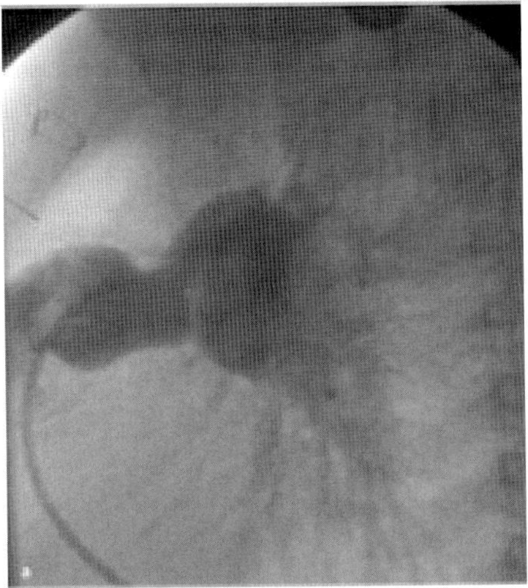

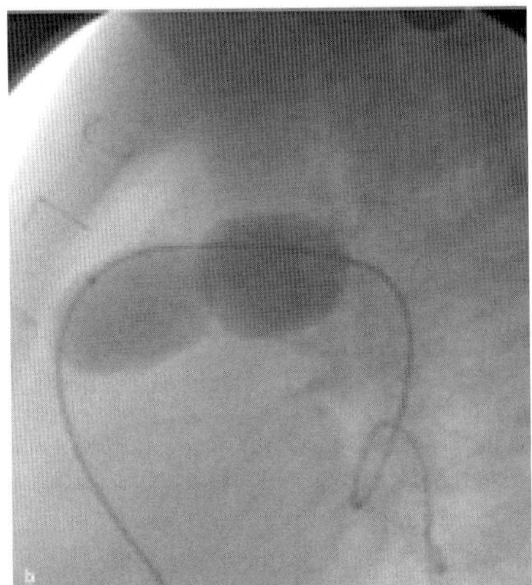

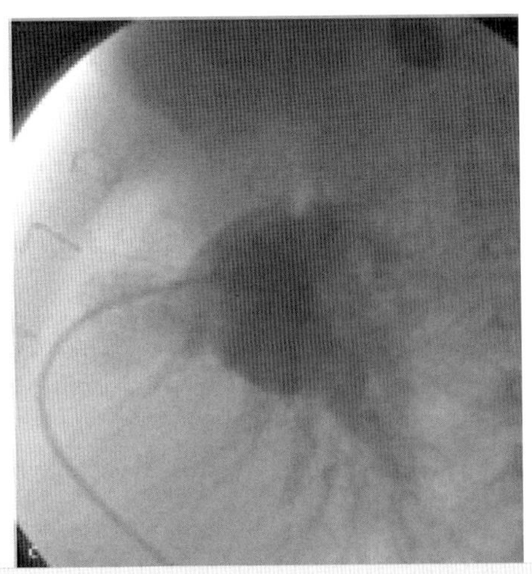

Fig. 24.9 Balloon dilation of supravalvular pulmonary stenosis in angiography. **a** Supravalvular stenosis due to membranous narrowing after implantation of a valved xenograft (Venpro). Gradient around 60 mmHg. **b** Balloon dilation with a 24-mm balloon. **c** The membrane has disappeared. Residual gradient around 15 mmHg systolic.

► **Risks/patient information.** The risk is below 1%, rupture of the pulmonary artery (stent implantation), emergency surgery (minimal risk), pneumectomy, dissection, tamponade, death, development of tricuspid regurgitation, infection/endocarditis, lung embolism, post-embolic pneumonia, reperfusion edema, chronic cough.

► **Procedure.** An antegrade approach via femoral vessels is undertaken, also feasible via the jugular vein.

► **Cardiac catheterization/treatment.** Angiography of the right ventricle, probing of the pulmonary artery, selective PA angiography, measurement of the stenosis, pressure measurement, switch to exchange wire, balloon dilation of the stenosis and pulmonary artery branches (► Fig. 24.11), check of the pressure in the pulmonary artery and right ventricle, repeat PA angiography to rule out dissection, possibly stent implantation; if unsuccessful possibly high-pressure balloon, possibly cutting balloon.

► **Monitoring.** Routine monitoring, chest X-ray to document the changed perfusion conditions, echocardiography, MRI later.

► **Heparinization/medication.** Same as for valvular pulmonary stenosis.

► **Echocardiography after cardiac catheterization.** Pulmonary regurgitation, tricuspid regurgitation, mean and maximum residual gradient, right ventricular function, pressure in the right ventricle.

24.2.2 Interventions in the Atrial Area

The atrial septum is technically easy to access and for this reason the atrial septum has long been the target of a number of different interventions. Many congenital heart defects have components in the atrial area (e.g., ASD and patent foramen ovale). This explains the wide range of closure systems available on the market for this indication. In addition, the targeted closure of defects in the atrial area, but also the creation of atrial shunts can achieve significant hemodynamic changes that have a positive effect on various diseases and heart defects. The usual interventions in the atrial area are presented below.

Rashkind Balloon Atrial Septostomy

► **Indication.** The necessity of a nonrestrictive communication in the atrial area to achieve a sufficient left-to-right shunt or right-to-left shunt. The indications are:

- Insufficient mixing of oxygenated and nonoxygenated blood (e.g., TGA)

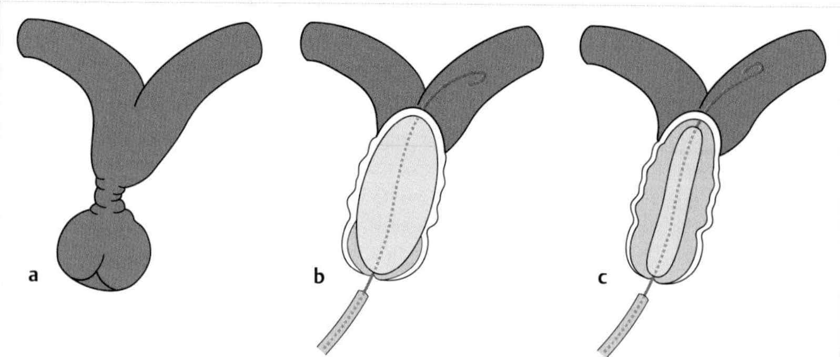

Fig. 24.10 Schematic diagrams of a balloon dilatation of a supravalvular pulmonary stenosis. **a** Initial situation. **b** The balloon catheter is advanced up to the stenosis and inflated. **c** After dilation, the balloon is deflated and the catheter is retrieved.

- Restriction at the atrial level necessitating a right-to-left shunt (e.g., tricuspid atresia, Ebstein anomaly)
- Restriction at the atrial level necessitating a left-to-right shunt (e.g., mitral atresia, hypoplastic left heart syndrome)

► **Echocardiography.** Assessment of the septal anatomy, PFO, gradient, ventricular function.

► **Risks/patient information.** The risk is less than 1%; rupture of the septum is intended. Possible complications are perforation, dissection, tamponade, death, air embolism, myocardial ischemia, arrhythmia, AV block, mitral regurgitation or tricuspid regurgitation, infection, lesion of the venae cavae or pulmonary veins.

► **Procedure.** An antegrade approach via the femoral vein or the umbilical vein is performed. The procedure is almost always performed solely under echocardiography guidance in the intensive care unit under sedation and without general anesthesia.

► **Cardiac catheterization/treatment.** Transseptal probe with the Rashkind balloon, inflation of the balloon and sudden pull-back to the inferior vena cava, rapid advancement into the right atrium, deflation. Repeat the maneuver until maximal balloon filling is achieved, a shunt of 5 to 6 mm has developed, and oxygen saturation has increased (► Fig. 24.12).

► **Monitoring.** Repeat echocardiography, routine monitoring in the intensive care unit, documentation of oxygen saturation over 24 hours.

► **Heparinization.** Administration of 100 IU/kg as an intravenous bolus during the cardiac catheterization, then 400 IU kg/d as a continuous infusion until the morning of the second day.

► **Echocardiography after cardiac catheterization.** Size of the defect, mean and maximum residual gradient, lesion of other anatomical structures (pulmonary vein, AV valves), pericardial effusion.

Blade Septostomy

► **Indication.** The indications are similar to those for a Rashkind balloon atrial septostomy, but a blade septostomy is usually performed in older patients. The septum is more rigid in these patients, so the balloon atrial septostomy is no longer technically possible. The septum is therefore cut using a special catheter with a retractable small blade at its tip.

- Insufficient mixing of oxygenated and nonoxygenated blood (e.g., TGA)
- Restriction at the atrial level in a necessary right-to-left shunt (e.g., tricuspid atresia, Ebstein anomaly)
- Restriction at the atrial level in a necessary left-to-right shunt (e.g., mitral atresia, hypoplastic left heart syndrome)
- A new communication at the atrial level is created as an overflow valve (e.g., pulmonary hypertension).

► **Echocardiography.** Visualization of the septal anatomy, gradient, left ventricular and right ventricular function.

► **Risks/patient information.** The overall risk is less than 5%; rupture/incision of the septum is intended. Possible risks are perforation, dissection, tamponade, death, air embolism, myocardial ischemia, arrhythmia, AV block, mitral or tricuspid regurgitation, infection, lesion of the venae cavae or pulmonary veins. In blade septostomy for pulmonary hypertension, acute massive cyanosis with decompensation may develop.

► **Procedure.** An antegrade approach via the femoral vein is undertaken.

► **Cardiac catheterization/treatment.** Transseptal probe, opening of the blade possibly under TEE guidance, pull-back to the inferior vena cava.

► **Monitoring, heparinization, and postinterventional echocardiography checkups.** The same as in a Rashkind balloon atrial septostomy.

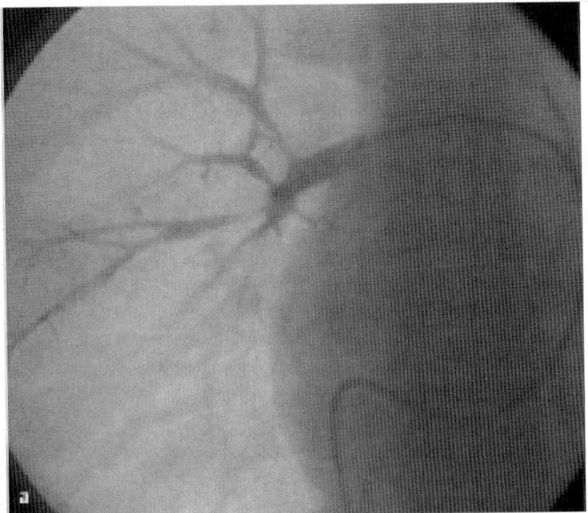
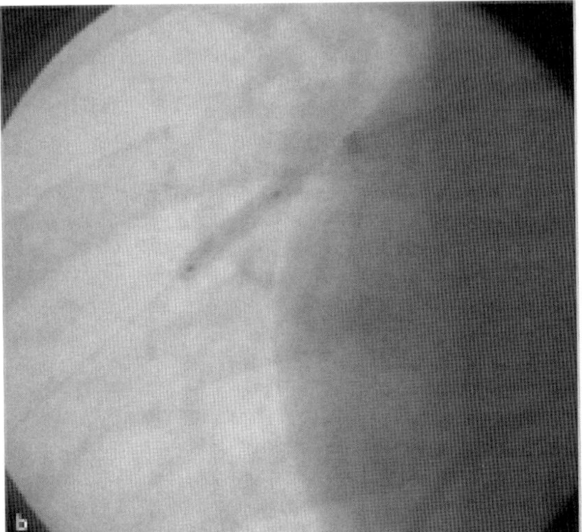
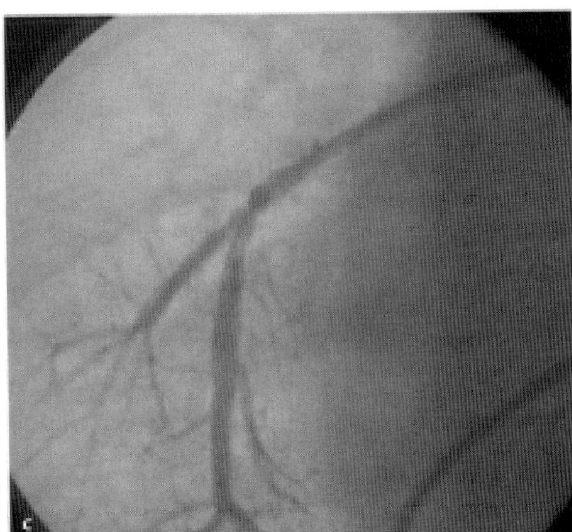

Fig. 24.11 Balloon dilation of a severe stenosis in the right middle lobe. The stenosis is visualized by selective PA angiography (**a**). After balloon dilation (**b**), with cutting balloon angioplasty, the patency of the previously stenotic area can be detected (**c**).

24.2.3 Interventional Catheterization Closure Procedures

Closure of a Patent Foramen Ovale

► **Indication.** Closure of a confirmed communication at the atrial level based on adequately confirmed paradoxical embolism or cyanosis with right ventricular anomaly (e.g., Ebstein anomaly). Indications are:

- Paradoxical embolism cerebrovascular accident/stroke
- Particular forms of migraine
- Professional divers, decompression sickness (risk of gas embolism in systemic circulation)
- Cyanosis—for example, in Ebstein anomaly or a small right ventricle (after pulmonary atresia or critical pulmonary stenosis)

► **Preliminary examinations.** Neurological investigation of suspected paradoxical embolism, bubble contrast studies including echocardiography, detailed coagulation diagnostics, echocardiography, TEE, possibly MRI.

► **Echocardiography.** Visualization of the precise septal anatomy including TEE.

► **Risks/patient information.** The risk is minimal. Thrombosis, embolism, displacement of the umbrella, umbrella embolism, myocardial ischemia, arrhythmia, AV block, development of AV valve regurgitation, residual defect.

► **Procedure.** An antegrade approach via the femoral vein is undertaken, insertion of the umbrella after measuring the patent foramen ovale, TEE guidance.

► **Cardiac catheterization/treatment.** Transseptal probing, measurement of the patent foramen ovale by balloon sizing, selection of the suitable closure material—today there are numerous manufacturers (e.g., Occlutech, Amplatzer, Cardia, Helex, PFM, etc.) Insert the occluding material. Routine TEE guidance with contrast echo, release the closing material (► Fig. 24.13). Usually performed under sedation without endotracheal anesthesia.

► **Heparinization.** Administration of 100 IU/kg as an intravenous bolus during the cardiac catheterization, then 400 IU/kg/d as a continuous infusion until the morning of the second day; aspirin/clopidogrel/warfarin may be given depending on the indication or underlying disease and coagulation disorder.

► **Echocardiography after cardiac catheterization.** Residual shunt, valve anatomy and function.

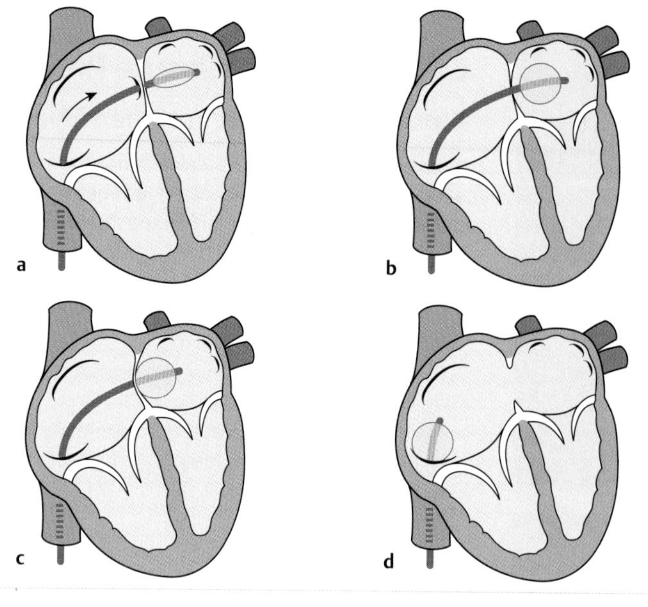

Fig. 24.12 Rashkind balloon atrial septostomy. First the catheter is advanced into the left atrium (**a**) and the balloon is then inflated (**b**). After the catheter is placed at the septum (**c**) it is pulled back into the right atrium abruptly while inflated (**d**).

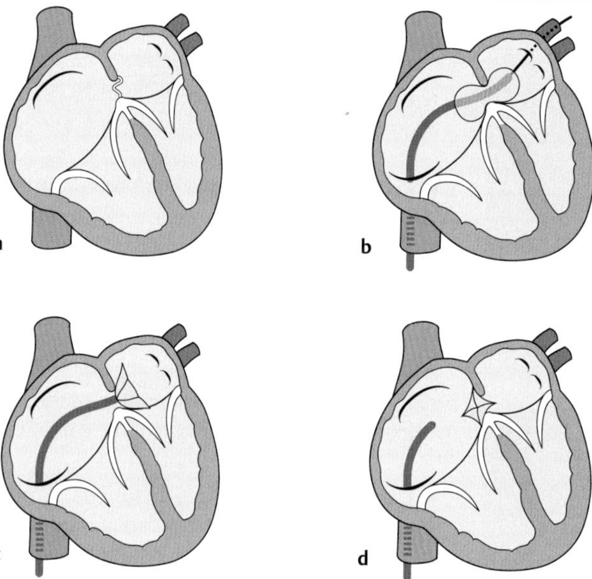

Fig. 24.13 Closure of a patent foramen ovale with an umbrella occluder. **a** Untreated patent foramen ovale. **b** First the size of the foramen is measured with a balloon and then the suitable umbrella size is selected. **c** The left atrial segment of the umbrella is opened. **d** The umbrella is detached from the catheter and the right atrial segment of the umbrella is opened.

Closure of an Atrial Septal Defect

▸ **Indication.** Closure of an ASD II is indicated if right ventricular overload is confirmed based on shunt volume and/or sufficient confirmation of paradoxical embolism (see also PFO closure) or cyanosis with a right ventricular anomaly. Indications are:

- Right ventricular overload (size above normal, flat or paradoxical septal movement)
- Defect size clearly over 6 mm
- Shunt over 1.5:1
- Paradoxical embolism/cerebrovascular accident/stroke
- Cyanosis—for example, due to Ebstein anomaly or a small right ventricle (after pulmonary atresia, or critical pulmonary stenosis)

▸ **Preliminary examinations.** Based on echocardiography alone, if necessary neurologic investigations, bubble contrast studies, detailed coagulation diagnostics, echocardiography, TEE, possibly MRI.

▸ **Echocardiography.** Visualization of the septum anatomy: cranial and caudal septal borders, length of the septum, the distance to the valves, aorta, and posterior septal wall. TEE is often necessary, which can be performed during the cardiac catheterization.

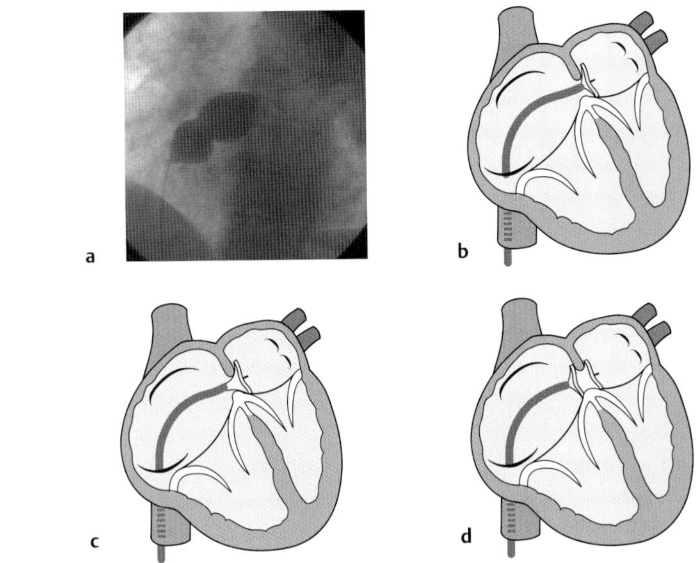

Fig. 24.14 Closure of ASD II with double-disc device. **a** First the size of the defect is measured with a balloon under fluoroscopy guidance. **b** The left atrial segment of the device is opened. **c** The middle segment that stents the ASD is opened. **d** The right atrial segment is opened.

► **Risks/patient information.** The risk is minimal. Thrombosis, embolism, displacement of the umbrella, umbrella embolism, myocardial ischemia, arrhythmia, AV block, development of AV valve regurgitation, residual defect. There is discussion about a minimal potential risk of erosion of the aorta by the device disks in patients with deficient aortic rims; this problem seems device-related (i.e. very stable left sided discs) and is under discussion.

► **Procedure.** An antegrade approach via the femoral vein is undertaken, insertion of the device after measuring the defect, TEE guidance. Usually performed under sedation without endotracheal anesthesia.

► **Cardiac catheterization/treatment.** Transseptal probing, measurement of the defect by balloon sizing and selection of the appropriate device. Insertion of the device under TEE guidance, testing of the stability of the position by a "wiggle manoever", afterward repeat TEE/ECHO control and then release of the device. (► Fig. 24.14).

► **Heparinization.** Administration of 100 IU/kg as an intravenous bolus during the cardiac catheterization, then 400 IU/kg/d in a continuous infusion until the morning of the second day. Aspirin/clopidogrel/warfarin may be given depending on the indication or underlying disease and coagulation disorder.

► **Echocardiography after cardiac catheterization.** Assessment of the residual shunt, valve anatomy and function.

Note

An ASD I or sinus venosus defect cannot be closed by interventional catheterization.

Closure of a Ventricular Septal Defect

► **Indication.** As for surgery, the indication for closure of the VSD is confirmed volume overload (significant shunt), the corresponding clinical symptoms (failure to thrive, pulmonary impairment, heart failure), as well as all other indications that apply to surgical closure. Endocarditis prophylaxis has also been discussed as an indication. Currently, children should at least weigh about 10 kg, that is, be around 1 year old. Muscular and subaortic defects can also be treated by interventional catheterization. Indications include:

- Left ventricular overload (size n/t beyond normal)
- Left atrial overload
- Frequent pulmonary infections
- New development of aortic regurgitation as a result of the VSD

► **Preliminary examinations.** Same as preparation for surgery, ECG (no more than 2 months old), echocardiography.

► **Echocardiography.** Visualization of the septal anatomy, distance of the cranial septal borders to the aortic valve, distance from the tricuspid valve, size of the left ventricle, size of the left atrium. Cardiac catheterization with the option of TEE guidance, possibly 3D echocardiography.

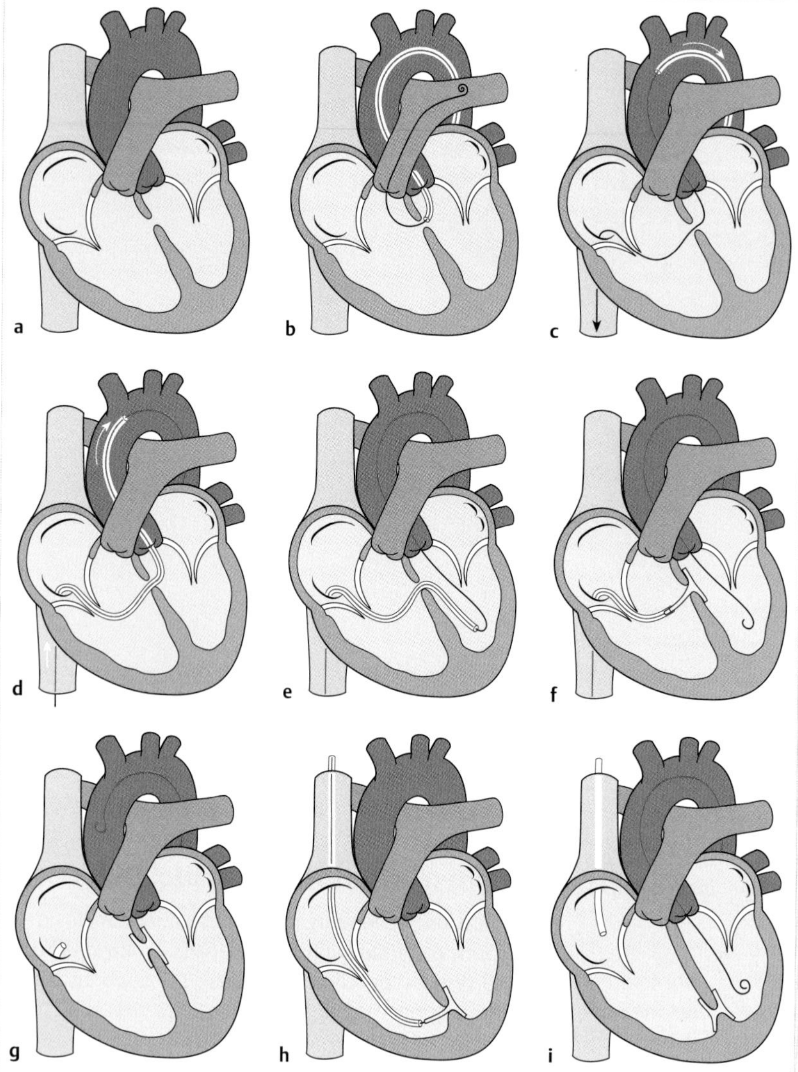

Fig. 24.15 Catheter interventional VSD closure. Procedure for a subaortic VSD (**a–g**) and a muscular VSD (**h–i**).
a Untreated subaortic VSD. **b** The VSD is probed with a wire. **c** A wire loop is made (venous-arterial). **d** The sheath is advanced. **e** The sheath is placed in the left ventricle. **f** The left ventricular disc is opened. **g** The device is detached after opening the right ventricular disc. **h** The left ventricular disc is opened in a muscular VSD via the jugular vein. **i** The device is detached in the muscular VSD.

► **Risks/patient information.** The risk is low for a strict indication (< 5%). Thrombosis, embolism, displacement of the umbrella, umbrella embolism, myocardial ischemia, tricuspid or aortic regurgitation, residual defect, hemolysis, surgery to remove the umbrella. Significant risks include arrhythmias, bundle branch block, and AV block necessitating the implantation of a pacemaker in double-disc devices. The risk of AV block seems minimal if VSD coils are used for closure.

► **Procedure.** Usually possible in sedation without endotracheal anesthesia, an antegrade approach via the femoral or jugular vein for a muscular VSD, possibly two venous accesses. Arterial puncture. After measuring the defect in the echocardiography, the device is inserted under ECO guidance (TEE if needed). The current umbrella models have a higher risk for an AV block; newer developments (coils) are now available with a reduced risk for AV block.

► **Cardiac catheterization/treatment.** First the size of the VSD is measured, and suitable closure material is selected. The VSD is probed from the left ventricle and the wire is placed in the pulmonary artery or vena cava. A veno-arterial loop is created and then the delivery sheath is advanced across the VSD. The device is inserted and the correct position checked by angiography, echocardiography or TEE; then the device is detached (► Fig. 24.15, ► Fig. 24.16).

► **Monitoring.** Aside from the routine investigations, additional one-off urine test for hemolysis, ECG monitoring over 24 hours, print-out of the monitor trend (AV block, bundle branch block?), chest X-ray in two planes to

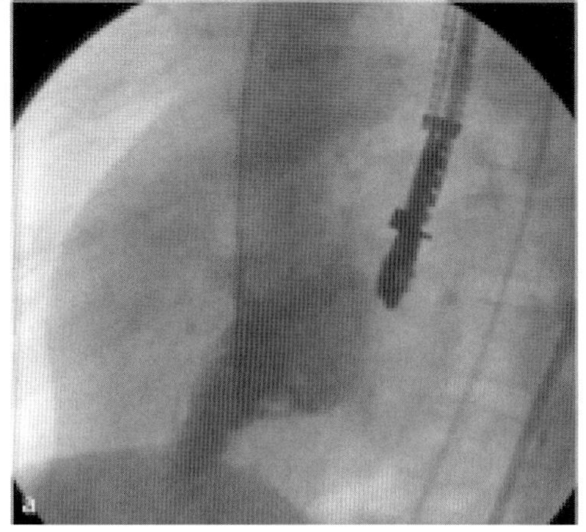

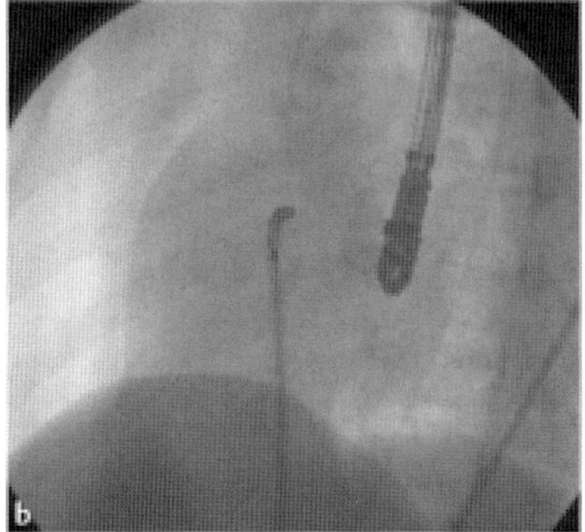

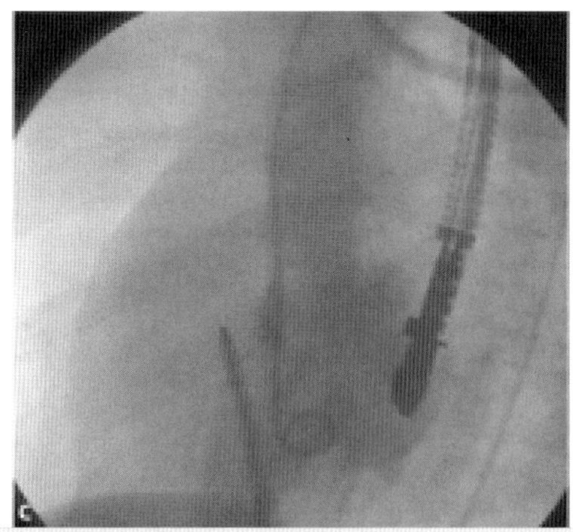

Fig. 24.16 Angiographic documentation of the interventional closure of a subaortic VSD. Contrast medium is injected into the left ventricle through a retrograde catheter. The contrast medium passes into the right ventricle across the subaortic VSD (a). The defect is then probed and closed with a double-disc device (b). After the device is detached from the catheter, contrast medium is again injected into the left ventricle and no longer passes into the right ventricle (c). The procedure is simultaneously documented with transesophageal echocardiography. The TEE probe can be seen at the left in the angiographic images.

document the position and configuration of the closure material. Echocardiography monitoring.

► **Heparinization/medication.** As for a valvular aortic stenosis.

► **Echocardiography after cardiac catheterization.** Residual shunt, valve anatomy and function, size of the left and right ventricle.

Closure of a Patent Ductus Arteriosus

► **Indication.** Closure of the PDA (► Fig. 24.17) if volume overload (significant shunt) is confirmed or the corresponding clinical symptoms (failure to thrive) are present as well as all other indications that apply to surgical closure. Other indications currently discussed are endocarditis and endarteritis prophylaxis. The closure is technically simple and involves only a minimal risk. With the currently available materials, children weighing from 2 kg and above with a large PDA can be treated safely. Indications are:

- Left ventricular overload (size far beyond normal)
- Left atrial overload
- Frequent pulmonary infections
- PDA with murmur

A silent PDA should not be closed at all and the children declared as healthy. Otherwise, a PDA should be closed after the age of 2 years if it is not hemodynamically necessary to perform closure earlier.

► **Echocardiography.** Size and function of the left ventricle and left atrium, PDA ampulla, diameter of the aorta and the pulmonary artery, rule out coarctation of the aorta.

► **Risks/patient information.** The risk is minimal even in small children. Possible complications are vascular complications, thrombosis, embolism, displacement of the umbrella, umbrella embolism, residual defect, hemolysis.

► **Procedure.** Depending on the system to be implanted, an antegrade approach via the femoral vein is undertaken and arterial puncture to visualize the PDA, or if the PDA is small, possibly only an arterial access. There are numerous manufacturers of occluding systems, for example, PFM coils, Amplatzer or Occlutech PDA devices, Cook coils, etc.

► **Cardiac catheterization/treatment.** Aortic injection, measurement of the PDA, selection of the system depending on the shape, size and course of the PDA, implantation possibly via the pulmonary artery or the aorta, angiography guidance, detachment of the system, final check (► Fig. 24.18, ► Fig. 24.19, ► Fig. 24.20).

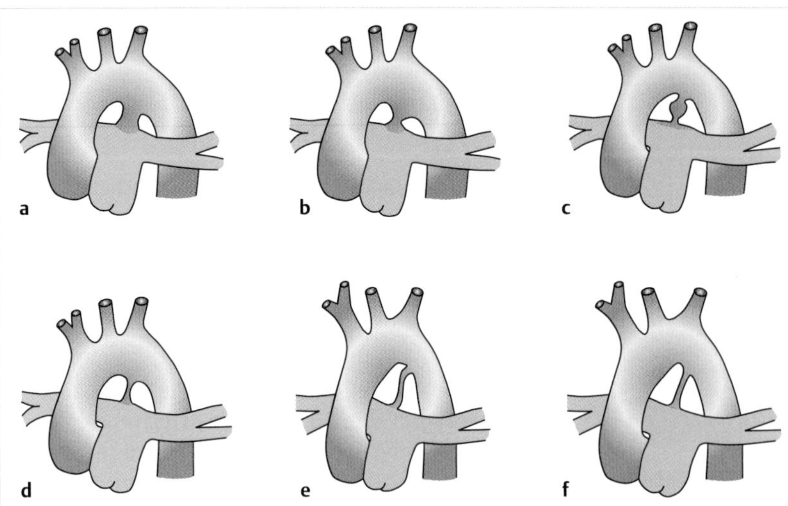

Fig. 24.17 a–f Examples of different PDA morphologies.

▶ **Echocardiography after cardiac catheterization.** Assessment of the residual shunt, rule out a new occurrence of coarctation of the aorta, stenosis of the left and right pulmonary artery, left ventricular and left atrial size and function.

Closure of Collateral Vessels

Therapeutic embolization with special coils or larger devices (occluders, plugs) is performed in the following situations:

- Additional hemodynamic stress with volume/pressure overload of a downstream vascular territory (e.g., aortopulmonary collaterals resulting in excessive pulmonary blood flow)
- Cardiac volume overload (AV fistula, shunts)
- Competitive blood flow so that normal function of the organ is no longer possible (e.g., aortopulmonary collaterals in Fontan circulation)
- Steal phenomenon (coronary collaterals)
- Other reasons for closure (e.g., preoperative embolization of a lung sequester or hemangioma)

Different systems are used for closure depending on the location and size of the collaterals. The range extends from a simple spiral coil to PDA or ASD occluders or specific vascular plugs.

Initially the coils occlude the vessels mechanically, sometimes with fibers attached to the coil. Then thrombosis develops in the upstream territory and finally fibrotic remodeling occurs. Coils may slip out of position or embolize, but can usually be recovered by catheterization. If not placed accurately, coils may also accidently occlude other vessels whose closure was not intended. Sometimes an occlusion test in advance with a balloon catheter is necessary.

Coil Occlusion of Aortopulmonary Collaterals

▶ **Indication.** Occlusion of collaterals if volume overload is confirmed (significant shunt) if the corresponding clinical symptoms (recurrent cough, failure to thrive) are present, and other indications, such as competing flows in Fontan hemodynamics (high CVP, protein-losing enteropathy, plastic bronchitis) or preoperatively for Fallotlike cardiac defects, for which a surgical correction is pending. Indications are:

- Ventricular overload (size beyond normal)
- Atrial overload
- Frequent pulmonary infections
- Competing perfusion of the dependent pulmonary circulation
- After opening a pulmonary atresia
- Fontan hemodynamics
- Preoperative (e.g., in tetralogy of Fallot, etc.)

▶ **Risks/patient information.** The risk is minimal: thrombosis, embolism, vascular complications, displacement of the coil, residual shunt, hemolysis, infarction in an unintended area.

▶ **Procedure.** Arterial puncture and angiographic visualization, then antegrade approach via afferent vessels. There are numerous manufacturers, for example, Amplatzer, PFM, Cook coils.

▶ **Cardiac catheterization/treatment.** Arterial injection and measurement of the collaterals to be occluded via angiography. The suitable occluding system is selected and inserted in the vessel. The system is detached and checked by angiography (▶ Fig. 24.21).

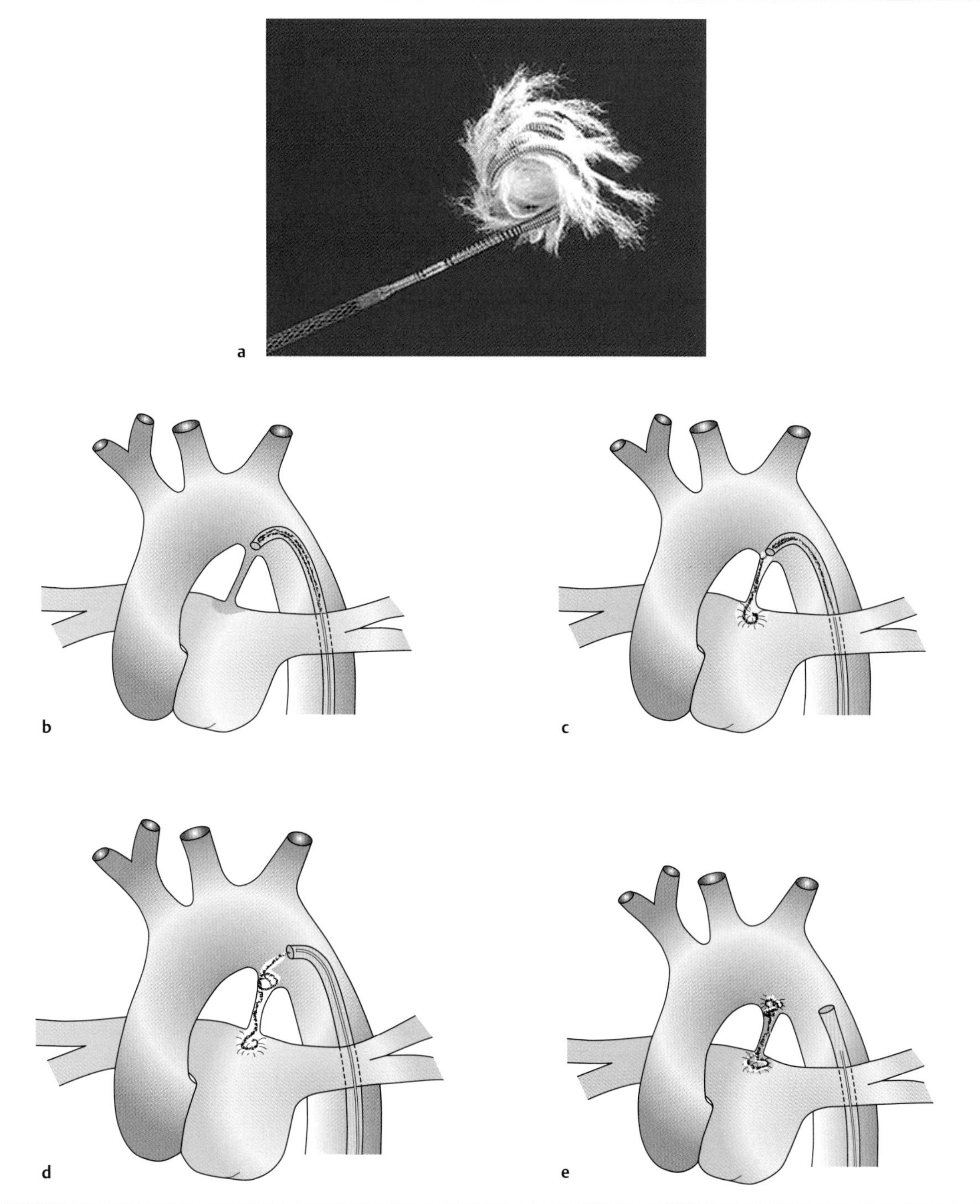

Fig. 24.18 Closure of a PDA with a Cook coil via the aorta. **a** Cook coil. **b** First the PDA is probed retrograde. **c** The Cook coil is advanced to the PDA while still extended in the insertion sheath. **d** The coil opens only after leaving the sheath, taking on its typical twisting shape. **e** Finally the coil is detached from the catheter and the final position and closure is documented.

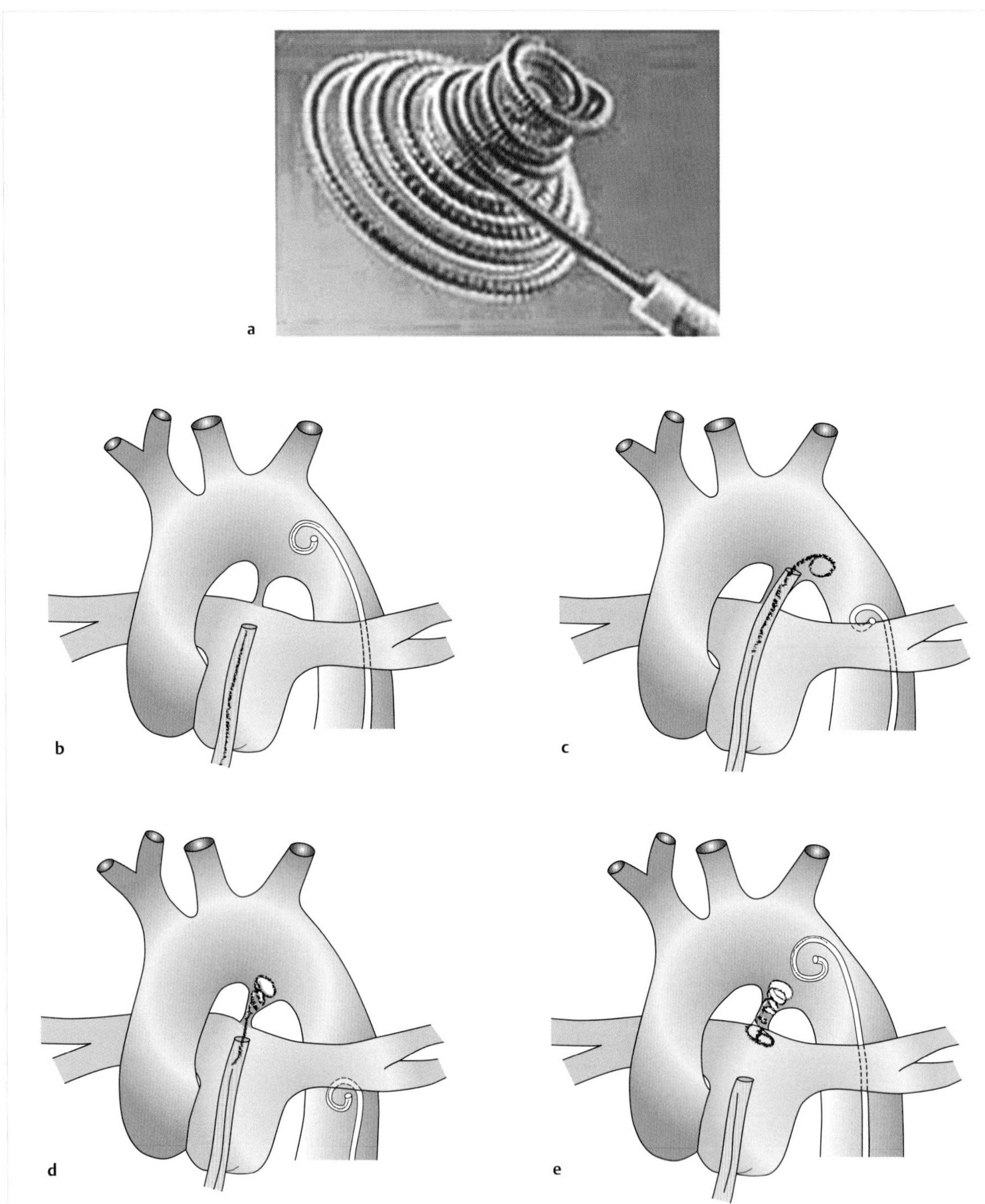

Fig. 24.19 Closure of a PDA with a PFM Nit-Occlud system via the pulmonary artery.
The PDA is probed with the insertion catheter containing the PFM Duct-Occlud system (**a**) via the pulmonary artery (**b, c**). A pigtail catheter is simultaneously advanced into the aorta for the angiographic visualization before and after the closure of the PDA. After the delivery catheter is withdrawn, the coil opens up and closes the PDA (**d**). Finally, the device is detached from the insertion system and the result and position confirmed.(**e**).

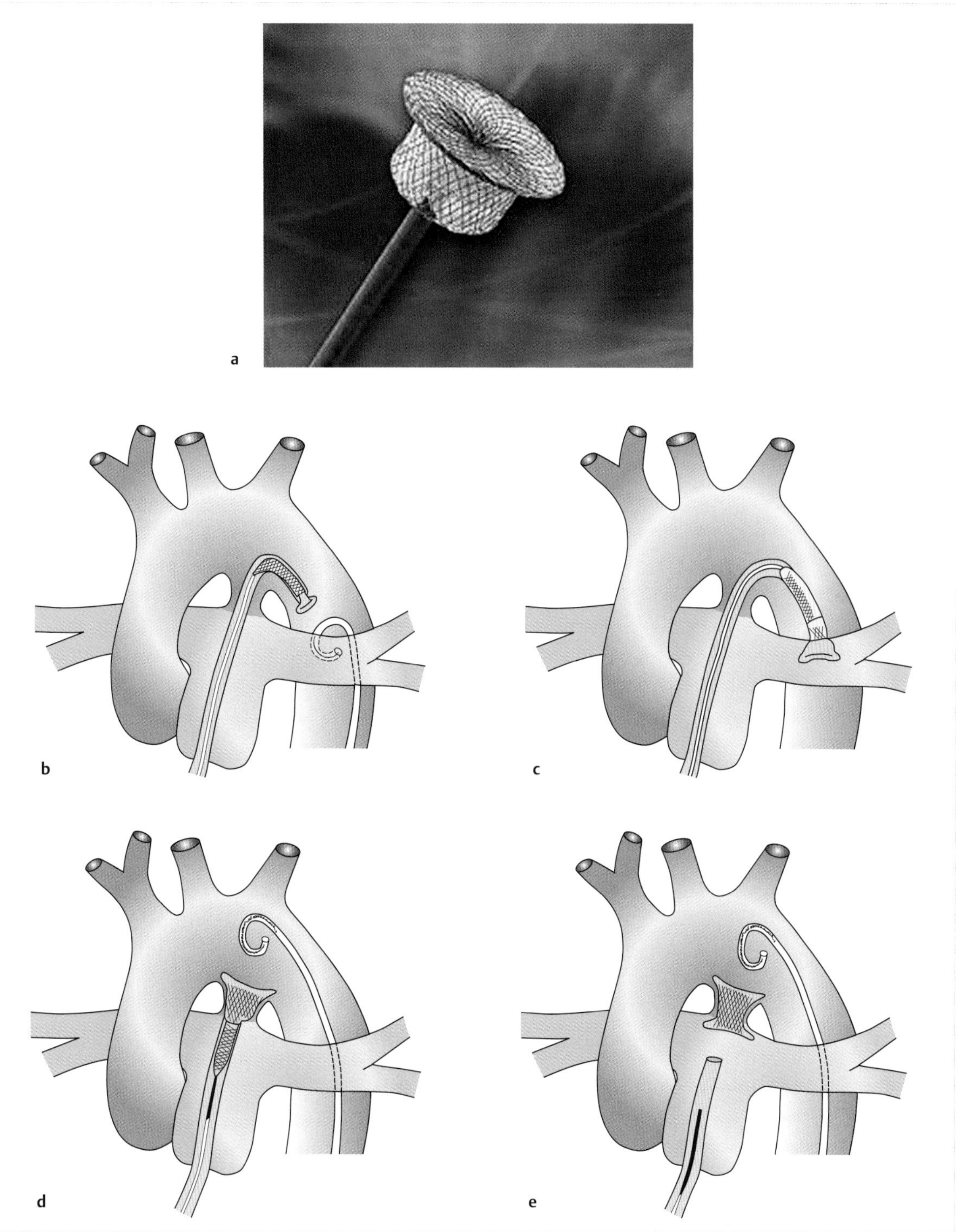

Fig. 24.20 Closure of a PDA with an Amplatzer PDA system (ADO) via the pulmonary artery. **a** Amplatzer PDA system (ADO). **b** The PDA is probed with the delivery sheath via the pulmonary artery. The pigtail catheter in the aorta is needed for the angiography. **c** After withdrawing the sheath, the aortic segment of the device opens first. **d** Now the device is pulled back into the PDA until the open aortic collar of the device is pulled against the PDA orifice. The pulmonary segment opens after the sheath is withdrawn further. **e** Finally the device is detached from the insertion system and the final position and closure are is documented.

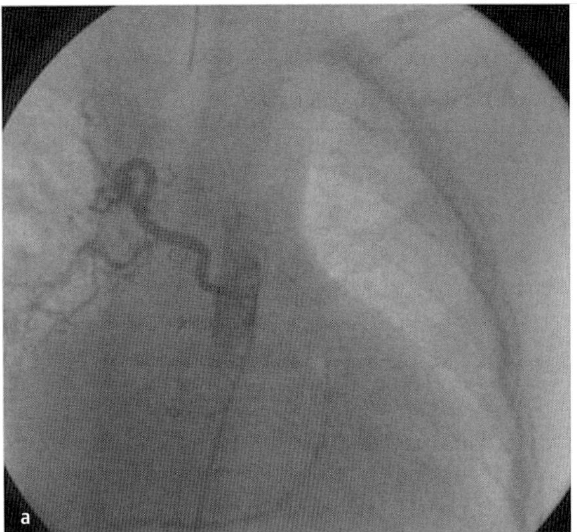

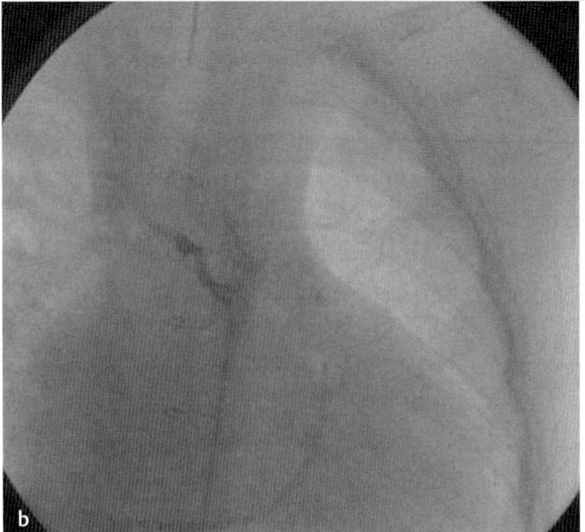

Fig. 24.21 Closure of small aortopulmonary collateral.
After contrast medium is injected in the thoracic aorta, the aortopulmonary collateral is visualized (**a**). The final control angiography after successful catheter interventional closure of the collaterals shows that flow of the contrast medium stops in the area of the device (**b**).

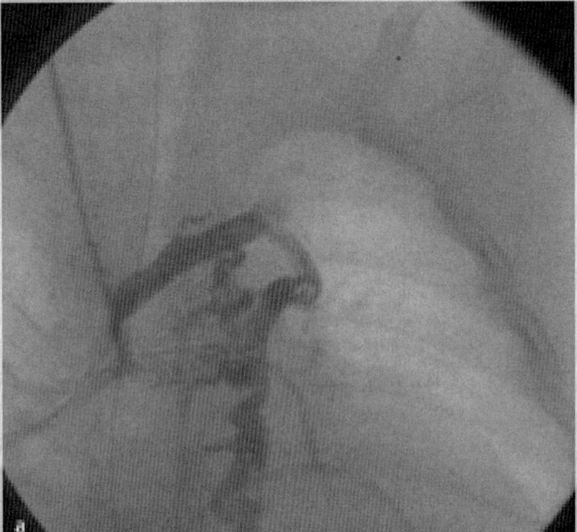

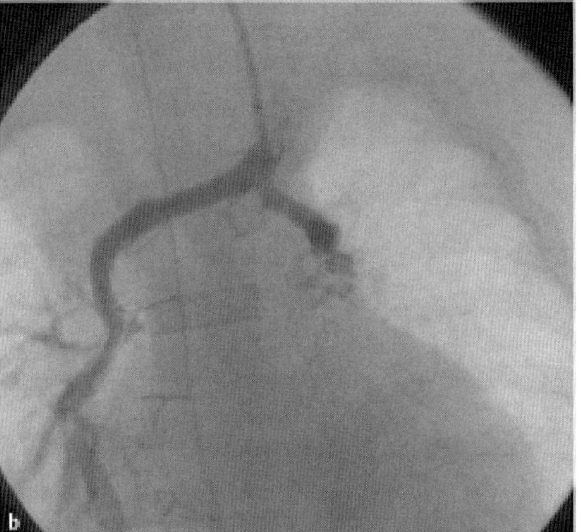

Fig. 24.22 Occlusion of a veno-venous collateral from the supply area of the left subclavian vein in a patient after upper cavopulmonary anastomosis.
The contrast medium injected into the left subclavian vein shows a veno-venous collateral (**a**). The corkscrew course of the collateral is typical. After the coil is inserted into the collateral by interventional catheterization, flow of the contrast medium is stopped, indicating the successful closure of the collateral (**b**).

Coil Occlusion of Venous Collaterals

► **Indication.** Occlusion of collaterals if a significant shunt is confirmed, the corresponding clinical symptoms (cyanosis) are present, and other indications such as competing blood flow, signs of impairment of the Fontan hemodynamics (increasing cyanosis, decreasing physical exercise capacity) are present. Indications include:

- Cyanosis
- Frequent pulmonary infections
- Decreased physical exercise capacity
- Impaired Fontan hemodynamics

► **Risks/patient information.** The risk is minimal: thrombosis, embolism, vascular complications, displacement of the coil, residual shunt, hemolysis, accidental infarction in an unintended area, possibly puncture at unusual locations.

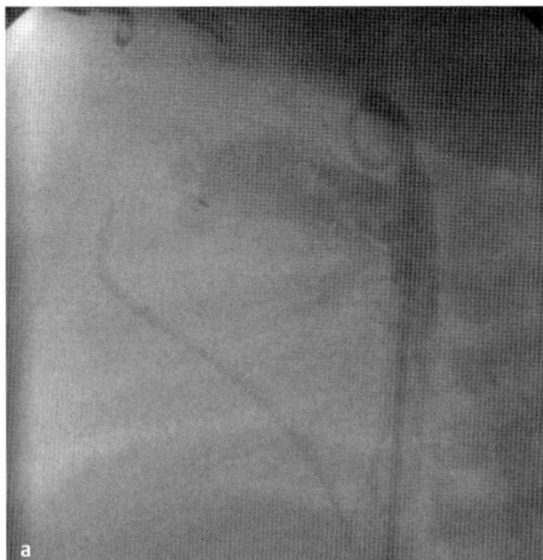

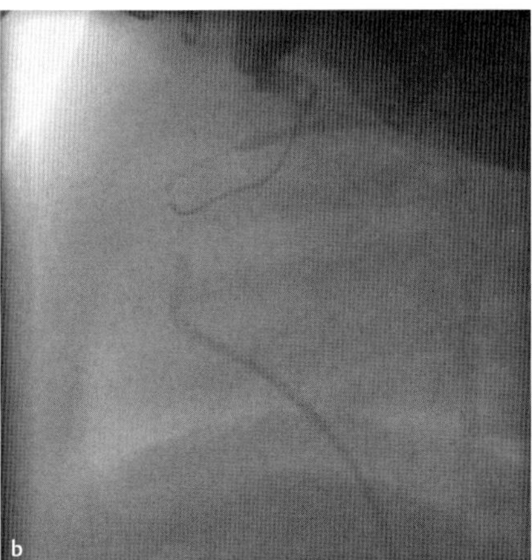

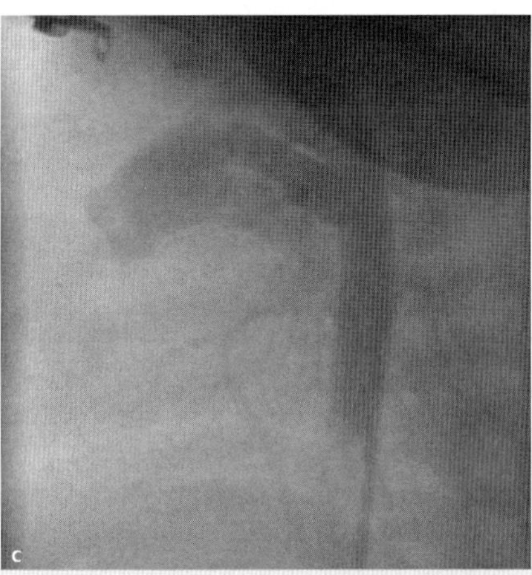

Fig. 24.23 Stent implantation in the PDA after opening a membranous pulmonary atresia and insufficient saturation. **a** The first injection of contrast medium into the aorta shows the long ductus through which the pulmonary artery is filled. In addition, the radiofrequency perforation catheter is seen in the pulmonary artery just above the opened pulmonary valve. **b** A balloon catheter with a stent is placed in the ductus. The balloon catheter and stent are not yet opened. **c** After expanding the balloon, the stent is opened in the ductus and ensures a continuous connection between the aorta and the pulmonary artery.

► **Procedure.** An antegrade approach via afferent vessels after angiographic visualization is undertaken, insertion of a suitable occluder system after measurement via angiography. Numerous manufacturers, e.g., Amplatzer, PFM, Cook coils.

► **Cardiac catheterization/treatment.** Injection into the upstream vessel, measurement of the collaterals, selection of the system, insertion into the main vessel, control angiography, detachment of the device, final angiography (► Fig. 24.22).

24.2.4 Stent Implantation in a Patent Ductus Arteriosus

► **Indication.** In ductal-dependent pulmonary perfusion (e.g., pulmonary atresia, severe pulmonary stenosis) or ductal-dependent systemic perfusion (i.e. HLHS), where blood flow depends on a patent ductus arteriosus, the decision can be taken to maintain patency of the PDA via stent implantation. The indications are handled differently; however, close consultation with the pediatric cardiac surgeon is always necessary. Depending on the clinical features, the risk is relatively high. The indications include:

- Ductal-dependent pulmonary circulation
- Ductal-dependent systemic circulation
- Indication for an aortopulmonary shunt
- As an interim measure until the definitive correction/ palliation (e.g., after opening a pulmonary atresia)

► **Preliminary examinations.** Usually the patient is in an intensive care setting, often ventilated, sometimes a critically ill neonate. ECG, detailed echocardiography, chest X-ray, preparation for surgery.

► **Echocardiography.** PDA diameter, detailed anatomy of the PDA, function of the right and left ventricle, aortic isthmus, diameter of the pulmonary artery and aorta.

► **Preparation.** Same as for cardiopulmonary bypass surgery, possibly implantation of an arterial catheter (umbilical) and a central venous catheter in advance, possibly catecholamines, if possible reduce prostaglandin treatment so that the PDA can start to constrict.

► **Risks/patient information.** The risk is high because a critically ill child is usually involved: rupture of the PDA, fatal blood loss during the procedure (low risk), acute PDA occlusion/thrombosis, renewed cardiac catheterization or emergency surgery with shunt implantation, myocardial ischemia, arrhythmia, infection or endocarditis, perfusion disorder or vessel occlusion of arterial puncture, repeat cardiac catheterization necessary after a short time for PDA stenosis or coarctation of the aorta.

► **Procedure.** If there is ductal-dependent systematic circulation, an antegrade approach via the pulmonary artery should be attempted if possible, otherwise a retrograde approach via an arterial puncture is undertaken, possibly from the axillary artery or the carotid artery.

► **Cardiac catheterization/treatment.** Left ventricle/ right ventricle or ascendogram, measurement of the PDA, probing of the PDA, switch to an exchange wire, then—depending on the stent—insertion of the long transport sheath, then stent implantation with the help of repeated control via hand angiography to ensure correct placement (► Fig. 24.23), ascendogram (patent ductus arteriosus?), re-dilation if necessary, switch the catheter to central venous catheter or arterial catheter.

► **Monitoring.** Continue intensive care, taper catecholamine treatment, discontinue prostaglandin, carry out regular echocardiography checkups.

► **Heparinization.** Administration of 100 IU/kg as an intravenous bolus during the cardiac catheterization, then 400 IU/kg/d as a continuous infusion until the morning of the second day, thereafter according to intensive care aspects.

► **Echocardiography after cardiac catheterization.** Stent position, mean and maximum residual gradient, function of the right and left ventricle, width of the aortic isthmus, anatomy of the right and left pulmonary artery.

24.2.5 Percutaneous Implantation of a Pulmonary Valve

► **Indication.** The percutaneous implantation of a pulmonary valve is currently performed for a stenotic and/ or incompetent pulmonary valve if there has been a relevant pressure overload of the right ventricle (stenosis

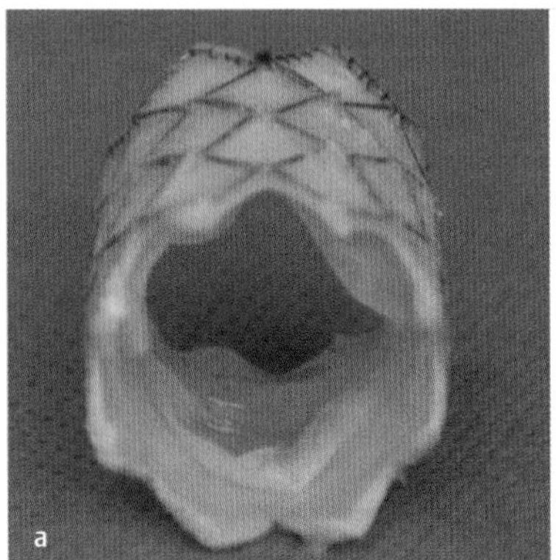
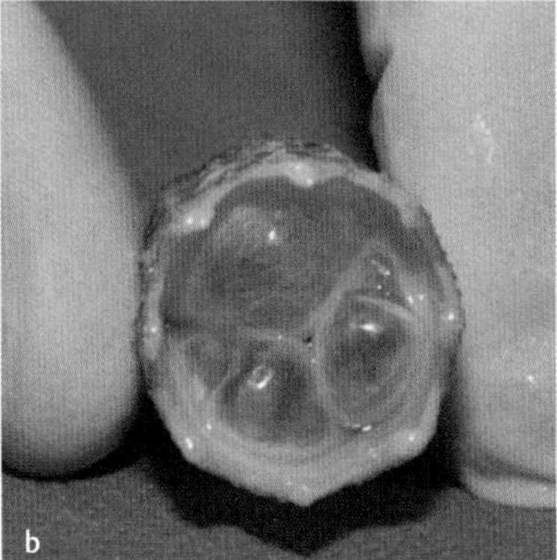
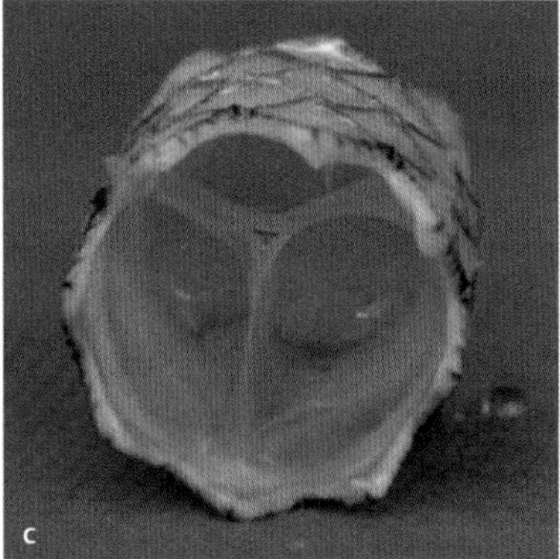

Fig. 24.24 Open Melody valve (**a**) and closed in flow direction (**b**) and closed in counter-flow direction (**c**).

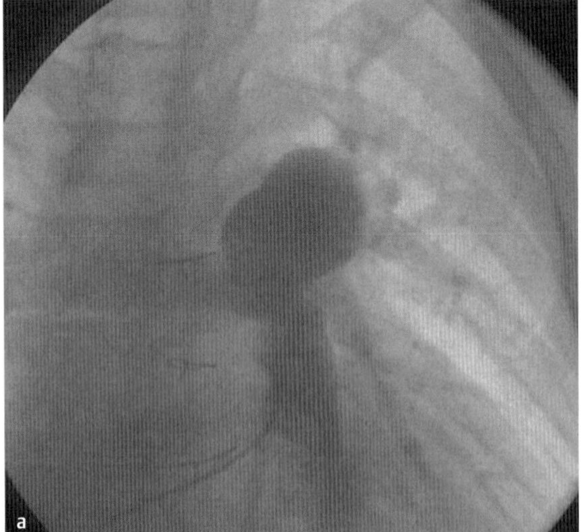
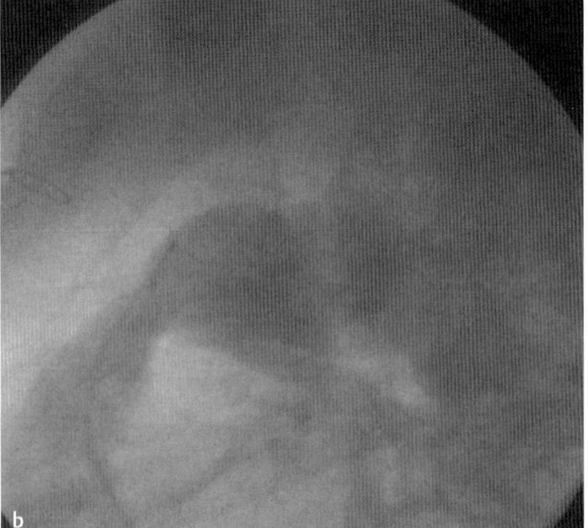

Fig. 24.25 Angiographies of the chest anteroposterior (**a**) and lateral (**b**) after implantation of a valved xenograft (Venpro). Supravalvular stenosis due to membranous narrowing, gradient around 60 mmHg. Additional significant regurgitation.

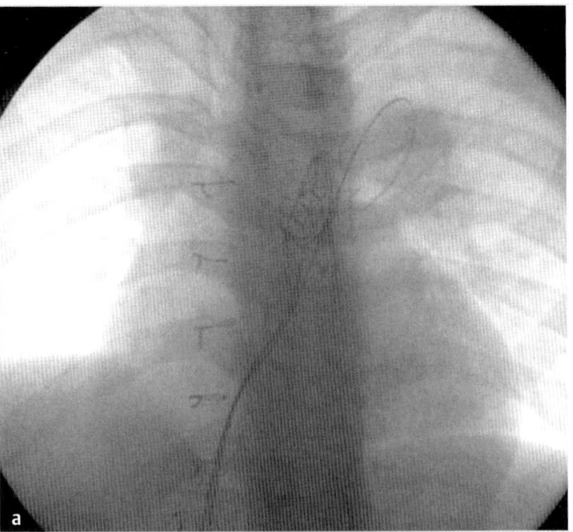

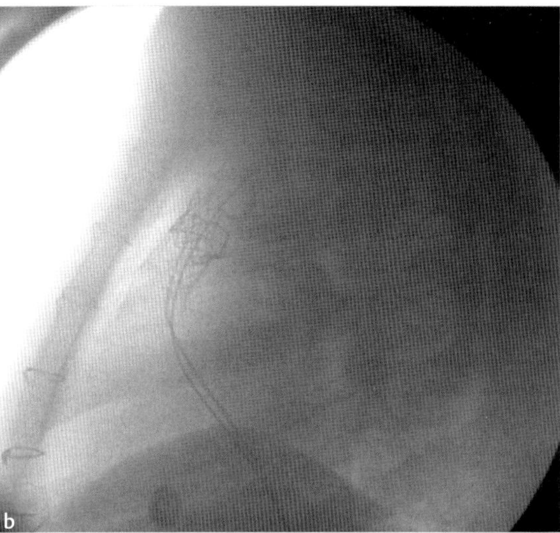

Fig. 24.26 Preparation of the right ventricular outflow tract by implantation of two stents. Angiographies of the chest anteroposterior (**a**) and lateral (**b**).The stents eliminate the stenosis (gradient-free right ventricular outflow tract), stabilize the right ventricular outflow tract as a tube, and provide necessary support for the valve to be implanted.

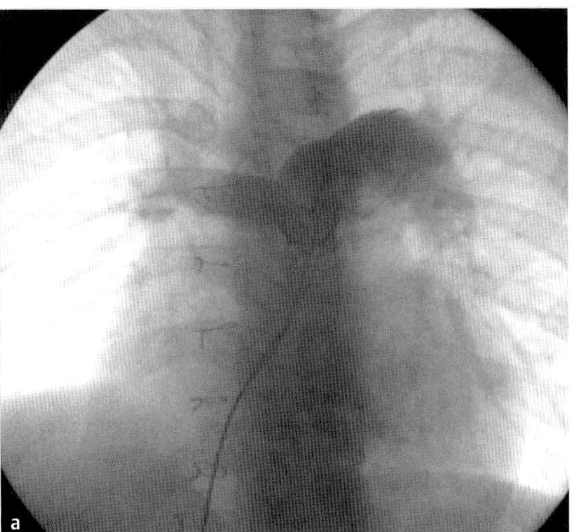

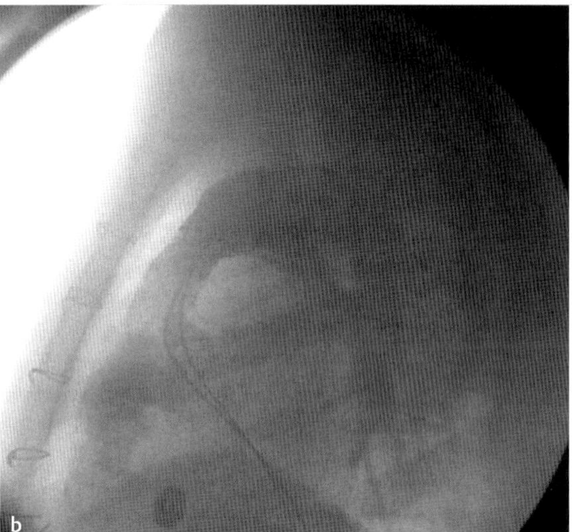

Fig. 24.27 Angiographic visualization anteroposterior (**a**) and lateral (**b**) after stent implantation. The right ventricular outflow tract is patent, however, with no valvular function (severe regurgitation).

component) or significant volume overload (pulmonary regurgitation). The currently approved valves consist of a commercially available stent and a biological valve (e.g., Melody valve, Edwards SAPIEN or XT valve). These valves are approved for postoperative stenosis after implantation of a conduit, homograft, or xenograft (e.g., after Fallot operation, Ross procedure, truncus) (▶ Fig. 24.24, ▶ Fig. 24.25, ▶ Fig. 24.26, ▶ Fig. 24.27, ▶ Fig. 24.28). Due to the relatively large implantation instruments, the procedure is currently not possible on patients weighing less than 20 to 30 kg. Generally, the right ventricular outflow tract is first stabilized with one or more stents and then the valve is inserted. The same indications are applicable as for surgery:

- Gradient dependency (Doppler gradient over 50 mmHg)
- Cardiac decompensation or decreased right ventricular function
- Increasing cardiac overload, pressure in the right ventricle over 50 to 60 mmHg
- Relevant pulmonary regurgitation (volume of the right ventricle > 160 mL/kg body weight/m^2)

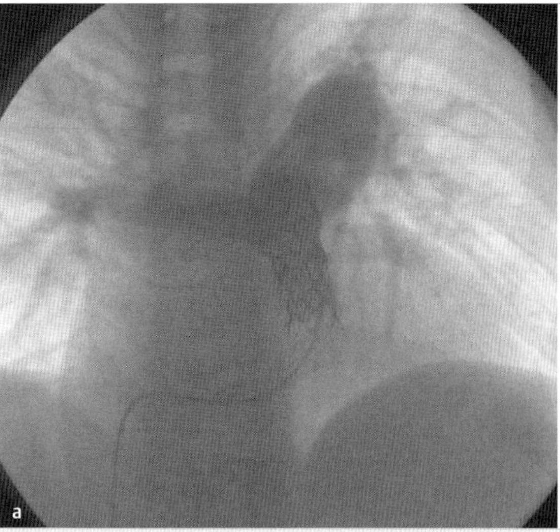

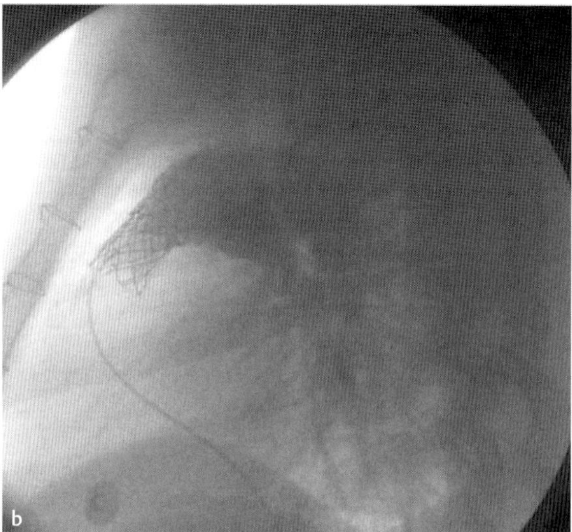

Fig. 24.28 After implantation of a Melody valve there is no regurgitation. Angiography anteroposterior (**a**) and lateral (**b**).

- Intermittent peripheral edema as a sign of a right heart failure
- Progressive deterioration of physical exercise capacity

▶ **Preliminary examinations.** ECG not older than 2 months, 24-hour Holter ECG if the ECG is abnormal, exercise ECG, cardiopulmonary exercise test in larger, cooperative children, optional MRI with 3D reconstruction.

▶ **Echocardiography.** Valve annulus diameter, pulmonary regurgitation? Anatomy of the valve, mean and maximum residual gradient, diameter of the left and right pulmonary artery, function of the right ventricle, right ventricular systolic pressure, tricuspid regurgitation, ASD or patent foramen ovale, subvalvular stenosis, other stenoses.

▶ **Risks/patient information.** The risk is moderate (< 5%): rupture or dissection of the pulmonary artery, coronary ischemia and myocardial ischemia (therefore clarify the relationship between the right ventricular outflow tract and coronary arteries), perforation of the pulmonary artery, death, arrhythmia, AV block, tricuspid regurgitation, infection, endocarditis, and, rarely, valve displacement.

▶ **Procedure.** An antegrade approach via the femoral vessels is undertaken, also possible via the jugular vein.

▶ **Cardiac catheterization/treatment.** Angiography of the right ventricle and the pulmonary artery, check of right ventricular pressure and pulmonary artery pressure, measurement of the valve annulus and the right ventricular outflow tract and pulmonary artery, probing of the pulmonary artery to test the later location, balloon dilation with simultaneous coronary angiography, change to extra stiff wire, pre-stenting of the pulmonary artery, often with a covered stent if there is a considerable mismatch, angiography of the pulmonary artery for positioning, implantation of the valve. High-pressure balloons are often necessary to obtain satisfactory results for homograft stenoses or if there is considerable calcification.

▶ **Echocardiography after cardiac catheterization.** Documentation of pulmonary regurgitation, mean and maximum residual gradient, right ventricular function, right ventricular systolic pressure, tricuspid regurgitation.

25 Postoperative Pediatric Cardiac Treatment

25.1 Hemodynamic Monitoring

The most important instrumental methods used for hemodynamic monitoring in the cardiac or cardiac surgery intensive care unit are presented below.

25.1.1 Noninvasive Blood Pressure Measurement

In intensive care, blood pressure is generally monitored automatically and noninvasively using the oscillometric technique. In seriously ill patients and small children, conventional measurement techniques using the Riva–Rocci method or auscultation of the Korotkoff sounds often lead to false low values.

The devices available for oscillometric measurement automatically measure the blood pressure at freely selected intervals and, in addition to systolic and diastolic pressure, also indicate the mean pressure and pulse rate.

To take the measurement, the blood pressure cuff is inflated to a suprasystolic level and then vented gradually. As long as the cuff pressure is above the systolic blood pressure, no blood flows in a distal direction under the cuff. As soon as there is blood flow under the cuff, pressure oscillations are conducted and registered. The cuff pressure is then equivalent to the systolic blood pressure. When the oscillations reach their maximum, the cuff pressure has reached the mean pressure. However, the diastolic pressure is difficult to determine using the oscillatory method, so it is calculated from the systolic pressure and the mean pressure in most devices.

Oscillometric blood pressure monitoring is sufficient for hemodynamically relatively stable patients and correlates well with arterial blood pressure measurements.

25.1.2 Arterial (Direct) Pressure Measurement

In invasive measurement of arterial blood pressure, a cannula is inserted into an artery and the blood pressure in the artery is determined using a pressure transducer. Invasive arterial blood pressure monitoring is indicated when the following measures are necessary:

- Continuous blood pressure monitoring (e.g., cardiac decompensation, shock, management of catecholamine treatment)
- Frequent checks of blood gases (e.g., in a difficult ventilation situation)

Another advantage of direct blood pressure measurement is that the pressure curve provides information on the volume status. The mean pressure is also indicated in addition to the systolic and diastolic pressure.

The following vessels are theoretically suitable for arterial blood pressure measurement:

- Radial artery (site of first choice)
- Femoral artery
- Brachial artery
- Axillary artery
- Dorsalis pedis artery
- Umbilical artery in neonates

► **Allen test.** Before cannulation of the radial artery, the Allen test is recommended. To check for adequate collateral circulation, first of all the radial and the ulnar arteries are both compressed manually until the hand becomes pale. Then the compression of the ulnar artery is released while the radial artery remains compressed. If there is sufficient collateral circulation, the hand will become pink again within a few seconds, although the radial artery is still compressed. The radial artery may be cannulated only if the Allen test is positive.

► **Arterial puncture.** The arterial puncture is made under sterile conditions. It is easiest using the Seldinger technique. To prevent thrombi, the arterial access is continuously flushed, sometimes with a heparin solution.

► **Measurement.** Before starting the measurement, a zero adjustment and calibration are needed. The pressure transducer must be at heart (atrial) level. This is for patients who are lying down, around the middle of the thorax. The tubing should be as short as possible and rigid.

A typical arterial pressure curve is shown in ► Fig. 25.1. The incisure is termed a dicrotic notch. The dicrotic wave arises at the transition from the systole to the diastole as a result of the Windkessel function after the valve closes. The area under the curve is proportional to the stroke volume (► Fig. 25.1 a).

Special Features of Measurements

► **Flat pressure curve.** The pressure curve may be flattened by excessive damping (► Fig. 25.1 b). The most common causes are air bubbles in the tubing or tubes that are too soft.

► **Overshooting.** If there is too little damping in the system, there is a conspicuously sharp pressure curve "overshoot" (► Fig. 25.1 c), which overestimates systolic blood pressure.

► **Hypovolemia.** If ventilated patients develop pronounced breath-synchronous fluctuations of the arterial pressure curve, it suggests an intravascular volume deficiency. During mechanical inspiration, the venous flow to the heart is throttled despite the only relatively low intrathoracic pressure increase, which also reduces the heart's stroke volume (▶ Fig. 25.2). The opposite occurs during expiration.

▶ **Complications.** Typical complications of arterial blood pressure measurement are:

- Infections
- Hemorrhages and hematoma in the vicinity of the puncture site
- Vascular complications: arterial vasospasms, dissection, aneurysms, AV fistula
- Nerve damage at cannulation
- Arterial (air) embolism

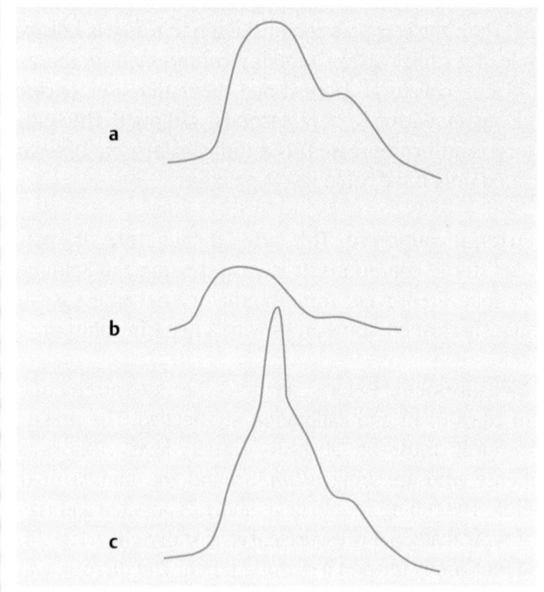

Fig. 25.1 Different arterial blood pressure curves. The stroke volume is proportional to the area under the systolic segment of the curve. **a** Optimal arterial pressure curve. **b** Excessive damping. **c** Overshoot.

- Vasospasms up to necrosis due to accidental arterial injection of drugs

> **Note**
>
> Caution: Never inject drugs into arterial accesses.

25.1.3 Central Venous Pressure

The central venous pressure (CVP) is the blood pressure in the vena cava at the transition to the right atrium. It is used to assess intravascular volume and right ventricular function.

The CVP is measured using a central venous catheter (CVC), through which it is also possible to apply medication, hyperosmolar infusions, and rapid volume substitution. The CVC should be located with the tip at the connection of the venae cavae to the right atrium. The CVC can be advanced via either the inferior or the superior vena cava. Typical access sites are:

- Superior vena cava: internal jugular vein, subclavian vein, external jugular vein (as flow-directed catheter), basilic vein (as flow-directed catheter)
- Inferior vena cava: femoral vein, umbilical vein (neonates)

The CVC is transferred via a tubing system to a pressure transducer that allows electronic measurement. Alternatively, a riser tube can also be used to measure CVP. Before measuring, a zero adjustment must be made. The pressure transducer or the zero point of the riser tube must be at the level of the heart (atrium).

▶ **Contraindications.** Contraindications for the insertion of a CVC are coagulation disorders and inflammatory skin changes at the puncture site.

▶ **Complications.** Typical complications from a CVC are infections, thromboses along the course of the catheter, and puncture-related problems such as compression of the artery, air embolism, vascular or nerve damage,

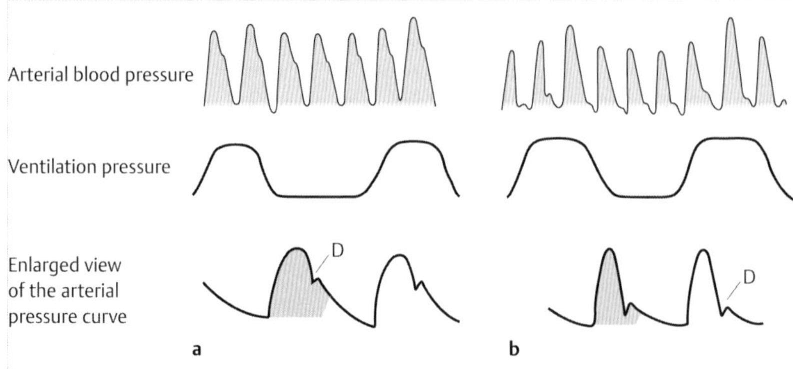

Fig. 25.2 Arterial pressure curve in normovolemia and hypovolemia.[24] **a** Normovolemia: The arterial pressure fluctuates only slightly depending on the respiratory cycle. The dicrotic notch (D) is high. **b** Hypovolemia: There is a pronounced drop in arterial pressure after inspiration and an increase after expiration. The dicrotic notch is low.

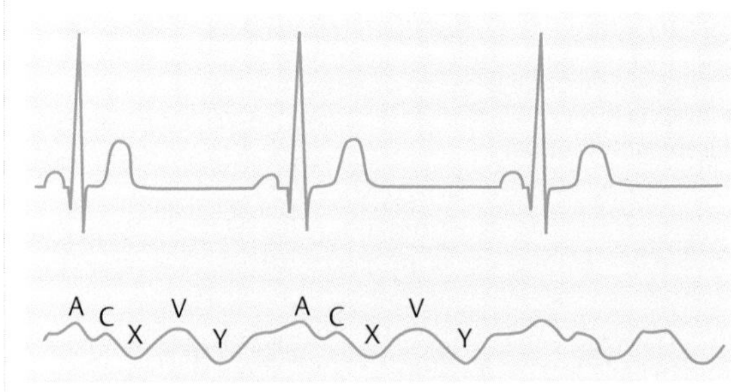

Fig. 25.3 Normal curve of central venous pressure (bottom) in relation to the ECG (top).
A wave: contraction of the right atrium (ventricular diastole)
C wave: protrusion of the tricuspid valve into the right atrium during contraction of the right ventricle
X wave: relaxation of the atrium and downward movement of the tricuspid valve (atrial diastole)
V wave: filling of the right atrium while the tricuspid valve is still closed (ventricular systole)
Y wave: opening of the tricuspid valve

pneumothorax, hematothorax, pericardial tamponade, AV fistulas, injury to the cervical sympathetic trunk in jugular vein punctures, or arrhythmia when the catheter is advanced into the right atrium or ventricle.

CVP Curve

The CVP curve has pressure fluctuations that are synchronous with heart action. There are three maximum pressures and two minimum pressures (▸ Fig. 25.3):

- A wave: contraction of the right atrium (ventricular diastole)
- C wave: protrusion of the tricuspid valve into the right atrium during contraction of the right ventricle
- X wave (atrial diastole): relaxation of the atrium and downward movement of the tricuspid valve
- V wave: filling of the right atrium while the tricuspid valve is still closed (ventricular systole)
- Y wave: opening of the tricuspid valve

The A wave and V wave are the most important in clinical routine.

Lack of coordination between the A wave and the V wave occurs in rhythm disorders in which there is no orderly sequence of atrial and ventricular contractions (so-called lack of atrioventricular synchonicity, e.g., 3rd degree AV block, junctional ectopic tachycardia).

Excessively high A waves suggest increased resistance during atrial emptying (tricuspid stenosis, pulmonary hypertension, reduced right ventricular compliance). A high V wave occurs in relevant tricuspid valve insufficiency.

The normal CVP value is around 5 mmHg (1–10 mmHg). The CVP is considered to be a parameter for right heart preload. The changes over time are more important than the absolute value. It should also be noted that if compliance of the right ventricle is reduced, there is no longer a linear relationship between the intravascular volume and the CVP, so volume therapy can no longer be reliably managed based on the CVP (e.g., after correction of a tetralogy of Fallot).

The CVP is elevated in the following situations:

- Hypervolemia
- Right heart failure, global heart failure
- Reduced right ventricular compliance
- Pulmonary hypertension
- Low cardiac output
- Pericardial effusion/tamponade
- Tension pneumothorax
- High PEEP (> 15 mmHg)

Causes of low CVP:

- Hypovolemia
- Shock
- High cardiac output

25.1.4 Pulmonary Artery Catheter

The pressure in the pulmonary artery, CVP, pulmonary capillary wedge pressure, and mixed venous oxygen saturation can be measured directly using a pulmonary artery catheter. In addition, the cardiac output can be calculated using the thermodilution method.

The pulmonary artery catheter (also called the Swan–Ganz catheter after its developers) consists of a distal and a proximal port and a balloon tip and a thermistor (▸ Fig. 25.4).

Like a CVC, the pulmonary artery catheter is inserted using the Seldinger technique into a large vein (right internal jugular vein, subclavian vein) and advanced so the tip with the distal port is located in the vicinity of the main pulmonary artery. Then the balloon tip is inflated so the balloon is carried by the bloodstream. During this flow-directed placement of the catheter, a continuous pressure curve is recorded that has a characteristic profile depending on the location of the catheter (▸ Fig. 25.5).

The correct location of the proximal port is in the right atrium, so the CVP is measured via this port. There is also a temperature sensor (thermistor) at the tip of the catheter that is connected by a wire to the monitor. The thermistor is used to measure cardiac output using the thermodilution method (see Cardiac Output below).

Most pulmonary artery catheters also have another port that ends in the region of the proximal segment and can be used for applying medication.

A pulmonary artery catheter can be indicated in the following situations:

- Severe left heart failure
- Cardiomyopathy
- Pulmonary hypertension
- Shock

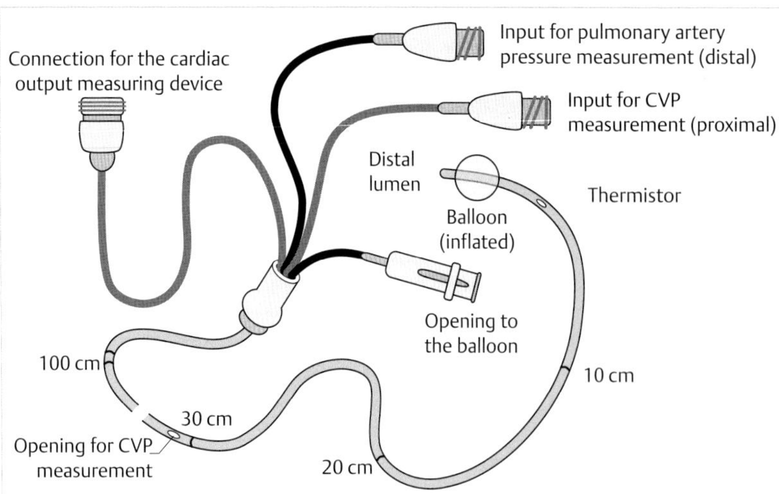

Fig. 25.4 Pulmonary artery catheter.

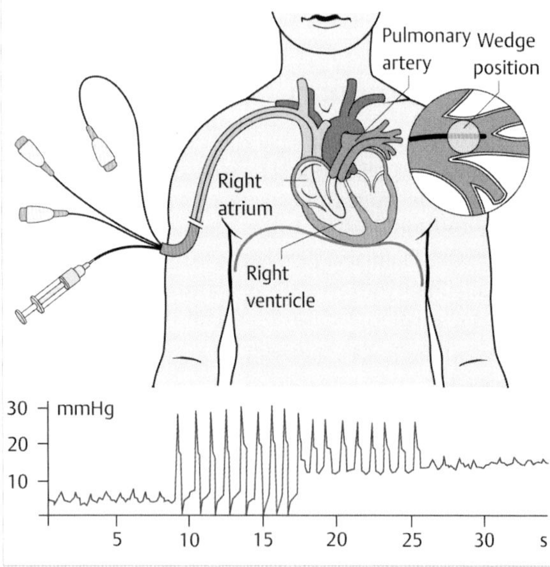

Fig. 25.5 Typical pressure curve using a flow-directed pulmonary artery catheter.[24]

- Sepsis
- Acute lung failure
- Acute pulmonary embolism

Generally speaking, the indication for a pulmonary artery catheter has become increasingly more restrictive as other methods are available, especially for measuring cardiac output (e.g., PiCCO system).

Contraindications:

- Tricuspid or pulmonary stenosis
- Tumor or thrombus in the right atrium or ventricle
- Severe coagulation disorders
- Severe arrhythmias
- Newly placed pacemaker electrodes (risk of dislocation)

► **Cardiac output.** Cardiac output is determined using the thermodilution method: an ice-cold solution of NaCl 0.9% is injected as quickly as possible into the right atrium and carried by the bloodstream to the pulmonary artery, where the change in temperature (result of dilution and warming by the blood) is measured by the thermistor. The cardiac output is then calculated using the area under the temperature–time curve (Stewart–Hamilton equation).

► **Central venous pressure.** The proximal port of the pulmonary artery catheter is located in the right atrium, so the CVP can be measured from this port.

► **Pulmonary capillary wedge pressure.** The pulmonary capillary wedge pressure (PCWP) is determined by inflating the balloon at the tip of the catheter and letting it be carried by the bloodstream until it is wedged into a branch of the pulmonary artery, occluding it completely. According to the principle of the static water column, the pressure in the occluded pulmonary artery capillary is equivalent to the pressure in the left atrium and thus also to the left ventricular end-diastolic pressure (LVEDP). The condition for these measurements is, of course, that there are no stenoses between the wedged pulmonary artery capillary, the left atrium, and the left ventricle. The left atrial pressure and the LVEDP are measures for left ventricular preload. The normal wedge pressure is 9 ± 4 mmHg.

After measuring, the balloon is deflated and the catheter tip is pulled back into the main pulmonary artery so that there is no risk of occluding the pulmonary artery capillary bed, which may lead to a pulmonary embolism.

► **Pulmonary artery pressure.** The pulmonary artery pressure is measured at the distal tip of the catheter. The normal pressure is less than 22 mmHg. The diastolic pulmonary artery pressure is normally approximately equivalent to the wedge pressure. The pulmonary artery pressure is elevated in patients with pulmonary hypertension or a pulmonary embolism, for example.

► **Calculated values.** The values described above can be used to calculate the following parameters:

$$\text{Cardiac index} = \frac{\text{Cardiac output (L/min)}}{\text{Body surface area (m}^2\text{)}}$$

Normal value: 2.5 to 4 l/min/m^2 body surface area (BSA).

$$\text{Systemic vascular resistance} = \frac{(\text{MAP} - \text{CVP}) \times 80}{\text{Cardiac output}}$$

Normal value for adults: 900 to 1400 dyn × s × cm^{-5}; for children: 15 to 30 Wood units × m^2 BSA

MAP: mean arterial pressure (in mmHg)

CVP: central venous pressure (in mmHg)

$$\text{Pulmonary vascular resistance} = \frac{(\text{MPAP} - \text{PCWP}) \times 80}{\text{Cardiac output}}$$

Normal value for adults: 150 to 250 dyn × s × cm^{-5}; for children: 1 to 3 Wood units × m^2 BSA (considerably higher in neonates)

MPAP: mean pulmonary artery pressure (in mmHg)

PCWP: pulmonary capillary wedge pressure (in mmHg)

The factor 80 is used to convert the conventional unit (Wood units) to the SI unit (dyn × s × cm–5). However, Wood units are still often used for children and related to the body surface area.

► **Mixed venous oxygen saturation** (**MVO$_2$**). Oxygen saturation in the pulmonary artery is termed mixed venous oxygen saturation. The term "mixed venous" is used because venous blood from the superior and inferior venae cavae is present as a mix in the pulmonary artery.

If the arterial saturation is 100%, the normal level for mixed venous saturation is approximately 75%. Due to the relatively high oxygen consumption in the central nervous system, the central venous saturation in the superior vena cava is about 72%, while saturation in the inferior vena cava is around 80%.

The mixed venous oxygen saturation reflects the oxygen consumption of the blood and is correlated with cardiac output. In patients with congestive heart failure and low cardiac output, the body is required to "extract" as much oxygen as possible from the low blood supply. This results in low mixed venous saturation in heart failure patients.

Elevated mixed venous saturation is a typical finding in septic patients in whom AV shunts are typically opened. The oxygen uptake in the tissue then sinks and the mixed venous oxygen saturation increases.

In practice, instead of measuring mixed venous oxygen saturation, which requires a pulmonary artery catheter, the central venous saturation is often measured via a CVC that is already inserted. In most cases, the two findings correlate quite well.

25.1.5 PiCCO System

A PiCCO (pulse contour cardiac output) system is a method for monitoring the hemodynamic situation. The principle of this method is determination of the stroke volume of the heart by analyzing the arterial blood pressure curve. Taking the heart rate into consideration, PiCCO is used to determine cardiac output. Beforehand, cardiac output must be determined using the thermodilution method (see Cardiac Output above) and the arterial pulse contour analysis must be calibrated to this measurement. In addition to cardiac output, other volumetric data such as extravascular lung fluid (measure for impending pulmonary edema), global end-diastolic volume (end-diastolic volume of all four heart chambers), and the intrathoracic blood volume can be determined. The PiCCO system thus makes it possible to make a differentiated assessment of the hemodynamic situation and manage the corresponding treatment.

The conditions for installing a PiCCO system are a central venous and an arterial access. A pulmonary artery catheter is not required.

25.2 Postoperative Intensive Therapy

The following remarks apply primarily to the postoperative transfer of the patient from the cardiac surgical operating room and the early postoperative period in the intensive care unit (ICU).

25.2.1 Basics

The job of the intensive care physician starts before the operated child is admitted to the ICU, as detailed information on the child is needed in advance. He or she must be aware of and understand the hemodynamics of the heart defect, complicating concomitant diseases, the planned surgical procedure, and possible perioperative and postoperative complications.

The intensive care physician should be familiar with the major steps of the surgery; they include opening the thorax and the mediastinum, arterial and venous cannulation for the cardiopulmonary bypass, initiation of cardiopulmonary bypass, cardioplegic arrest, and finally the restoration of cardiac function at the end of the operation and decannulation and closure of the thorax.

Regular observership in the cardiac surgical operating theater is mandatory in order to gain a better understanding of the surgical processes.

25.2.2 Preparation of the Bed

Before the patient is transferred to the ICU, preparation of the bed must be completed. This preparation includes the following:

- Preparation of the ventilation equipment and setting to patient-specific parameters (see Chapter 25.2.4) and check of the ventilation bag and mask. In addition, it must be determined whether NO ventilation is possible/necessary with the ventilation equipment.
- Medication plan: The prepared medication plan should include the medication and dosages for postoperative treatment (antibiotics, sedation, catecholamines, vasodilators, diuretics, infusions). The perfusors and flushing solutions are purged and primed before the patient is transferred to the ICU.
- Monitoring: The bedside monitor is checked beforehand and the patient-specific alarms are set.
- Administrative tasks: An X-ray order for the first postoperative X-ray and lab order for the first laboratory tests should be prepared.

25.2.3 Postoperative Transfer of the Patient to the ICU

The checklist in ▸ Table 25.1 contains the questions that the intensive care physician should discuss with the surgeons, anesthesiologists, and cardiac technicians at transfer.

25.2.4 Initial Examination after Transfer to the ICU

Immediately after the patient is admitted to the ICU, the most important clinical parameters must be tested:

- Respiration: How are thorax movements? Symmetrical lung expansion? Oxygen saturation? FiO_2?
- Circulation: Palpation of peripheral pulses, check of pressure parameters on the monitor (arterial blood pressure, CVP, possibly pulmonary artery pressure, possible LA pressure), check of capillary filling time (normal < 2–3 s).
- Diuresis: Is the urine bag filled? Is the urine clear? Does the patient appear edematous or rather dehydrated?
- Bleeding: How much do the drainages produce? Is the secretion dark red (venous blood), bright red (arterial blood), clear (serous), warm (fresh) or cold (older)?
- Neurology: Pupil status, spontaneous movements.
- Body temperature.

After the gross examination, the patient is connected to the bedside monitor. The arterial and central venous accesses are connected with the pressure transducers, set to zero, and activated. The patient is also connected to the ventilation equipment and the drainages to suction (suction generally around 15 cm H_2O). In addition, the external pacemaker is checked for proper function.

The first blood gas analysis including electrolyte status provides information on the ventilation situation, the hemodynamic status (lactate), and electrolyte metabolism (especially potassium). A six-lead standard ECG is recorded, a chest X-ray arranged, and an initial exploratory echocardiography made carried out.

Table 25.1 Checklist for postoperative transfer

Surgical aspects
• What was the intraoperative finding? • What surgical technique was performed? • What drainages were placed intraoperatively (e.g., pleural drainage, mediastinal drainage)? • What is the assessment of the postoperative result? • Was an intraoperative transesophageal echocardiography performed and what was the finding (residual gradient, valve insufficiency, residual shunt, myocardial function)? • Did any intraoperative arrhythmias occur? How were they treated? • Did any intraoperative bleeding problems occur? How were they treated?
Anesthesiology aspects
• Tube position and size, and brand • Ventilation situation (FiO2, tidal volume, rate, peak pressure, and PEEP) • Central venous catheter: location, size, lumen • Arterial accesses: location, size • Was an LA or pulmonary artery catheter placed? • Anesthetics and cardiac medication used (catecholamines, vasodilators, antiarrhythmics) and their dosages • Heparinization and current coagulation levels • Use of blood products (packed red cells, platelet concentrates, fresh frozen plasma)
Cardiopulmonary bypass
• Bypass time • Aortic clamp time • Cardiac arrest time • Minimum temperature during bypass • Was hemofiltration performed at the end of the bypass?

25.2.5 Further Postoperative Treatment

▸ **Fluid intake.** In all operations involving cardiopulmonary bypass, capillary leak occurs following the procedure, so the amount of free water intake must be limited postoperatively. Fluid intake is generally reduced to 30 to 50% of the normal maintenance amount on the first postoperative day and then increased day by day to 50, 75, and finally 100%.

Patients who underwent the operation without cardiopulmonary bypass (e.g., resection of an aortic coarctation, PDA ligature) usually do not require a restriction of fluid intake.

▸ **Ventilation.** Practically all patients are ventilated when they arrive in the ICU. Lung function is affected by numerous preoperative, intraoperative, and postoperative factors. Important examples are listed below:

- Preoperative factors:
  - Pre-existing pulmonary hypertension
  - Pre-existing excessive pulmonary blood flow
  - External compression of the airways, for example, due to vascular rings or prominent pulmonary arteries
- Intraoperative factors:
  - Edema tendency due to the bypass
  - Atelectasis due to surgical manipulation in the thorax or lack of ventilation during the bypass
- Postoperative factors:
  - Swollen mucosa
  - Atelectasis
  - Lung edema as a result of a postoperative increased lung perfusion, for example, after a shunt procedure or operative opening of circulation in the lungs in pulmonary atresia ("reperfusion edema")
  - Deteriorated respiratory mechanism due to postoperative diaphragmatic paresis
  - Pain-related reduction of respiratory capacity
  - Drugs causing respiratory depression
  - Pneumothorax, pleural effusions

▸ **Settings of the ventilation device.** The following values can be used as references for the age-specific respiratory rate:

- Neonates: 40/min
- Infants: 25 to 30/min
- Toddlers: 25/min
- School-age children: 20/min
- Adolescents: 15/min

For volume-controlled ventilation, markedly lower rates are usually used (e.g., 20/min for neonates).

To prevent and treat atelectasis, the tidal volume is usually set to 10 to 15 mL/kg. A relatively long inspiration time is usually selected initially. The PEEP is around 5 to 10 mmHg and an FiO_2 value is selected at which oxygen saturation of over 95% can be achieved.

The following situations are important departures from this procedure:

- *Univentricular heart:* For univentricular hearts, the balance between systemic and pulmonary circulation is very important. At an oxygen saturation of around 75 to 85%, a balance between systemic and pulmonary perfusion is achieved (Qp/Qs = 1:1). Therefore, the target oxygen saturation is approximately 80%.
- *Fontan circulation:* Theoretically, a high PEEP increases the intrathoracic pressure and thus reduces passive blood flow to the pulmonary vascular system. A lower PEEP level (ca. 5 mmHg) is therefore often recommended for Fontan patients. On the other hand, a higher PEEP also increases the residual functional capacity, so better lung perfusion can be achieved via the Euler–Liljestrand reflex.
- *Pulmonary hypertension:* A low pCO_2, a high pH, and a high FiO_2 reduce pulmonary vascular resistance, so mild hyperventilation with oxygen saturation around 100% should be attempted to treat pulmonary hypertension (target pCO_2: 30–35 mmHg).

▸ **Infection prophylaxis.** Postoperative antibiotic prophylaxis is almost always instigated for children after cardiac surgery. The antibiotics used and the duration of antibiotic treatment are the subject of some controversy, however. Second-generation cephalosporins are frequently used, for example, cefazolin 100 mg/kg/d in three single doses. For an uncomplicated postoperative course, many centers perform antibiotic prophylaxis for 3 days, although hardly any evidence-based data for this procedure are available.

▸ **Sedation.** In most centers, a combination of an opioid (morphine, fentanyl) and a benzodiazepine (midazolam) is administered intravenously continuously in the initial postoperative period. Propofol is often used in older children who are sedated for only a short period.

▸ **Analgesia.** A combination of nonsteroidal analgesics (paracetamol, ibuprofen) and opioids (morphine, fentanyl) is usually used for analgesia. Patient-controlled analgesia with a PCA pump is also available for older children (who can already play a video game).

▸ **Kidney function.** Kidney function nearly always deteriorates in patients who have undergone cardiac surgery. The use of the cardiopulmonary bypass leads to intraoperative fluid loading and inflammatory reactions that cause fluid retention. A negative fluid balance is therefore targeted postoperatively.

Urine excretion reflects the heart's ejection fraction and kidney function. Urine excretion of at least 2 mL/kg/h is desired. After cardiac surgery, patients most often have *prerenal* kidney failure (low cardiac output, capillary leak,

Table 25.2 Typical postoperative problems and the most common causes

Problem	Common causes
Blood pressure too high	Pain, fear, catecholamines, excessive fluid volume, result of the abrupt drug discontinuation (beta blockers, ACE inhibitors); typical postoperative problem after correction of an aortic coarctation. Rare causes: cerebral seizures, hypoglycemia (counter-regulation)
Blood pressure too low	Low cardiac output: limited myocardial function, pericardial effusion, arrhythmia (junctional ectopic tachycardia [JET], AV block), excessive drainage loss, hemorrhage, excessive diuresis; vasodilators, anaphylaxis, sepsis, shock, pneumothorax, fluid deficit.
Central venous pressure (CVP) too low	Fluid deficit (excessive drainage losses, hemorrhage, excessive diuresis, volume intake too low)
CVP too high	Agitated patient (reaction to wake-up, insufficient sedation in ventilated patients); impaired right ventricular function (typical example: the stiff, muscular right ventricle in Fallot patients is initially dependent on a high preload even after correction). In patients with univentricular hearts, a high CVP suggests poor systemic ventricular or a relevant AV valve insufficiency. Other causes are a pericardial tamponade or pneumothorax.
Arterial saturation too low	Atelectasis, hypoventilation, technical problems with the ventilation device, disconnected/ obstructed tube, pneumothorax, pleural effusion, pneumonia, pulmonary edema, pulmonary hemorrhage, secretion, right-to-left shunt
Arterial saturation too high	In patients with univentricular hearts, saturation over 85% suggests an imbalance between pulmonary and systemic perfusion: excessive blood flow to the lungs and diminished supply to the systemic circulation
Bradycardia	Sinus bradycardia, AV block
Tachycardia	Narrow QRS complexes: sinus tachycardia, supraventricular tachycardia, JET Wide QRS complexes: ventricular tachycardia
Increase in lactate	Poor systemic perfusion, seizures, intestinal ischemia

volume deficit). A low systemic blood pressure and, in case of ascites, high intra-abdominal pressure lead to a low perfusion pressure in the kidneys. Examples of renal kidney failure are renal vein thrombosis or iatrogenic kidney damage (aminoglycosides, cyclosporine A). Postrenal kidney failure can be caused by obstructions in the region of the efferent urinary tract (e.g., obstruction of the urinary catheter or the urethra).

Suitable diuretics in the postoperative phase are primarily loop diuretics. They are administered as a bolus or as a continuous infusion if the response is inadequate. The combination with theophylline sometimes enhances the effect.

If excretion is insufficient or the fluid balance is clearly positive, peritoneal dialysis should be initiated early.

25.2.6 Common Postoperative Problems and Complications

Typical postoperative problems and their most common causes are summarized in ▶ Table 25.2.

Low Cardiac Output

Numerous factors can lead to myocardial dysfunction and low cardiac output postoperatively. They include an inflammatory reaction to cardiopulmonary bypass, myocardial ischemia as a result of the intraoperative clamping of the aorta, intraoperative hypothermia, a reperfusion edema, or—if one was performed—a ventriculotomy, coronary ischemia, inadequate cardioplegia, or an infection.

▶ **Symptoms.** Typical signs of low cardiac output are:
- Tachycardia
- Oliguria
- Delayed capillary filling time
- Hypotension
- Reduced mixed venous saturation (a difference between arterial and mixed venous saturation of less than 20 to 25% suggests sufficient cardiac output and adequate oxygen supply)
- Metabolic acidosis, high lactate level

▶ **Treatment.** The treatment of low cardiac output includes eliminating the underlying cause and the following measures depending on the hemodynamic situation:
- Inotropic support (catecholamines, phosphodiesterase inhibitors, intravenous calcium)
- Chronotropic support (pacemaker therapy, positive chronotropic drugs)
- Afterload reduction (sodium nitroprusside, milrinone)
- Volume substitution (in case of deficiency)

- Mechanical circulatory support
- Ventilation
- Sedation, cooling (reduction of oxygen consumption)

Pulmonary Hypertensive Crisis

Postoperatively, in certain situations, there may be a critical increase in pulmonary arterial pressure or pulmonary vascular resistance. The result is a standstill of the transpulmonary blood flow with congestion in the right atrium and ventricle and drop in pressure in the left atrium and ventricle. Ultimately, cardiac output collapses. The following patients are at a particularly high risk for this type of crisis:

- Patients with already increased pulmonary vascular resistance preoperatively
- Neonates within the first days of life
- Patients with pulmonary venous hypertension (e.g., within the context of a total anomalous pulmonary venous connection or mitral stenosis)
- Older children with a still uncorrected shunt defect that led to an increase in pulmonary vascular resistance (e.g., complete AV canal, large VSD)

The following factors increase pulmonary vascular resistance:

- Hypoxia
- Acidosis
- High partial pressure of carbon dioxide
- Polycythemia
- Atelectasis
- Agitation

The following factors reduce pulmonary vascular resistance:

- Oxygen administration
- Alkalosis
- Hyperventilation
- NO inhalation
- Recruitment of atelectatic lung segments

The treatment or prophylaxis of a pulmonary hypertensive crisis includes the following measures:

- Sufficient analgesia and sedation or relaxation
- Oxygenation
- Optimizing the ventilation situation (adequate PEEP)
- Slightly alkaline pH level (target pH 7.4–7.5) and mild hyperventilation
- Pharmacological vasodilators (NO, iloprost, prostacyclin)
- Avoidance of unnecessary manipulations such as too frequent suctioning

Specific Early Postoperative Problems

Cardiac defects or surgery-specific postoperative problems and complications are summarized in ▶ Table 25.3.

Postoperative Features of Heart Defects with a Univentricular Heart

The large group of heart defects with a univentricular physiology poses great challenges to postoperative intensive care. These defects include patients with a hypoplastic left heart syndrome, tricuspid atresia, or a double-inlet left ventricle.

The most important principles in the postoperative treatment of these patients are presented below.

As an example, the three-stage surgical procedure for a patient with a hypoplastic left heart syndrome is explained. Palliation in a Fontan procedure is made with the goal of achieving complete separation of the pulmonary and systemic circulation. The lungs are perfused passively from the venae cavae without any pumping chamber in between. The single ventricle supplies the systemic circulation. The three stages are:

- Norwood procedure
- Superior cavopulmonary anastomosis (Glenn procedure, "hemi Fontan")
- Total cavopulmonary anastomosis (Fontan procedure)

Norwood Procedure

The Norwood procedure is the first step for patients with a hypoplastic left heart syndrome toward separation of the circulatory systems by a Fontan procedure. There are several modifications of this surgical procedure. The goal is to form a neo-aorta from the pulmonary artery and the hypoplastic aorta that can supply the systemic circulation with blood without a pressure gradient. To do this, the pulmonary artery and the hypoplastic aorta are anastomosed distal to the valves. Additional patch material is usually required for the reconstruction of the aortic arch. In this manner, a strong single vessel for systemic perfusion is created from the aorta and the pulmonary artery. Prior to this, the pulmonary artery is transected shortly before the pulmonary artery bifurcation. In addition, pulmonary perfusion is ensured via an aortopulmonary shunt.

To achieve the unobstructed outflow from the pulmonary veins, an atrial septectomy is also performed. There is a balance between the pulmonary and systemic circulatory systems when arterial saturation is between 75% and 85% (Qp/Qs = 1).

Typical problems after a Norwood procedure are low cardiac output and hypoxemia.

▶ **Low cardiac output.** As a result of the long bypass time or prolonged circulatory arrest, a systemic inflammatory response syndrome (SIRS) occurs. Myocardial function is usually markedly impaired so that a certain amount of catecholamine support is always needed postoperatively. Other causes of poor systemic perfusion are increased pulmonary perfusion at the expense of systemic perfusion (Qp/Qs > 1; leading symptoms: arterial

Table 25.3 Specific early postoperative problems and complications[20]

Cardiac defect/operation	Specific early postoperative problems and complications
ASD closure	Sinus node dysfunction, excessive diuresis, left heart failure / pulmonary edema in older children and adults
VSD closure	Pulmonary hypertensive crisis, complete AV block, JET, residual shunt
AV canal correction	Pulmonary hypertensive crisis, complete AV block, JET, AV valve stenosis or incompetence
PDA ligation	Injury to the recurrent laryngeal nerve (vocal cord paralysis) or the thoracic duct (chylothorax), accidental ligation or injury to surrounding vessels (especially left pulmonary artery, aorta)
Truncus arteriosus correction	Pulmonary hypertensive crisis, truncus valve stenosis or incompetence, right ventricular dysfunction
Aortopulmonary window (correction)	Pulmonary hypertensive crisis, coronary ischemia
Anomalous pulmonary venous connection (correction)	Pulmonary hypertensive crisis, atrial arrhythmia, residual stenosis of the pulmonary veins or pulmonary vein anastomosis with the left ventricle, high left ventricular filling pressure due to the relatively small left atrium and ventricle
Fallot correction	Right ventricular dysfunction (poor compliance of the hypertrophic ventricle), JET, complete AV block, residual pulmonary stenosis, residual VSD, pulmonary insufficiency after a transannular patch
Pulmonary atresia with intact ventricular septum	Right ventricular dysfunction, myocardial ischemia due to right ventricle-dependent coronary circulation, circular shunting due to creation of an aortopulmonary shunt and opening of right ventricular outflow tract
Aortic stenosis correction	Residual stenosis, disruption of left ventricular diastolic function, aortic insufficiency, AV block
Ross procedure	Coronary ischemia
Konno procedure	Coronary ischemia, obstruction of the right ventricular outflow tract, arrhythmias (e.g., AV block), mitral regurgitation
Subaortic stenosis (resection)	Residual stenosis, mitral valve injury, (ventricular) arrhythmia
Coarctation of the aorta (resection)	Residual obstruction, paraplegia, post-coarctectomy syndrome, unmasking an aortic valve stenosis, injury to the recurrent laryngeal nerve, chylothorax
Interrupted aortic arch (correction)	Residual obstruction, compression of the left main bronchus by the aorta, injury to the recurrent laryngeal nerve, chylothorax
Mitral stenosis correction	Pulmonary hypertensive crisis, residual stenosis, mitral regurgitation, left ventricular dysfunction
Creation of an aortopulmonary shunt	Imbalance between systemic and pulmonary perfusion, shunt leak, shunt thrombosis
Pulmonary artery banding	Cyanosis, insufficient banding (excessive pulmonary blood flow), Qp-Qs mismatch
Norwood I procedure	Low cardiac output, imbalance between systemic and pulmonary perfusion, residual obstruction of the aortic arch, AV valve insufficiency, SIRS
Upper cavopulmonary anastomosis	Cyanosis, hypertension, edema/congestion of the upper half of the body
Fontan completion	Ascites, pleural effusions, edema, cyanosis, low cardiac output, arrhythmias
TGA (switch operation)	Coronary ischemia, left ventricular dysfunction, neo-aortic insufficiency, peripheral pulmonary stenosis
TGA (Mustard/Senning atrial baffle procedure)	Pulmonary or systemic venous obstruction, atrial arrhythmias
Bland–White–Garland syndrome (correction)	Myocardial dysfunction, mitral regurgitation

saturation > 85%, tachycardia, hypotension, oliguria, metabolic acidosis). An attempt is made to treat these cases by reducing the afterload of the systemic circulation and increasing pulmonary resistance.

AV valve insufficiency or arrhythmias can also cause low cardiac output.

▶ **Hypoxemia.** Hypoxemia can be the result of an imbalance between pulmonary and systemic circulations to the detriment of the pulmonary circulation—for example, in an obstruction of the aortopulmonary shunt or increased pulmonary resistance.

Other causes are pulmonary problems such as a pleural effusion or pneumonia. Peripheral cyanosis occurs with low cardiac output or increased oxygen consumption (leading symptom: reduced systemic venous saturation).

Superior Cavopulmonary Anastomosis

The aim of an upper cavopulmonary anastomosis is to allow passive blood flow from the upper half of the body into the pulmonary circulation. The superior vena cava is anastomosed with the pulmonary artery and the systemic venous blood from the upper half of the body then flows passively to the lungs without an intermediate pumping chamber and is oxygenated there. The systemic venous blood from the lower half of the body does not reach the lungs, but is mixed with the pulmonary venous blood in the heart and pumped into the systemic circulation. The systemic circulation thus contains mixed blood.

The cardiac load is also reduced and normalized by the creation of the upper cavopulmonary anastomosis, as the pulmonary circulation and systemic circulation are now connected in series. The Qp/Qs ratio is then 0.6 to 0.7; oxygen saturation is 75 to 85%. The ratio of pulmonary to systemic perfusion can be still higher in younger children. In comparison with older children, the head and upper limbs are still relatively large in young children, so there is a higher proportion of systemic venous blood from the upper half of the body that reaches the lungs via the cavopulmonary anastomosis and is oxygenated there.

Typical postoperative problems are increased pressure in the superior vena cava, hypertension, and hypoxemia.

▶ **Elevated pressure in the superior vena cava.** In an superior cavopulmonary anastomosis, the superior vena cava is anastomosed directly with the pulmonary circulation. Elevated pressure in the superior vena cava thus suggests an obstruction in the area of the cavopulmonary anastomosis or pulmonary circulation or elevated pulmonary vascular resistance.

The transpulmonary gradient (difference in pressure between the superior vena cava and atrium) should be less than 10 mmHg. High pressure in the superior vena cava can restrict cerebral outflow and lead to edema in the upper half of the body (superior vena cava syndrome).

After a superior cavopulmonary anastomosis, patients should therefore be positioned with the upper body elevated and quickly extubated. Elevated intrathoracic pressure from mechanical ventilation additionally hinders passive blood flow from the superior vena cava into the pulmonary circulation.

▶ **Hypertension.** Temporary hypertension during the first few postoperative days is not unusual. It may be caused by the elevation of intracranial pressure that is necessary to maintain adequate cerebral perfusion pressure. Aggressive lowering of the blood pressure should therefore be avoided.

▶ **Hypoxemia.** Saturation levels below 75% following an upper cavopulmonary anastomosis can be caused by a reduction of pulmonary perfusion due to an obstruction in the area of the anastomosis or pulmonary vessels. Another possible explanation is that blood from the upper half of the body is conducted past the alveoli of the lungs, for example, if there are venovenous collaterals (connections between the systemic and pulmonary veins) or arteriovenous collaterals (connections between the pulmonary arteries and veins).

In the early postoperative phase, arterial saturation can often be improved by attempting mild hypoventilation. The blood can also be slightly alkalized by administering sodium bicarbonate (target pH > 7.4). Slightly elevated pCO_2 (> 50 mmHg) causes vasodilatation of the cerebral vessels so more blood flows to the brain. Since this allows relatively more blood to reach the upper half of the body, more blood is conducted through the upper cavopulmonary anastomosis into the lungs and becomes oxygenated.

Total Cavopulmonary Anastomosis (Fontan Procedure)

In a Fontan procedure (total cavopulmonary anastomosis) the pulmonary and systemic circulation are completely separated by anastomosing the inferior vena cava with the pulmonary circulation. A tunnel is created that connects the inferior vena cava with the pulmonary artery. This tunnel passes either through the atrium or alternatively outside the heart (extracardiac tunnel). Sometimes a small shunt is left between the Fontan tunnel and the atrium that functions as an overflow valve if the resistance in the pulmonary circulation is too high and not all of the systemic venous blood can enter the pulmonary circulation. In these cases, there is a right-to-left shunt across the Fontan fenestration. This can have the disadvantage that arterial saturation is then reduced.

When the Fontan circulation is completed, all of the systemic venous blood (with the exception of the coronary sinus) flows passively into the pulmonary circulation without passing through a pumping chamber. The oxygenated blood is pumped through the univentricular heart into the systemic circulation.

Typical postoperative problems are low cardiac output, hypoxemia, effusions, and thrombosis.

► **Low cardiac output.** Low cardiac output can occur due to low preload (hypovolemia), increased pulmonary resistance, or an obstruction in the area of the systemic venous outflow (tunnel stenosis, anastomosis stenosis). Poor ventricular function or AV valve insufficiency and arrhythmias can also cause low cardiac output.

► **Arrhythmias.** Atrial arrhythmias may occur as a result of the sometimes elaborate manipulations in the atrial region. For example, sinus node dysfunction is typical. A pacemaker (atrial stimulation) sometimes becomes necessary.

► **Hypoxemia.** Cyanosis can be the result of a relevant right-to-left shunt across a tunnel fenestration. Pulmonary problems (pleural effusion, pneumonia) can also lead to hypoxemia. Peripheral cyanosis is the result of reduced cardiac output. Reduced pulmonary perfusion, as well as arteriovenous or venovenous collaterals can also cause hypoxemia.

► **Effusions.** Effusions (pleural effusion, ascites) can be the result of elevated venous pressure and may lead to considerable postoperative complications.

► **Thromboses.** Fontan patients are at an increased risk of developing venous thromboses. This risk is increased especially if there is low cardiac output. Most centers therefore recommend anticoagulation for Fontan patients. There is no uniform opinion with respect to the duration or the form of anticoagulation (vitamin K antagonists or platelet aggregation inhibitors).

While many different anticoagulation regimens are used in small children (no anticoagulation, aspirin, warfarin/phenprocoumon), there is a general consensus that anticoagulation is obligatory in patients after puberty and immediately after surgery.

25.3 Postpericardiotomy Syndrome

25.3.1 Basics

Definition

The postpericardiotomy syndrome is an inflammatory reaction of the pericardium and pleura, probably with an immunological cause. The leading symptom is pericardial effusion. The postpericardiotomy syndrome typically occurs following open-heart surgery. The pericardial effusion is usually detected 1 to 6 weeks after the operation and is associated with fever. In rare cases, a postpericardiotomy syndrome can also be triggered by interventional cardiac catheterization, implantation of pacemaker wires, or blunt trauma to the chest.

Epidemiology

The frequency of postpericardiotomy syndromes after operations in which the pericardium was opened ranges, according to the literature, from 2% to 30%. Children under 2 years old are only rarely affected.

Etiology

The exact cause of postpericardiotomy syndrome is unclear. An immunological cause has been suggested. It is probably an inflammatory reaction to myocardial or pericardial damage. Viral infections may play a role in triggering it. There is probably a pathomechanism similar to the one responsible for the Dressler syndrome following a myocardial infarction.

25.3.2 Diagnostic Measures

Symptoms

The leading symptom of the postpericardiotomy syndrome is pericardial effusion. Fever is often present. There may also be other nonspecific symptoms such as fatigue, chest pain, or joint pain. Occasionally, pleural effusions also develop. A very rare, but greatly feared, complication is a pericardial tamponade.

The symptoms typically appear 1 week after surgery at the earliest. On average, the symptoms begin around 4 weeks after surgery, but they can occur as late as a few months postoperatively in rare cases.

Echocardiography and Laboratory

The pericardial effusion can be reliably visualized by echocardiography. The laboratory tests often show elevated inflammatory markers.

Differential Diagnosis

In the differential diagnosis, primarily infection must be ruled out as the cause of the fever and the pericardial effusion. Other causes of postoperative pericardial effusion are a hemopericardium or chylopericardium.

25.3.3 Treatment

Bed rest is recommended until the fever is reduced. Pharmacological treatment consists mainly of anti-inflammatory drugs and diuretics. Nonsteroidal anti-inflammatory drugs (NSAIDs) can be given, such as ibuprofen (30–

40 mg/kg/d in 3 to 4 single doses) or aspirin (50–75 mg/kg/d in 3 single doses) each for 4 to 6 weeks. If the patient does not respond adequately to NSAIDs, treatment is sometimes supplemented by steroids (e.g., prednisolone 2 mg/kg/d in 2 single doses, then gradually tapered off over 2–4 weeks). Diuretics are often used if there is pericardial effusion but are rarely effective. A pericardial drainage is needed if there is hemodynamically relevant pericardial effusion or a pericardial tamponade.

25.3.4 Prognosis

This is generally a self-limiting disease. The average duration of the disease is 2 to 3 weeks, but a recurrence is not uncommon. A pericardial tamponade as a result of a post-pericardiotomy syndrome is very rare.

25.4 Chylothorax

25.4.1 Basics

Definition

Chylothorax results from an accumulation of lymphatic fluid in the pleural cavity. It is usually caused by trauma or leakage of the thoracic duct or its numerous branches.

Anatomy

The thoracic duct runs dorsal to the esophagus between the thoracic aorta and the spine (▶ Fig. 25.6). At the level of the 4th thoracic vertebra, the thoracic duct changes course and passes between the left subclavian artery and the left common carotid artery to the left subclavian–jugular confluence (left subclavian vein and internal jugular vein). Numerous variants of the course of the thoracic duct have been described, which is why intraoperative injuries occasionally occur.

The thoracic duct drains lymphatic fluid from a large part of the body, including from the entire left half of the body, the abdominal organs, and the lower limbs.

The composition of lymphatic fluid is very similar to that of plasma. It contains less protein, but more lipids, stemming mainly from the intestine. Medium-chain triglycerides, however, are metabolized directly in the liver and portal vein system and are not drained through the lymphatic vessels. Due to the high lipid content, the lymphatic fluid is milky white.

Etiology

A chylothorax in childhood most commonly occurs as a result of a cardiac or pediatric surgical procedure. Due to the location of the thoracic duct, which is between the aorta and the esophagus and in the area of the head and neck vessels, injuries occur especially during the following operations: arterial switch procedure, resection of an aortic coarctation, ligation of a patent ductus arteriosus, and correction of an esophageal atresia.

Other causes are:

- Thromboses of the superior vena cava, the innominate vein, or the right subclavian vein (e.g., as a result of a central venous catheter)
- Increase in central venous pressure (e.g., associated with Fontan hemodynamics)
- Lymphatic anomalies in genetic syndromes: for example, Noonan syndrome (chylothorax often already present at birth), triploid syndromes
- Chest or neck trauma
- Malignant lymphomas

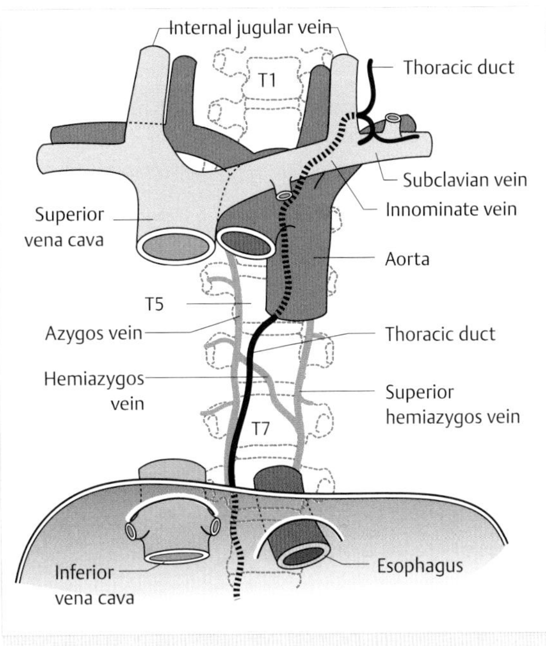

Fig. 25.6 Normal course of the thoracic duct.

25.4.2 Diagnostic Measures

Symptoms

In chylothorax, the initial clinical symptoms are the typical findings of a pneumothorax (dyspnea, weak breath sounds). When the effusion is aspirated, a cloudy, milky white secretion is typically drained, provided the child has already ingested at least a small amount of fatty food orally.

Laboratory

The diagnosis is made based on the clinical symptoms. Laboratory tests are not generally needed, but may be useful if the finding is unclear. The following findings in the pleural fluid suggest a chylothorax if there has already been at least minimal oral fat intake:

- Triglyceride concentration over 1.1 mmol/L (96 mg/dL)
- Absolute cell count over 1000/µL with more than 80% white blood cells
- Chylomicrons detected in the lipid electrophoresis (proof, but not necessarily required)

25.4.3 Treatment

Chylothorax is normally treated conservatively. Most patients can be cured by conservative measures, but the course is often very prolonged and can take weeks to months.

Conservative Treatment

The treatment principle is to reduce chyle production and thus relieve the fluid transport via the thoracic duct. This should have a favorable effect on the healing process of an injury to the thoracic duct.

▶ **Diet.** Initially a fat-free diet and then an MCT diet (medium-chain triglycerides). Medium-chain triglycerides are metabolized directly by the liver and the portal vein system and therefore do not strain the thoracic duct. If the diet is successful, it is continued for at least 1 to 2 more months. Then a normal diet is gradually reintroduced.

▶ **Total parenteral nutrition.** If the diet is unsuccessful, total parenteral nutrition is instituted. Since the lipids are given entirely parentally, the choice of fats is not important. If treatment is successful a normal diet is gradually reintroduced.

▶ **Somatostatin.** There is some data on treatment of chylothorax with the hormone somatostatin or its synthetic analogue octreotide. Somatostatin probably works via vasoconstriction in the area of the splanchnic nerve. The main side effects that have been observed are blood sugar imbalance, diarrhea, nausea, and impaired liver function. Treatment lasts around 3 weeks. The dosage of somatostatin is 3.5 to 7 (up to 10) µg/kg/h or 1 to 4 µg/kg/h for octreotide. Both drugs are administered in a continuous infusion.

Note

Calorie intake must be greater than the age-appropriate level, as the chylothorax causes high losses of lipids and proteins. Particularly significant are the losses of coagulation factors and immunoglobulins and if the amounts lost are high, corresponding substitution (e.g., at weekly intervals) must be considered.

Surgical Treatment

If all conservative treatment fails, the last treatment options are surgical procedures, including:

- Ligation of the thoracic duct
- Pleurodesis
- Pleuroperitoneal shunting
- Pleurectomy

25.4.4 Prognosis

The success rate in children under conservative treatment is between 70% and 80%. The disadvantages of conservative treatment are long hospitalization, inadequate weight gain, and the risk of infections (immunoglobulin deficiency). In general, the chances of success are lower if there are central venous thromboses or elevated central venous pressure.

26 Operations with Cardiopulmonary Bypass

Synonym: extracorporeal circulation

26.1 Basics

26.1.1 Principle of the Cardiopulmonary Bypass Machine

The cardiopulmonary bypass machine assumes the pumping function of the heart and the central task of the lungs, gas exchange, during open-heart surgery.

▸ **Function.** The cardiopulmonary bypass machine consists mainly of a pump, an oxygenator, a heat exchanger, and a reservoir (▸ Fig. 26.1). The principle is simple: the venous blood is drained from the heart through a system of tubes via a cannula in the right atrium or cannulas in the superior and inferior vena cava. The blood accumulates in a reservoir together with the blood suctioned from the surgical field. The blood is conducted to an oxygenator by a roller or centrifugal pump. A membrane oxygenator is usually used. The blood is oxygenated and carbon dioxide is removed by diffusion. A heat exchanger is also attached that can warm or cool the blood in order to affect the body temperature as desired.

To prevent embolisms, the blood is passed through a filter before being pumped back into the systemic circulation via the aortic cannula.

Because the blood is in continuous contact with foreign surfaces during bypass, anticoagulation with heparin is essential. At the end of the operation, the heparin is neutralized with protamine.

During cardiopulmonary bypass, the body temperature is usually cooled down to 25 to 28°C. This reduces the body's demand for oxygen and increases the ischemia tolerance time of the myocardium.

▸ **Cardioplegia.** After a gradual increase, the entire cardiac output is pumped through the cardiopulmonary bypass machine. The heart initially continues to beat as the coronaries are still perfused. The coronary arteries continue to receive blood until the aorta is clamped off proximal to the aortic cannula (▸ Fig. 26.2). In addition, a cardioplegic solution is injected into the aortic root and the heart stops beating. Most intracardiac operations are performed on a bloodless and nonbeating heart. The cardioplegic solution, which contains potassium, magnesium, and buffer substances, is also used for cardioprotection. The cardioplegic solution is usually reapplied every 20 to 30 minutes during the operation to achieve optimal cardioprotection.

▸ **Transition to normal circulation.** The heart does not begin to beat again until the myocardium is again perfused with blood and a normal membrane potential can be established after the aortic clamp has been opened. The heart either resumes activity spontaneously or the rhythm must be restored electrically. Later, the temperature of the blood and body is gradually warmed up again. The activity of the cardiopulmonary bypass machine is reduced in parallel.

Especially in neonates and small children, a modified ultrafiltration of the blood is also performed during this phase. This withdraws water from the circulatory system, increases hematocrit, and removes inflammatory mediators. Ultrafiltration has a favorable effect on postoperative course, which can otherwise often be complicated by a considerable capillary leak.

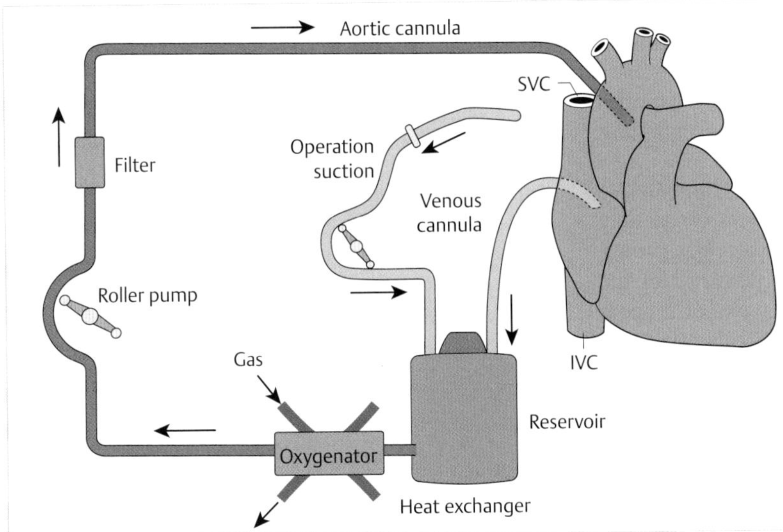

Fig. 26.1 Cardiopulmonary bypass setup.
SVC, superior vena cava; IVC, inferior vena cava.[4]

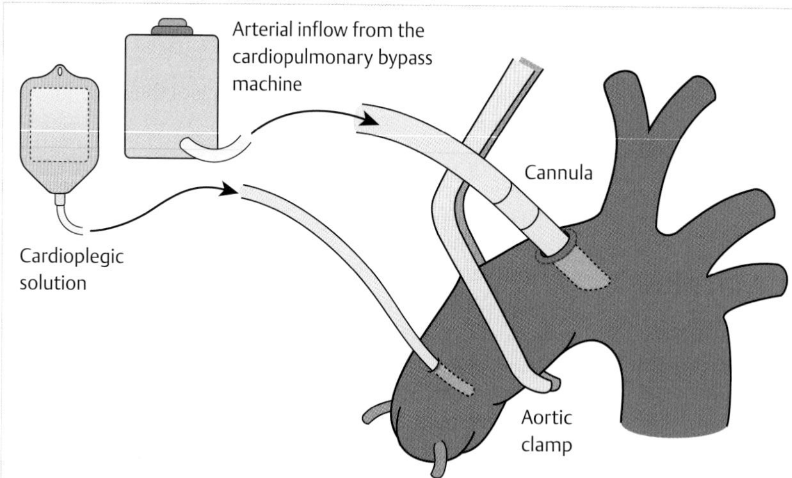

Fig. 26.2 Clamping the aorta and instillation of the cardioplegic solution.[4]

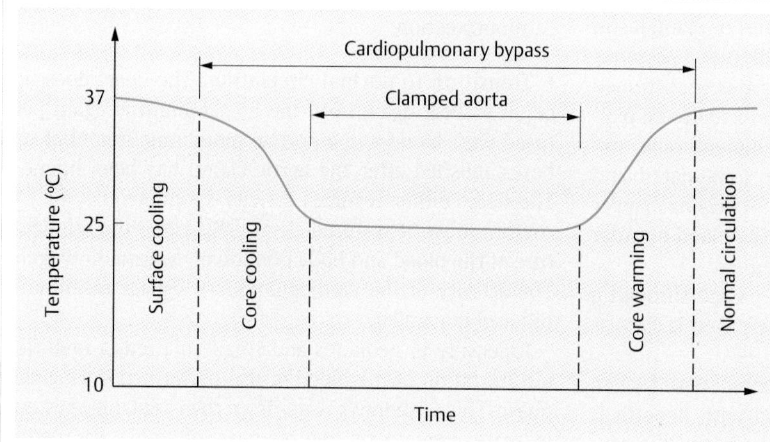

Fig. 26.3 Temperature curve during the different phases of an operation with the cardiopulmonary bypass machine in mild hypothermia.[4]

► **Circulatory arrest in deep hypothermia.** Circulatory arrest is sometimes needed, especially in neonates or small infants. Some procedures that necessitate this are operations on the aortic arch distal to the aortic cannula, for example, in a Norwood procedure or the correction of a hypoplastic aortic arch or a total anomalous pulmonary venous connection. In these procedures, using the cardiopulmonary bypass machine would result in a continuous flow of blood to the operation field, making the correction impossible. In these cases, the cardiopulmonary bypass machine is either switched off entirely or only minimal blood flow via a cannula in the right carotid artery is maintained for the selective perfusion of the head. To protect the organism, the body is cooled down to a temperature of 14–20°C during circulatory arrest (► Fig. 26.3, ► Fig. 26.4). In this way, neurological damage can be reduced surprisingly well. However, the risk of later neurological damage increases when the arrest lasts more than 45 to 60 minutes.

► **Side effects of extracorporeal circulation.** Extracorporeal circulation triggers a number of systemic reactions in the organism that have a decisive effect on the postoperative course, including:

- Increased risk of hemorrhage as a result of activating the coagulation and fibrinolytic system
- Hemolysis as a result of the shear forces that act on the red blood cells by the roller pumps and suctioning
- Activation of the complement system, activation of inflammatory mediators and neutrophils resulting in systemic inflammatory response syndrome (SIRS)
- Capillary leak and generalized tendency for edema
- Myocardial dysfunction, impaired myocardial contractility
- Impaired renal function

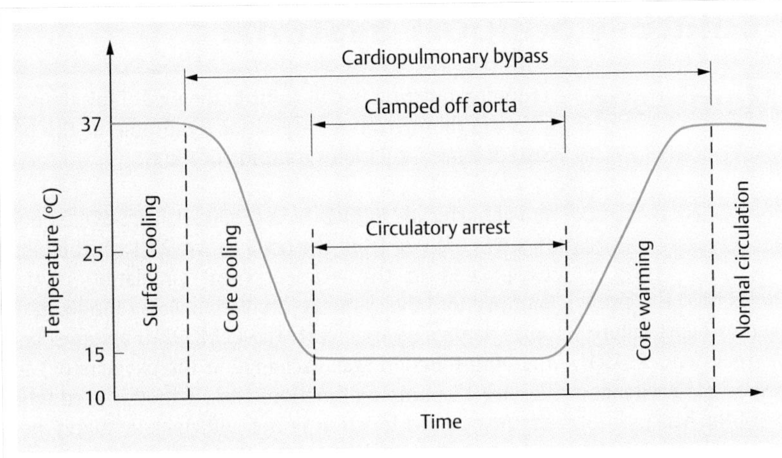

Fig. 26.4 Temperature curve during the different phases of an operation with circulatory arrest in deep hypothermia.[4]

27 Mechanical Circulatory Support Systems

27.1 Extracorporeal Membrane Oxygenation

27.1.1 Basics

Principle of ECMO

Extracorporeal membrane oxygenation (ECMO) is a procedure for patients with severe lung and/or heart failure who do not respond to conventional treatment. ECMO makes it possible to temporarily take over gas exchange from the lungs or the pumping function of the heart.

An ECMO system is similar in structure to a cardiopulmonary bypass machine: venous blood is drained from the body, pumped to an oxygenator, brought to a certain temperature in a heat exchanger, and then returned oxygenated to the body.

ECMO is a temporary measure to bridge the time until lung and/or cardiac function recovers or until definitive treatment, such as transplantation, is possible. The duration of the use of ECMO is between one day and several weeks.

▸ **Venovenous ECMO.** In this case, the blood oxygenated in the extracorporeal circulation is returned to the patient's venous circulation (▸ Fig. 27.1 a). In order to reach the pulmonary and systemic arterial circulation, the oxygenated blood must be pumped by the heart. Adequate cardiac function is thus a prerequisite for venovenous ECMO. This method is therefore used when lung function is considerably impaired, but the heart's pumping function is still sufficiently good. Typical examples are the meconium aspiration syndrome or the persistent fetal circulation syndrome or ARDS.

▸ **Venoarterial ECMO.** In venoarterial ECMO, venous blood is drained from the body (▸ Fig. 27.1 b). The blood oxygenated in the extracorporeal circulation is then pumped into the systemic circulation via a cannula in the aorta, bypassing the heart. The ECMO thus assumes both the lung function (gas exchange in the oxygenator) and the heart's pumping function. This method is used when the myocardial function is not sufficient to supply both pulmonary and systemic circulation (e.g., after cardiac surgery or fulminant myocarditis). The disadvantage of venoarterial ECMO is that the aorta must be cannulated, which has considerably higher risks (hemorrhage, systemic embolism) than the cannulation of veins only.

Epidemiology

ECMO has now been used in over 20,000 neonates around the world. Since ventilation options have been improved (high-frequency ventilation, inhaled NO, surfactant) the number of ECMOs performed for pulmonary indications has decreased but the number of ECMOs for cardiac indications has increased.

Indications

ECMO is indicated when there is a serious impairment of lung or cardiac function that is reversible or can be

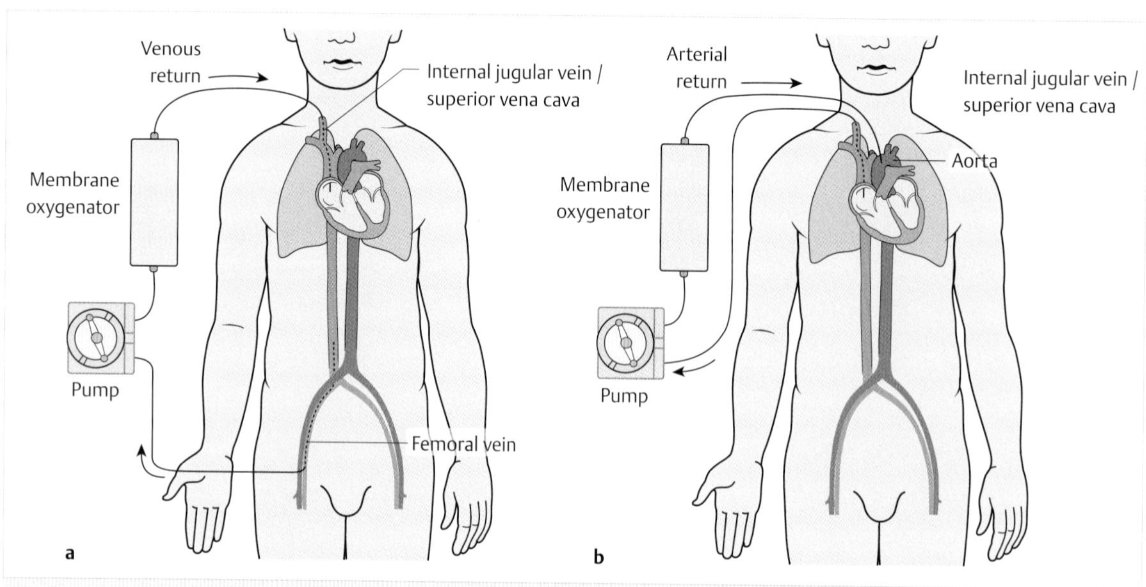

Fig. 27.1 Extracorporeal membrane oxygenation (ECMO). **a** Venovenous ECMO. **b** Venoarterial ECMO.

successfully treated within a few days up to a maximum of weeks. The severity of the disease and the mortality risk must be weighed against the risks of ECMO when the indication is made.

Typical indications for ECMO are:

- Cardiac surgery patients who cannot be weaned from the cardiopulmonary bypass machine (e.g., due to a severe temporary ventricular function disorder or pulmonary hypertension)
- Severe congenital heart defects that need to be stabilized until the definitive operation (e.g., hypoplastic left heart syndrome, total anomalous pulmonary venous connection with pulmonary venous obstruction)
- Cardiocirculatory arrest in the hospital requiring resuscitation: while continuing resuscitation, ECMO can be implanted, thus improving the chances of survival
- Interim measure until a heart or heart/lung transplant
- Lung failure: neonates with severe pulmonary disorders (meconium aspiration, persistent pulmonary hypertension) with an oxygenation index over 0.4 (oxygenation index = mean airway pressure × FiO_2/PaO_2)
- Interim measure until implantation of a cardiac assist device

Contraindications

Contraindications for ECMO are disorders that would entail the serious impairment of quality of life despite successful ECMO therapy. A high-grade cerebral hemorrhage is a contraindication, as is a body weight of neonates/infants less than 1,800 to 2,500 g.

27.1.2 Performing ECMO

In infants and neonates, usually the right neck vessels are cannulated for implanting the ECMO cannulas: the jugular vein for a venovenous ECMO and the jugular vein and carotid artery for a venoarterial ECMO. For a venovenous ECMO, blood drainage and return occur jointly via the jugular vein in a double-lumen catheter or separately via the additional cannulation of the femoral vein. If venoarterial ECMO is begun in cardiac surgery, the right atrium and ascending aorta are usually cannulated.

As preparation, the ECMO system is filled with a priming solution (such as Ringer solution, human albumin).

For a venoarterial ECMO, the cardiac output is rapidly taken over almost completely by the ECMO system when it is put into operation. A standard value for cardiac output in childhood is 100 to 150 mL/kg/min (ca. 200 mL/kg/min for neonates). The ECMO flow can be controlled via central venous oxygen saturation, for which a normal level of 70 to 75% is targeted. For a venoarterial ECMO, arterial oxygen saturation should also reach normal levels (> 95%).

Either roller pumps or centrifugal pumps can be used for the extracorporeal circulation. In a centrifugal pump, a kind of propeller (like in a turbine) ensures continuous blood flow. The blood pressure amplitude is eliminated when cardiac output is completely taken over by the ECMO.

For ECMO that is initiated due to pulmonary failure, an attempt is made to eliminate damaging effects on the lungs. Therefore, high ventilation pressure and high oxygen concentration (oxygen toxicity) are avoided. In some cases, application of surfactant may have a positive effect on recovery of the lungs.

The oxygen content of the blood can be increased by either increasing the blood flow through the oxygenator or by increasing the oxygen content of the gas that flows through the oxygenator (sweep gas). Carbon dioxide is exchanged almost exclusively by the flow of sweep gas. Increasing this flow leads to greater elimination of carbon dioxide.

▶ **Ventilation.** The goal is to set ventilation so carefully that the lungs can regenerate, while preventing atelectasis. To do this, a low respiratory rate (e.g., 5/min), a long inspiration time (e.g., 2 s), limit to peak pressure (e.g., 15–20 mmHg, PEEP around 10–15 mmHg), and low oxygen supply (e.g., FiO_2 0.3) are used. When lung function improves, the flow of sweep gas in the ECMO can be reduced.

▶ **Anticoagulation.** Heparin is used for anticoagulation. The heparin effect is checked using the activated clotting time (ACT), which can be determined quickly in a bedside test. An ACT of around 180 s is usually targeted.

As a result of the contact with the foreign body surfaces of the ECMO system, there is also a drop in platelets. Platelet levels of 50,000/µL should be maintained.

▶ **Renal function.** Hemofiltration can be readily integrated into the ECMO system. It is frequently needed for ECMO patients, as the high volume demand as a result of SIRS under ECMO therapy often leads to serious edema. In addition, patients occasionally have kidney failure with oligouria or anuria due to impaired renal perfusion and hypoxia even before the ECMO implantation.

▶ **Weaning.** The weaning process from the ECMO begins as organ function increasingly recovers. The cardiac output pumped by the ECMO is gradually reduced. Catecholamines are almost always needed for cardiac support. Parallel to reducing the ECMO, mechanical ventilation is again intensified, as oxygenation must now be assumed mainly by the lungs. In some systems, it is possible to "short circuit" the extracorporeal circulation on a trial basis by connecting the two cannulas so the blood can be diverted past the ECMO pump and oxygenator to flow back to the body.

If the neck vessels were cannulated, the jugular vein is usually ligated when the ECMO cannulas are removed, while an attempt is made to reconstruct the carotid artery.

There is thus far no consensus as to when ECMO should be discontinued if the organ fails to recover or the prognosis is unfavorable. The decision must be made on a case-by-case basis.

27.1.3 Complications

The most common complications are listed below. The most significant are bleeding complications.

- Hemorrhage (cerebral hemorrhage, gastrointestinal bleeding, bleeding at cannulation sites or surgical incisions)
- Infections
- Hemolysis
- Drop in platelets
- Thrombi in the extracorporeal circulation
- Air embolism
- Technical complications (oxygenator failure, ruptured tube, pump failure)

27.1.4 Prognosis

The survival rate under ECMO treatment depends to a great extent on the underlying disease. The survival rate is best for neonates with a meconium aspiration syndrome (> 90%). The survival rate is 50 to 60% for acute respiratory distress syndrome (ARDS) in pediatric patients. Children in whom ECMO was initiated due to a cardiac indication have the poorest chance of survival (survival rate between 40% and 50%).

27.2 Circulatory Support Systems

27.2.1 Basics

Definition

Mechanical circulatory support systems (artificial heart, ventricular assist device) are mechanical pump systems that take over the heart's pumping function if ventricular function is inadequate. The goal is to ensure sufficient perfusion of the organs and relieve the heart. The systems are only an interim measure in childhood to bridge the time until the myocardium recovers or until definitive treatment is possible (i.e., usually until transplantation).

The most important mechanical circulatory support systems used in childhood are described briefly below. Extracorporeal membrane oxygenation (ECMO) is discussed separately in Chapter 27.1.

Principle

The principle of a ventricular assist device is that a pumping chamber is connected in parallel or in series with the cardiac chambers. Left ventricular assistance alone or biventricular assistance can be provided. In most cases it is sufficient to provide left ventricular assistance alone, as the right ventricular dysfunction is generally the result of increased afterload (lung congestion due to left heart failure). Right ventricular assistance is needed if the right ventricular myocardium is already damaged (e.g., due to severe myocarditis) or if pulmonary hypertension is present.

In left ventricular assist devices, the inflow cannula of the pump is implanted in the apex of the left ventricle. The blood drained from the left ventricle into the pumping chamber is then returned to systemic circulation via the outflow cannula, which is implanted in the ascending aorta. The assistance of the pumping chamber relieves the left ventricle.

In right ventricular assist devices, the right ventricle or the right atrium and the pulmonary artery are cannulated in a similar manner.

▸ **Extracorporeal systems.** In extracorporeal systems, the pumping chamber is outside the body. Only the inflow and outflow cannulas penetrate the thorax wall.

▸ **Completely implantable systems.** In completely implantable devices, the pumping chamber is completely implanted in the body. Only the wire for the control unit and energy supply leads out of the body. Completely implantable devices are currently available only as left ventricular assist devices.

▸ **Pulsatile pumping chambers.** Pulsatile pumping chambers have a pneumatic drive. The pumping chamber is divided by a membrane into two sections. The compression of gas in one section of the chamber causes the membrane to protrude into the other section and this generates pressure that drives the blood out of the pumping chamber (systole). During diastole, suction acts on the membrane, which causes the pumping chamber to be filled with blood again. Valves ensure that the blood flow moves in one direction only (▸ Fig. 27.2). Various sizes of pumping chambers are available depending on the size of the patient.

▸ **Nonpulsatile pumping chambers.** These devices generate a nonpulsatile flow using impeller turbines or centrifugal pumps. These pumps are driven by electric or magnetic power. Sometimes these come in the form of portable battery-run devices.

▸ **Anticoagulation.** Due to contact with foreign body surfaces, anticoagulation is needed for all systems to prevent thrombi. Usually a vitamin K antagonist (phenprocoumon, warfarin) is used. Usually, a platelet aggregation inhibitor (aspirin, clopidogrel) or platelet adhesion inhibitor (dipyramidole) is given in addition. Practically all modern devices have heparin-coated surfaces in the pumping chamber and tubes.

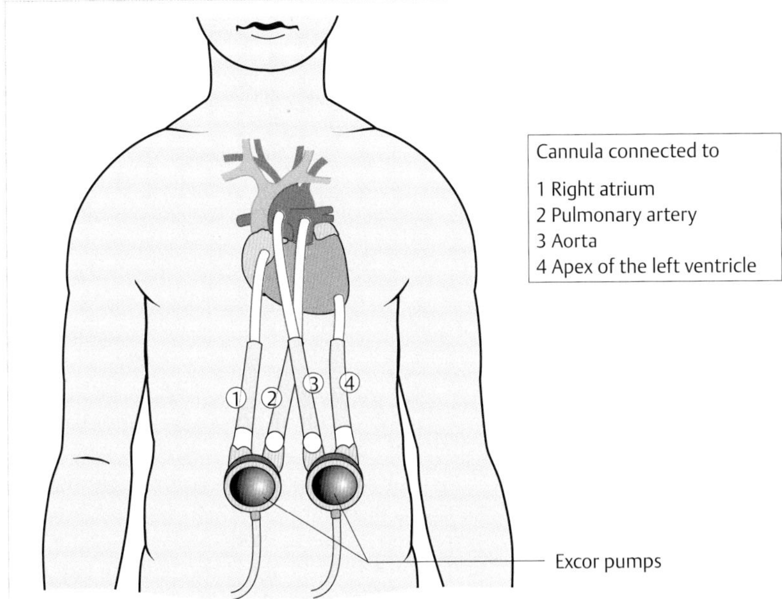

Fig. 27.2 Principle of a biventricular pulsatile mechanical circulatory support system with an extracorporeal pumping chamber (Berlin Heart Excor, biventricular assistance).

► **Indications.** Circulatory support systems are indicated when there is no hope of improvement through conventional treatment for terminal heart failure. There can be two goals for the use of the system:

- Interim measure until heart transplantation
- Interim measure until the myocardium recovers (e.g., after myocarditis)

In childhood, a circulatory support system is most often used due to a dilated cardiomyopathy in the stage of terminal heart failure to bridge the time on the waiting list for a donor heart.

Contraindications

In principle, the same contraindications apply to implantation of a circulatory support system as to heart transplantation, as a heart transplant is almost always the definitive treatment that is aimed for and no recovery of the myocardium is expected. In addition, the following contraindications also apply:

- Multiple organ failure, severe kidney or liver damage (however, early-stage organ failure is usually reversible with implantation of a mechanical circulatory support system. Sometimes early-stage organ damage as a result of heart failure is considered to be the right time for the implantation of the device)
- Septic shock
- Severe bleeding or coagulation disorders

27.2.2 Complications

The most important complications are thrombi, hemorrhage, infections, and relatively rare technical malfunctions.

27.2.3 Prognosis

The prognosis depends to a great extent on whether the device is implanted in time. The survival rate is reduced if right ventricular assistance in the form of a biventricular assist device is required in addition to left ventricular assistance.

28 Initial Treatment of Critically Ill Neonates with Cardiac Defects

In this chapter, the general features, clinical symptoms, and treatment principles for congenital heart defects that become symptomatic in neonates are discussed. In addition, the specific measures for the initial treatment of the most common defects are presented.

28.1 Basics

28.1.1 Epidemiology

The incidence of congenital heart defects is said to be 6 to 11 per 1,000 live births. Nearly half of these children require surgery or interventional catheterization within the first year of life.

28.1.2 Symptoms

The different congenital heart defects typically become manifest at different times. Important times at which congenital heart defects become symptomatic are the closure of the ductus arteriosus for ductal-dependent cardiac defects or the drop in pulmonary vascular resistance for shunt defects.

> **Note**
>
> **Leading symptoms of congenital heart defects in neonates are:**
> - Heart failure or cardiogenic shock (usually in the first or second week of life if there is left heart obstruction; for shunt defects typically not until after the drop in pulmonary resistance at the age of 2 to 8 weeks)
> - Cyanosis

Other symptoms that indicate a congenital heart defect in neonates are a murmur or arrhythmia (rarely as the primary symptom of a congenital heart defect).

► **Heart failure.** The characteristic signs of heart failure in neonates are:

- Tachypnea, dyspnea, thoracic retractions, possibly pulmonary edema
- Tachycardia
- Hepatomegaly
- Difficulty feeding, failure to thrive, increased sweating
- Pallor, prolonged capillary refill time
- Shock

The symptoms of heart failure in neonates are similar to the clinical symptoms of sepsis. Many neonates with heart failure are therefore first treated for suspected sepsis.

Especially cardiac defects with left heart obstruction (hypoplastic left heart syndrome, critical aortic stenosis, or coarctation of the aorta) can become manifest as early as the first 2 weeks of life with the clinical symptoms of cardiogenic shock.

► **Cyanosis.** The hyperoxia test is used to distinguish between cardiac and pulmonary cyanosis. In patients with pulmonary cyanosis, the oxygen saturation increases markedly after oxygen is given, while oxygen saturation usually does not significantly improve in those with cyanotic heart defects. Both pre- and postductal oxygen saturation should be measured. Cardiac cyanosis is the result of either reduced lung perfusion due to a right-to-left shunt or intracardiac mixing of systemic and pulmonary venous blood. Cyanosis can also very rarely be caused by methemoglobinemia. Cyanosis caused by the central nervous system must also be considered (e.g., central apnea in premature neonates or after cerebral hemorrhage).

> **Note**
>
> If there is not an adequate increase in oxygen saturation in a cyanotic neonate in the hyperoxia test, a congenital heart defect with ductal-dependent lung perfusion must be assumed. If the diagnosis cannot be immediately confirmed or ruled out by echocardiography, an attempt at treating it with intravenous prostaglandin E_1 is justified.

► **Heart murmur.** A heart murmur in a neonate is always suggestive of a congenital heart defect. Innocent murmurs are less common in this age group than in older children. While stenoses of the semilunar valves or AV valve insufficiency can already be detected immediately after birth due to a loud systolic murmur, the typical VSD murmur, for example, cannot be auscultated until after the pulmonary resistance has dropped and the pressure gradient between the left and right ventricles increases. It should also be noted that there may be no indicative heart murmur in some critical heart defects (e.g., d-TGA simplex, coarctation of the aorta).

► **Arrhythmias.** Arrhythmias are relatively rarely the first symptom of a congenital heart defect. An AV block, for example, occurs frequently in association with an l-TGA. Supraventricular tachycardias due to accessory conduction pathways occur more frequently with an Ebstein anomaly.

Table 28.1 Classification of congenital heart defects which become symptomatic in the neonatal period

Group	Examples
• Cardiac defects with ductal-dependent systemic circulation (left heart obstructions)	Critical aortic stenosis, hypoplastic left heart syndrome, interrupted aortic arch, critical coarctation of the aorta
• Cardiac defects with ductal-dependent pulmonary circulation (right heart obstructions)	Critical pulmonary stenosis, pulmonary atresia with intact ventricular septum, pulmonary atresia with VSD, pronounced form of tetralogy of Fallot, severe Ebstein anomaly, tricuspid atresia with pulmonary atresia or high-grade pulmonary stenosis
• Cardiac defects with parallel circulation	d-TGA
• Cardiac defects with complete intracardiac mixing of blood	Truncus arteriosus communis, total anomalous pulmonary venous connection, univentricular heart
• Cardiac defects with a large left-to-right shunt	Large VSD, complete AVSD, large PDA, aortopulmonary window
• Cardiac defects with severe valve incompetence	Severe mitral regurgitation, severe tricuspid regurgitation (Ebstein anomaly), aortico-left ventricular tunnel.

28.1.3 Hemodynamic Situation

The congenital heart defects that become symptomatic in neonates can be divided into six groups (▶ Table 28.1).

A ductal-dependent defect is a congenital heart defect in which survival depends on the persistence of a patent ductus arteriosus. Ductal-dependent systemic circulation must be distinguished from ductal-dependent pulmonary circulation. In ductal-dependent systemic circulation, there is a high-grade obstruction of the left heart. To ensure sufficient systemic perfusion, the systemic circulation must be supplied with blood from the pulmonary circulation across the patent ductus arteriosus.

In ductal-dependent pulmonary circulation, there is a corresponding high-grade right heart obstruction. Perfusion of the pulmonary circulation depends on blood supply from the aorta across the patent ductus arteriosus.

In parallel circulations (d-TGA), survival depends on shunts (especially a sufficiently large atrial shunt) between the two circulations.

In cardiac defects with complete intracardiac mixing of blood, cyanosis is often only relatively mild, as excessive pulmonary blood flow is often present simultaneously, which leads to pulmonary recirculation of the saturated blood. Heart failure usually develops as a result of the excessive pulmonary blood flow.

Cardiac defects with a large left-to-right shunt usually do not become symptomatic until the age of about 4 to 6 weeks when the pulmonary resistance has dropped and the shunt between the left and right heart increases. If left heart obstruction is also present (e.g., coarctation of the aorta), the symptoms develop as early as the first week of life.

Cardiac defects with predominant severe valve incompetence are rare diseases. In tricuspid valve diseases, these patients have a duct dependent pulmonary circulation. In left sided valve affection these children present in a low cardiac output state.

28.1.4 Diagnostic Measures

Oxygen Saturation

Oxygen saturation should be measured both preductally (right hand) and postductally (lower limb). If there is ductal-dependent systemic circulation, the (postductal) oxygen saturation measured in the legs is lower than the (preductal) saturation in the right hand.

Because the brachiocephalic trunk (except in the rare cases of a lusoria artery) branches off from the aortic arch well before the ductus arteriosus, it is safe to assume that the saturation measured in the right hand is equivalent to preductal saturation.

Blood Gas Analysis

Metabolic acidosis is the typical finding of severe heart failure and cardiogenic shock.

Hyperoxia Test

Note

If possible, an echocardiography examination is preferable to a hyperoxia test. One reason is that a hyperoxia test is associated with diagnostic uncertainty. On the other hand, in ductal-dependent defects, the ductus arteriosus can theoretically close when oxygen is administered. In addition, by lowering the pulmonary resistance as a result of administering oxygen to a patient with a shunt defect, pulmonary blood flow can increase and exacerbate heart failure.

The hyperoxia test is used to distinguish between cardiac or pulmonary central cyanosis. The cyanotic patient is allowed to breathe 100% oxygen for a few minutes. In pulmonary cyanosis, the cyanosis disappears or is clearly reduced and there is a relevant increase in arterial partial oxygen pressure. In cardiac cyanosis, the partial oxygen pressure remains largely unchanged, as the cardiac right-to-left shunt or inadequate pulmonary perfusion cannot be compensated by the administration of oxygen.

Pulse and Blood Pressure in all Limbs

A difference in blood pressure between the right arm (preductal) and the lower limbs (postductal) or pulses in the lower limbs that cannot be palpated are leading findings of coarctation of the aorta or an interrupted aortic arch.

Note:

In a large patent ductus arteriosus, there may be no difference in blood pressure between the upper and lower halves of the body even with relevant coarctation of the aorta or interrupted aortic arch.

Echocardiography

Echocardiography is the diagnostic method of choice. It allows all significant cardiac defects that become symptomatic in the neonatal period to be reliably diagnosed.

28.1.5 Treatment

The treatment principles for the various groups of congenital heart defects are presented below. The specific treatments of the individual heart defects in the neonatal period are then described.

▸ **Cardiac defects with ductal-dependent systemic circulation.** In ductal-dependent systemic circulation, an attempt must be made to allow as much blood flow as possible from the pulmonary circulation to reach the systemic circulation via the patent ductus arteriosus. The treatment principles of ductal-dependent systemic circulation are:

- Maintain patency of the ductus arteriosus with a prostaglandin E_1 infusion (initial dosage 50 to 100 ng/kg/min).
- Lower systemic resistance:
  - Reduce afterload: for example, with sodium nitroprusside infusion.
  - If catecholamines are needed: Give milrinone and/or dobutamine (vasodilatative effects); avoid vasoconstrictive catecholamines (noradrenaline).
- Increase pulmonary resistance, increase pulmonary artery pressure:
  - Avoid additional oxygen.
  - Aim for mild metabolic acidosis (pH 7.35).
  - Aim for mild hypoventilation (pCO_2 around 60 mmHg).
- In case of pulmonary edema, give intravenous furosemide, apply high PEEP; reduce prostaglandin E_1 to a minimum (e.g., 10 ng/kg/min)

Note

The uncritical administration of oxygen and hyperventilation in patients with ductal-dependent systemic circulation can lead to acute decompensation of the hemodynamic situation.

▸ **Cardiac defects with ductal-dependent pulmonary circulation.** In ductal-dependent pulmonary circulation, the situation is reversed. The following measures can be useful to allow as much blood as possible to flow from the systemic circulation to the pulmonary circulation via the patent ductus arteriosus:

- Maintain patency of the ductus arteriosus with a prostaglandin E_1 infusion (initial dosage 50 to 100 ng/kg/min).
- Lower pulmonary resistance:
  - Increase FiO_2.
  - Aim for mild metabolic alkalosis (use buffering is necessary) (pH 7.45–7.5).
  - Adjust ventilation for mild hyperventilation (pCO_2 around 35 mmHg).
- Increase systemic resistance, increase systemic pressure by:
  - noradrenaline infusion,
  - possibly also adrenaline infusion.
- Maintain rather high dosage of prostaglandin E_1.

Excursus: Prostaglandin

Prostaglandin E_1 is given to maintain patency or reopen the ductus arteriosus in neonates with a ductal-dependent defect. Due to its short half-life, it must be administered continuously intravenously. The initial dosage is between 50 and 100 ng/kg/min. Depending on the effect, the dosage can then be gradually reduced to a minimum of 5 to 10 ng/kg/min.

The most common adverse effects are:

- Apnea (administer in readiness for intubation)
- Bradycardia
- Vasodilatation, hypotension
- Edema
- Fever
- Cortical hyperostosis, periostitis only after long-term administration

Practical tip: When using prostaglandin, a second venous access should always be available to ensure the ability to administer prostaglandin immediately via the other access if the first one is dislocated. The second access can also be used for volume substitution in case of acute hypotension.

▸ **Cardiac defects with parallel circulations.** The only example of this kind of heart defect is a d-TGA. Its treatment is described in the specific treatment section.

▸ **Cardiac defects with complete intracardiac mixing of blood.** The different cardiac defects in this group are also described in the specific treatment section.

▸ **Cardiac defects with a large left-to-right shunt.** When the pulmonary resistance drops, the left-to-right shunt and pulmonary blood flow increase. Heart failure develops, which must be treated conservatively (diuretics, ACE inhibitors, beta blockers, possibly digoxin or catecholamines) until corrective surgery is performed. To prevent lowering the pulmonary resistance and thus increasing excessive pulmonary blood flow, no additional oxygen should be administered.

▸ **Cardiac defects with severe valve incompetence.** In left-sided lesions, inotropic support (dubutamine, milrinone) together with adequate afterload reduction (sodium nitroprusside infusion) should be installed. In right-sided lesions, lowering the pulmonary vascular resistance together with inotropic support (milrinone) should be achieved (i.e. additional oxygen).

28.1.6 Specific Treatment of the Most Common Symptomatic Heart Defects in the Neonatal Period

Critical Aortic Stenosis

Hemodynamic Situation

Due to the obstruction in the region of the aortic valve, the left ventricle cannot pump sufficient cardiac output for the systemic circulation. The systemic circulation is supplied with blood from the pulmonary artery via the patent ductus arteriosus. Left ventricular hypertrophy and possibly fibroelastosis have already developed in utero. It is often associated with other left heart obstructions (mitral stenosis, coarctation of the aorta, hypoplastic aortic arch). If a heart murmur is not already detected in the child, many critical aortic stenoses manifest in shock.

In a patient with critical aortic stenosis with ductal-dependent systemic circulation, a shunt at the atrial level is necessary to allow the oxygenated pulmonary venous blood to reach the systemic circulation via the right atrium, the right ventricle, the pulmonary artery, and the patent ductus arteriosus. If the shunt at the atrial level is not large enough, a balloon atrial septostomy (Rashkind maneuver) may be necessary.

Initial Treatment

- Shock therapy, including intubation and ventilation (high PEEP if there is pulmonary edema)
- Prostaglandin E_1: initial dosage 50 to 100 ng/kg/min
- Oxygen: cautiously administered or not at all (lowers pulmonary resistance and thus increases pulmonary blood flow)
- Possibly furosemide, to lower preload or for pulmonary edema
- Possibly catecholamines (dobutamine, adrenaline), possibly milrinone depending on blood pressure and myocardial function. (If there is a subvalvular stenosis, catecholamines should be administered with particular caution due to a possible increase of the obstruction.)
- Possibly reduce afterload (e.g., sodium nitroprusside).
- Aim for moderate metabolic acidosis (target pH 7.35).
- Administer as little volume as possible; preferably only after cardiac function has recovered or is assessed to be stable in echocardiography.

Further Procedure

Ensure prompt transfer to a pediatric cardiac center for interventional catheterization and performance of balloon valvuloplasty or surgical commissurotomy; possibly carry out an emergency Rashkind maneuver if there is a restrictive foramen ovale.

Coarctation of the Aorta

Hemodynamic Situation

In a critical coarctation of the aorta, the lower half of the body is supplied with blood from the pulmonary artery via the patent ductus arteriosus. When the ductus arteriosus closes, dramatic hypoperfusion distal to the aortic isthmus occurs. The left ventricle is suddenly forced to pump against the pronounced obstruction. Rapid decompensation usually occurs. Associations with other left heart obstructions or a VSD are not infrequent.

Initial Treatment

- Shock therapy, including intubation and ventilation (high PEEP if there is pulmonary edema)
- Prostaglandin E_1: initial dosage 50 to 100 ng/kg/min
- Oxygen: administered cautiously or not at all (lowers pulmonary resistance and thus increases pulmonary blood flow)
- Possibly furosemide to lower preload or for pulmonary edema
- Possibly catecholamines (dobutamine, adrenaline), possibly milrinone depending on blood pressure and myocardial function
- Possibly reduce afterload (e.g., sodium nitroprusside).
- Aim for moderate metabolic acidosis (target pH 7.35).
- Administer as little volume as possible; preferably only after cardiac function has recovered or is assessed to be stable in echocardiography.

Further Procedure

Prompt transfer to a pediatric cardiac center for surgical correction, which is generally attempted after the hemodynamic situation has been stabilized. In exceptions, primary interventional catheterization for stabilization until surgery may be indicated (e.g., for patients in poor general condition with necrotic enterocolitis).

Interrupted Aortic Arch

Hemodynamic Situation

In an interrupted aortic arch, perfusion of the lower half of the body depends entirely on a patent ductus arteriosus. A VSD is nearly always associated with an interrupted aortic arch and other left heart obstructions occur occasionally. In an interrupted aortic arch, oxygen saturation should be measured preductally (right hand), as the preductal saturation reflects the situation in the CNS and coronary arteries. The levels measured in the lower limbs correspond with pulmonary arterial saturation.

Initial Treatment

- Shock therapy, including intubation and ventilation (high PEEP if there is pulmonary edema)
- Prostaglandin E_1: initial dosage 50 to 100 ng/kg/min
- Oxygen: administered cautiously or not at all; target saturation at the right hand (preductal) 95%
- Possibly furosemide to lower preload or for pulmonary edema
- Possibly catecholamines (dobutamine, adrenaline), possibly milrinone depending on blood pressure and myocardial function
- Possibly reduce afterload (e.g., sodium nitroprusside).
- Aim for moderate metabolic acidosis (target pH 7.35).
- Administer as little volume as possible; preferably only after cardiac function has recovered or is assessed to be stable in echocardiography.

Further Procedure

Prompt transfer to a pediatric cardiac center for surgical correction.

Hypoplastic Left Heart Syndrome

Hemodynamic Situation

In a hypoplastic left heart syndrome, both the pulmonary and systemic systems are supplied by the right ventricle. Retrograde coronary perfusion takes place across the ductus arteriosus with mixed blood from the pulmonary artery. Within the first few hours of life, the drop in pulmonary resistance causes the blood from the pulmonary artery to flow primarily into the pulmonary circulation and the systemic circulation—and thus the coronary arteries as well—are increasingly less perfused. Severe heart failure develops, which occasionally results in shock. There is severe metabolic acidosis in the blood gas analysis, but due to pulmonary recirculation; cyanosis should however be detected during routine neonatal pulse oximetry screening. the oxygen saturation is often only moderately reduced. The higher the oxygen saturation is, the more the ratio of pulmonary to systemic perfusion changes are in favor of pulmonary perfusion.

Thereafter the patent ductus arteriosus has a tendency to close. This leads to additional severe impairment of perfusion of the whole body, especially the coronaries and the heart, the brain, and the abdominal organs, and subsequently to severe shock with profound metabolic acidosis.

It is important to note that oxygenated pulmonary venous blood from the left atrium can reach the systemic circulation only across a sufficiently large shunt to the right atrium and then across the right ventricle, pulmonary artery, and patent ductus arteriosus.

Initial Treatment

- Shock treatment, including intubation and ventilation (but avoid ventilation if possible, as long as the pH is balanced); hyperventilation must be avoided
- If possible avoid intubation and ventilation; extubate early after initial stabilization.
- Prostaglandin E_1: initial dosage 50 to 100 ng/kg/min
- Avoid administering oxygen (additionally reduces pulmonary resistance and thus systemic perfusion), target saturation 70 to 85%.
- Possibly furosemide may be used to lower preload or for pulmonary edema.
- Catecholamine treatment is often required, but should be administered with restraint (can increase the myocardial oxygen consumption), give milrinone if needed.
- Possibly reduce afterload (e.g., sodium nitroprusside).
- Aim for moderate metabolic acidosis (over-buffering) (target pH 7.35).
- Administer as little volume as possible; preferably only after cardiac function has recovered or is assessed to be stable in echocardiography.

Further Procedure

If there is a restrictive atrial defect (leading symptom: seriously ill child, severe cyanosis, oxygen saturation < 65%), an emergency balloon atrial septostomy (Rashkind maneuver) is needed.

After stabilization, the patient should be transferred quickly to a pediatric cardiac center for surgery (usually a Norwood procedure as the first step of three-stage Fontan palliation).

Critical Pulmonary Stenosis

Hemodynamic Situation

A critical pulmonary stenosis is a high-grade obstruction of the pulmonary valve with hypoxemia. Hypoxemia is caused because the right ventricle cannot deliver the blood flow adequately into the pulmonary circulation, and hypoxia occurs due to a right-to-left shunt across the foramen ovale. The right ventricle is usually clearly hypertrophic and the right ventricle and tricuspid valve are sometimes also hypoplastic. The pulmonary circulation is supplied with blood from the aorta via the patent ductus arteriosus.

Initial Treatment

- Prostaglandin E_1 infusion: initial dosage 50 to 100 ng/kg/min
- Generous oxygen therapy (lowers pulmonary resistance)
- Aim for mild metabolic alkalosis (over-buffering) (pH 7.45–7.5)
- Possibly ventilation and mild hyperventilation (pCO_2 around 35 mmHg)
- Possibly effect increase in systemic resistance (adrenaline or noradrenaline)

Further Procedure

Rapid transfer to a pediatric cardiac center for interventional catheter balloon valvuloplasty.

Pulmonary Atresia with Intact Ventricular Septum

Hemodynamic Situation

In pulmonary atresia with intact ventricular septum, the right ventricle cannot drain the intraventricular blood volume normally to the pulmonary arteries. The blood from the right ventricle either flows back into the right atrium due to tricuspid regurgitation, or the right ventricle is connected with the coronary arteries via myocardial sinusoids. In the latter case, the coronary arteries are frequently atretic or stenotic and coronary perfusion may depend on blood flow from the right ventricle. There is suprasystemic pressure in the right ventricle. The right ventricle is hypoplastic to various degrees. The pulmonary circulation is supplied with blood from the aorta via the ductus arteriosus.

Initial Treatment

- Prostaglandin E_1 infusion: initial dosage 50 to 100 ng/kg/min
- Generous oxygen administration (lowers pulmonary resistance)
- Aim for mild metabolic alkalosis (over-buffering) (pH 7.45–7.5)
- Possibly ventilation and mild hyperventilation (pCO_2 around 35 mmHg)
- Possibly effect increase in systemic resistance (adrenaline or noradrenaline)

Further Procedure

Rapid transfer to a pediatric cardiac center. Cardiac catheterization is almost always needed to rule out myocardial sinusoids and coronary anomalies. Sometimes it is possible to open the right ventricular outflow tract by interventional catheterization or implant a stent into the ductus arteriosus, otherwise interim palliative surgery (opening the right ventricular outflow tract, aortopulmonary shunt) must be performed quickly.

Tricuspid Atresia

Hemodynamic Situation

In tricuspid atresia, there is no continuity between the right atrium and ventricle, so the right atrium can only drain into the left atrium only across a right-to-left shunt at the atrial level. The right ventricle is usually perfused from the left ventricle across a VSD that is almost always present. The right ventricle can be hypoplastic to various extents. Because of the complete mixing of blood, oxygen saturation is identical in the aorta and pulmonary artery. Stenosis and even atresia of the pulmonary artery occur frequently and have a decisive effect on the blood flow to the pulmonary circulation. If there is atresia or a high-grade stenosis of the pulmonary artery, perfusion of the lungs depends on a patent ductus arteriosus. The great vessels can be in normal position or transposed.

If there is no pulmonary stenosis and blood flow to the pulmonary circulation is unobstructed, the main symptom is heart failure (tachypnea, hepatomegaly, pallor, possible pulmonary edema), but this constellation is much less common.

Initial Treatment

For high-grade pulmonary stenosis or atresia (leading symptom: cyanosis):

- Prostaglandin E_1 infusion: initial dosage 50 to 100 ng/kg/min
- Generous oxygen therapy (lowers pulmonary resistance)
- Aim for mild metabolic alkalosis (over-buffering) (pH 7.45–7.5)
- Possibly ventilation and mild hyperventilation (pCO_2 around 35 mmHg)
- Possibly effect increase in systemic resistance (adrenaline or noradrenaline)

If there is no pulmonary stenosis (leading symptom: heart failure):

- Anticongestive treatment (diuretics, possibly catecholamines)
- Restrictive oxygen therapy
- Restrictive volume therapy

Further Procedure

Rapid transfer to a pediatric cardiac center. If there is a restrictive atrial shunt (rare), an interventional catheter balloon atrial septostomy (Rashkind maneuver) is needed. Otherwise, if lung perfusion is low, an aortopulmonary shunt is placed as a palliative measure. The separation of circulations is performed in a Fontan procedure.

Tetralogy of Fallot

Hemodynamic Situation

In tetralogy of Fallot, pulmonary blood flow and thus cyanosis are determined by the extent of the obstruction of the right ventricular outflow tract. In most cases, this obstruction is only mild at birth, but becomes more significant due to the increase in the infundibular stenosis during the first few weeks of life. If there is pronounced stenosis of the right ventricular outflow tract (functional pulmonary atresia), the children may already develop symptoms with cyanosis or cyanotic spells in the neonatal period.

Initial Treatment

- For functional pulmonary atresia, prostaglandin E_1 infusion: initial dosage 50 to 100 ng/kg/min
- Generous oxygen therapy (lowers pulmonary resistance)
- Aim for mild metabolic alkalosis (over-buffering) (pH 7.45–7.5)
- Generous volume treatment
- Possibly ventilation and mild hyperventilation (pCO_2 around 35 mmHg)
- Possibly effect increase in systemic resistance (noradrenaline; caution: catecholamines and digoxin increase the infundibular stenosis)

Treatment of a Cyanotic Spell

- Immediate sedation (e.g., ketamine IV 1–3 mg/kg, alternatively opiates, benzodiazepines)
- Oxygen therapy
- Increase of systemic resistance by pressing the child's flexed knee against the chest ("jack-knife position"), possibly infusion of vasoconstrictors (noradrenaline)
- Generous volume bolus (e.g., 20–50 mL/kg)
- Compensation of metabolic acidosis by buffering
- Possibly beta blockers (e.g., propranolol IV 0.01–0.1 mg/kg very slowly under monitor guidance)

Further Procedure

Rapid transfer to a pediatric cardiac center. In some cases, early surgical correction is attempted. In special situations (e.g., very small children) an aortopulmonary shunt is first placed as a palliative measure to ensure lung perfusion. In case of pulmonary valve stenosis, balloon dilation can initially improve lung perfusion. This measure is not likely to be successful for infundibular stenoses.

In such patients, interventional placement of a stent in the right ventricular outflow tract underneath the pulmonary valve has become an excellent palliative treatment option.

Pulmonary Atresia with Ventricular Septal Defect

Hemodynamic Situation

From the hemodynamic aspect, this disease is an extreme form of tetralogy of Fallot. Lung perfusion is dependent on a patent ductus arteriosus or aortopulmonary collaterals.

Initial Treatment

- Prostaglandin E_1 infusion: initial dosage 50–100 ng/kg/min
- Generous oxygen therapy (lowers pulmonary resistance)
- Aim for mild metabolic alkalosis (over-buffering) (pH 7.45–7.5)
- Generous volume therapy
- Possibly ventilation and mild hyperventilation (pCO_2 around 35 mmHg)
- Possibly effect increase in systemic resistance (adrenaline or noradrenaline)

Further Procedure

Rapid transfer to a pediatric cardiac center. If there is only membranous valvular atresia, an attempt can be made to open the valve by interventional catheterization, possibly placing a stent in the right ventricular outflow tract across the pulmonary valve area or in the ductus arteriosus to achieve catch-up growth of the pulmonary vessels, which are almost always hypoplastic.

Otherwise, an aortopulmonary shunt is placed first as surgical palliation. After catch-up growth of the pulmonary vascular system, continuity between the pulmonary vessels and the right ventricle is created later (e.g., with a valved conduit).

Ebstein Anomaly

Hemodynamic Situation

A pronounced Ebstein anomaly is already symptomatic in the neonatal period. In Ebstein anomaly, there is apical displacement of the tricuspid valve into the right ventricle. There is usually severe tricuspid regurgitation and only a slight flow from the functionally small right ventricle to the pulmonary artery. The right atrium is markedly to massively dilated. Cyanosis occurs due to a right-to-left shunt at the atrial level.

The disease is often complicated by accessory pathways and Wolf–Parkinson–White syndrome.

Initial Treatment

- If there is insufficient antegrade flow through the pulmonary artery (leading symptom: severe cyanosis), prostaglandin E_1 infusion: initial dosage 50–100 ng/kg/min
- Generous oxygen therapy (lowers pulmonary resistance)
- Aim for mild metabolic alkalosis (over-buffering) (pH 7.45–7.5)
- Possibly ventilation and mild hyperventilation (pCO_2 around 35 mmHg)
- Possibly effect increase in systemic resistance (noradrenaline)
- If there is heart failure, possibly catecholamines and diuretics
- If there is supraventricular tachycardia, it should be terminated with a vagal maneuver, adenosine, amiodarone, possibly cardioversion (Chapter 18)

Further Procedure

Rapid transfer to a pediatric cardiac center. The goal of surgical treatment is to reconstruct the tricuspid valve. If there is insufficient lung perfusion, it may be necessary to place an aortopulmonary shunt as a palliative measure. If there is pronounced hypoplasia of the right ventricle, the only option may be univentricular Fontan palliation. The overall prognosis is poor for children who become symptomatic in the neonatal period.

d-Transposition of the Great Vessels

Hemodynamic Situation

In d-TGA, the pulmonary and systemic circulations are connected in parallel instead of in series: the systemic venous blood is pumped back into the aorta and the oxygenated pulmonic venous blood is pumped back to the pulmonary artery. Survival is possible only if there are shunts between the two circulatory systems. The most important is a shunt at the atrial level (patent foramen ovale or ASD), so oxygenated blood can reach the right ventricle and thus the systemic circulation across the left-to-right shunt. A patent ductus arteriosus has a favorable effect on oxygenation because blood flows from the aorta into the pulmonary circulation and increases lung perfusion. As a result of the increased pulmonary venous blood flow, the pressure in the left ventricle is increased, so the left-to-right shunt at the atrial level increases and more oxygenated blood can reach the systemic circulation.

Oxygen therapy acts indirectly by lowering pulmonary resistance and thus increasing pulmonary perfusion and left atrial pressure (caution: uncontrolled administration of oxygen can also lead to closure of the ductus arteriosus).

In addition to improving the mixing of blood between the two circulations, especially in "poor mixers," an attempt should be made to improve mixed venous saturation. Venous saturation is largely equivalent to systemic arterial saturation if there is poor mixing between the circulations.

If there is an associated large VSD, cyanosis is usually less pronounced.

Initial Treatment

- Prostaglandin E_1 infusion: initial dosage 50 to 100 ng/kg/min
- Generous volume therapy
- Aim for mild metabolic alkalosis (over-buffering) (pH 7.45–7.5, lowers pulmonary resistance)
- Oxygen therapy for severe cyanosis in neonates (caution: induces closure of the ductus arteriosus)
- Possibly consider intubation, ventilation, and relaxation (lowers oxygen consumption and therefore increases mixed venous saturation. On the other hand, ventilation increases the intrathoracic pressure, which can hinder mixing of the blood)
- Consider giving catecholamines (improve cardiac output and thus mixed venous saturation)
- Generous treatment of anemia with a transfusion (improves oxygen supply)

Further Procedure

Rapid transfer to a pediatric cardiac center. If there is a restrictive shunt at the atrial level, an interventional catheter balloon atrial septostomy (Rashkind maneuver) should be performed as soon as possible. The surgical treatment of choice today is an arterial switch operation (Jatene procedure) within the first 2 weeks of life.

Truncus Arteriosus Communis

Hemodynamic Situation

In a truncus arteriosus communis, only one vessel arises from the heart. The systemic and pulmonary circulation and the coronaries are supplied with blood from this common trunk. A ventricular septal defect is almost always present. The trunk vessel contains mixed blood. Since the blood follows the path of least resistance and tends to flow into the pulmonary circulation, there is often excessive pulmonary blood flow after the drop in pulmonary resistance between the second and eighth week of life. Clinical signs of heart failure are already present in the first weeks of life. Due to pulmonary recirculation, there is often only very mild cyanosis, although the trunk vessel contains only mixed blood.

In addition the common truncal valve can be stenotic or-more often- incompetent, so that regurgitation may substantially aggravate the hemodynamic situation.

Initial Treatment

- Do not administer oxygen uncritically! (Oxygen lowers pulmonary resistance and thus increases blood flow to the pulmonary circulation, leading to excessive pulmonary blood flow and increasing heart failure.)
- Treatment of heart failure: diuretics, possibly catecholamines (dobutamine) or phosphodiesterase inhibitor (milrinone), afterload reducer (ACE inhibitor, possibly sodium nitroprusside)
- In association with an interrupted aortic arch: prostaglandin E_1 infusion: initial dosage 50 to 100 ng/kg/min

Further Procedure

Elective transfer to a pediatric cardiac center. The definitive correction with a Rastelli procedure is generally performed within the first weeks of life owing to heart failure.

Total Anomalous Pulmonary Venous Connection

Hemodynamic Situation

In a total anomalous pulmonary venous connection, all pulmonary veins drain into the systemic venous system and from there into the right atrium. The perfusion of the systemic circulation thus depends on a right-to-left shunt at the atrial level that is necessary for survival. Depending on the anomalous connection of the pulmonary veins, we distinguish between supracardiac, cardiac, infracardiac, and mixed forms.

It is particularly important that an infracardiac total anomalous pulmonary venous connection is regularly associated with an obstruction of the pulmonary veins.

In a total anomalous pulmonary venous connection without obstruction of the pulmonary vein, the hemodynamic situation is similar to that of a large ASD (volume overload of the right atrium, ventricle, and pulmonary circulation).

Initial Treatment

Total anomalous pulmonary venous connection with obstruction of the pulmonary vein:

- Oxygen therapy
- For pulmonary edema, intubation and ventilation with a high PEEP
- Lower pulmonary resistance: hyperventilation, possibly inhaled NO or prostacyclin IV, generous buffering (target pH 7.45–7.5), increase oxygen supply
- Diuretics, possibly catecholamines for low cardiac output (caution: catecholamines can exacerbate pulmonary edema)

Further Procedure

A total anomalous pulmonary venous connection with obstruction of the pulmonary vein is an absolute cardiac surgery emergency that must be surgically corrected immediately. In individual cases, dilation with or without stent implantation can eliminate the stenosis of the pulmonary vein so the operation can then be performed after the child is stabilized.

If there is a restrictive atrial shunt or if surgical correction is not possible immediately, an interventional catheter balloon atrial septostomy (Rashkind maneuver) may be considered.

Complete Atrioventricular Septal Defect

Hemodynamic Situation

In a complete atrioventricular septal defect (AVSD, AV canal), segments of the atrial and ventricular septum in the region of the AV valves are absent. The development of the AV valves is also impaired. The result is a large left-to-right shunt that increases within the first weeks of life when the pulmonary resistance drops. The situation can be complicated by AV valve insufficiency. Children with a complete AVSD usually develop heart failure when the pulmonary resistance drops after 2 to 8 weeks of life.

> **Note**
>
> An AVSD is frequently associated with trisomy 21. All neonates with trisomy 21 should therefore have an echocardiography at an early age.

Initial Treatment

- Avoid oxygen (excessive pulmonary blood flow is increased)
- Pharmacological treatment of heart failure: diuretics, ACE inhibitors, beta blockers, possibly digoxin, possibly catecholamines

Further Procedure

Elective transfer to a pediatric cardiac center. The corrective surgery is generally performed at the age of 4 to 6 months, possibly sooner if conservative heart failure treatment is unsuccessful.

29 Heart Transplantation

29.1 Basics

Heart transplantation has become an established treatment for children with terminal heart failure. In some centers, heart transplants are performed even on neonates with complex congenital heart defects. In childhood, heart transplants are most often performed on patients with a dilated cardiomyopathy. In children under 1 year old, the indication for heart transplantation is a hypoplastic left heart syndrome.

Lifelong immunosuppressive therapy is required after a heart transplant. Transplants are also considerably limited due to the global lack of donor organs.

In Germany, donor organs are assigned via Eurotransplant in Leiden (Netherlands). Besides Germany, Austria, the Benelux countries, Croatia, and Slovenia are linked with this central registry for organ donors and recipients. There are also links with other European centers.

29.1.1 Epidemiology

More than 75,000 heart transplants have now been performed across the world. Children are involved in around 10% of all heart transplants. Every year, around 400 children receive heart transplants.

29.1.2 Indications

A heart transplant is considered the last treatment option for terminal heart failure when other measures are not likely to succeed. For complex congenital heart defects, it may be an alternative to surgical palliation. According to clinical aspects, a heart transplant is generally indicated if the estimated survival time is less than 6 to 12 months.

Possible indications for heart transplantation in childhood include the following:

- Cardiomyopathies:
  - Dilatated cardiomyopathy (most frequent indication for heart transplantation in childhood)
  - Hypertrophic cardiomyopathy
  - Restrictive cardiomyopathy
  - Endocardial fibroelastosis
  - Arrhythmogenic right ventricular cardiomyopathy
- Congenital heart defects:
  - Hypoplastic left heart syndrome
  - Shone complex (extreme form)
  - Complete AVSD with hypoplastic left ventricle
  - Single ventricle with subaortic obstruction
  - Severe forms of Ebstein anomaly
  - Pulmonary atresia with intact ventricular septum and pronounced coronary fistulas/sinusoids
  - Bland–White–Garland syndrome with extensive infarction
  - Irreversible failure of the systemic ventricle following an atrial baffle procedure or Fontan procedure
- Cardiac tumors (obstructive, nonresectable tumors)
- Malignant arrhythmias (untreatable by pharmacological means or intervention, e.g., associated with arrhythmogenic right ventricular dysplasia)
- Coronary anomalies (severe changes, e.g., after Kawasaki syndrome)

29.1.3 Contraindications

The list of contraindications for a heart transplant is continuously evolving. Some of the contraindications listed below are relative contraindications. From the surgical perspective, for a heart transplant due to a congenital heart defect, it is important that the pulmonary veins are sufficiently large. In addition, for a total anomalous pulmonary vein connection, pulmonary venous confluence must be present that can be anastomosed with the left atrium of the donor heart.

Absolute or relative contraindications are:

- Severe fixed increase in pulmonary resistance
- Diffuse hypoplasia of the pulmonary arteries
- Total anomalous pulmonary vein connection without a pulmonary venous confluence
- Ectopia cordis
- Active systemic Infection
- HIV infection or chronic active hepatitis B or C
- Irreversible liver or kidney dysfunction
- Multiple organ failure
- Untreatable malignant disease
- Drug dependency
- Systemic diseases that impair the recovery or survival after the transplantation (e.g., neuromuscular diseases)
- Severe malformation syndromes
- Severe diseases of the CNS
- Lack of compliance by the patient or family
- Weight less than 1,800 g
- Preterm infants born before the 36th week of gestation

29.1.4 Diagnostics of the Organ Recipient

The diagnostic measures for the recipient before the heart transplant include the following examinations:

- Routine blood tests: blood count, blood sugar, electrolytes including magnesium, phosphate, urea, creatinine, uric acid, protein, INR, PTT, AT III, AST, ALT, γGT, LDH, AP, CK, CRP, iron, ferritin, transferrin, cholesterol, triglycerides, carnitine, T3, fT4, TSH, BGA
- Auto-antibodies: ANA, smooth muscles, heart muscle, cardiolipin antibodies

- Thrombophilia screening
- Infection serology: CMV, EBV, HSV, hepatitis A, hepatitis B, hepatitis C, Coxsackie, adenovirus, influenza/parainfluenza virus, HIV, measles, mumps, rubella, varicella, Candida, Aspergillus, toxoplasmosis.
- HLA typing and HLA antibody screening
- Cytoimmunological examination
- Urine status
- Metabolism screening
- Stool test for pathogens
- Tuberculin test
- ECG
- Echocardiography
- Chest X-ray
- Cardiac catheterization including coronary angiography and biopsy
- Abdominal ultrasonography, also cranial ultrasound for infants
- Cranial MRI
- ENT examination and dental status (to rule out a source of infection)

29.1.5 Diagnostics of the Organ Donor

The organ donor must fulfill the German Medical Association's criteria for brain death. The current criteria can be seen at www.baek.de.

The transplantation is generally between compatible blood types. However, even ABO-incompatible hearts have now been successfully transplanted—especially in children under age 1 year, in whom antibodies against the blood type characteristics have not yet formed. The significance of the human leukocyte antigens (HLAs) is not fully understood. Prospective HLA matching is not yet carried out, although a total HLA mismatch is considered to be a risk factor. Donor and recipient hearts should be of approximately the same size. A weight difference of up to 20% between donor and recipient is tolerable. Larger donor hearts are better tolerated than smaller. To prevent long ischemia times, the time between explantation and implantation should not exceed 4 (–8) hours. After explantation, the organ is stored in a cardioplegic solution at 4°C. The donor should be stabilized in intensive care until explantation (e.g., maintain adequate blood pressure, balance fluids and electrolytes, avoid hypoxia and anemia).

Exclusion criteria for organ donors (from Overbeck 2007):

- Malignant disease (except primary brain tumors)
- Active bacterial, viral, or mycotic infections
- Positive HIV serology
- Diffuse coronary sclerosis
- Documented heart attack
- Treatment-resistant ventricular arrhythmias
- CO poisoning

Relative exclusion criteria:

- Positive HBsAg or HBc test
- Severe chest trauma
- Prolonged hypotension
- High catecholamine use
- Prolonged hypoxia
- Known cardiac diseases (except patent foramen ovale, ASD II, PDA)

29.1.6 Surgical Procedure

Orthotopic heart transplantation is the usual procedure. A surgical technique is used that was described in 1960 by Lower and Shumway. In this procedure, the diseased heart is excised, leaving the posterior walls of the right and left atria, which are anastomosed with the donor heart. The stump of the aorta and pulmonary artery of the donor heart are anastomosed end-to-end with the respective vessels of the recipient (▶ Fig. 29.1).

A modification of this surgical technique is required in a hypoplastic left heart syndrome because the aorta of the recipient must be augmented with a long segment of the donor aorta (▶ Fig. 29.2).

29.1.7 Postoperative Treatment

Immunosuppressive Treatment

Immunosuppressive treatment is begun a few hours before the transplantation and must be continued lifelong (▶ Table 29.1). In most centers, a combination treatment with cyclosporine A, azathioprine, and steroids is carried out initially. In some centers, induction therapy with anti-lymphocyte antibodies (OKT3, ATG) is also started in the early postoperative period.

The most important immunosuppressants are listed below.

Calcineurin Inhibitors

▸ **Cyclosporine A.** The introduction of cyclosporine A in the 1980s led to the decisive breakthrough in immunosuppressive treatment after a heart transplant. Cyclosporine is a fungal metabolite. It inhibits the production and release of interleukin 1 from activated macrophages and interleukin 2 from activated T helper cells. Cyclosporine is broken down mainly in the liver. A serious side effect of calcineurin inhibitors is nephrotoxicity, which leads to progressive chronic renal failure in many patients. In addition, hypertension requiring treatment often develops (especially in a combination therapy with steroids). Neurotoxicity can lead to tremor and paresthesia. Moreover, hypertrichosis, gingival hyperplasia, and neurodermitis are frequent. At therapeutic dosages, no bone marrow depression occurs, but the therapeutic range is narrow and laboratory controls are required. Interactions

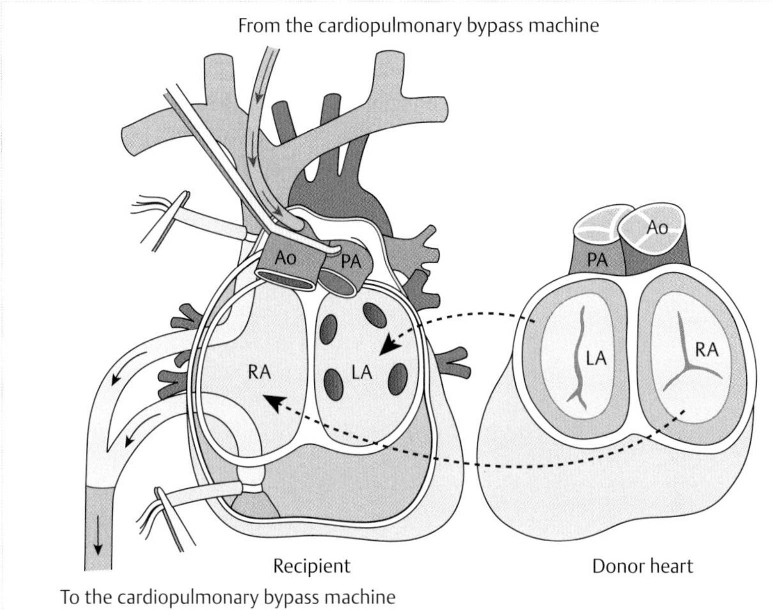

Fig. 29.1 Orthotopic heart transplantation. In the usual surgical technique, the posterior walls of the recipient are left and anastomosed with the atria of the donor heart. The stumps of the aorta and pulmonary artery of the donor heart are anastomosed end-to-end with the respective vessels of the recipient.
RA, right atrium; LA, left atrium; PA, pulmonary artery; Ao, aorta.

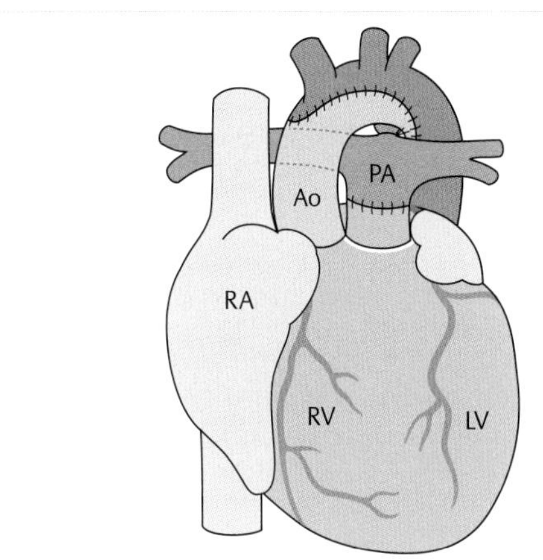

Fig. 29.2 Heart transplantation in a hypoplastic left heart syndrome. Since the recipient's ascending aorta is markedly hypoplastic, it must be augmented using the ascending aorta of the donor.
RA, right atrium; RV, right ventricle; LV, left ventricle; PA, pulmonary artery; Ao, aorta.

Table 29.1 Immunosuppressive therapy for heart transplants (example)

Initial therapy	
Cyclosporine A	Preoperative: 5–6 mg/kg/d continuously IV until operation Postoperative: 1–3 mg/kg/d continuously IV Later 5–10 (–30) mg/kg/d orally depending on the level measured *
Azathioprine	Preoperative: 3–4 mg/kg Postoperative: 1–2 mg/kg/d in two single doses
Prednisolone	< 10 kg: 3 × 12.5 mg/kg/d for 3 days 10–30 kg: 3 × 125 mg/d for 3 days 30–60 kg: 3 × 250 mg/d for 3 days > 60 kg: 4 × 250 mg/d for 3 days
Maintenance therapy	
Cyclosporine A	5–10 mg/kg/d orally depending on level measured *
Azathioprine	1–2 mg/kg/d orally
Prednisolone	1 mg/kg/d orally, gradual reduction to 0.1 mg/kg/d

* Target levels: perioperative 300–350 ng/mL; 3–6 months after heart transplantation 200–250 ng/mL; 6–12 months after heart transplantation 150–200 ng/mL; more than 12 months after heart transplantation 100–150 ng/mL.

with other drugs are common—for example, elevation of the serum level of cyclosporine A during simultaneous treatment with erythromycin, itraconazole, ketoconazole, amphotericin B, oral contraceptives, and some calcium antagonists; whereas the serum level of cyclosporine A can drop under treatment with phenytoin, carbamazepine, or barbiturates.

► **Tacrolimus (FK 506).** Tacrolimus has a mode of action similar to that of cyclosporine A, but its immunosuppressive effect is significantly stronger. The range of side effects is comparable with cyclosporine A (nephro- and neurotoxic), but hypertrichosis and gingival hyperplasia are not typical side effects. Tacrolimus is therefore an option if hypertrichosis or gingival hyperplasia has occurred under cyclosporine.

Antimetabolites

► **Azathioprine.** Azathioprine is metabolized in the liver to 6-mercaptopurine and affects protein biosynthesis as an antimetabolite. It has some selective anti-T cell activity. Over time, the dosage is usually controlled so that the white blood cell count is between 4 and 6/nL.

► **Mycophenolate.** Mycophenolate leads to selective proliferation inhibition of lymphocytes via a reversible inhibition of inosine monophosphate dehydrogenase. The most important side effects are diarrhea, vomiting, and leukopenia. It is not nephrotoxic and does not cause hypertension. In some centers, it is used as an alternative to azathioprine.

► **Steroids.** Steroids act primarily by inhibiting the cytokine interleukin 1. In this way they inhibit the cellular and humoral immune response.

Lymphocyte Antibodies

► **OKT 3.** OKT 3 is a murine monoclonal antibody against the CD3 antigen of human T cells, which it blocks. However, prior to this, cytokine is released. OKT 3 is therefore often poorly tolerated. Fever and chills are common. Hypersensitivity reactions up to anaphylactic shock may occur. For this reason, OKT 3 is not administered until after prophylaxis with a steroid and antihistamine as well as pretesting with a lower dose. It is used mainly for acute steroid-resistant rejection reactions, in some centers during induction therapy as well.

► **Antithymocyte globulin.** This is a polyclonal antibody from rabbits against human T cells. The range of side effects and indications are similar to those of OKT 3.

Infections

Infections are the most common cause of death in the first year following a heart transplant. The appropriate hygiene measures must be maintained immediately postoperatively in the ICU (airlock, sterile gowns, mask, cap).

In the early phase, nosocomial infections must be especially considered (e.g., catheter infections with *Staphylococcus* species or infections with gram-negative pathogens such as Enterobacter and Klebsiella). Later, opportunistic infections (CMV, HSV, Aspergillus, Pneumocystis carinii) play an important role.

The most important infections in transplanted patients include those with the cytomegalovirus (CMV), which can arise either as a primary infection (e.g., from blood products or a CMV-positive organ donor) or as reactivation of a previous CMV infection in the recipient. A CMV infection typically occurs 1 to 3 months after the transplantation ("40-day fever"). The highest risk is for CMV-negative recipients of an organ from a CMV-positive donor. Because of the significance of opportunistic infections, infection prophylaxis against CMV, Candida, and Pneumocystis carinii infections in the initial period after the transplantation is justified (► Table 29.2).

Rejection

Forms of Rejection

Different types of rejection reactions are distinguished depending on the time they become manifest and their course.

► **Hyperacute rejection reaction.** A hyperacute rejection reaction occurs within the first hours or days after the heart transplantation. The cause is presensitization of the recipient (e.g., formation of preformed cytotoxic antibodies after transfusions). The prognosis is very poor. These antibodies can be detected early in preoperative laboratory tests (panel reactive antibody).

► **Acute rejection.** Acute rejection is a process mediated by T cells that is almost always caused by insufficient immunosuppression.

Table 29.2 Example of infection prophylaxis following heart transplantation

Pathogen	Medication	Dosage
CMV	CMV immunoglobulin	100–400 mg/kg 2 × per week in the first 2 weeks after the heart transplant
• For a CMV-positive recipient	CMV immunoglobulin	100 mg/kg 2–3 × per week in the first weeks after the heart transplant
• For a CMV-positive donor	Ganciclovir or acyclovir	• Ganciclovir: 10 mg/kg in 2 single doses per day for 23 weeks or • Acyclovir: 30 mg/kg in 2 single doses per day for 3 months
Candida	Amphotericin B suspension	6 single doses per day orally for 6 months
Pneumocystis carinii	Cotrimoxazole	2 × per week for 1 year, dosage depends on age: • Up to 5 months: 40 mg Trimethoprim p.o. • 6 months to 5 years: 80–120 mg Trimethoprim p.o. • 6–12 years: 160–320 mg Trimethoprim p.o.

▶ **Chronic rejection.** Chronic rejection manifests as transplant vasculopathy associated with intima thickening of the coronary vessels. Transplant vasculopathy has a decisive effect on the long-term survival after a heart transplant. The fact that patients do not have any typical symptoms of angina pectoris due to the denervation of the donor heart makes it difficult to make the clinical diagnosis in time. Treatment approaches are calcium antagonists or HMG-CoA reductase inhibitors and newer immunosuppressants. Sometimes a new transplant is needed.

Diagnostic Measures

The gold standard for rejection diagnostics is an endomyocardial biopsy, but rejection can often be reliably assessed using endocardiography parameters. If a myocardial biopsy is not performed, the severity of rejection must be estimated based on the clinical picture and examination findings.

Typical signs of acute rejection are:

- Fever, pallor, discomfort, edema, gallop rhythm
- ECG: low voltage, arrhythmias, AV block, bundle branch block, repolarization disturbances
- Echocardiography: impaired systolic and/or diastolic function, myocardial thickening, mitral regurgitation, pericardial effusion
- Laboratory: elevated white blood cells, conspicuous cytoimmunological finding

Treatment

The treatment of rejection depends on the histological severity of the reaction (classification according to Billingham et al. 1990)[51]. A minimal rejection reaction does not require treatment. For mild rejection, the previous immunosuppressive therapy is optimized. Moderate to severe rejection requires treatment with high-dose steroids, if unsuccessful, supplemented with OKT 3 or ATG (▶ Table 29.3).

Aftercare

Even long after surgery, the patient must remain in close contact with the transplant center. In addition to the clinical examination, regulatory laboratory tests (including blood count, drug levels, CMV/EBV serology, kidney enzymes) and ECG and echocardiography are carried out.

The children may usually return to kindergarten or school 3 months after a heart transplant. Vaccinations should have been completed before the heart transplantation; otherwise they may be completed 6 months after the transplant. However, live vaccines (measles, mumps, rubella, varicella, oral polio) are contraindicated. After contact with measles, varicella, or herpes zoster, the respective immunoglobulins are given; in case of varicella or herpes zoster, possibly acyclovir in addition. After contact with herpes simplex, oral acyclovir is also used. One year after a heart transplant, many centers perform cardiac catheterization including coronary angiography. If the findings are unremarkable, the next examinations are conducted in 2 to 3 years. In most centers, routine myocardial biopsies are no longer performed in children.

Table 29.3 Example of treatment of acute rejection following heart transplantation

Prednisolone	• < 10 kg: 3 × per day 12.5 mg/kg IV for 3 days • 10–30 kg: 3 × 125 mg/d IV for 3 days • 30–60 kg: 3 × 250 mg/d IV for 3 days • > 60 kg: 4 × 250 mg/d IV for 3 days • Possibly followed by 1 mg/kg/d, gradual reduction to 0.5 mg/kg/d and then ever more gradually to 0.1 mg/kg/d
OKT 3 or ATG	If steroid therapy is unsuccessful

29.1.8 Prognosis

The 1-year survival rate is now around 80 to 90%. The mean survival time is currently 12 to 15 years. Physical capacity is good in most heart transplant patients (NYHA class I). The morbidity after heart transplantation is affected to a considerable extent by adverse effects of the immunosuppression (infections, nephrotoxicity, hypertension, malignant disease).

▶ **Risk of malignant disease.** Around 2 to 10% of children who have had a heart transplant develop malignant diseases under immunosuppression. The most common is posttransplant lymphoproliferative disease (PTLD), which involves lymphomas associated with an EBV infection. Some of the patients respond to a reduction of immunosuppression, depending on the histological finding, otherwise chemotherapy is needed.

29.1.9 Heart–Lung Transplantation

The combined heart–lung transplantation is a treatment option for some patients. The indications include complex cyanotic defects with underdeveloped pulmonary circulation or shunt defects with an irreversible increase in pulmonary resistance (Eisenmenger reaction). However, there are only a few centers with experience. The 5-year survival rate is about 50%. The 5-year survival rate is even lower for patients for whom the indication for a heart–lung transplant was made because of a congenital heart defect.

30 Vaccinations for Pediatric Patients with Cardiac Disease

Theoretically, the current vaccination schedule of the German Vaccination Committee (STIKO) also applies to children with congenital heart defects. The current recommendations are available on the Internet (www.rki.de). National vaccination guidelines should be applied according to local standards for each country.

However, some special aspects should be observed for children with heart disease and these are discussed briefly below. For detailed recommendations, the reader is referred to the official STIKO publications and the respective Summary of Product Characteristics.

▸ **RSV prophylaxis.** Passive immunization with palivizumab is recommended for children under age 2 years with a hemodynamic heart defect at the beginning of the respiratory syncytial virus (RSV) season (dosage: 15 mg/kg every 4 weeks during the RSV season). The RSV season begins between October and December and ends between March and May in the Northern Hemisphere.

▸ **Flu vaccine.** For children, adolescents, and adults with chronic cardiovascular disease, the STIKO recommends an annual flu shot, optimally between September and November. Vaccination is approved over age 6 months.

▸ **Oral anticoagulation.** Patients who take phenprocoumon or warfarin should not have intramuscular injections due to the risk of muscular bleeding. The vaccine is usually injected subcutaneously in this case.

▸ **Congenital asplenia.** For patients with congenital asplenia (e.g., in a heterotaxy syndrome), vaccinations against pneumococci, meningococci, and Haemophilus influenzae type b (Hib) are particularly important.

The Hib vaccination is given according to the regular vaccination schedule. For the pneumococci immunization, the usual procedure of general basic immunization applies (three basic vaccinations with the pneumococcal conjugate vaccine in the first year of life and booster in the second year). At the age of 2 to 5 years, the children are given another supplementary vaccination with pneumococcal conjugate vaccine. After age 5 they are then given the polysaccharide vaccine. Other boosters may be considered—for children under age 10 at intervals of at least 3 years and for adults at intervals of 5 years. There may be pronounced reactions to the vaccination, however, so a risk–benefit assessment must be made on a on a case-by-case basis (e.g., taking the current vaccine titer into consideration).

In addition, all patients under age 2 years should also be vaccinated with the conjugated meningococcal C vaccine. Afterward, supplementary immunization with the meningococcal polysaccharide vaccine against serotypes A, C, W135, and Y is recommended at an interval of 6 to 12 months after reaching age 2 years. It should be noted that most meningococcal infections in Germany, Austria, and Switzerland are caused by serotype B, for which there is no approved vaccine yet.

▸ **DiGeorge syndrome.** The DiGeorge syndrome is common in patients with conotruncal heart defects such as tetralogy of Fallot, truncus arteriosus communis, or pulmonary atresia. The range of immune deficiency due to hypoplasia or aplasia of the thymus in patients with a DiGeorge syndrome is wide. It extends from patients that have no T cell abnormalities to patients with a low T cell count but largely normal T cell function (partial DiGeorge syndrome) to patients who have almost no T cells, (complete DiGeorge syndrome). The respective immunological examinations should always be ordered if there is a suspicion of a DiGeorge syndrome.

For inactivated vaccines, the regular vaccination schedule applies to DiGeorge patients. The annual flu shot is also recommended. The success of the vaccination should be checked by monitoring the titer. Before vaccinating with live vaccines, a basic immunological examination is recommended. Live vaccinations should be given only after consultation with an immunologist. In addition, RSV prophylaxis is recommended for the winter months. Varicella immunoglobulin is indicated for patients exposed to chickenpox.

▸ **Before and after cardiac surgery.** For elective surgery, a minimum waiting period of 3 days should be maintained after immunization with inactivated vaccines and a minimum period of 14 days after live vaccines. This makes it possible to distinguish between possible reactions to immunization and complications of surgery. These minimum waiting periods also apply to vaccinations given after surgery. For urgent or vital indications, however, neither vaccination nor surgery should be postponed.

Immunoglobulins, which are also components of fresh frozen plasma, block the proliferation of live vaccine viruses. For this reason, an interval of 3 months between administration of immunoglobulin products and vaccination with live vaccines is recommended.

To reduce the risk of a hepatitis B infection through transfusions, the hepatitis B immunization should be completed before cardiac surgery if possible.

► **Heart transplantation.** Before a heart transplant, basic immunization should be completed if possible. It may be recommended to give the vaccinations as soon as possible—ahead of the normal vaccination schedule (e.g., starting hepatitis B in the neonatal period; MMR and varicella after 9 months; diphtheria, pertussis, tetanus, polio, Hib as early as 6 weeks). An annual flu shot is also recommended for transplant patients.

After transplantation, live vaccines are contraindicated under immunosuppression treatment (exceptions must be cleared with the immunologist on a case-by-case basis). Under high-dose steroids, it should be noted that an adequate antibody titer is not reached after vaccinations. The success of the vaccination should be checked by determining the titer for patients undergoing immunosuppression treatment.

31 Pharmacological Treatment

▶ Table 31.1 provides an overview of commonly used drugs in pediatric cardiology.

Antiarrhythmic agents, immunosuppressants after heart transplantation, and drugs for the treatment of pulmonary hypertension are listed in separate tables in the respective chapters.

Table 31.1 Overview of commonly used drugs in pediatric cardiology

Drug	Indication/effect	Mechanism of action	Dosage	Adverse effects	Remarks
Inotropic and vasoactive drugs					
Dobutamine	Acute heart failure Increases myocardial contractility and cardiac output	Strong β1 and mild β2/α1 stimulation Improves contractility and reduces systemic resistance	Continuous infusion: 2–**5–10**–15 (–30) μg/kg/min	Sinus tachycardia, proarrhythmogenic, palpitations, hypertension, headache, vomiting, paresthesia	Incompatible with alkaline solutions, sodium bicarbonate, furosemide, ethacrynic acid, heparin, cefazolin, penicillin Compatible with other vasoactive agents, lidocaine, and muscle relaxants
Dopamine	Should no longer be used	Moderate α_1, α_2, and β_1 and mild β_2 stimulation, DA1 and DA2 stimulation (dose-dependent)	Continuous infusion: 1–5 mg/kg/min: increases renal and mesenteric blood flow 5–15 μg/kg/min: increases renal blood flow and heart rate, positive inotropic > 15 μg/kg/min: systemic vasoconstriction	Sinus tachycardia, proarrhythmogenic, systemic and pulmonary vasoconstriction, palpitations, headache, vomiting, suppression of the neuroendocrine axis, increased sepsis rate	Incompatible with alkaline solutions Compatible with other vasoactive agents, lidocaine, muscle relaxants. and KCl No renal protective effect
Dopexamine	Acute heart failure Increases myocardial contractility, reduces afterload, improves renal and mesenteric blood flow	Strong β_2 stimulation, moderate DA1, DA2, and β_1 stimulation	Continuous infusion: 0.5–6 μg/kg/min	Similar to dobutamine, also hyperglycemia, hypokalemia, neutropenia, thrombocytopenia	Do not mix with other vasoactive substances
Epinephrine (adrenaline)	Asystole, bradycardia, shock, severe hypotension, acute heart failure	α_1, β_1, and β_2 stimulation Low dose: Vasodilatation (β_2 effect) High dose: Vasoconstriction (α_1 effect)	Asystole, bradycardia: 0.01 mg/kg (0.1 mL/kg of 1:10,000 diluted solution) IV, intraosseous or intratracheal, if necessary, repeat every 3–5 min If ineffective or for intratracheal administration, increase up to 0.1–0.2 mg/kg (0.1–0.2 mL/kg of 1:1,000 diluted solution) Continuous infusion: 0.1–1 μg/kg/min	Sinus tachycardia, proarrhythmogenic, hypertension, agitation, tremor, nausea, vomiting, deterioration of renal and mesenteric blood flow, increase in intraocular pressure, hyperglycemia, leukocytosis	Increases myocardial oxygen consumption (caution with myocardial ischemia) Incompatible with alkaline solutions Compatible with other vasoactive drugs and muscle relaxants

Table 31.1 continued

Drug	Indication/effect	Mechanism of action	Dosage	Adverse effects	Remarks
Orciprenaline	Bradycardia	ß1 and ß2 stimulation	Continuous infusion: 0,1-0,5 μg/kg/min	Similar to epinephrine	Increases myocardial oxygen consumption (caution with myocardial ischemia)
Isoprenaline (Isoproterenol)	AV block, bradyarrhythmia, shock (vasoconstrictive), bronchospasm, acute pulmonary hypertension	β_1 and β_2 stimulation (positive inotropic and chronotropic effect, pulmonary and systemic vasodilation)	Continuous infusion: 0.05–5 μg/kg/min	Similar to epinephrine	Contraindications: digitalis poisoning, low diastolic blood pressure, uncorrected Fallot tetralogy (drop in peripheral resistance), subaortic stenosis (increases the gradient)
Noradrenaline (norepinephrine)	Vasoplegic or cardiogenic shock in combination with dobutamine, dopamine, or epinephrine, possibly for Fallot crisis	Strong α_1 and weaker β_1 stimulation, pronounced systemic vasoconstriction, less pronounced inotropic and chronotropic effects	Continuous infusion: 0.05–2 μg/kg/min	Sinus tachycardia, reflex bradycardia, proarrhythmogenic, hypertension, chest pain, headache, hyperglycemia, mesenteric vasoconstriction, severe peripheral vasoconstriction	Combination with dobutamine, dopamine or epinephrine
Amrinone (Inamrinon)	Acute heart failure (especially after cardiopulmonary bypass and in cardiomyopathy); adjuvant for pulmonary hypertension	Phosphodiesterase inhibitor (increases cAMP) Positive inotropic effect, relaxation of smooth muscle cells ("inodilator"), reduces myocardial oxygen consumption	IV bolus of 0.75 mg/kg over 3 min Maintenance dose: • Neonates: 3–5 μg/kg/min IV • Older children: 5–10 μg/kg/min IV	Hypotension, thrombocytopenia, tachyarrhythmia, hepatotoxicity, nausea, vomiting, fever	Do not dissolve in glucose solution (infusion with glucose solutions possible using a Y connector) Incompatible with sodium bicarbonate and furosemide Caution: may have a negative inotropic effect in neonates
Enoximone	Same as amrinone	Same as amrinone	Initially 0.5 mg/kg as short infusion over at least 10 min, maintenance dose: 2.5 - 10 μg/kg/min IV	Similar to amrinone	Do not dissolve in glucose solution; incompatible with other solutions.
Milrinone	Same as amrinone	Same as amrinone	Initially 50 μg/kg as short infusion over at least 15 min (in case of hypotension if necessary administer a volume bolus and reduce infusion rate, possibly without the bolus) Maintenance dose: 0.25–1 μg/kg/min IV	Arrhythmia, hypotension, hypokalemia, thrombocytopenia	

Table 31.1 continued

Drug	Indication/effect	Mechanism of action	Dosage	Adverse effects	Remarks
Vasopressin	Cardiac arrest, ventricular fibrillation or pulseless tachycardia, that cannot be ended by defibrillation Vasoplegic shock that is unresponsive to volume or catecholamines Diabetes insipidus, massive hemorrhage of the gastrointestinal tract	Binds to AVPR1 receptors, activates phospholipase C, and increases intracellular calcium concentration Vasoconstriction, may also increase sensitivity of catecholamines	Cardiac arrest, ventricular fibrillation, pulseless tachycardia: 0.4 U/kg IV, if unsuccessful, other measures including epinephrine Vasoplegic shock: 0.0002–0.003 U/kg/min	Hypertension, bradycardia, arrhythmia, thrombosis, angina pectoris, cardiac arrest, bronchospasm, dizziness, headache, seizures, water intoxication, hyponatremia	Little experience in use during resuscitation in children
Levosimendan	Decompensation or impending heart failure, also perioperative	Calcium sensitizer, new group of "inodilators," binds to troponin C, provides a more effective contraction without increasing the intracellular calcium concentration	Initially 12 µg/kg over 1 h Maintenance dose: 0.1–0.2 µg/kg/min (usually over 24 h)	Symptomatic hypotension (rare), palpitations, flush, headache, dizziness, vomiting	Can be used with other inotropic drugs, no deterioration of diastolic function
Calcium chloride	Symptomatic hypocalcemia, hypermagnesemia, hyperkalemia, poisoning with calcium antagonists, tetany, cardiac arrest in connection with the above-mentioned electrolyte imbalance, reduced cardiac contractility due to low concentration of ionized calcium (especially after heart surgery)	Essential among other things for the function of nerve, muscle, and skeletal systems, as well as for the action potential	Symptomatic hypocalcemia: 10–20 mg/kg IV slowly Cardiac arrest, electromechanical decoupling, poisoning with calcium antagonists: 20 mg/kg IV slowly, if necessary repeat after 10 min Symptomatic hyperkalemia: 25 mg/kg IV slowly	Sinus bradycardia, vasodilatation, hypotension, arrhythmias, dyspnea, dizziness, hypokalemia, hypomagnesemia, hypophosphatemia	Special caution for simultaneous use of digitalis Hemodynamic monitoring required
Vasodilators					
Captopril	Hypertension, chronic heart failure, afterload reduction	ACE inhibitor, blocks the conversion of angiotensin I to angiotensin II, which is a competent vasoconstrictor	Preterm neonates: initially 0.01 mg/kg orally 2–3 × daily as a test dose, then increase depending on the effect Neonates: initial test dose 2–3 × 0.05–0.1 mg/kg orally, then increase to max. 1–4 × 0.5 mg/kg Older children: initial test dose 0.15–0.5 mg/kg orally, depending on the effect, increase to 2.5–6 mg/kg/d in 2–4 single doses	Hypotension, tachycardia, dry cough, airway obstruction, cholestasis, increased renal retention parameters, proteinuria, hyperkalemia (particularly with simultaneous use of spironolactone), neutropenia, agranulocytosis, angioedema	Monitor blood pressure 1–3 h after the first dose Determine dose individually, choose lowest dose that achieves the desired effect Low doses especially in patients with impaired renal function, diuretic medication, and fluid restriction, as well as in severe heart failure or in arterial obstruction (coarctation of the aorta, aortic stenosis)

Table 31.1 continued

Drug	Indication/effect	Mechanism of action	Dosage	Adverse effects	Remarks
Enalapril	Hypertension, chronic heart failure, afterload reduction	ACE inhibitor	Neonates: initial test dose 0.1 mg/kg orally 1 × daily, adjust dose and interval every 3–5 days depending on the effect (max. 2 doses/d) Older children: initial test dose 0.05–01 mg/kg orally 1–2 × daily, increase according to effect up to 0.5 mg/kg/d in 1–2 single doses for 2 weeks	Similar to captopril	Similar to captopril
Lisinopril	Hypertension, chronic heart failure, afterload reduction	ACE inhibitor	Children under 6 years: no dose information Children over 6 years: initial test dose 0.07 mg/kg orally 1 × daily (max. 5 mg), increase dose 1–2 x weekly until the desired effect is achieved (no experience with doses above 0.61 mg/kg/d, or over 40 mg/d)	Similar to captopril	Similar to captopril
Losartan	Arterial hypertension, protective for renal impairment and hypertension	Angiotensin II antagonist	Children under 6 years: no data Children 6–16 years: 1 × 0.7 mg/kg, max. 50 mg/d	Hypotension, tachycardia, orthostatic hypotension, hypoglycemia, hypokalemia, anemia, fever	Do not use in pregnancy or lactation
Nifedipine	Arterial hypertension, hypertrophic cardiomyopathy	Calcium antagonist	Neonates and infants: no data Older children: hypertensive crisis: 0.25–0.5 mg/kg/dose orally or sublingually every 4–6 h (max. 10 mg/dose) Hypertrophic cardiomyopathy: 0.6–0.9 mg/kg/d orally in 3–4 single doses Hypertension long-term treatment: initially 0.25–0.5 mg/kg/d orally in 1–2 single doses, increase according to effect to max. 3 mg/kg/d	Hypotension, tachycardia, flush, headache, respiratory distress, nausea, increase in liver enzymes, cholestasis, arthritis, thrombocytopenia, leukocytopenia, anemia, dermatitis	Caution with heart failure or aortic stenosis
Amlodipine	Arterial hypertension (pulmonary hypertension)	Calcium antagonist	Initially 0.05–0.13 mg/kg/d, depending on the effect increase every 5–7 days by 25–50% No experience in children with doses over 5 mg/d	Flush, palpitations, edema, hypotension, chest pain, vasculitis, headache, dizziness, abdominal pain, increase in liver enzymes, thrombocytopenia, leukocytopenia	
Nitroglycerin	Hypertensive crisis, improves coronary blood flow and myocardial perfusion after cardiac surgery	NO donor, improves coronary perfusion and myocardial oxygen consumption	Continuous infusion: initially 0.25–0.5 µg/kg/min, increase by 0.5–1 mg/kg/min every 3–5 min until the desired effect is achieved, maximum dose is usually 5 mg/kg/min	Hypotension, reflex tachycardia, flushing, headache (common), nausea	Caution in hypovolemia IV solution is not compatible with other drugs Leaves deposits on plastic, therefore, apply solution in glass bottle and do not infuse via PVC tubes

Table 31.1 continued

Drug	Indication/effect	Mechanism of action	Dosage	Adverse effects	Remarks
Sodium nitroprusside	Treatment of hypertension and afterload reduction in ICU patients	NO donor, vasodilation (stronger effect in arterial vessels than in venous vessels)	Continuous infusion: initially 0.5–1 µg/kg/min, depending on effect gradual increase to max. 5 µg/kg/min	Hypotension, reflex tachycardia, palpitations, central nervous system symptoms, nausea	Most potent antihypertensive drug. Continuous blood pressure and heart rate monitoring required. Rapid onset and short duration of action. Sensitive to light (infuse protected from light). Cyanide is produced during prolonged administration or with higher doses (it blocks intracellular respiration), therefore nitroprusside should be infused with sodium thiosulfate (10 times the nitroprusside dose), which detoxifies cyanide
Phenoxybenzamine	Arterial hypertension (particularly with pheochromocytoma), afterload reduction and vasodilation after cardiac surgery (e.g., Norwood procedure)	Long-acting, irreversible α_1 and α_2 blockade Systemic (and pulmonary) vasodilation ("chemical sympathectomy")	Orally: 0.2–1 mg/kg every 12–24 h IV: 1 mg/kg over 2 h, then 0.5 mg/kg over 1 h every 6–12 h May be increased to 1–2 mg/kg 1–2 × daily	Tachycardia, arrhythmias, hypotension, nausea, miosis, fatigue, nasal congestion	In case of overdose, supplement volume and if necessary noradrenaline (possibly vasopressin). Epinephrine is contraindicated (leads to vasodilatation via β stimulation if an α blockade is present!)
Phentolamine	Arterial hypertension (particularly in pheochromocytoma), afterload reduction and vasodilation after cardiac surgery	Long-acting, reversible α_1-and α_2 blockade Systemic vasodilation	0.02–011 mg/kg IV over 10–30 min, then continuous IV 5–50 µg/kg/min	Similar to phenoxybenzamine	Same as phenoxybenzamine
Prostaglandin E_1 (Alprostadil)	Maintains patency of the ductus arteriosus in ductal-dependent perfusion	Vasodilation through direct effect on the smooth muscle cells of blood vessels and especially on the ductus arteriosus	Continuous infusion: initially 0.05–0.1 µg/kg/min then reduce gradually and continue with the lowest effective dose	Apnea, flushing, bradycardia, hypotension, fever, edema, hypocalcemia, hypokalemia, hyperkalemia, hypoglycemia Platelet function disorder, cortical hyperostosis after prolonged use	

Table 31.1 continued

Drug	Indication/effect	Mechanism of action	Dosage	Adverse effects	Remarks
Hydralazine	Arterial hypertension	Peripheral vasodilator	Orally: 0.75–1 mg/kg/d in 2–4 single doses (max. 25-mg/dose), increase over 3–4 weeks to max. 5 mg/kg/d in infants and up to max. 7.5 mg/kg/d in older children (max. 200 mg/d) IV: initially 0.1–0.2 mg/kg/dose every 4–6 h	Hypotension, tachycardia, palpitations, lupuslike symptoms after prolonged use	
Diuretics					
Furosemide	Reduces edema in heart failure, renal or hepatic diseases, hypertension	Loop diuretic	Premature/neonates: • Orally: 1–4 mg/kg 1–2 × daily • IV: 0.25–2 mg/kg 1–2 × daily Older children: • Orally: 1–6 mg/kg/d in 2–4 single doses • IV: 0.25–2 mg/kg 2–4 x daily • Continuous infusion: 0.05–0.1–0.4 mg/kg/h IV	Hypokalemia, hyponatremia, hypercalciuria, nephrocalcinosis, hyperuricemia, ototoxicity (enhanced by aminoglycosides or ethacrynic acid), hypochloremic alkalosis, agranulocytosis, thrombocytopenia, deterioration of glucose tolerance, azotemia, delayed ductal closure in preterm infants	Monitor serum electrolytes, renal function, and blood pressure
Ethacrynic acid	Same as furosemide	Loop diuretic	Orally: 1 mg/kg every 24–48 h (max. 3 mg/kg/d) IV: 0.5–1 mg/kg every 8–12 h	Similar to furosemide	No proven additional diuretic effect
Hydrochlorothiazide	Reduces edema in heart failure, bronchopulmonary dysplasia, nephrotic syndrome, hypertension	Thiazide diuretic, inhibits NaCl transport system in the proximal part of the distal tubule	Under 6 months: 2–4 mg/kg/d orally in 1–2 single doses (max. 37.5 mg/d) Over 6 months: 2 mg/kg/d orally in 1–2 single doses (max. 200 mg/d)	Hypokalemia, hyponatremia, hypochloremic alkalosis, hyperuricemia, hyperglycemia, azotemia, cholestasis, leukocytopenia, thrombocytopenia	
Spironolactone	Reduces edema in congestive heart failure, liver failure, nephrotic syndrome, hypertension, hypokalemia, primary hyperaldosteronism	Potassium-sparing diuretic, aldosterone antagonist	1–4 mg/kg/d orally in 1–2 single doses (higher for primary hyperaldosteronism)	Hyperkalemia (especially in combination with ACE inhibitors), hyponatremia, gynecomastia, amenorrhea, agranulocytosis	Combination with loop or thiazide diuretics useful
Mannitol	Treatment of oliguria or anuria in renal failure, reduction of intracranial pressure in brain edema	Osmotic diuretic	Test dose: 0.2 g/kg (max. 12.5 g) over 3–5 min; the target is diuresis of at least 1 mL/kg/h over 1–3 h, otherwise discontinue Initial dose: 0.5–1 g/kg IV over 20 min as a 20% solution Maintenance dose: 0.25–0.5 mg/kg IV every 4–6 h	Volume overload, congestive heart failure, pulmonary edema, electrolyte shifts, hyperosmolality	First test dose; if diuresis does not increase, volume shift from intra- to extracellular may occur. Monitor diuresis, balance, serum electrolytes, renal function, serum and urine osmolality (for intracranial pressure treatment, serum osmolality of 310–320 mosm/kg should be targeted)

Table 31.1 continued

Drug	Indication/effect	Mechanism of action	Dosage	Adverse effects	Remarks
Beta blockers for congestive heart failure• Start with low doses and increase slowly under careful observation for adverse effects • Do not use beta blockers in hemodynamically unstable patients • Start beta blockers only as a supplement to existing medication with ACE inhibitors, diuretics, and possibly digoxin • If possible, use only beta blockers that have been adequately studied in heart failure (e.g., carvedilol, metoprolol) • Do not discontinue beta blockers abruptly after long-term treatment • Do not combine beta blockers with catecholamines or phosphodiesterase inhibitors when changing the IV treatment to oral treatment in acute heart failure					
Metoprolol	Additional treatment for heart failure	Cardioselective beta blocker	Initially 2 × 0.1–0.2 mg/kg orally Gradual increase to 2 × 0.25–1 mg/kg orally	Deterioration of heart failure, bradycardia, AV block, Raynaud symptoms, bronchospasm, psoriasis-like symptoms, hypoglycemia, hypertriglyceridemia, fatigue	No data for neonates
Carvedilol	Additional treatment for heart failure	Nonselective beta and α_1 blocker (additional vasodilation)	Initially 2 × 0.03–0.08 mg/kg orally (max. 3.125 mg/dose) Gradual increase every 2–3 weeks to 2 × 0.3–0.95 mg/kg orally (max. 25 mg/dose)	Same as metoprolol	Under 3.5 years, possibly higher dose required (increased carvedilol elimination in this age group), no data on neonates
Propranolol	Additional treatment for heart failure	Nonselective beta blocker	Initially 2 × 0.5 mg/kg orally Increase every 2–4 weeks by 0.25 mg/kg/dose up to max. 2 × 1.5 mg/kg orally	Same as metoprolol	
Antithrombotics					
Alteplase (RTPA)	Acute pulmonary embolism, systemic thrombosis, acute myocardial infarction, acute ischemic cerebrovascular accident, thrombotic occlusion of central venous catheters (CVCs)	Plasminogen activator which amplifies the conversion of mainly fibrin-bound plasminogen to plasmin (local fibrinolysis)	Systemic thrombosis: initially 0.5 mg/kg as a bolus over 30 min, maintenance dose 0.1–0.2 mg/kg/h CVC blockage: weight < 10 kg: 0.5 mg, > 10 kg: add 1 mg diluted in 0.9% NaCl slowly to the catheter, leave to interact for 1–2 h, then aspirate alteplase (do not inject into the patient) and rinse the catheter	Bleeding, drop in blood pressure, fever, nausea, arrhythmia	Contraindications: active bleeding, brain tumor, aortic dissection, AV anomalies, aneurysms, tendency to bleed, severe hypertension during lysis Maintain fibrinogen concentration over 100 mg/dL during thrombolysis Monitor signs of bleeding and fibrinogen Short plasma half-life (ca. 6 min) Heparinization after lysis
Acetylsalicylic acid (ASA)	Thrombosis prophylaxis (e.g., endovascular stents, aortopulmonary anastomosis, upper cavopulmonary anastomosis or Fontan circulation), Kawasaki syndrome	Prostaglandin synthesis inhibitors Irreversible inhibition of platelet aggregation	Platelet aggregation inhibition: 3–10 mg/kg/d orally (max. 325 mg) Aortopulmonary shunt, endovascular stent: 1–5 mg/kg/d orally Fontan circulation: 5 mg/kg/d orally Kawasaki syndrome (Chapter 16.5)	Bleeding tendency, leukocytopenia, thrombocytopenia, hepatotoxicity, tinnitus, urticaria, Reye syndrome	

Table 31.1 continued

Drug	Indication/effect	Mechanism of action	Dosage	Adverse effects	Remarks
Heparin	Prophylaxis and treatment of thromboembolism	Amplification of AT-III effect	Systemic heparinization (target PTT 60–80 s): 100 IU/kg as an IV bolus, maintenance dose 400 IU/kg/d	Bleeding, thrombocytopenia (heparin-induced thrombocytopenia), osteoporosis after long-term high-dose treatment, allergic reactions	Attenuated heparin effect in AT-III deficiency (lower AT-III level in premature infants and neonates) Monitor PTT 4 h after initiation of treatment and every 4 h after changing the dose Antidote: protamine Heparin-induced thrombocytopenia II: 5–20 days after the start of heparin treatment (in case of re-exposure possibly immediately) drop in platelets below 100/nL, risk of thromboembolism; discontinue heparin immediately on suspicion, continue anticoagulation with lepirudin or argatroban
Enoxaparin	Prophylaxis and treatment of thromboembolism	Low molecular weight heparin (inactivated factor Xa and IIa)	Infants < 2 months: • Prophylaxis: 2 × 0.75 mg/kg SC • Treatment: 2 × 1.5 mg/kg SC Children > 2 months: • Prophylaxis: 2 × 0.5 mg/kg SC • Treatment: 2 × 1 mg/kg SC	Similar to heparin	Monitoring and determination of the anti-factor-Xa level 4 h after administration Target levels: • Prophylaxis: 0.2–0.4 U/mL • Treatment: 0.5–1 U/mL
Protamine	Heparin antagonist (e.g., following cardiopulmonary bypass surgery)	Forms an inactive complex with heparin	1 mg (= 100 IU) of protamine antagonizes approximately 100 IU of heparin (max. dose 50 mg)	Bradycardia, drop in blood pressure, acute pulmonary hypertension, pseudo-allergic reactions, rebleeding tendency 8–18 h after application	Onset of action after about 5 min
Tranexamic acid	Bleeding after cardiac surgery	Antifibrinolytic, competitive inhibition of plasminogen activation	3 × 10–15 mg/kg IV	Drop in blood pressure in rapid IV injection, thromboembolism, nausea	Dose reduction in renal failure

Table 31.1 continued

Drug	Indication/effect	Mechanism of action	Dosage	Adverse effects	Remarks
Warfarin	Prophylaxis and treatment of thromboembolism (e.g., atrial fibrillation, artificial heart valves, upper cavopulmonary anastomosis, Fontan circulation, venous thrombosis, clotting disorders)	Inhibition of vitamin K-dependent coagulation factors (II, VII, IX, X), as well as protein C and S	Regimen to achieve an INR of 2–3: Initially 0.2 mg/kg orally (in Fontan patients or liver disorders 0.1 mg/kg) Adjust dose on day 2–4: • INR 1.1–1.3: repeat dose • INR 1.4–3: half of the initial dose • INR 3.1–3.5: one quarter of the initial dose • INR > 3.5: pause until INR is < 3.5, then continue with half of the last dose Dose adjustment during maintenance therapy: • INR 1.1–1.4: increase dose by ~ 20% • INR 1.5 to 1.9: increase dose by ~ 10% • INR 2–3: do not change dose • INR 3.1 to 3.5: reduce dose by ~ 10% • INR > 3.5: Pause if INR is < 3.5, continue with ~ 20% reduced dose	Bleeding tendency, skin necrosis, fever, hair loss	Monitoring with INR Antidote: Vitamin K and FFP (particularly in patients with artificial heart valves, very careful dosing to prevent excessive reaction). In insufficient INR possibly overlap treatment with heparin until a more effective INR is achieved
Analgesia, sedation					
Propofol	Induce and maintain anesthesia, sedation	Interaction with GABA, hypnotic, no analgesia	Induction of anesthesia: • < 6 years: 2.5–3.5 mg/kg IV • 6 years: 1.5–2.5 mg/kg IV Maintaining anesthesia: • after the first bolus of 12–18 mg/kg/h continuous IV • then reduce dose to 7.5–9 mg/kg/h within the next 30 min • Sedation: (0.3–)1.5–6 mg/kg/h continuous IV (titrate according to effect and accompanying analgesics/sedatives)	Respiratory depression, apnea, hypotension (decrease in peripheral resistance, negative inotropy), pain on injection (oil-in-water emulsion), histamine release, stimulation (myoclonus, rarely seizures), QT prolongation, arrhythmias (especially bradycardia), in long-term use very rarely propofol infusion syndrome (severe metabolic acidosis, rhabdomyolysis, renal failure, arrhythmias, heart and circulatory failure)	Rapid awakening after discontinuation. For prolonged use monitor pH, lactate, and CK (propofol infusion syndrome). Injection pain can be reduced by additional administration of opioids, ketamine or lidocaine. Available as a 0.5%, 1%, and 2% solution
Etomidate	Induction of anesthesia, sedation (should no longer be used)	Hypnotic, no analgesia	0.15–0.3 mg/kg IV	Little cardiovascular effect, respiratory depression, pain on injection, myoclonia, nausea/vomiting	Duration of action about 5 min CAUTION: Adrenal insufficiency possible after only a single dose!

Table 31.1 continued

Drug	Indication/effect	Mechanism of action	Dosage	Adverse effects	Remarks
Ketamine	Deep conscious sedation, status asthmaticus First choice drug in all patients with cardiorespiratory instability or heart failure	"Dissociative anesthesia" (loss of consciousness despite eyes open, analgesia, amnesia), bronchodilation	IV 0.5–5 mg/kg Continuous sedation: 5–20 μg/kg/min in a continuous IV IM: 5–10 mg/kg Oral: 5–15 mg/kg	Sympathomimetic (increase in heart rate and blood pressure), respiratory depression, nightmares (< 10%), hallucinations during the recovery phase (hence combination with benzodiazepines), hypersalivation, increased defense reflexes in the nasopharyngeal space (caution: laryngospasm), increase in intraocular pressure	Ketamine is a racemate, the S(+) enantiomer (ketanest S) has a higher analgesic and anesthetic effect and a shorter recovery period. Only 70% the dose of ketamine is required, especially in hemodynamically unstable patients (sympathomimetic effect)
Morphine	Severe pain	Opiate	0.01–0.1 mg/kg IV, IM, SC every 3–6 h	Respiratory depression, miosis, nausea, vomiting, development of tolerance, muscle rigidity (rigid chest wall), central sympatholytic (small decrease in heart rate, blood pressure, cardiac output, and oxygen consumption)	
Fentanyl	Severe pain	Opiate Significantly more analgesic than morphine	IV, IM: 1–4 g/kg, if necessary, repeat every 30–60 min Continuous infusion: 2–4 μg/kg/h (ventilation: 5–10 μg/kg/h)	Similar to morphine, significant respiratory depression	
Piritramide	Severe pain	Opiate Slightly less analgesic than morphine, longer duration of action	0.05–0.1 mg/kg IV, IM, SC every 4–8 h	Similar to morphine	
Pethidine	Severe pain	Opiate Less analgesic than morphine	IV: 0.5–1 mg/kg every 3–6 h IM: 0.5–2 mg/kg Oral: 0.6–1.2 mg/kg	Similar to morphine Little miosis	Frequently used in postoperative "shivering"
Tramadol	Severe pain	Opiate Less analgesic than morphine	1 mg/kg IV, oral every 2–4–6 h	Similar to morphine, rarely respiratory depression and cardiovascular effects, often nausea, vomiting	Orally available, not subject to the BtMVV (German Narcotics Act)
Naloxone	Effects of opiate overdose	Opiate antagonist	0.01 mg/kg IV, IM, SC, if no effect, repeat every 2–3 min	Tachycardia, arrhythmia, sweating, tremor, cerebral seizures	Endotracheal administration also possible; for this purpose dilute naloxone with 0.9% NaCl. Doses for endotracheal application are 2–10 times the IV dose

Table 31.1 continued

Drug	Indication/effect	Mechanism of action	Dosage	Adverse effects	Remarks
Paracetamol	Mild to moderate pain, fever reduction	Nonsteroidal anti-inflammatory drug (NSAID), prostaglandin synthesis inhibitor	IV, oral: 10–15 mg/kg every 4–6 h Rectal: 20–30 mg/kg every 6 h	Hepatotoxic, nephrotoxic, hemolysis in glucose-6-phosphate dehydrogenase deficiency, rarely gastrointestinal problems	No relevant inhibition of platelet aggregation
Ibuprofen	Mild to moderate pain, fever reduction	Nonsteroidal anti-inflammatory drug (NSAID), prostaglandin synthesis inhibitor	Oral: 4–10 mg/kg every 3–8 h	Gastrointestinal disorders, dizziness, tinnitus	Dosage for pharmacological PDA closure, see Chapter 15.5
Metamizole	Moderate to severe pain, fever reduction	Nonsteroidal anti-inflammatory drug (NSAID), prostaglandin synthesis inhibitor	Oral, rectal: 15 mg/kg every 6 h IBV (short infusion): 10–15 mg/kg every 4 h	Agranulocytosis, leukocytopenia, allergic reactions, hypotension (especially too rapid IV injection), hemolysis in glucose-6-phosphate dehydrogenase deficiency	Also spasmolytic effect
Midazolam	Sedation, anxiolysis, cerebral seizures	Short-acting benzodiazepine	Sedation: 0.1–0.2 mg/kg IV, IM; 0.2–0.4 mg/kg intranasally Premedication: 0.5 mg/kg orally	Respiratory depression, hypotonia, paradoxical excitement, drop in blood pressure	
Chloral hydrate	Sedation, cerebral seizures	Sedative, anticonvulsant	Neonates: • 25 mg/kg orally, rectally for sedation. (Repeat only with great caution because of accumulation) Older children: • sedation/anxiolysis: 25–50 mg/kg/d in 3–4 single doses orally, rectally • sedation before nonpainful procedures: 50–100 mg/kg orally, 30–100 mg/kg rectally; if necessary repeat after 30 min (max. dose 120 mg/kg or 1 g in infants and 2 g in older children)		

Part V

Appendix

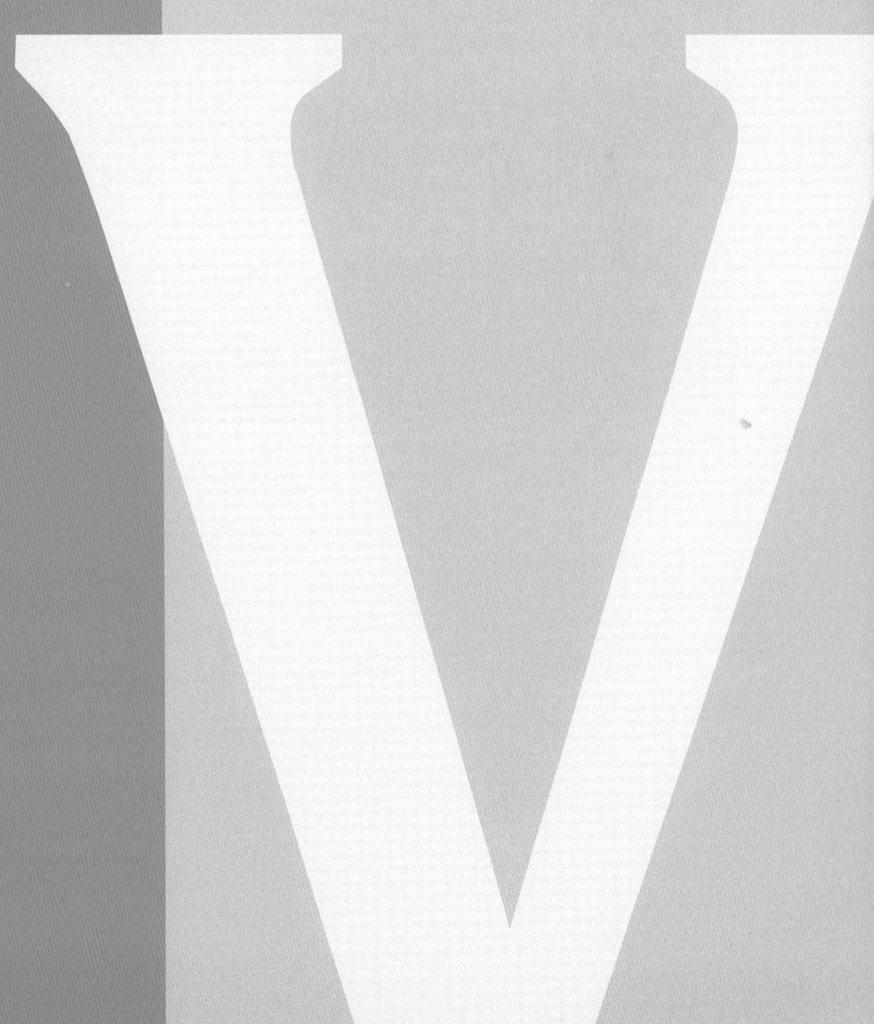

32 Tables

32.1 Normal Values for M-mode Echocardiography

Normal values for M-mode echocardiography, based on body weight (▶ Table 32.1) and body surface area (▶ Table 32.2). The mean value is in the middle row; the value above that is –2 SD, and the value below is + 2 SD.

AoD: Aortic diameter
Wt.: Weight
IVSd: Interventricular septum end-diastolic
IVSs: Interventricular septum end-systolic
LAD: Left atrial diameter
LVEDd: Left ventricular diameter end-diastolic
LVEDs: Left ventricular diameter end-systolic
LVPWd: Left ventricular posterior wall end-diastolic
LVPWs: Left ventricular posterior wall end-systolic
PAD: Pulmonary artery diameter
RVAWd: Right ventricular anterior wall end-diastolic
RVDd: Right ventricular diameter end-diastolic

Table 32.1 Normal values for M-mode echocardiography based on body weight (Kampmann et al. 2000)[77]

Wt. (kg)	RVAWd (mm)	RVDd (mm)	IVSd (mm)	IVSs (mm)	LVEDd (mm)	LVEDs (mm)	LVPWd (mm)	LVPWs (mm)	PAD (mm)	AoD (mm)	LAD (mm)
2.0	1.3	4.0	2.1	2.4	15.0	9.7	1.9	2.8	6.2	6.9	8.3
	2.4	8.4	3.5	4.4	17.1	11.0	2.7	4.5	9.3	8.2	11.5
	3.5	12.8	4.7	6.4	19.2	12.3	3.5	6.2	12.4	9.5	14.7
2.5	1.4	4.0	2.1	2.4	15.0	9.2	2.2	2.9	6.8	7.4	8.5
	2.5	8.4	3.5	5.0	18.1	11.7	3.2	5.0	11.0	8.8	12.1
	3.6	12.8	4.7	7.6	21.1	14.2	4.2	7.1	15.2	10.2	15.6
3.0	1.4	4.1	2.3	2.5	15.1	9.2	2.4	3.1	7.0	7.5	9.4
	2.5	8.5	3.6	5.1	18.2	11.7	3.5	5.1	11.0	9.1	12.6
	3.6	12.9	4.9	7.7	21.3	14.2	4.6	7.1	15.0	10.7	15.8
3.5	1.5	4.1	2.3	2.5	15.4	9.5	2.5	3.3	8.0	7.5	10.2
	2.6	8.6	3.7	5.3	18.8	11.9	3.6	5.4	11.2	9.3	13.2
	3.7	13.1	5.1	8.1	22.2	14.3	4.7	7.5	14.4	11.1	16.2
4.0	1.5	4.1	2.4	2.6	16.5	10.2	2.6	3.5	9.3	7.6	10.5
	2.6	8.6	3.8	5.4	19.9	12.7	3.7	5.7	12.5	9.6	13.7
	3.7	13.1	5.2	8.2	23.3	15.2	4.8	7.9	15.7	11.6	16.9

Table 32.2 Normal values for M-mode echocardiography based on body surface area (Kampmann et al. 2000)[77]

BSA (m^2)	RVAWd (mm)	RVDd (mm)	IVSd (mm)	IVSs (mm)	LVEDd (mm)	LVEDs (mm)	LVPWd (mm)	LVPWs (mm)	PAD (mm)	AoD (mm)	LAD (mm)
0.25	1.4	4.2	2.4	2.5	16.4	10.2	2.6	3.7	9.6	8.0	10.5
	2.6	8.7	3.8	5.2	20.0	13.2	3.6	5.7	12.8	10.4	14.0
	3.8	13.2	5.2	7.9	23.6	16.2	4.6	7.7	16.0	12.8	17.5
0.275	1.4	4.2	2.4	2.6	17.0	10.4	2.7	3.9	9.6	8.6	11.5
	2.6	8.7	3.8	5.4	21.2	13.6	3.8	5.9	13.6	11.1	15.1
	3.8	13.2	5.2	8.2	25.4	16.8	4.9	7.9	17.6	13.6	18.7
0.30	1.6	4.2	2.5	3.0	18.0	10.8	2.8	4.2	10.3	9.0	11.5
	2.7	8.7	3.9	5.8	22.9	14.8	4.1	6.3	14.5	11.3	15.3
	3.8	13.2	5.3	8.6	25.8	18.8	5.4	8.4	18.7	13.6	19.1
0.35	1.6	4.3	2.5	3.0	19.0	10.8	2.8	4.4	11.0	10.0	12.0
	2.7	8.8	3.9	5.8	23.6	14.8	4.1	6.6	15.0	12.0	16.3
	3.8	13.3	5.3	8.6	27.2	18.8	5.4	8.8	19.0	14.0	20.6
0.40	1.6	4.4	2.6	3.2	21.0	12.0	2.9	4.5	11.5	10.9	13.0
	2.7	8.9	4.1	6.2	26.0	16.1	4.2	6.8	15.4	12.9	16.8
	3.8	13.4	5.6	9.2	31.0	20.1	5.5	9.1	19.3	14.9	20.6
0.45	1.65	4.5	2.6	3.3	22.0	13.0	3.1	5.0	12.8	11.9	13.8
	2.75	9.0	4.2	6.3	27.1	17.0	4.6	7.3	17.2	14.1	17.8
	3.85	13.5	5.8	9.3	32.1	21.0	6.1	9.6	21.6	16.3	21.8
0.50	1.65	4.8	2.7	3.5	23.4	14.0	3.1	5.2	13.6	12.2	14.5
	2.75	9.3	4.3	6.6	29.0	18.0	4.6	7.5	18.3	14.9	18.7
	3.85	13.8	5.9	9.7	34.6	22.0	6.1	9.8	23.0	17.7	22.9
0.55	1.65	5.0	3.1	3.7	25.6	15.0	3.3	5.7	14.6	12.6	15.3
	2.75	9.5	4.6	6.8	31.0	19.3	4.8	8.0	19.6	15.2	19.7
	3.85	14.0	6.1	9.9	36.4	23.6	6.3	10.3	24.6	17.8	24.1
0.60	1.7	5.2	3.3	3.8	26.0	15.4	3.3	5.7	15.3	12.8	16.1
	2.8	9.6	4.8	6.9	31.6	19.9	4.8	8.0	20.3	15.6	20.1
	3.9	14.0	6.3	10.0	37.2	24.4	6.3	10.3	25.3	18.4	24.1
0.65	1.7	5.5	3.3	3.8	27.2	15.7	3.4	5.8	15.4	13.2	16.1
	2.8	9.9	4.8	6.9	33.2	20.4	4.9	8.2	20.4	16.2	20.8
	3.9	14.3	6.3	10.0	39.2	25.1	6.4	10.6	25.4	19.2	25.5
0.70	1.7	5.7	3.5	4.2	27.4	16.1	3.5	6.1	15.8	13.5	16.2
	2.8	10.1	5.0	7.2	33.9	21.3	5.2	8.7	20.8	16.9	21.2
	3.9	14.5	6.5	10.2	40.4	26.5	6.9	11.3	25.8	20.3	26.2
0.80	1.7	5.8	3.6	4.4	29.6	17.7	3.6	6.2	15.8	14.5	16.5
	2.8	10.5	5.2	7.5	35.8	22.7	5.7	9.1	20.8	17.9	22.5
	3.9	15.2	6.8	10.6	42.0	27.7	7.8	12.0	25.8	21.3	28.5

Table 32.2 continued

BSA (m^2)	RVAWd (mm)	RVDd (mm)	IVSd (mm)	IVSs (mm)	LVEDd (mm)	LVEDs (mm)	LVPWd (mm)	LVPWs (mm)	PAD (mm)	AoD (mm)	LAD (mm)
0.90	1.7	6.4	3.8	4.9	31.0	18.0	3.7	6.8	16.7	15.1	17.0
	2.8	11.0	5.6	8.3	37.1	23.6	5.9	9.5	22.5	18.7	23.2
	3.9	15.6	7.4	11.7	43.2	29.2	8.1	12.2	28.3	22.3	29.4
1.00	1.7	6.4	4.0	5.1	31.7	18.6	3.7	6.8	17.8	16.3	19.2
	2.8	11.2	5.8	8.4	38.5	24.4	5.9	9.5	24	19.9	25
	3.9	16.0	7.6	11.7	45.3	30.2	8.1	12.2	30.2	23.5	30.8
1.10	1.8	7.4	4.3	5.4	32.5	19.6	3.9	7.0	17.8	17.5	19.5
	2.9	11.8	6.2	9.0	39.4	25.2	6.3	10.3	24	20.9	25.2
	4.0	16.2	8.1	12.6	46.3	30.8	8.7	13.6	30.2	24.3	30.9
1.20	1.8	7.6	4.7	5.4	35.5	21.5	4.0	7.6	18.3	17.5	20.9
	2.9	12.4	6.5	9.0	41.7	27.1	6.6	10.7	24.3	21.0	26.0
	4.0	17.2	8.3	12.6	47.9	32.7	9.2	13.8	30.3	24.5	31.1
1.30	1.9	8.5	4.8	5.4	35.8	21.5	4.3	8.1	18.8	17.5	21.7
	3.0	13.5	6.6	9.0	42.4	27.1	6.9	11.0	24.6	21.7	27.3
	4.1	18.5	8.4	12.6	49.0	32.7	9.5	13.9	30.4	25.9	32.9
1.40	1.9	9.0	4.9	5.8	37.3	22.0	4.3	8.5	21.4	17.9	22.8
	3.0	14.0	6.7	9.2	43.3	27.6	6.9	11.5	26.8	22.7	28.2
	4.1	19.0	8.5	12.6	49.3	33.2	9.5	14.5	32.2	27.5	33.6
1.50	1.9	10.0	5.2	5.8	39.0	22.5	4.9	8.5	21.8	18.2	23.7
	3.1	15.6	7.4	9.5	45.4	28.6	7.7	12.0	27.4	23.6	29.9
	4.3	21.2	9.6	13.2	51.8	34.7	10.5	15.5	33.0	29.0	36.1
1.75	1.9	10.3	5.6	5.8	36.8	23.4	5.1	9.5	22.5	18.2	23.8
	3.1	16.5	8.0	9.8	46.8	29.8	8.1	12.8	28.5	24.4	30.4
	4.3	22.7	10.4	13.8	54.8	36.2	11.1	16.1	34.5	30.6	37.0
2.00	1.9	11.5	6.8	6.5	45.4	25.6	5.1	9.6	23.5	23	23.7
	3.1	17.5	9.3	10.3	53.4	34.4	8.1	14.2	29.5	27.4	32.5
	4.3	23.5	11.8	14.1	61.4	43.2	11.1	18.8	35.5	31.8	41.3

32.2 Aortic Root Diameter in 2D Echocardiography

► Table 32.3 shows an overview of the diameter of the aortic root in 2D echocardiography depending on body length. The 95% confidence interval is indicated in parentheses.

Ratio of the diameter of the sinus of Valsalva / aortic valve annulus 1.37 (1.18–1.56)

Ratio of the ascending aorta / aortic valve annulus 1.16 (0.97–1.35)

Table 32.3 Diameter of the aortic root in 2D echocardiography (Sheil ML et al. 1995)[99]

Body length (cm)	50	60	70	80	90	100	110	120	130	140	150	160	170	180	190
Aortic valve annulus (mm)	7 (4–10)	8 (5.5–11.5)	9.5 (6.5–13)	10.5 (7–13.5)	12 (8.5–14.5)	13 (9.5–16)	14 (11–17)	15 (12–18)	16.5 (13.5–19)	17 (14–20)	18.5 (15.5–21.5)	19 (16.5–23)	20.5 (17.5–24)	21.5 (18.5–24.5)	23 (19.5–25.5)
Sinus of Valsalva (mm)	9 (5–13.5)	11 (7–15)	13 (8–17)	14 (10–18.5)	15.5 (12–20)	17.5 (13.5–22)	19 (15–23.5)	20.5 (16.5–25)	22.5 (18–26.5)	24 (20–27.5)	26 (21.5–29.5)	27.5 (23–31.5)	29 (25–33)	30 (26–34.5)	32 (28–36)
Ascending aorta (mm)	7.5 (3–11.5)	9 (5–12.5)	10.5 (6.5–14)	12 (8–15.5)	13.5 (9.5–17)	15 (11–18.5)	16.5 (12.5–20)	18 (14–21.5)	19 (15–22.5)	20.5 (17–24)	21.5 (18–25.5)	23 (19.5–27)	24 (21–28)	26 (22–30)	27.5 (23.5–32)

32.3 Diameter of the Mitral and Tricuspid Valve Annulus

► Table 32.4 shows an overview of the diameter of the mitral and tricuspid valve annulus in 2D echocardiography. The 95% confidence interval is indicated in parentheses.

Table 32.4 Diameter of the mitral and tricuspid valve annulus in 2D echocardiography (King DH et al. 1985)

BSA (m^2)	0.2	0.25	0.3	0.4	0.5	0.6	0.7	0.8	0.9	1.0	1.2	1.4
Wt. (kg)	2	3	4	7	10	13	16	19	23	28	37	46
Mitral valve (parasternal long axis)	10 (7–13)	12 (9–15)	13 (10–16)	16 (13–19)	18 (15–21)	19 (16–23)	21 (18–24)	22 (18–26)	23 (19–26)	24 (20–27)	25 (22–28)	26 (23–30)
Mitral valve (apical or subcostal four-chamber view)	12 (7–17)	15 (10–20)	17 (12–22)	20 (16–25)	23 (18–28)	25 (20–31)	27 (22–32)	29 (23–35)	31 (25–36)	32 (26–37)	35 (28–40)	36 (31–42)
Tricuspid valve (apical or subcostal four-chamber view)	12 (8–17)	15 (10–19)	17 (12–22)	21 (16–26)	23 (18–29)	26 (20–31)	27 (22–33)	29 (33–36)	31 (24–37)	32 (25–38)	34 (25–42)	36 (28–44)

32.4 Normal ECG Values for Children and Adolescents

Table 32.5 Normal ECG values for children and adolescents (from Davignon A et al. 1979–80)[60]

	0–3 days	3–30 days	1–6 months	6–12 months	1–3 years	3–5 years	5–8 years	8–12 years	12–16 years
Heart rate (bpm)	90–160	90–180	105–185	110–170	90–150	70–140	65–135	60–130	60–120
PQ interval in lead II (ms)	80–160	70–140	70–160	70–160	80–150	80–160	90–160	90–170	90–180
QRS duration in lead V_5 (ms)	25–75	25–80	25–80	25–75	30–75	30–75	30–80	30–85	35–90
QRS axis	60–195°	65–185°	10–120°	10–100°	10–100°	10–105°	10–135°	10–120°	10–130°
QRS in lead V_1									
Q (mV)	0	0	0	0	0	0	0	0	0
R (mV)	0.5–2.6	0.3–2.3	0.3–2.0	0.2–2.0	0.2–1.8	0.1–1.8	0.1–1.5	0.1–1.2	0.1–1.0
S (mV)	0–2.3	0–1.5	0–1.5	0–1.8	0.1–2.1	0.2–2.1	0.3–2.4	0.3–2.5	0.3–2.2
QRS in lead V_6									
Q (mV)	0–0.2	0–0.3	0–0.25	0–0.3	0–0.3	0.02–0.35	0.02–0.45	0.01–0.3	0–0.3
R (mV)	0–1.1	0.1–1.3	0.5–2.2	0.5–2.3	0.6–2.3	0.8–2.5	0.8–2.6	0.9–2.5	0.7–2.4
S (mV)	0–1.0	0–1.0	0–1.0	0–0.8	0–0.6	0–0.5	0–0.4	0–0.4	0–0.4

32.5 Normal Values for the Corrected QT Interval

The frequency-corrected QT interval (QTc) is calculated using the Bazett formula:

$$QT_C = \frac{\text{QT time}}{\sqrt{\text{RR interval}}}$$

Table 32.6 Normal values for the frequency-corrected QT interval (QTc)

	Normal value	Borderline prolonged QTc interval	Prolonged QTc interval
Children and adolescents under age 15	< 0.44 s	0.44–0.46 s	> 0.46 s
Men	< 0.43 s	0.43–0.45 s	> 0.45 s
Women	< 0.45 s	0.45–0.46 s	> 0.46 s

32.6 Classification of Sports

Table 32.7 Type and intensity of exercise in various sports (from Mitchell JH et al. 2005)[86]

	Low dynamic demand	Moderate dynamic demand	High dynamic demand
Low static demand	• Billiards • Golf • Bowling	• Dancing • Ping pong • Tennis (doubles) • Volleyball • Hiking	• Badminton • Field hockey * • Jogging • Running (distance) • Squash * • Cross-country skiing (classic style) • Tennis (singles) • Race walking
Moderate static demand	• Motorcycling*/** • Equestrian*/** • Riflery • Sailing** • Diving*/**	• Mountain hiking • Fencing • Figure skating* • Field events (jumping) * • Synchronized swimming ** • Taekwondo *	• Aerobics • Basketball * • Ice hockey * • Soccer * • Handball * • Inline skating */** • Sprints • Bike racing */** • Cross-country skiing (skating style) • Swimming**
High static demand	• Gymnastics */** • Weight lifting* • Gymnastics • Martial arts * • Sport climbing */** • Field events (throwing) • Windsurfing */**	• Downhill skiing */** • Snowboarding */** • Judo * • Karate * • Weight training, bodybuilding * • Wrestling*	• Boxing * • Speed ice skating • Canoeing** • Mountain biking */** • Rowing**

* Increased risk of injury (relevant e.g. for patients with pharmacological anticoagulation)
** Increased risk if syncope occurs

References

[1] Allen HD, et al. Moss and Adams' heart disease in infants, children, and adolescents including the fetus and young adult. Philadelphia: Lippincott Williams & Wilkins; 2008

[2] Apitz J. Pädiatrische Kardiologie. Darmstadt: Steinkopff; 2002

[3] Borth-Bruns T, Eichler A. Pädiatrische Kardiologie. Berlin, Heidelberg: Springer; 2004

[4] Chang AC, et al. Pediatric cardiac intensive care. Philadelphia: Lippincott Williams & Wilkins; 1998

[5] Claussen CD, et al. Pareto-Reihe Radiologie Herz. Stuttgart: Thieme; 2007

[6] Cloherty JP, Eichenwald EC, Stark AR. Manual of neonatal care. Philadelphia: Lippincott Williams & Wilkins; 2008

[7] Deutsche Gesellschaft für pädiatrische Infektiologie (DGPI). DGPI Handbuch. Stuttgart: Thieme; 2009

[8] Driscoll DJ. Fundamentals of Pediatric Cardiology. Philadelphia: Lippincott Williams & Wilkins; 2006

[9] Everett AD, Lim DS. Illustrated field guide to congenital heart disease and repair. 2nd ed. Charlottesville: Scientific software solutions; 2005

[10] Fröhlig G, et al. Herzschrittmacher- und Defibrillator-Therapie. Stuttgart: Thieme; 2006

[11] Gatzoulis MA, et al. Adult congenital heart disease: a practical guide. Oxford: Blackwell; 2005

[12] Goldberg SJ, et al. Doppler Echocardiography. Philadelphia: Lea & Febiger; 1985

[13] Gupta R. Step-by-step fetal echocardiography. New York: McGraw-Hill; 2008

[14] Gutheil. Herz-Kreislauf-Erkrankungen im Kindes- und Jugendalter. Stuttgart: Thieme; 1990

[15] Gutheil H. EKG im Kindes- und Jugendalter. Stuttgart: Thieme; 1998

[16] Hamm CW. Willems P. Checkliste EKG. Stuttgart: Thieme; 2007

[17] Hansmann G. Neugeborenen-Notfälle. Stuttgart: Thieme; 2004

[18] Hausdorf G, Keck EW. Pädiatrische Kardiologie. Munich, Jena: Urban & Fischer; 2002

[19] Hausdorf G. Intensivbehandlung angeborener Herzfehler. Darmstadt: Steinkopff; 2000

[20] Helfaer MA, Nichols DG. Roger's handbook of pediatric intensive care. Philadelphia: Lippincott Williams & Wilkins; 2009

[21] Hombach V, Grebe O, Botnar RM. Kardiovaskuläre Magnetresonanztomographie. Stuttgart: Schattauer; 2005

[22] Keane JF, Lock JE, Fyler DC. Nadas' pediatric cardiology. Philadelphia: Saunders Elsevier; 2006

[23] Kerbl R, et al. Checkliste Pädiatrie. Stuttgart: Thieme; 2007

[24] Kretz FJ, Becke K. Anästhesie und Intensivmedizin bei Kindern. Stuttgart: Thieme; 2007

[25] Lederhuber HC. Basics Kardiologie. Munich: Urban & Fischer; 2005

[26] Mewis C, Riessen R, Spyridopoulos I. Kardiologie compact. Stuttgart: Thieme; 2006

[27] Munoz R, et al, Eds. Handbook of pediatric cardiovascular drugs. London: Springer; 2008

[28] Obladen M, Maier RF. Neugeborenenintensivmedizin. Heidelberg: Springer; 2006

[29] Park MK. Pediatric cardiology for practitioners. Philadelphia: Mosby Elsevier; 2008

[30] Reinhard D. Therapie der Krankheiten im Kindes- und Jugendalter. Berlin, Heidelberg, New York: Springer; 2004

[31] Reynolds T. The pediatric echocardiographer's pocket reference. Phoenix: Arizona Heart Institute; 2002

[32] Roos R, Proquitté H, Genzel-Boroviczény O. Checkliste Neonatologie. Stuttgart: Thieme; 2008

[33] Rühle KH. Praxisleitfaden der Spiroergometrie. Stuttgart, Berlin, Cologne: Kohlhammer; 2001

[34] Schmaltz AA. Leitlinien zur Diagnostik und Therapie in der Pädiatrischen Kardiologie. Munich, Jena: Elsevier, Urban & Fischer; 2007

[35] Schmaltz AA, Singer H. Herzoperierte Kinder und Jugendliche. Stuttgart: WVG; 1994

[36] Schmid C, Asfour B. Leitfaden Kinderherzchirurgie. Darmstadt: Steinkopff; 2009

[37] Schumacher G, Hess J, Bühlmeyer K. Klinische Kinderkardiologie. Heidelberg: Springer; 2008

[38] Schuster HP, Trappe HJ. EKG-Kurs für Isabel. Stuttgart: Enke; 1997

[39] Stierle U, Niederstadt C. Klinikleitfaden Kardiologie. Munich, Jena: Urban & Fischer Verlag; 2003

[40] Striebel HW. Operative Intensivmedizin. Stuttgart: Schattauer; 2008

[41] Taketomo CK, Hodding JH, Kraus DM. Pediatric dosage handbook international. Hudson Lexi-Comp;2006

[42] Walsh EP, Saul JP, Triedman JK. Cardiac arrhythmias in children and young adults with congenital heart disease. Philadelphia: Lippincott Williams & Wilkins; 2001

[43] Wilkenshoff U, Kruck I. Handbuch der Echokardiographie. Stuttgart: Thieme; 2008 1.2 Overview Articles

[44] Alsoufi B, Bennetts J, Verma S, Caldarone CA. New developments in the treatment of hypoplastic left heart syndrome. Pediatrics 2007; 119: 109–117

[45] Arslan-Kirchner M, von Kodolitsch Y, Schmidtke J. Genetische Diagnostik beim Marfan-Syndrom und verwandten Erkrankungen. Dtsch Arztebl 2008; 105: 483–491

[46] Baddour LM, Wilson WR, Bayer AS et al; Committee on Rheumatic Fever, Endocarditis, and Kawasaki Disease; Council on Cardiovascular Disease in the Young; Councils on Clinical Cardiology, Stroke, and Cardiovascular Surgery and Anesthesia; American Heart Association; Infectious Diseases Society of America. Infective endocarditis: diagnosis, antimicrobial therapy, and management of complications: a statement for healthcare professionals from the Committee on Rheumatic Fever, Endocarditis, and Kawasaki Disease, Council on Cardiovascular Disease in the Young, and the Councils on Clinical Cardiology, Stroke, and Cardiovascular Surgery and Anesthesia, American Heart Association: endorsed by the Infectious Diseases Society of America. Circulation 2005; 111: e394–e434

[47] Bald M. Arterielle Hypertonie. Pädiatrie up2date 2007; 3: 209–228

[48] Bauer J et al. Herztransplantation bei Neugeborenen und Säuglingen. Dtsch Arztebl 1997; 94: A-3178–A-3182

[49] Bauer J et al. Morbidität nach Herztransplantation. Monatsschr Kinderheilkd 2007; 155: 1040–1047

[50] Bauersfeld U, Pfammatter JP, Jaeggi E. Treatment of supraventricular tachycardias in the new millennium—drugs or radiofrequency catheter ablation? Eur J Pediatr 2001; 160: 1–9

[51] Billingham ME, Cary NR, Hammond ME et al; The International Society for Heart Transplantation. A working formulation for the standardization of nomenclature in the diagnosis of heart and lung rejection: Heart Rejection Study Group. J Heart Transplant 1990; 9: 587–593

[52] Brickner ME, Hillis LD, Lange RA. Congenital heart disease in adults. First of two parts. N Engl J Med 2000; 342: 256–263

[53] Brickner ME, Hillis LD, Lange RA. Congenital heart disease in adults. Second of two parts. N Engl J Med 2000; 342: 334–342

[54] Brignole M, Alboni P, Benditt DG et al; Task Force on Syncope, European Society of Cardiology. Guidelines on management (diagnosis and treatment) of syncope-update 2004. Executive Summary. Eur Heart J 2004; 25: 2054–2072

[55] Brugada R, Hong K, Cordeiro JM, Dumaine R. Short QT syndrome. CMAJ 2005; 173: 1349–1354

[56] Buchhorn R. Medikamentöse Therapie der Herzinsuffizienz bei Kindern mit angeborenen Herzfehlern. Dtsch Arztebl 2002; 39: 2555–2559

[57] Burns JC, Glodé MP. Kawasaki syndrome. Lancet 2004; 364: 533–544

[58] Cachat F, Di Paolo ER, Sekarski N. Behandlung der arteriellen Hypertonie im Kindesalter: Aktuelle Empfehlungen. Paediatrica 2004; 15: 35–43

[59] Chaoui R, Heling K, Mielke G, Hofbeck M, Gembruch U. Qualitätsanforderungen der DEGUM zur Durchführung der fetalen Echokardiografie. Ultraschall Med 2008; 29: 197–200

[60] Davignon A, Rautaharju P, Barselle E et al. Normal ECG standards for infants and children. Pediatr Cardiol 1979–80; 1: 123–134

[61] Dalla Pozza R. Synkope im Kindes- und Jugendalter. Monatsschr Kinderheilkd 2006; 154: 583–593

[62] Dannecker G., Kawasaki-Syndrom DG. Monatsschr Kinderheilkd 2006; 154: 872–879

[63] Derrick G, Cullen S. Transposition of the great arteries. Curr Treat Options Cardiovasc Med 2000; 2: 499–506

[64] Dubowy KO, Baden W, Camphausen C et al. Vorschlag für ein einheitliches spiroergometrisches Laufbandprotokoll der Deutschen Gesellschaft für pädiatrische Kardiologie (P50). Z Kardiol 2002; 91: 767

[65] Ehl P. DiGeorge-Syndrom. Allergologie 2004; 11: 473–476

[66] Ewert P. Interventioneller Verschluss von Vorhofseptumdefekten (ASD) und persistierender Foramen ovale (PFO). Der Kardiologe 2008; 2: 39–48

[67] Fuchs AT et al. Kreislaufunterstützungssysteme bei Kindern und Jugendlichen. Monatsschr Kinderheilkd 2003; 151: 669–682

[68] Gabriel H. Sport bei Patienten mit angeborenen Herzfehlern. Journal für Kardiologie 2005; 12: 170–173

[69] Golka T et al. „Noncompaction" des Kammermyokards (spongiöses Myokard). Monatsschr Kinderheilkd 1999; 147: 42–44

[70] Haas NA et al. Nierenarterienstenose im Kindesalter. Monatsschr Kinderheilkd 2004; 152: 62–71

[71] Haas NA, Plumpton K, Justo R, Jalali H, Pohlner P. Postoperative junctional ectopic tachycardia (JET). Z Kardiol 2004; 93: 371–380

[72] Hager A, Hess J. Lebensqualität nach Operation angeborener Herzfehler. Monatsschr Kinderheilkd 2006; 154: 639–643

[73] Hager A. Impfkalender für Patienten mit angeborenem Herzfehler. Monatsschr Kinderheilkd 2006; 154: 263–266

[74] Hirth A, Reybrouck T, Bjarnason-Wehrens B, Lawrenz W, Hoffmann A. Recommendations for participation in competitive and leisure sports in patients with congenital heart disease: a consensus document. Eur J Cardiovasc Prev Rehabil 2006; 13: 293–299

[75] Hofbeck M, Apitz C. Herzgeräusche. Pädiatrie update 2007; 2: 105–123

[76] Humpl T. Myokarditis im Kindesalter. Pädiat Prax 2009/2010; 74: 431–439

[77] Kampmann C, Wiethoff CM, Wenzel A et al. Normal values of M mode echocardiographic measurements of more than 2000 healthy infants and children in central Europe. Heart 2000; 83: 667–672

[78] Kaulitz R, Ziemer G, Hofbeck M. [Atrial isomerism and visceral heterotaxy] Herz 2004; 29: 686–694

[79] Kay JD, Colan SD, Graham TP, Jr. Congestive heart failure in pediatric patients. Am Heart J 2001; 142: 923–928

[80] Keane MG, Pyeritz RE. Medical management of Marfan syndrome. Circulation 2008; 117: 2802–2813

[81] Khalid O, Luxenberg DM, Sable C et al. Aortic stenosis: the spectrum of practice. Pediatr Cardiol 2006; 27: 661–669

[82] Kosch A, von Kries R, Nowak-Göttl U. Thrombosen im Kindesalter. Monatsschr Kinderheilkd 2000; 148: 387–397

[83] Lai WW, Geva T, Shirali GS et al; Task Force of the Pediatric Council of the American Society of Echocardiography; Pediatric Council of the American Society of Echocardiography. Guidelines and standards for performance of a pediatric echocardiogram: a report from the Task Force of the Pediatric Council of the American Society of Echocardiography. J Am Soc Echocardiogr 2006; 19: 1413–1430

[84] Lawrenz W. Sport und körperliche Aktivität für Kinder mit angeborenen Herzfehlern. Deutsche Zeitschrift für Sportmedizin 2007; 9: 334–337

[85] McLeod KA. Syncope in childhood. Arch Dis Child 2003; 88: 350–353

[86] Mitchell JH, et al. 36th Bethesda Conference. Task Force 8. Classification of sports. J Am Coll Cardiol 2005; 1364–1367

[87] Monagle P, Chan A, Massicotte P, Chalmers E, Michelson AD. Antithrombotic therapy in children: the Seventh ACCP Conference on Antithrombotic and Thrombolytic Therapy. Chest 2004; 126 Suppl: 645S–687S

[88] Müther S, Dähnert I. Das Heterotaxiesyndrom. Z Herz Thorax Gefäßchir 2000; 14: 134–136

[89] Naber CK et al. S2-Leitlinien zur Diagnostik und Therapie der infektiösen Endokarditis. Chemotherapie Journal 2004; 6: 227–237

[90] Newburger JW, Takahashi M, Gerber MA et al; Committee on Rheumatic Fever, Endocarditis and Kawasaki Disease; Council on Cardiovascular Disease in the Young; American Heart Association; American Academy of Pediatrics. Diagnosis, treatment, and long-term management of Kawasaki disease: a statement for health professionals from the Committee on Rheumatic Fever, Endocarditis and Kawasaki Disease, Council on Cardiovascular Disease in the Young, American Heart Association. Circulation 2004; 110: 2747–2771

[91] Nora JJ, Nora AH. The evolution of specific genetic and environmental counseling in congenital heart diseases. Circulation 1978; 57: 205–213

[92] Olschewski H, Hoeper MM, Borst MM et al. Diagnostik und Therapie der chronischen pulmonalen Hypertonie. Pneumologie 2006; 60: 749–771

[93] Paul T, Bertram H, Kriebel T, Windhagen-Mahnert B, Tebbenjohanns J, Hausdorf G. Supraventrikuläre Tachykardien bei Säuglingen, Kindern und Jugendlichen: Diagnostik—Medikamentöse und interventionelle Therapie. Z Kardiol 2000; 89: 546–558

[94] Schickendantz S, Sticker EJ, Bjarnason-wehrens B et al. Bewegung, Spiel und Sport mit herzkranken Kindern. Dtsch Arzteblatt 2007; 104: A563–A569

[95] Schmaltz AA. Dilatative Kardiomyopathie im Kindesalter. Monatsschr Kinderheilkd 1997; 145: 218–224

[96] Schmaltz AA. Dilatative Kardiomyopathie im Kindesalter. Z Kardiol 2001; 90: 263–268

[97] Schranz D. Pulmonale Hypertonie im Kindesalter. Intensivmedizin update 2 2006; 2: 177–193

[98] Schwartz PJ, Moss AJ, Vincent GM, Crampton RS. Diagnostic criteria for the long QT syndrome. An update. Circulation 1993; 88: 782–784

[99] Sheil ML, Jenkins O, Sholler GF. Echocardiographic assessment of aortic root dimensions in normal children based on measurement of a new ratio of aortic size independent of growth. Am J Cardiol 1995; 75: 711–715

[100] Simonneau G, Galiè N, Rubin LJ et al. Clinical classification of pulmonary hypertension. J Am Coll Cardiol 2004; 43 Suppl S: 5S–12S

[101] Soergel M, Kirschstein M, Busch C et al. Oscillometric twenty-four-hour ambulatory blood pressure values in healthy children and adolescents: a multicenter trial including 1141 subjects. J Pediatr 1997; 130: 178–184

[102] Thumfart J, Gellermann J, Querfeld U. Therapie der arteriellen Hypertonie im Kindes- und Jugendalter. Monatsschr Kinderheilkunde 2008; 156: 1121–1131

[103] Towbin JA, Lowe AM, Colan SD et al. Incidence, causes, and outcomes of dilated cardiomyopathy in children. JAMA 2006; 296: 1867–1876

[104] Trappe HJ, Schuster HP. Brugada-Syndrom. Intensivmed 2000; 37: 680–687

[105] Von Kodolitsch Y et al. Das Marfan-Syndrom. Pädiat Prax 2009; 73: 93–107

[106] Yetman AT, McCrindle BW. Management of pediatric hypertrophic cardiomyopathy. Curr Opin Cardiol 2005; 20: 80–83

[107] Zuber M, et al. Mitralklappenprolaps und Mitralklappenprolapssyndrom. Schweiz Med Forum 2006; 6: 664–667

[108] Blume ED, Altmann K, Mayer JE, Colan SD, Gauvreau K, Geva T. Evolution of risk factors influencing early mortality of the arterial switch operation. J Am Coll Cardiol 1999; 33 (6): 1702–1709

[109] Goor DA, Lillehhei CW. Congenital malformations of the heart. New York, Grune and Stratton, 1975

[110] Jaoude S, Leclercq JF, Coumel P. Progressive ECG changes in arrhythmogenic right ventricular disease. Eur Heart J 1996; 17: 1717–1722

[111] Wernowsky G, Mayer JE, Jonas RA, et al. Factors influencing early and late outcome of arterial switch operation for transposition of the great arteries. J Thorac Cardiovasc Surg 1995; 109: 289–302

[112] Wilde AAM, Antzelevitch C, Borggrefe M, et al. Diagnostic criteria for the Brugada Syndrome. A consensus report. Eur Heart J 2002; 23: 1648–1654

[113] Sohn DW, Chai IH, Lee DJ, Kim HC, Kim HS, Oh BH, Lee MM, Park YB, Choi YS, Seo JD, Lee YW. Assessment of mitral annulus velocity by Doppler tissue imaging in the evaluation of left ventricular diastolic function. JACC 1997; 30: 474–480

[114] Ziegler RF. Electrocardiographic studies in normal infants and children. Philadelphia: Charles C. Thomas; 1951

[115] Cui W, Roberson DA, Zen Z, et al. Systolic and diastolic time intervals measured from Doppler tissue imaging: normal values and Z-score tables, and effects of age, heart rate and body surface area. J Am Soc Echocardiogr 2008; 21: 361–370

[116] Wasserman K, Hansen JE, Sue DY, et al. Principles of Exercise Testing and Interpretation. 4th ed. Philadelphia, Lippincott Williams & Wilkins, 2005

[117] Eidem BW, Cetta F, O'Leary PW (Editors). Echocardiography in Pediatric and Adult Congenital Heart Disease. Philadelphia, Lippincott Williams & Wilkins, 2009

Internet

www.emedicine.com
www.uptodate.com

Index

Page numbers in *italics* refer to illustrations and those in **bold** refer to tables

Abbreviations used in subentries: ASD - atrial septal defect; AV - atrioventricular; AVRT - atrioventricular re-entrant tachycardia with accessory pathway; IART - intra-atrial re-entrant tachycardia; LV - left ventricle; PAPVC - partial anomalous pulmonary venous connection; PDA - patent ductus arteriosus; RV - right ventricle; TAPVC - total anomalous pulmonary venous connection; VSD - ventricular septal defect

Index subentry 'Diagnostic measures' includes all imaging modalities and other investigations, symptoms and differential diagnosis.

Index subentry 'Prognosis, clinical course' includes long-term prognosis, outpatient checkups, follow-up, exercise capacity, lifestyle and adolescents'.

B

C

D

E

R

S

T

U

V

W

X

Y

Z